900 Lomaland Drive, San Diego, CA 92106-2899

Essentials of
Psychiatric Nursing

Essentials of Psychiatric Nursing

Cecelia Monat Taylor, Ph.D., R.N.

**Professor and Chair,
Department of Nursing,
Co-Chair, Health Science Division,
The College of St. Scholastica,
Duluth, Minnesota**

FOURTEENTH EDITION

with 54 Illustrations

Mosby

St. Louis Baltimore Boston Chicago London Madrid Philadelphia Sydney Toronto

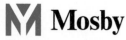

Dedicated to Publishing Excellence

Managing Editor: Jeff Burnham
Developmental Editor: Jolynn Gower
Associate Developmental Editor: Linda Caldwell
Project Manager: Patricia Tannian
Manuscript Editor: Roger McWilliams
Senior Book Designer: Gail Morey Hudson
Manufacturing Supervisor: John Babrick
Cover Design: Teresa Breckwoldt

FOURTEENTH EDITION

Copyright © 1994 by Mosby–Year Book, Inc.

Previous editions copyrighted 1940, 1944, 1949, 1953, 1958, 1962, 1966, 1970, 1974, 1978, 1982, 1986, 1990

Printed in the United States of America
Composition by Graphic World, Inc.
Printing/binding by R.R. Donnelley & Sons Company

Mosby–Year Book, Inc.
11830 Westline Industrial Drive, St. Louis, Missouri 63146

Library of Congress Cataloging in Publication Data

Taylor, Cecelia Monat.
    Essentials of psychiatric nursing.—14th ed. / Cecelia Monat
Taylor.
        p.   cm.
    Rev. ed. of: Mereness' essentials of psychiatric nursing. 13th ed.
/ Cecelia Monat Taylor.
    Includes bibliographical references and index.
    ISBN 0-8016-7814-5
    1. Psychiatric nursing.   I. Taylor, Cecelia Monat.   Mereness'
essentials of psychiatric nursing.   II. Title.
    [DNLM: 1. Psychiatric Nursing.   WY 160 T239m 1994]
RC440.M38   1994
610.73′68—dc20
DNLM/DLC
for Library of Congress   93-6324
93 94 95 96 97 / 9 8 7 6 5 4 3 2 1   CIP

To

Dorothy A. Mereness

Ed.D., R.N., F.A.A.N.

1910-1991

Dr. Mereness was a pioneer in psychiatric nursing
and collaborator, coauthor, or sole author of
this textbook from the third to the tenth editions (1949-1978).

She was also a dear friend, teacher, and mentor to
scores of psychiatric nurses.

Contributors

Ruth E. Davidhizar, D.N.S., R.N., C.S.

Assistant Dean and Chair,
Division of Health Professions,
Bethel College,
Mishawaka, Indiana

Sharon Evers, M.S.N., R.N., C.S.

Associate Professor, Department of Nursing,
Columbus College,
Columbus, Georgia

Christine S. Fawcett, M.S., R.N., C.S.

Psychiatric Mental Health Nurse and Consultant,
Philadelphia, Pennsylvania

Joyce N. Giger, Ed.D., R.N., C.S.

Chair and Professor, Department of Nursing,
Columbus College,
Columbus, Georgia

Charlotte Ingram, M.S.N., R.N., C.S.

Assistant Professor, Department of Nursing,
Columbus College,
Columbus, Georgia

Kem B. Louie, Ph.D., R.N., C.S., F.A.A.N.

Director of the Graduate Program and Associate
Professor, Department of Nursing,
College of Mount Saint Vincent,
Riverdale, New York

Barbara L. MacDermott, M.S., R.N.

Associate Professor and Assistant Dean (Retired),
College of Nursing, Syracuse University,
Syracuse, New York

**Beatrice C. Yorker, J.D., M.S., R.N.,
F.A.A.N.**

Department Chair and Associate Professor,
Department of Psychiatric Mental Health Nursing,
School of Nursing, Georgia State University,
Atlanta, Georgia

Reviewers

Betty J. Craft, M.P.N., R.N.

Assistant Professor,
Psychiatric Mental Health Nursing,
College of Nursing,
University of Nebraska Medical Center,
Omaha, Nebraska

Janet Dahm, M.S., R.N.

Associate Professor of Nursing,
St. Xavier University,
Chicago, Illinois

Patricia O. Dardis, M.S., R.N., C.S., F.N.P.

Assistant Professor, School of Nursing,
University of North Dakota,
Jamestown, North Dakota

Susan Dewey-Hammer, M.N., R.N.

Assistant Professor, Department of Nursing,
Suffolk Community College,
Selden, New York

Joan Elberg, M.A., R.N.

Instructor, Department of Nursing,
Iowa Central Community College,
Fort Dodge, Iowa

Sarah Fishman, Ph.D., R.N., C.S.

Adjunct Professor, College of Nursing,
Florida Atlantic University,
Boca Raton, Florida

Carolyn Anne Green, M.S.N., Ed.D., R.N.

Professor, Department of Nursing,
Solano Community College,
Suisun City, California

Sandra Halsey, M.S.N., R.N.

Associate Professor, Department of Nursing,
Sinclair Community College,
Dayton, Ohio

Alison Harrigan, M.S.N., R.N.C.

Instructor, Department of Nursing,
University of Akron,
Akron, Ohio

Arlene Hurwitz, Dr. P.H., R.N.

Associate Professor, School of Nursing,
City College, City University of New York, New York,
New York

Ann Isaacs, M.S., R.N.

Associate Professor, Department of Nursing,
Luzerne County Community College,
Nanticoke, Pennsylvania

Alexander H. Jennings, M.N. Ed., R.N.

Assistant Professor,
College of Health Sciences,
Gannon University,
Erie, Pennsylvania

Jo Anne McDaniel

Instructor, Nursing Department,
Jefferson College,
Hillsboro, Missouri

Marie McGillicuddy, Ph.D., R.N.

Assistant Professor, Department of Nursing,
Hostos Community College,
Bronx, New York

Constance O'Kane, M.S., R.N.

Associate Professor, Nursing Faculty,
Division of Mathematics, Health, and Natural
Sciences, College of the Mainland,
Texas City, Texas

Lynne G. Pearcey, Ph.D., R.N., C.N.A.A.

Dean and Professor, School of Nursing,
The University of North Carolina at Greensboro,
Greensboro, North Carolina

Anita Throwe, M.S., R.N., C.S.

Associate Professor, College of Nursing,
Medical University of South Carolina,
Florence, South Carolina

Preface

The fourteenth edition of this classic textbook was written within the context of revolutionary changes in the health care delivery system, including nursing. Not a day passed without a news report referring to the health care reform expected to be announced by the Clinton administration. Many of these reports cited the potentially pivotal role of nurses who are educationally and experientially prepared for advanced practice. Along with changes at the federal level, most state governments were either studying or had already enacted health care reform measures. Although it is too early to know with certainty what role nursing will ultimately assume in a reformed health care system, assuredly the roles of all health care professionals (and consumers) will change.

Concurrently, massive changes in the mental health delivery system continue to occur. State-supported hospitals for mental health care have been closed or dramatically downsized in all states. Persons with an acute mental illness are receiving short-term treatment in community-based general hospitals; those with a chronic mental illness are being discharged from state hospitals to community-based care. In addition, progress continues in discovering biological bases for the major mental illnesses.

Unfortunately, it is not certain that the anticipated health care reform on either the federal or the state level will adequately provide for the continued community care of persons with a chronic mental illness. It is even less certain how nursing will meet the increased needs of those with a mental illness. I make this statement because many nursing programs are devoting less and less time to learning experiences with persons who have a mental illness during a time when there is more to learn than ever before. For example, reason dictates that the challenges of understanding the biological bases of such illnesses as schizophrenia would lead nurse educators to lengthen the course in psychiatric nursing. Such is not the case! I am fully aware that resources, including time, are finite and there are multiple, competing claims for them. Nevertheless, I continue in the belief that all nurses should have sound theoretical and experiential preparation in the care of persons with a mental illness. At the same time it is important to emphasize that students of nursing who are preparing for beginning professional practice should not be expected to become psychiatric nursing specialists. Instead they should be encouraged to use knowledge learned during earlier learning experiences and in turn to apply skills gained during the psychiatric nursing experience to the care of all persons. As a result, this edition retains material on concepts basic to psychiatric nursing, which includes topics such as personality development and the process of communication, the understanding of which is integral to the effective practice of nursing in any setting and with any client.

CONTENT

The content of this edition has been strengthened with three new chapters and expanded coverage of important topics. Chapter 2, Psychiatric Nursing in the Hospital, and Chapter 3, Psychiatric Nursing in the Community, were thought to be necessary in light of the changing sites and nature of mental health care. Chapter 10 is a totally new chapter on psychopharmacology that was added because of the increasing reliance on pharmaceutical treatment of mental illness and the major role of the nurse in this treatment modality. Coverage of substance abuse and family abuse and violence has been expanded. Nursing care has also been expanded by including more nursing interventions with rationales and clinical examples throughout.

Although the entire book was reorganized and all chapters were revised, the greatest revisions were made in Section Four, The Consumers of Psychiatric Nursing. Causative factors of each disorder are included in each chapter and a description of client behaviors is aligned with the diagnostic criteria of the **DSM-III-R** and **NANDA** diagnoses. Anticipated changes in the **DSM-IV** have been noted as warranted.

FEATURES

Pedagogical changes in this edition include a list of **key terms** and **chapter outlines** at the beginning of each chapter and a list of **key points** at the end of every chapter. **Key interventions** are also cited for all chapters in Section Four. In addition, each chapter in Section Four has several vignettes depicting **clinical examples** of the behaviors discussed. The **case study** and nursing care plan at the end of each chapter in Section Four have been retained with the addition of a **rationale** for each objective of care.

The design of this edition has been enhanced with many new **illustrations, tables,** and **boxes** that support the narrative and with the use of a new two-color design throughout.

The list of suggested sources of additional information at the end of each chapter has been enlarged to reflect the latest information available, regardless of its source. Older, classic references have been retained when they contain currently applicable information.

I believe this edition of *Essentials of Psychiatric Nursing* continues to provide accurate and useful information to entry-level students of psychiatric nursing. I trust that both students and teachers will find the format esthetically pleasing.

TEACHING-LEARNING PACKAGE

An expanded package of supplements is available with the text to facilitate the teaching-learning process. An expanded and updated *Instructor's Resource Manual* includes new student worksheets with a variety of activities, including clinical examples with critical thinking questions for classroom or self-paced use by students. The new test bank includes 500 test items in NCLEX format, with 150 new test items added. Qualified adopters of the textbook may receive a set of 50 transparency acetates.

Two new documents designed to enhance student learning are also available with this edition: the *Student Learning Guide for Essentials of Psychiatric Nursing* and the *Quick Reference for Psychiatric Nursing.* Both these ancillaries were written by Marianne Miles, Ph.D., R.N., and are closely correlated with the text.

TERMINOLOGY AND LANGUAGE

Because I have become sensitized to the overwhelming stigma experienced by those with a mental illness (and those who care for them), I have replaced the term "mentally ill" with the phrase "those with a mental illness" throughout this text. I believe that the former term implies that all that is necessary to know about a person is that he or she has a mental illness, whereas the latter phrase conveys that there is more to the individual than his or her mental illness. I suspect some readers will find this new terminology cumbersome at first. I trust everyone will become quickly accustomed to it and will adopt its use in both conversation and writing.

Every effort has been made to delete evidence of sexism from this text. The term "client" is used instead of "patient" in keeping with the current thinking that health care consumers have rights, responsibilities, and a participatory role in their own care. In the same spirit, in this edition the objectives and outcome criteria in the nursing care plans are worded in client-centered language.

ACKNOWLEDGMENTS

As the reader will note on the dedication page of this text, Dr. Dorothy A. Mereness, a pioneer in psychiatric nursing, died in 1991 at the age of 80. Current students are unlikely to recognize her name, much less know of her achievements and dedication to psychiatric nursing. Some teachers of psychiatric nursing will have known her through this text and other publications. A few may have had the privilege to know her personally. However, all psychiatric nurses have benefited from her wisdom and professional leadership. Dorothy's death is a great loss to me personally. I knew her well, but I doubt I fully appreciate the extent of her contributions to the profession or to my own personal and professional development. Nevertheless, I feel blessed that our lives were intertwined for so many years. I am sure she would be pleased that this text continues to be useful to students of psychiatric nursing.

The contributors to this edition deserve a great deal of thanks and acknowledgment for sharing their expertise within a short timeframe. Their chapters place this text on the cutting edge of essential knowledge in psychiatric nursing.

Special thanks are due Henry (Hank) Visalli, M.S., R.N., Clinical Specialist at Mohawk Valley Psychiatric Center, Utica, New York. Hank cheerfully and expertly searched the literature for recent publications that provided the bases for this revision. The clients and staff of Mohawk Valley Psychiatric Center also are acknowledged for providing me with the reality of psychiatric nursing in the 1990s. I miss you all and thank you for the growth-producing experiences you provided.

I particularly enjoyed renewing my relationship with Marianne (Mandy) Miles, who wrote the *Student Learning Guide* and the *Quick Reference* that accompany this edition. I was pleased to be one of Mandy's instructors at Syracuse University and now am honored to be among her colleagues.

This edition was written with the support and encouragement of the administration, faculty, and staff of The College of St. Scholastica. These people create and sustain a nurturing environment in which my aspirations and those of other faculty and students are valued and therefore achievable. I feel fortunate to be among you.

Only those who have written a textbook can fully appreciate the role and influence of the editor. I was particularly fortunate that Jeff Burnham served in this capacity for this edition of *Essentials of Psychiatric Nursing.* Jeff cajoled, supported, encouraged, and assisted me in the tedious process of this revision. He is truly an expert in this process and I thank him!

Finally, for those faculty who have used this text since 1974, I want to update you on the progress of my daughter Corliss. Corliss was 3 years old when I first officially participated in the revision of this text. In fact, you can find some pictures of her in the tenth edition! Corliss graduated from college with a baccalaureate degree in May 1993 and will begin graduate studies in September 1993. I trust I can report that she has a salaried position when I write the acknowledgments for the fifteenth edition of this text!

Even though the preface is in the front of the book, it is written last. As a closing thought, I commend the book's content to you in the wish that it may enlighten and inspire you to provide the best possible care to those who are among the most vulnerable in our society, those with a mental illness.

Cecelia M. Taylor

Contents

Detailed Contents

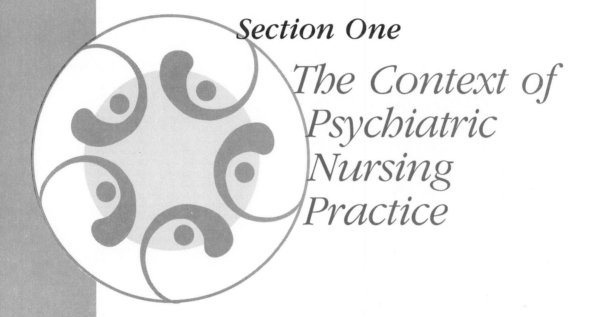

Section One

The Context of Psychiatric Nursing Practice

Chapter 1

The Mental Health Delivery System and Health Care Team

LEARNING OBJECTIVES

After studying this chapter, the student will be able to:

* State the primary mode of mental health treatment during key periods from prehistoric times to the present.

* Identify the advantages and the disadvantages of the state mental hospital delivery system of the late nineteenth and early twentieth centuries.

* Cite the major federal legislation affecting mental health delivery in the public sector.

* Discuss the relationship between the fiscal constraints of the 1980s and 1990s and the availability of mental health services in both the public and the private sectors.

* Explain the importance of including the client and the family as integral members of the treatment team.

* Differentiate among the roles and functions of the psychiatrist, psychologist, psychiatric social worker, activity therapist, and psychiatric case manager.

KEY TERMS
Philippe Pinel
York Retreat
Benjamin Rush
Eastern Psychiatric Hospital
Dorothea Dix
Institutionalization
Clifford Beers
Sigmund Freud
National Mental Health Act
Mental Health Study Act
Community Mental Health Centers Act
President's Commission on Mental Health
Interdisciplinary mental health team
National Alliance for the Mentally Ill
Nurse
Psychiatrist
Psychologist
Social worker
Activity therapist
Psychiatric case manager

Human beings have always been concerned about behavior that is different from what is usually encountered in their society. At times the source of this concern has been compassion; at other times concern has stemmed from fear. At the same time, the labels applied to those who behave in a deviant manner have varied throughout the ages and include such terms as *witch,* *sinner, lunatic, insane,* and *mentally ill.* The systems devised by the society to care for these persons have been strongly influenced by the prevailing beliefs about the cause and nature of the deviant behavior. The responsibility for provision of care has shifted among the various subsystems of society, ranging from the family to the community as a whole to specialized agents of

Table 1-1.   Historical overview of events related to mental health treatment

DATES	EVENTS
Ancient times	Primitive people perceived their bodies as the dwelling place of the soul, and illness was seen as the result of malevolent spirits projecting some noxious object into the body. Indian and Chinese philosophers saw all life as a whole, and the spirit was unseparated from the rest of the person.
400-300 BC	Plato contended that human beings possess a spirit with direct access to the realm of the nonphysical, seen in prophecy and healing. Aristotle distinguished between experiences that involved physical activities (sensations, appetites, passions) and those that involved activity of the soul (thinking).
1600s-1700s	Descartes' suggestion that the body and mind were two different entities encouraged the establishment of medical systems in which physical problems were solved by dealing exclusively with the body and mental problems were approached by dealing with the mind. Repressive measures by the Church of England led a small religious group to separate from the main church to seek religious freedom. This group of separatists, known as Puritans, believed that an austere life released their soul from bondage to the body and permitted union with a divine being.
1800s	William James proposed relationships between experiences that involved emotional stimulus, emotional behavior (visceral reactions, overt actions), and emotional experience.
1960s	The emergence of mass society, identified by such factors as depersonalization, mechanization, and loss of individuality and privacy, has promoted the view that people are a mass target of influence rather than individual human beings.
1970s	The women's movement contributed to altering sex role differentiation, particularly in areas of work and education. Dramatic changes were seen in childrearing practices, male and female roles, and concerns about the environment and the structure of society.
1980s	Research indicated that intellectual capacity is not predetermined, that individuals use less than half their brains, and that the decline in intellectual functioning can be prevented.
1990s	Current health care models recognize the interrelationships of the mind, body, and environment.
Future	As the elderly population increases, nurses will need to provide holistic care to this population in an era of decreased funding.

From Rawlins RP and others: *Mental health–psychiatric nursing,* ed 3, St Louis, 1993, Mosby–Year Book.

society such as the religious, political, and legal subsystems. The factors influencing this evolution are multiple and complex but include such variables as population density, availability of resources, religious beliefs and social practices, and the prevailing body of knowledge about human behavior (Table 1-1).

The following section is a history of the treatment of persons with a mental illness. It is presented in the belief that the contemporary system of mental health delivery can be understood best if one appreciates its historical roots.

HISTORICAL PERSPECTIVE

Prehistoric times

The treatment of persons exhibiting deviant behavior during prehistoric times probably consisted of tribal rites designed to alter behavior. If these measures proved unsuccessful, the individual likely was abandoned to die of starvation or attack by wild animals. Critics of contemporary community-based mental health care point to the many persons with a mental illness left to fend for themselves on the streets and in single-room occupancy dwellings of large cities as reflecting a slightly more sophisticated parallel to the measures used by primitive peoples of ancient times.

Early Greek and Roman era

The Golden Age of Greece was noted for its humane regard for sick persons. For hospitals, the Greeks used temples that had an abundance of fresh air, pure water, and sunshine. Theatricalism, riding, walking, and listening to the sound of a waterfall were all recommended as methods to lift the mood. Despite this humane attitude, the treatment at times was harsh; even in the best of the Greek temples, starving, using chains, and flogging were advocated "because with these it was believed that when those who refused food began to eat, frequently the memory was also refreshed thereby."

Little information exists about the Roman era in reference to mental illness. Galen, a Greek who practiced in Rome, based his treatment on the teachings of his Greek predecessors. Other physicians of the Roman era treated persons with a mental illness by bleeding, purging, and giving sulfur baths.

Middle Ages

With the collapse of Greek and Roman civilizations, the care of sick persons, along with other cultural developments, underwent an almost complete eclipse. The treatment of persons with a mental illness was left to priests, and superstitious beliefs flourished. Insane persons were flogged, fettered, scourged, and starved in the belief that the devils that possessed them could be driven out.

Positive areas in this tragic picture included some monasteries or shrines where this technique of "exorcising" the evil spirit was performed by the gentle laying on of hands instead of the whip. Members of the nobility, self-appointed ascetics, and holy men of varying degrees of sincerity practiced this art, which at least was not physically cruel.

Sixteenth century

Although the treatment of persons with a mental illness in the Middle Ages was not commendable, these persons fared even more poorly in the period that followed. When the church and the monastery gave up the care of insane persons, it was gradually taken over by the so-called almshouse, the contract house, and the secular asylum. The more violent persons were placed in jails and dungeons. In the sixteenth century, Henry VIII officially dedicated Bethlehem Hospital in London as a lunatic asylum. It soon became the notorious "Bedlam," whose hideous practices were immortalized by Hogarth, the famous cartoonist. There keepers were allowed to exhibit the most boisterous patients for 2 pence a look, and the more harmless inmates were forced to seek charity on the streets of London as the "Bedlam beggars" of Shakespeare's *King Lear.*

Out of the tradition and belief in the "holy" or "royal" touch" arose several great shrines, of which the one at Gheel in Belgium is most famous. This legend tells of a king living in Ireland who was married to a beautiful woman and who became the father of an equally beautiful daughter. The good queen developed a fatal illness, and at her deathbed the daughter dedicated herself to a life of purity and service to poor persons and those with a mental illness. The widowed king was overcome with grief and announced to his subjects that he must at once be cured of his sorrow by marrying the woman in his kingdom who most resembled the dead queen. No such person was found. However, the devil came and whispered to the king that there was such a woman, his own daughter. The devil spurred the king to propose marriage to the girl, but she was appropriately outraged and fled across the English Channel to Belgium. There the king overtook her and, with Satan at his elbow, slew the girl and her faithful attendants. In the night an angel came, recapitated the girl's body, and concealed it in the forest near the village of Gheel. Years later, five persons with a mental illness spent the night with their keepers at a small wayside shrine near this Belgian village. According to the legend, all recovered overnight. Here must be the place where the dead girl, reincarnated as St. Dymphna, was buried, and here was the sacred spot where her cures were effected.

In the fifteenth century, pilgrimages to Gheel from every part of the civilized world were organized for persons with a mental illness. Many pilgrims remained in Gheel to live with the local people, and in the passing years these pilgrims were accepted into the homes. Thus the first colony for persons with a mental illness, and the only one that has been consistently successful, was formed. In 1851 the Belgian government took charge of this colony. It continues to the present. Hundreds of individuals with a mental illness live in private homes, work with the townspeople, and have no particular restriction of freedom, except to refrain from visiting public places and using alcohol and to report regularly to the supervising psychiatrist. Despite the success of the Gheel colony and its great humanizing value, most attempts at duplicating it elsewhere have been total or partial failures.

Seventeenth century

Superstition about mental illness reached a horrible peak in the seventeenth century. God and Satan were still thought to be engaged in a ceaseless battle for possession of one's soul. The year after the *Mayflower* sailed into Plymouth Harbor, Burton published his classic work *Anatomy of Melancholy,* wherein he stated that "witches and magicians can cure and cause most diseases." To seek out and execute witches became a sacred religious duty. At least 20,000 persons were said to have been burned in Scotland alone during the seventeenth century. One can easily see why Cotton Mather precipitated the witch mania in Salem, Massachusetts, since he was merely subscribing to the beliefs prevalent in his day.

In those dark days, society was interested in its own self-security, not in the welfare of persons with a mental illness. The almshouses were a combination of jail and asylum, and within their walls petty criminals and persons with a mental illness were herded indiscriminately. In the seventeenth and eighteenth centuries the dungeons of Paris were the only places where persons who were violent and mentally ill could be committed. Drastic purgings and bleedings were the favorite therapeutic procedures of the day, and "madshirts" and the whip were applied religiously by the cell keepers.

Eighteenth century

The political and social reformations in France toward the end of the eighteenth century influenced the hospitals and jails of Paris. In 1792 **Philippe Pinel** (1745-1826), a young physician who was medical director of the Bicêtre asylum outside Paris, was given permission by the Revolutionary Commune to liberate the inmates of two of the largest hospitals, some of whom had been in chains for 20 years. Had his experiment proved a failure, he might have been guillotined. Fortunately, his experiment succeeded, and by his act he proved conclusively the fallacy of inhumane treatment of persons with a mental illness. The reforms instituted by Pinel were continued by his pupil Esquirol, who founded 10 asylums and was the first regular teacher of psychiatry. The Quakers, under the Brothers Tuke, at this time had established the **York Retreat** and effected the same epoch-making reforms in England.

In America the Pennsylvania Hospital was completed in 1756 under the guidance of Benjamin Franklin. One of the first two patients admitted was described as a "lunatic." Although patients with a mental illness were relegated to the cellar, they were assured clean bedding and warm rooms. **Benjamin Rush** (1745-1813), a prime humanitarian and the "father of American psychiatry," began his duties at the Pennsylvania Hospital in 1783.

Rush believed that the phases of the moon influenced behavior (the lunar theory of insanity) and invented an inhumane restraining device called the "tranquilizer." At the same time, however, he insisted on more humane treatment of patients and, as such, stands as a prominent transitional figure between the old era and the new.

Nineteenth century

The first public psychiatric hospital in America was built in Williamsburg, Virginia, in 1773 and is known today as the **Eastern Psychiatric Hospital** (Figure 1-1). Nevertheless, most states were still without special institutions for persons with a mental illness in the first quarter of the nineteenth century.

The poorhouse or almshouse was still popular, but it invariably became a "catchall" for all types of offenders, and people who were mentally ill received the harshest treatment. Most shocking to people of today was placing poor and mildly demented persons on the auction block, where those with the strongest backs and the weakest minds were sold to the highest bidder, with the returns from the sale assigned to the township treasury.

About 1830 a vigorous movement for the construction of suitable state hospitals spread simultaneously through several states. The excellent results obtained by private institutions such as the Hartford Retreat, founded in 1818, probably served as an object lesson. Horace Mann took an enthusiastic interest in the plight of persons with a mental illness, and the advantages of a state hospital system were publicized to promote construction of such institutions.

However, it remained for a sickly, 40-year-old schoolteacher to expose the sins of the poorhouse. From that day in 1841 when **Dorothea Lynde Dix** (1802-1887) described the hoarfrost on the walls of the cells of the East Somerville jail in Massachusetts to the day when she retreated into one of the very hospitals she was instrumental in creating, she effected reforms that shook the world. She so aroused the public conscience that millions of dollars were raised to build suitable hospitals, and 20 states responded directly to her appeals. She played an important part in the founding of St. Elizabeth's Hospital in Washington, D.C., directed the opening of two large institutions in Canada, completely reformed the asylum system in Scotland and in several other foreign countries, and rounded out a most amazing career by organizing the nursing forces of the northern armies during the Civil War. A resolution presented by the U.S. Congress in 1901 characterized her as

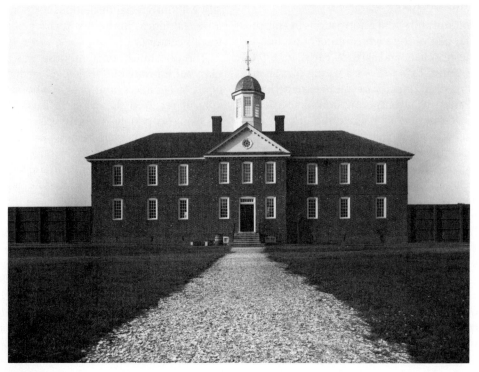

Figure 1-1

Eastern Psychiatric Hospital in Williamsburg, Virginia, was built in 1773 and is regarded as the first American public psychiatric hospital.

Courtesy Colonial Williamsburg Foundation.

"among the noblest examples of humanity in all history."

The state hospital system that rapidly developed throughout many states was limited almost solely to large institutions built in remote rural areas of the state and designed according to architectural plans developed by Dr. Thomas Kirkbride. The location of these institutions was determined by many considerations. For example, it was believed that the tranquil environment of the country would be soothing to disturbed individuals, rural land was inexpensive to purchase, and the remoteness of the setting effectively protected society from the inmates, both physically and emotionally.

The design of the institution resulted from a genuine desire to provide a homelike environment that would also be safe. However, because of the remoteness of the setting, the staff had to live in adjoining quarters, and the institution had to produce its own food, heat, and other necessities. What evolved was a self-contained community where patients who were able worked on the farm; in the kitchen, laundry, and machine shop; and on the grounds and wards. For some patients, this responsibility proved therapeutic because it provided meaningful activity, thereby increasing their sense of self-esteem and group cohesiveness. In some state hospitals, selected patients were invited to share the Sunday dinner with the hospital superintendent. Many, if not all, were more comfortable than if they had remained in their local community. On the other hand, abuses occurred. At the very least, even the most able patients were taken advantage of, since they were not paid for their labor. In addition to exploitation and perhaps related to it, a negative outcome of the state hospital system was the syndrome of **institutionalization.** This syndrome is discussed further in Chapter 2.

By the middle of the nineteenth century the asylum, "the big house on the hill" surrounded by its landscaped park and topped by high towers and domes, became a familiar landmark. Although such matters as management, housing, and feeding of the patients were slowly attaining decent humanitarian standards, as late as 1840 no clear classification of mental disorders existed. A German teacher, Dr. Heinroth, was still advancing the theory that insanity and sin were identical. Not until 1845 was the first authentic textbook on mental disease published, aligning the treatment of mental illness with the treatment of other illnesses.

This self-contained state hospital system of mental health delivery, with all its advantages and disadvantages, might well have continued had it not been for the waves of immigrants to the United States in the midnineteenth century. The effect of this "population explosion" was an enlargement of the cities so that the state hospitals were no longer so geographically remote. In addition and perhaps more important, the system was confronted with huge numbers of individuals who were believed to need mental health care. Because the cultural backgrounds and language of the immigrants were sufficiently different from those of the mainstream population, the behavior of many immigrants was poorly tolerated by society, and the census of the state hospitals swelled. This made it impossible to continue the humane treatment delivered earlier, and by the twentieth century the state hospital system had turned into an inefficient, expensive, and inhumane system able to do little

more than protect inmates from one another and from society.

Twentieth century

Overt change in the state hospital system of mental health care began in 1908 when **Clifford Beers,** a psychiatric patient who was hospitalized several times, wrote a book entitled *A Mind That Found Itself.* Having a vivid, colorful temperament, Beers had unlimited enthusiasm, which he directed to founding the National Committee for Mental Hygiene. Under the momentum of his leadership the movement became worldwide, and for the first time, prevention of mental illness and early intervention were emphasized.

Simultaneously with the mental hygiene movement came the astounding contributions of **Sigmund Freud** (1856-1939), which revolutionized the orthodox concepts of the mind, proposed a new technique for exploring it, and brought the subject of human behavior to the attention of the public. In addition, many other theorists made major contributions to the understanding of human behavior, although they were not as well known as Freudian concepts.

Mental health delivery in the public sector

One of the most progressive actions the United States has ever taken in relation to mental illness was the passage of the **National Mental Health Act** in 1946. Other accomplishments included the establishment of the National Institute of Mental Health (NIMH). A similar act was passed about the same time in Canada, and it had a similar effect in moving Canada into the forefront in the field of mental health. Both these acts provided for financing research and training programs. Through their enactment the governments expressed their belief that it was necessary to acquire more knowledge concerning the cause, prevention, and treatment of mental illness and that more professionally trained workers were needed to improve the care and treatment of persons with a mental illness. Financial support for the education of psychologists, psychiatric social workers, psychiatrists, and psychiatric nurses was provided in the United States for many years through the National Mental Health Act.

The National Mental Health Act grew out of U.S. experiences during World War II when more men in the armed forces were disabled by mental illness than by all the other problems related to military action. The many soldiers incapacitated by acute and chronic mental illness alerted the U.S. population to the need for many more trained professional workers in the field, for greater knowledge about the cause and prevention of mental illness, and for greatly improved treatment techniques.

Because of U.S. society's increased attention to the problem of mental illness, new methods for treating persons in need of mental health care were developed in the late 1940s and early 1950s. These methods included short-term and long-term treatment programs and crisis-oriented therapy. At about the same time, several new treatment methods were introduced into public psychiatric hospitals. Two of the most noteworthy programs were the *therapeutic community,* where the milieu was used as a specific therapeutic tool through examination of group processes and community self-regulation, and the *open-door hospital,* where the doors of the units were unlocked, allowing patients who were able to move freely within the hospital and the community. Interestingly, both these treatment modalities were first developed in England and were most successful with patients who were not severely or chronically ill.

Major changes in the care of persons with a severe and chronic mental illness were not possible until the development of psychotropic drugs, particularly the antipsychotic agents, which alter the chemistry of the brain and therefore the person's emotions and the behavior. These medications were first used experimentally in 1953. By 1956 the number of patients in the state mental hospitals was reported to have fallen slightly, instead of increasing as had been the case for decades. This phenomenon largely resulted because, with the help of these medications, more individuals could control their behavior and thus could spend time outside the hospital in the community. Without these medications, many individuals would never have been able to control their unusual behavior sufficiently to remain at home and receive continuing treatment on an outpatient basis.

In 1955 the U.S. Congress passed the **Mental Health Study Act.** This act provided funds for a 5-year study of the problem of mental illness in the United States. As a result of the act, the Joint Commission on Mental Illness was established. On Dec. 31, 1960, this commission submitted its final report to Congress, the Surgeon General of the Public Health Service, and the governors of the 50 states. The published report was entitled *Action for Mental Health* and was available to the public in 1961. It was widely read, provided the necessary stimulus for developing more effective services for people in need of psychiatric help, and was the basis for additional legislation.

A milestone in the U.S. public's developing awareness of the need for an improved approach to the problems of mental health and illness was reached on Feb. 5, 1963, when President John F. Kennedy delivered his special message to the Congress on mental illness and mental retardation. In this speech he mentioned a few goals: "Central to a new mental health program is comprehensive community care.... The mentally ill can achieve...a constructive social adjustment.... The centers will focus on community resources.... Prevention as well as treatment will be a major activity." In that same year, 1963, the **Community Mental Health Centers Act** was passed, followed in 1965 by the Staffing Act for the Community Mental Health Centers. These acts sought to revolutionize the provision of mental health care by emphasizing prevention and decentralized, local community treatment as opposed to institutional care for even those persons who manifest severe psychiatric difficulties. Federal funds to build and staff community mental health centers were appropriated and served as the force behind the rapid development of many such centers in a relatively short period. The first federally funded centers began operation in 1966, and thus began the deinstitutionalization of persons with a mental illness.

In 1975 the U.S. Congress enacted the Community Mental Health Centers Amendments. This law provided for the continuation of federal funds to community mental health centers but also designated specific guidelines for services that must be provided. A full range of inpatient, outpatient, and emergency services was specified in these guidelines. Certain population groups such as children and elderly persons were targeted as especially requiring services. Drug and alcohol abusers and addicts and persons being discharged from mental institutions also were included in the population groups given priority for services.

In 1977 President Jimmy Carter called for the development of a **President's Commission on Mental Health,** which was charged with identifying "the mental health needs of the nation." Nursing was represented on such a commission for the first time by Martha Mitchell, a nurse educator and clinical specialist in psychiatric–mental health nursing. The report of the 1977 commission recommended the development of a new federal grant program designed to strengthen existing community efforts and to develop new initiatives to address the mental health needs of communities. Special emphasis was placed on meeting the needs of underserved and high-risk populations and areas, such as elderly persons, children, persons with a chronic mental illness, cultural minorities, rural communities, and inner-city neighborhoods. The timely issue of the economics of mental health care was addressed by a recommendation that mental health coverage be included in all health insurance and

that this coverage not be limited to hospitalization. The commission also recommended that evaluation of federally funded community mental health centers be centralized.

In October 1980 Congress passed the Mental Health Systems Act. This legislation grew out of the commission's recommendations and addressed, among other issues, research and training priorities and clients' rights.

Unfortunately, before this legislation could be implemented, the political climate of the United States changed, and a conservative administration was elected to the White House. In 1981 the Congress passed the Reagan administration's Omnibus Budget Reconciliation Act. This legislation reallocated existing funding, resulting in a drastic curtailment of federal funding for all health services, including mental health care. Funds that remained for this purpose were distributed to the states in the form of "block grants" in the belief that it is both the right and the responsibility of the state government to determine priorities for finite resources and to distribute these funds. The one exception was the maintenance of federal funding for research, particularly biomedical research, into the causes and treatment of mental illness. Consequently, funding of publicly supported psychiatric hospitals and clinics became dependent primarily on state and local tax dollars, for which many other worthwhile claims existed.

Because of these severe fiscal constraints, many persons hospitalized because of mental illness, particularly elderly people, were transferred to nursing homes and other community institutions, where they were not provided with care appropriate to their needs. The federal Omnibus Budget Reform Act (OBRA) of 1987 was enacted in part to stem this practice.

During the Bush administration the U.S. economy became an increasing public concern, particularly in regard to the federal budget deficit, which had grown dramatically during the Reagan years. Simultaneously and somewhat a result of the federal response to the deficit, most, if not all, states found themselves in a deficit situation. As a means of curtailing government spending, most states instituted massive cutbacks in funding allocations for inpatient psychiatric care, often with promises that at least part of the money saved would be reinvested in community care for those persons with a mental illness. Often this promise was not realized. Therefore, state hospitals were downsized or closed, with many clients transferred to other facilities or discharged to the community, where local private and government agencies were not in any better fiscal position to provide care. Because of these fiscal realities, the deinstitutionalization of per-

sons with a severe, persistent mental illness, begun in the 1960s, was most fully achieved in the 1980s and 1990s. However, experience had shown that the level of funding required to operate fully a comprehensive community mental health center as originally conceived was now prohibitive. New models for delivering clinically effective and cost-efficient care in the public sector are needed. Their development represents one of the greatest challenges to U.S. society in the twenty-first century.

Table 1-2 identifies the loci of mental health care throughout history, and Table 1-3 outlines legislation on mental health care delivery in the public sector.

Table 1-2.   Locus of mental health care throughout history

	FAMILY/ COMMUNITY	RELIGIOUS ORDERS	PENAL INSTITUTIONS/ ALMSHOUSES	STATE MENTAL HOSPITALS	COMMUNITY MENTAL HEALTH CENTERS	PRIVATE HOSPITALS AND CLINICS	YET TO BE DETERMINED
Prehistoric times	X						
Early Greek and Roman eras		X					
Middle Ages		X					
Sixteenth, seventeenth, and eighteenth centuries			X				
Nineteenth century				X			
Twentieth century				X	X	X	
Twenty-first century	?	?	?	?	?	?	?

Mental health delivery in the private sector

Many private hospitals for the treatment of those with a mental illness were established even before the reforms of Dorothea Dix in the nineteenth century. Some, most notably the Hartford Retreat for the Insane in Connecticut, became models for other private and state hospitals during the nineteenth century. However, the number and size of private hospitals remained small, since very few individuals or families could afford to pay for the long-term treatment required by those who had a mental illness.

When third-party payment for psychiatric treatment became sporadically available in the 1960s, a few general hospitals began to include psychiatric care in their services. These psychiatric units were designed to provide care to those individuals who were acutely ill and needed short-term treatment. If recovery sufficient for discharge was not achieved within a short period, or if insurance reimbursement was depleted, the individual was often transferred to the state hospital.

Therefore, until the 1970s, most persons who needed inpatient treatment of a mental illness were hospitalized in a publicly supported facility, most often a state hospital. This situation began to change in the late 1970s, when most insurance companies and the federal govern-

Table 1-3. U.S. federal legislation affecting mental health care delivery in the public sector

YEAR	LEGISLATION	EFFECT
1946	National Mental Health Act	Established the National Institute of Mental Health (NIMH)
		Financed research and training programs
1955	Mental Health Study Act	Financed a 5-year study of mental illness in the United States
		Resulted in revolutionary report, *Action for Mental Health*
1963	Community Mental Health Centers Act	Emphasized prevention and decentralized, local community treatment
		Financed construction of community mental health centers
1965	Staffing Act for Community Mental Health Centers	Provided funding for staff for community mental health centers
1975	Community Mental Health Centers Amendments	Required inpatient, outpatient, and emergency services
		Specified target populations for priority services, including children, elderly persons, drug and alcohol abusers, and discharged persons with a mental illness
1980	Mental Health Systems Act	Designed to strengthen existing community efforts and to develop new initiatives
		Never implemented because of 1981 legislation
1981	Omnibus Budget Reconciliation Act	Drastically curtailed federal funding for health care services
		Allocated available funds as "block grants" to states
1987	Omnibus Budget Reform Act	Stopped warehousing of persons with a mental illness in nursing homes and other community institutions

ment agreed to include provisions for reimbursement for treatment of mental illness, particularly hospitalization, in their policies. As more and more employers provided this benefit to their employees, more people were able to secure treatment from the private sector, and an increasing number of free-standing private psychiatric hospitals and psychiatric units in general hospitals were developed. Although many of these hospitals provided a range of psychiatric services, many also restricted admission to those persons who were at low risk for violence to themselves or others and those who were hospitalized voluntarily. In addition, many institutions specialized in certain psychiatric disorders, such as depression or eating disorders. Therefore an ability to pay did not guarantee that one could be treated in the private sector.

Operationally, the emergence of privately funded psychiatric hospitals and units dramatically increased the disparity between socioeconomic groups and severity of illness; those who were most poor and most severely and chronically ill still had no choice but to receive services in the public sector. Many believe that this phenomenon increased the already great stigma associated with receiving psychiatric care in the public sector.

Ironically, the distinction between the public and private sectors is becoming blurred, since funding for all mental health care is becoming increasingly constrained in the 1990s and is likely to remain so for the foreseeable future. In addition, federal laws and most state regulations now require all private hospitals that receive public monies through reimbursement or other methods to admit involuntary clients.

INTERDISCIPLINARY MENTAL HEALTH TEAM

The **interdisciplinary mental health team** is no longer viewed as solely limited to professionals. A growing conviction exists that if treatment is to be effective, the team must include

the client and the family as integral members. This position reflects the belief that effective treatment of a person with a mental illness, especially one who has serious, persistent illness, must include the insights and experience of those who know him or her best—the client and those who have known him or her over a lifetime and who help manage the client's care on a daily basis, most often the family.

This awareness is more than a mere shift in treatment modality. Rather, it reflects a fundamental change in attitude toward those who have a mental illness and their families. Unfortunately, until recently, clients have been seen as culprits or victims because they and/or family members were mistakenly believed to be the cause of the illness. Therefore, clients needed to be protected from themselves and the family, and care had to be designed and delivered whether it was desired or even relevant to the client's situation. Consequently, the relationship between mental health professionals and the client and family was, at best, a patronizing one in which the professional was assumed by all to know best. At worst, an adversarial relationship existed.

The current collegial attitude about the role of the client and family in treatment is a result of increased scientific documentation that mental illness, particularly such serious and persistent mental illnesses as schizophrenia and the mood disorders, is a disease of the brain similar to other illnesses known to be diseases of other body organs. Even when this information became available to professionals, however, substantive changes in attitudes and practice did not occur until the relatives of those with a mental illness organized and, as a group, put public, visible pressure on professionals and policy makers to change policies and practices. This highly active, successful lay group is called the **National Alliance for the Mentally Ill** (NAMI).

It is not sufficient to say merely that clients and their families should be integrally involved in treatment decisions. Since most professionals practicing today were educated in the era when clients and their families were believed to be the cause of mental illness, it is understandable although not excusable that changes in practice are often only superficial. In addition, clients and their families sometimes do not wish to be involved, but rather are accustomed to having the burden of responsibility for care rest with the professional. Furthermore, the inclusion of clients and their families as equal members of the treatment team can raise some ethical, if not legal, issues. For example, what position should the professional take when clients insist that they do not want their parents to know the nature of their illness but at the same time insist on being discharged to their parents' home?

Nevertheless, most treatment facilities require that, at the very least, the client and family be invited to participate in treatment planning meetings. Most likely, the next generation of professionals will need to work with the next generation of clients and their families before the goal of NAMI for clients and their families to become fully empowered partners with professionals will be achieved.

Four health care professions constitute the core mental health disciplines: psychiatric nursing, psychiatry, clinical psychology, and psychiatric social work. They all emerged as specialties within their respective professions during the last half of the nineteenth century at the time when behaviorally disturbed persons were generally viewed as being ill rather than as being possessed by demons or morally corrupt. Because of the current knowledge explosion about the causes of mental illnesses, the educational preparation of all these specialists is undergoing significant change.

Psychiatric nursing

The first school of nursing in a psychiatric setting was established at McLean Hospital in 1882, 9 years after the first schools of nursing in the United States had been founded. Up to this time, poorly trained, nonprofessional workers had dominated the care of patients in psychiatric

institutions, and this school's purpose was to improve the care of patients by upgrading the skills of attendants. The first class of 15 women graduated in 1886. By 1917, 41 mental institutions were operating training schools for nurses. Unfortunately, the standards for admission and graduation established by most schools were much lower than those of schools of nursing in general hospitals. Beginning in 1906, nurse educators began to work toward establishing affiliations in psychiatric hospitals for students enrolled in schools of nursing in general hospitals, but not until 1955 did all schools of nursing offer an experience in psychiatric nursing as a required part of the curriculum. Schools of nursing in psychiatric hospitals no longer exist (Table 1-4).

Nurses are professionals whose initial educational preparation is through an associate degree, baccalaureate degree, or diploma program. After this preparation the nurse becomes licensed as a registered nurse through successful completion of state board examinations. Without additional educational or experiential preparation, this nurse can function as a generalist in any setting. An increasing number of nurses with baccalaureate degrees have continued their education to attain master's degrees in a particular clinical specialty. Nurses prepared as clinical specialists in psychiatric–mental health nursing at the graduate level have advanced preparation in promoting the mental health of individuals, groups, families, and communities, as well as in assisting these persons in increasing the effectiveness of their adaptations. The American Nurses' Association (ANA) administers an examination process whereby psychiatric nurse generalists and psychiatric clinical nurse specialists both can document their expertise and become certified at the appropriate level. Although no legal requirement to hold ANA certification exists at this time, many psychiatric nurses are choosing to earn this credential. In addition, third-party providers are increasingly using certification as one determinant of eligi-

Table 1-4. Peplau's history of psychiatric nursing

PERIOD	EVENTS
1773-1881	Psychiatric nursing did not exist as such.
	Psychiatric care was generally custodial and harsh.
1882-1914	Mental health nurses were trained and introduced into mental health facilities.
	New methods of treatment that avoided the use of restraints were used.
	The mental hygiene movement began and emphasized prevention and more humane treatment.
	Nurses played a subordinate and custodial role as managers of the ward and keepers of the keys; their primary function was to implement treatment programs devised by others.
	Psychiatric nurses' training did not include much psychology or psychiatry.
1915-1935	The number of undergraduate programs, including courses in psychiatric nursing, increased to half the existing programs by 1935.
	The first psychiatric nursing textbook was published.
	Some training at the postgraduate level for psychiatric nurses was given in psychiatric hospitals.
1936-1945	Three universities offered courses in postgraduate psychiatric nursing education.
	The establishment of the Mental Health and Psychiatric Nursing Project within the National League for Nursing Education brought psychiatric nursing into the mainstream of nursing.
1946-1959	Postgraduate education in psychiatric nursing was firmly established.
	The National League for Nursing assumed responsibility for the accreditation of psychiatric nursing curricula.

From Rawlins RP and others: *Mental health–psychiatric nursing,* ed 3, St Louis, 1993, Mosby–Year Book.

bility for reimbursement for services provided. The specific roles and functions of the psychiatric nurse generalist are discussed in detail in Section Two.

Psychiatry

Although the superintendents of the asylums were physicians, the specialty of psychiatry was not known until 1846, when the practice of hospitalizing persons with a mental illness made possible the systematic observation and study of mental disorders. Not until after World War I was the specialty given any significant attention in the curricula of medical schools.

Psychiatrists are physicians who have had several years of supervised residency training in the medical specialty of psychiatry. The law does not require licensing beyond that necessary for any physician, but the medical profession makes available a voluntary examination in this clinical specialty. Physicians who successfully complete this examination are "board certified" and identify themselves as such. This designation helps to assure the lay public of the services of a physician with advanced knowledge and experience in psychiatry. Psychiatrists function in private practice and treat hospitalized clients. In the latter instance the psychiatrist may be the leader of the treatment team, although the trend is toward the treatment team leader being the person who is most knowledgeable about the client, regardless of professional discipline. The psychiatrist's unique function is prescribing medications and administering other somatic treatments such as electroconvulsive therapy. In addition, the psychiatrist is the only professional equipped to make a medical diagnosis and is particularly skilled in identifying and treating persons whose problems have highly interrelated emotional and physiological components.

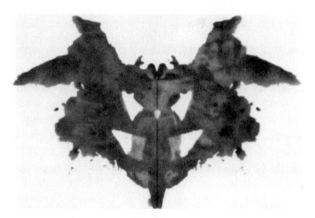

Figure 1-2
Rorschach test.
Courtesy Hans Huber Medical Publisher, Berne.

Clinical psychology

Unlike psychiatry, which had its origin in the practice setting, psychology began within the university as an academic, research-oriented discipline devoted to the scholarly study of human behavior. The first psychological clinic was established in 1896 at the University of Pennsylvania, followed shortly by the establishment of psychological laboratories in such hospitals for mentally disturbed persons as McLean Hospital in Massachusetts, St. Elizabeth's Hospital in Washington, D.C., and Boston Psychopathic Hospital.

Psychologists are professionals who have advanced education in the study of mental processes and the treatment of mental disorders. They are not physicians but hold doctoral degrees. As in the fields of nursing and medicine, psychology has become such a broad discipline that most psychologists specialize. Those who are most directly involved in the diagnosis of mental illness and in the treatment of those with a mental illness are called *clinical psychologists*. Those clinical psychologists concerned with the diagnosis of mental illness have developed expertise in the use of inferential tools designed to assist in the diagnostic process and assessment of treatment effects. Such tools are projective techniques best exemplified by the Rorschach test (Figure

1-2), personality inventories such as the Minnesota Multiphasic Personality Inventory, and intelligence tests. Only clinical psychologists are trained in the use and interpretation of these highly complex instruments. Other clinical psychologists have chosen to develop expertise in the treatment of persons with a mental illness. Since the education of these psychologists traditionally has been geared to the study of human behavior, they have been particularly effective when the problems of the individual or the family are psychogenic in origin and manifestation. Most clinical psychologists work in close collaboration with a psychiatrist, who assists in the treatment program if somatic therapies are indicated. Some states make legal certification mandatory for practice as a clinical psychologist.

Psychiatric social work

Social work began as an organized profession in the 1870s, but the specialty of psychiatric social work did not emerge until 1906 as a result of the aftercare movement, which was designed to provide adequate financial, medical, and moral assistance to patients released from mental hospitals. Mary C. Jarrett, believed to be the first psychiatric social worker, directed the first formal training course for psychiatric social workers at Smith College in 1918.

Social workers are health professionals, many of whom have educational preparation at the master's degree level. Although social workers are prepared to work with individuals and families who have a wide variety of physical, emotional, and social problems, some specialize in psychiatric social work. *Psychiatric social workers* are particularly skilled in assessing familial, environmental, and social factors that contribute to the dysfunctional behavior of the individual and the family. They also are major contributors to the planning and implementation of follow-up care.

Activity therapies

Although activity therapies are not considered a core mental health discipline, no discussion of the mental health care team would be complete without mention of them. The disciplines that make up the activity therapies include occupational therapy, recreational therapy, music therapy, rehabilitation counseling, educational therapy, and patient library services (bibliotherapy). Within these specialties, other services may be provided, such as dance therapy, drama therapy, art therapy, horticulture therapy, and manual arts therapy. The history of occupational therapy, the first of the activity therapies, is cited here because of its intimate connection with nursing.

The first book on the subject of occupational therapy was written by a nurse, Susan E. Tracy. This book, *Studies in Invalid Occupation,* was published in 1910. Tracy also gave the first course of instruction on the subject in 1906 at the Adams Nervine in Boston. As such, nurses were the first *occupational therapists,* although that term was not used until 1921.

Some physicians also saw the potential therapeutic benefit of a planned activities program. As early as 1892, Dr. E.N. Brush wrote that even the most simple, routine tasks keep the mind occupied, awaken new trains of thought and in-

terest, and divert clients from the delusions or hallucinations that harass and annoy them. Brush particularly advocated the use of outdoor activities in the belief that physical exertion has a beneficial effect on the client's emotional health. Since the nursing staff was responsible for initiating and supervising all client activities, a book titled *Occupation Therapy, a Manual for Nurses* was published in 1915. The author was Dr. William Rush Dunton, one of the earliest leaders in the field of occupational therapy. Dunton advised that the nurse "provide herself with an armamentarium which should consist at least of the following: playing cards, dominoes or card dominoes, cribbage board, scrap book with puzzles and catches, and one or more picture puzzles. . . . She is also urged to cultivate a particular craft in order that she may herself have a hobby and also that she may have special ability in instructing her client."*

All **activity therapists** are required to have at least a bachelor's degree in their field, and many have advanced degrees. A master's degree is required for entry into art therapy. Although each form of activity therapy has a specific focus, they share the principle that it is helpful to the emotionally disturbed person to be engaged in an activity that focuses on objects outside the self. The concept of *object relations* is fundamental in activity therapies. This concept includes not only the materials used in the therapy but also the setting, the therapist, and the other participants. These objects all have symbolic value, and through their use the individual expresses feelings, needs, and impulses. In this sense, all activity therapies are creative and therefore can be used in varying ways and for varied purposes. They are developed into a program based on psychodynamics but are highly individualized to meet the needs of the person for whom they are designed.

---

*Dunton, WR: *Occupation therapy, a manual for nurses,* Philadelphia, 1915, Saunders, p 8.

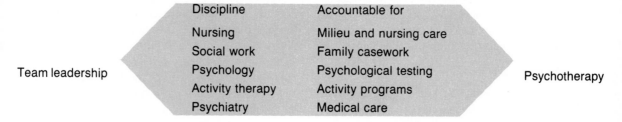

Discipline	Accountable for
Nursing	Milieu and nursing care
Social work	Family casework
Psychology	Psychological testing
Activity therapy	Activity programs
Psychiatry	Medical care

Team leadership   Psychotherapy

Figure 1-3

Roles assumed by mental health team members.

From Stuart GW, Sundeen SJ: *Principles and practice of psychiatric nursing,* ed 4, St Louis, 1991, Mosby–Year Book.

The following five goals are common to all activity therapies in a mental health setting:

1. *To provide opportunities for structured normal activities of daily living.* Activities are designed to help the clients deal with their basic problems. In addition, the activities permit the maintenance and reinforcement of the healthy aspects of the client's personality.

2. *To assist in diagnostic and personality evaluation.* As trained members of the health care team, activity therapists can assist with diagnostic and personality evaluations through their observations of clients as they participate in activities. In addition, the process of participation, such as the type of activity chosen and the interaction that occurs between the client and the therapist and between the client and other participants, gives the therapist much valuable information about the client's personality structure.

3. *To enhance psychotherapy and other psychotherapeutic measures.* The activity prescribed for the client often provides a nonverbal means for the client to express and resolve the feelings being discussed verbally in other settings. In addition, the interpersonal relationship established between the client and the therapist provides another vehicle for the provision of corrective emotional experiences.

4. *To assist the client in making the transition from the sick role to becoming a contributing member of society.* Some activities provide opportunity for work experience, often with the use of community resources. Through these activities the client is able to learn a skill that may be marketable. Other activities in this category focus on the development of the client's talents and interests so that he or she may learn to use time in satisfying ways.

5. *To assist the client to develop skills in relating and interacting with others in a cooperative manner.* This goal is most often achieved through group activities in which clients are helped to learn effective interpersonal behaviors as they interact about the topic of the activity. For example, a group activity designed to teach clients to cook can be a valuable opportunity to teach them not only how to cook but also how to share.

All activity therapies are designed to achieve a specified goal, and the therapist's role is to observe, direct, and guide the client in the activity. The therapist continuously assesses the client's reactions to the activity both as a means of providing information to other members of the treatment team and as a basis on which to alter the activity as the client's needs change.

Psychiatric case management

A new mental health worker, the **psychiatric case manager,** has developed over the last decade. Case management is both a treatment intervention and a delivery method that has become increasingly necessary for individuals whose needs are complex and long term, such as those with a serious, persistent mental illness. The case manager's role is based on the belief that to be successful in the community, the client needs continuity of care that is accessible and comprehensive. Because hospital stays are becoming shorter with the discharged client still needing varying degrees and types of care, many believe that a worker or group of workers is needed on whom the client can depend to help coordinate care and gain access to various types of care. It is believed that the availability of case manager services will prevent costly rehospitalization and increase the client's quality of life. In fact, the federal government has mandated that everyone with a serious, persistent mental illness who is eligible for publicly funded mental health services must receive case management services. At this point, results of studies are inconclusive about whether case management is successful in achieving the goals of clinically effective and cost-efficient community care.

Psychiatric case managers can and do have professional preparation in any one of the four core mental health disciplines, although the vast majority are nurses and social workers. In addition, most authorities agree that further training is necessary, including the development of skills in holistic, biopsychosocial assessment; counseling and teaching activities of daily living; negotiating the bureaucracy; and intervening in crises.

Although case management practice differs widely, it is generally agreed that the five core components of case management are (1) client identification and outreach, (2) assessment, (3) service planning, (4) monitoring of service delivery, and (5) advocacy. Furthermore, case management services are delivered in a variety of formats. In the caseworker model the case manager carries his or her own caseload of clients. In the paraprofessional-extender model the case manager supervises paraprofessionals who provide the direct care. In the team model a group of professionals and paraprofessionals functions as a team in providing services to each client. Regardless of model, the services delivered to the client are available 24 hours a day, 7 days a week.

It should be noted that anyone may legally call himself or herself a psychotherapist or psychoanalyst, and these designations do not guarantee a level of expertise. All reputable therapists and analysts, however, have years of advanced education and supervised clinical training in their particular discipline.

KEY POINTS

1. In prehistoric times, persons with deviant behavior were treated by tribal rites. If these failed, individuals were left to die of starvation or be attacked by wild beasts.
2. The early Greeks often used their temples to house persons who had a mental illness. Sometimes these people were treated with great kindness, whereas at other times treatment was harsh and barbaric.
3. In the Middle Ages the treatment of mental illness was left to priests. Both harsh and humane treatments were used to drive out the "evil spirit."
4. In the sixteenth century, persons with a mental illness were locked up in jails, dungeons, or lunatic asylums where curious people could pay to watch the "performance" of the sick inmates.
5. During the seventeenth century, society was interested in its own self-security, not in the welfare of persons with a mental illness. As a result, they were treated brutally and subjected to whippings and bleedings in the name of "treatment."

6. In 1792 Philippe Pinel was instrumental in demonstrating the error of treating persons with a mental illness inhumanely. His pupil Esquirol continued humane treatment and is regarded as the first teacher of psychiatry.

7. In 1756 Benjamin Franklin founded the Pennsylvania Hospital, where Benjamin Rush, the "father of American psychiatry," began working in 1783.

8. Eastern Psychiatric Hospital, Williamsburg, Virginia, was built in 1773 and is regarded as the first American public psychiatric hospital.

9. Dorothea Dix, an American schoolteacher in the mid-1800s, stirred public awareness of the evils of the poorhouse and raised money to build suitable hospitals for persons with a mental illness in parts of the United States, Canada, and Europe.

10. The state hospitals of the nineteenth century provided meaningful activity for some patients, thereby increasing their sense of self-esteem and group cohesiveness. The labor of others was exploited.

11. The first authentic textbook on psychiatric disorders was published in 1845; for the first time, discussion of mental illness paralleled that of other illnesses.

12. One of the most progressive actions the United States has ever taken in relation to mental illness was the passage of the National Mental Health Act in 1946.

13. Major changes in the care of persons with a severe and chronic mental illness were not possible until the development of psychotropic drugs, first used experimentally in 1953.

14. The Joint Commission on Mental Illness was established as a result of the Mental Health Study Act of 1955. This commission submitted a report entitled *Action for Mental Health,* which provided the necessary stimulus for developing more effective services for people in need of psychiatric help and served as the basis for additional legislation.

15. On Feb. 5, 1963, President John F. Kennedy delivered a special message to the Congress on mental illness and mental retardation and called for a focus on comprehensive community care and prevention as well as treatment.

16. The first federally funded community mental health centers began operation in 1966, beginning the deinstitutionalization of persons with a mental illness.

17. Additional federal funding for community mental health services was authorized during the 1970s. During the 1980s, however, federal funding was reallocated, resulting in a drastic curtailment of funding for all health services, including mental health services. Remaining funds were distributed to the states in the form of "block grants."

18. As a result of growing fiscal constraints in the 1980s and early 1990s, state hospitals were downsized or closed, and the deinstitutionalization of persons with a severe and persistent mental illness that began in the 1960s was most fully achieved.

19. The development of new models for delivering clinically effective, cost-efficient mental health care in the public sector represents one of the greatest challenges to U.S. society in the twenty-first century.

20. In the late 1970s, most insurance companies and the U.S. federal government agreed to include provisions for reimbursement for treatment of mental illness in their policies. As a result, more private psychiatric hospitals and psychiatric units in general hospitals were developed.

21. Currently, the distinction between the availability of mental health care in the public and private sectors is becoming blurred because funding for all mental health care is becoming increasingly constrained.

22. The interdisciplinary mental health team is no longer viewed as solely limited to professionals. A growing conviction exists that if treatment is to be effective, the team must include the client and family as integral members.

23. Four health care professions constitute the core mental health disciplines: psychiatric nursing, psychiatry, clinical psychology, and psychiatric social work.

24. Activity therapies include occupational therapy, recreational therapy, music therapy, rehabilitation

counseling, educational therapy, and patient library services (bibliotherapy). These therapies are considered essential to comprehensive mental health services.

25. Psychiatric case management is a relatively new discipline that is considered necessary for individuals whose needs are complex and long term, such as those with a serious, persistent mental illness.

SUGGESTED SOURCES OF ADDITIONAL INFORMATION

Adelson G, Leader M: The social worker's role: a study of private and voluntary hospitals, *Hosp Community Psychiatry* 31:776, November 1980.

Beers C: *A mind that found itself,* New York, 1948, Doubleday.

Chamberlain JC: The role of the federal government in the development of psychiatric nursing, *J Psychosoc Nurs Ment Health Serv* 21:11, April 1983.

Church O: From custody to community in psychiatric nursing, *Nurs Res* 36:48, January 1987.

Ebben P and others: Problems and issues in community mental health service delivery in the 1990s, *Community Ment Health J* 27:225, June 1991.

Joint Commission on Mental Illness and Health: *Action for mental health,* New York, 1961, Basic Books.

Kanter J: Clinical case management: definition, principles, components, *Hosp Community Psychiatry* 40:361, April 1989.

Kassis J and others: The family support group: families and professionals in partnership, *Psychosoc Rehabil J* 15:91, April 1992.

Mark B: From "lunatic" to "client": 300 years of psychiatric patienthood, *J Psychosoc Nurs Ment Health Serv* 18:32, March 1980.

Maurin JT: Case management: caring for psychiatric clients, *J Psychosoc Nurs Ment Health Serv* 28:6, July 1990.

The mental health disciplines: notes on the development of 13 disciplines that play important roles in the treatment of the mentally disabled, *Hosp Community Psychiatry* 27:495, July 1976.

Morrissey J, Goldman H: Cycles of reform in the care of the chronically mentally ill, *Hosp Community Psychiatry* 35:785, August 1984.

Mound B and others: The expanded role of nurse case managers, *J Psychosoc Nurs Ment Health Serv* 29:18, June 1991.

Petrila J, Sadoff R: Confidentiality and the family as caregiver, *Hosp Community Psychiatry* 43:136, February 1992.

Pittman D: Nursing case management: holistic care for the deinstitutionalized chronically mentally ill, *J Psychosoc Nurs Ment Health Serv* 27:23, November 1989.

Smoyak S: Psychosocial nursing in public versus private sectors: an introduction, *J Psychosoc Nurs Ment Health Serv* 29:6, August 1991.

Thompson J and others: Fifty years of psychiatric services: 1940-1990, *Hosp Community Psychiatry* 33:711, September 1982.

Two hundred years of mental health care in America, *Hosp Community Psychiatry* 27:443-537, July 1976.

Van Donogen C, Jambunathan J: Pilot study results: the psychiatric RN case manager, *J Psychosoc Nurs Ment Health Serv* 30:11, November 1992.

Chapter 2

Psychiatric Nursing in the Hospital

LEARNING OBJECTIVES
After studying this chapter, the student will be able to:

- Discuss changes in the site and nature of hospital care of persons with a mental illness.

- Differentiate between voluntary and involuntary admission for the treatment of mental illness.

- Describe the usual procedure for involuntary admission to a psychiatric hospital.

- Discuss the following client rights:
  1. The right to habeas corpus
  2. The right to treatment
  3. The right to informed consent
  4. The right to confidentiality-privacy
  5. The right to an independent psychiatric examination
  6. The right to refuse treatment
  7. The right to be free of restraints

- List five goals to be achieved during the process of admitting a person to an acute care setting.

- Discuss the factors to be considered when preparing a client for discharge from an acute care setting.

- State the overall mission of psychiatric rehabilitation.

- Explain why psychiatric rehabilitation is an appropriate intervention model for many clients residing in long-term care settings.

KEY TERMS
Action for Mental Health
Voluntary admission
Involuntary admission
Emergency commitment
Temporary commitment
Indefinite commitment
Criminal commitment
Guardian
Mental Health Systems Act Bill of Rights
Informed consent
Confidentiality
Target symptom

Until relatively recently the practice of psychiatric nursing in hospitals took place almost exclusively in institutions that were state supported. Now, with a major shift in the nature of the mental health care delivery system, individuals with a mental health problem who require hospitalization are treated in one or more of a variety of settings, including free-standing private and publicly supported hospitals and psychiatric units in general hospitals. Along with changes in the site of treatment, the nature of treatment has also changed. The individual admitted to the hospital no longer is destined to remain for months. Today the average length of stay for persons requiring acute care is less than 30 days. At the same time, many individuals still require long-term psychiatric care for various reasons. For some, this care is also provided in hospitals. With both short-term and long-term psychiatric hospitalization, the nurse's role has changed from what it was less than a decade ago. The nurse's role also differs depending on the type of hospital setting in which the nurse practices. This chapter discusses that role in both acute care and long-term care settings.

HISTORICAL PERSPECTIVE

As discussed in detail in Chapter 1, before the nineteenth century most people who had a mental illness were housed in poorhouses or almshouses. In the midnineteenth century the state hospital system for the care of those with a mental illness emerged. By the beginning of the twentieth century, society had seemingly agreed that it was the state government's role to care for those with a mental illness. As a result, one or more large state-supported hospitals existed in most states, and the vast majority of those persons who needed psychiatric care were hospitalized in these facilities (Figure 2-1). Several outstanding private psychiatric hospitals also existed. Unfortunately the services of these hospitals were available only to a small number of people who could afford to pay for what was frequently long-term care.

The state hospitals of the first half of the twentieth century provided asylum to a wide range of individuals, including those who were ill for the first time and those who had been ill for most of their lives. For all, however, the length of stay was months and years, not days or weeks, regardless of the individual's ability to be discharged. For most patients, this elongated length of stay resulted in a syndrome called *institutionalization*. Simply put, institutionalization is the result of the person adapting to the environment and becoming unable and/or unwilling to live in another environment. This syndrome is not unique to psychiatric hospitalization in state-supported facilities. However, it occurred frequently in these settings because of their geographical remoteness, self-contained nature, and many rigidly enforced rules and regulations designed to control and regulate the behavior of large groups of patients with the smallest number of staff. Therefore, clients learned the dependent sick role very well, and what became normal was to behave in a manner considered abnormal by the rest of society. Morale of both clients and staff was low, and little hope existed for positive change. To make matters worse, when positive change did occur, it often was viewed as a sign of pathology. For example, a client who questioned a rule was likely to be seen as overly suspicious or aggressive rather than as thoughtful, independent, and assertive.

In the 1960s a movement emerged to include psychiatric units in general hospitals. These units were designed to care for those who were in the acute phase of a mental illness and resulted from the combined result of the national report **Action for Mental Health,** fiscal constraints, and the development of medications that helped alleviate some of the most distressing symptoms of the major mental illnesses. These psychiatric units were most frequently found in large, urban general hospitals, particularly those associated

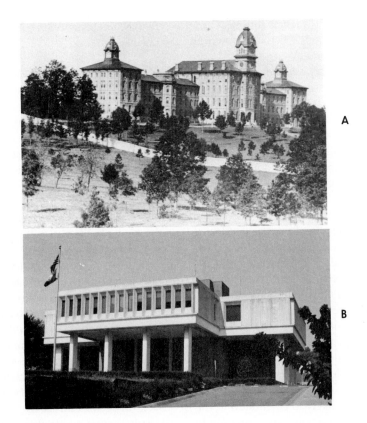

Figure 2-1

A, This photograph of the Arkansas Lunatic Asylum was taken in 1883 by L.W. Banks. **B,** Arkansas State Hospital in 1991.

A courtesy the Heiskell Library Collection at the *Arkansas Gazette.* From Rawlins RP and others: *Mental-health psychiatric nursing: a holistic life-cycle approach,* St Louis, 1993, Mosby–Year Book.

with medical schools. A positive outcome of these units was a reduction in the average length of stay, since patients were either discharged or transferred for continuing care to the state hospital. Therefore the feeling of hope for recovery in both clients and staff gradually increased, as did staff morale. It was also believed that once mental illness was treated as any other illness, the societal stigma associated with having a mental illness would be reduced. This hope has yet to be fully realized.

The demand for psychiatric services has escalated in the 1980s and 1990s. This demand, combined with increased insurance coverage for the treatment of mental illness, has resulted in the development of free-standing private psychiatric hospitals, the number of which has almost tripled since 1979. The number of psychiatric units in general hospitals has doubled during that time. In addition, many general hospitals not large enough or with insufficient resources to support a psychiatric unit have beds designated for persons with a mental illness. These are known as "scatter beds." Usually, however, the length of stay is short.

Very few state psychiatric hospitals still admit persons in the acute phase of mental illness, unless these persons need the type of treatment or protection that cannot be provided in the general hospital. Rather, most state hospitals have diminished dramatically in size and are becoming specialized in the care and rehabilitation of those individuals who are chronically ill and who have had unsuccessful past attempts to live and be treated in the community. This trend is so recent that many of these persons have the syndrome of institutionalization described earlier. As these persons are successfully rehabilitated or die, the need for state-supported psychiatric hospitals is likely to continue to diminish. It is predicted that in the future, those persons with an acute, first-time episode of mental illness either will be treated without hospitalization or, if hospitalization is necessary, will be treated in the general hospital and not develop the need for long-term care. Therefore the role of the state-supported psychiatric hospital is likely to be limited to the care of those very few persons who continue to require the asylum that only continuous institutionalization can provide. Thus, for the foreseeable future, the state government is likely to continue fulfilling its responsibility to provide for the care of those with a mental illness by regulating mental health services rather than providing them.

LEGAL ASPECTS OF PSYCHIATRIC HOSPITALIZATION

It is vital that nurses who work in psychiatric settings know and understand the legal parameters of treating persons with a mental illness in a hospital. Since these parameters are most often defined by state government, nurses need to be particularly knowledgeable about the laws of the state in which they practice. This section is a general discussion of those legal issues most

likely to be encountered in the practice of psychiatric nursing.

Methods of psychiatric admission

The detention of persons considered to have a mental illness is permitted by law, although the specifics of the law differ from state to state. However, all states assume the responsibility of segregating from society those persons whom psychiatrists deem dangerous or incompetent because of mental illness.

In 1953 the U.S. Public Health Service published the Draft Act Governing Hospitalization of the Mentally Ill. The following distinctions were suggested:

1. **Voluntary admission** is to be characterized by the individual's admission and discharge via his or her own signature.
2. **Involuntary admission** is undertaken by someone other than the client.

The least restrictive manner of obtaining treatment for mental illness is voluntary admission. Since many individuals with a mental illness lack insight concerning their behavior and will not seek hospitalization of their own will, voluntary hospitalization is not always possible. The nurse must realize that a combination of overt behaviors and legal status, not a diagnostic category, determines whether an individual can be treated voluntarily or involuntarily. Suicidal, violent, acute psychotic, and antisocial behaviors in persons unwilling to be treated are the usual reasons for involuntary admission to a hospital.

Three types of involuntary admission result in legal commitment to a psychiatric hospital. The first is an **emergency commitment,** in which the individual presents a "clear and present" danger to self or to others. The length of this hospitalization is limited; in most states it is only for 3 to 5 days. The second type of involuntary admission is **temporary commitment,** in which the individual can be involuntarily hospitalized for a longer period; in some states this is 6 months. The third type of commitment is called *extended* or **indefinite commitment,** which is valid for an unspecified period, usually subject to periodic judicial review. **Criminal commitment** is a form of extended or indefinite commitment allowing involuntary hospitalization of persons charged with crimes who are awaiting trial or who have been acquitted of a crime by reason of insanity.

In the past, only state hospitals and some private psychiatric hospitals would admit persons on an involuntary status. Psychiatric units in general hospitals, in particular, were willing to admit only those individuals who voluntarily chose to be treated and could control their behavior sufficiently to be treated safely on an unlocked unit. This situation resulted in obvious and dramatic differences between the client populations treated in psychiatric hospitals and those treated in psychiatric units in general hospitals. Most recently, however, the trend in a number of states is for psychiatric units to accept clients for treatment regardless of their admission status.

Commitment methods are not uniform among the states, but no one can be deprived of liberty without due process of law. In general, commitment proceedings consist of (1) application, (2) examination, (3) determination, and (4) detention if indicated. The action is usually initiated by relatives or friends, although any legally appointed officer of the law, members of charitable organizations, a public health official, or a private citizen may make the application, which will bring the matter to the attention of the proper court. In most states the court that settles matters of psychiatric commitment is the common pleas court or the probate court. Here the application is submitted, statements by interested parties are heard under oath, and all available information about the individual and his or her behavior is recorded.

Frequently the application must be accompanied by the certificates of one or more physicians, or the judge may appoint one or two physicians to conduct a psychiatric examination. Some states require that at least one physician be a psychiatrist. The testimony of lay witnesses

and of the examining physicians must be sufficient to convince a judge or jury that the person in question is potentially dangerous to self or others and needs to be segregated and treated.

The issue of commitment is more than simply a legal and psychiatric question. Ideally, it is an issue of freedom of choice. Each nurse must decide whether to take a stand for or against commitment. It is imperative that nurses know and understand the commitment procedures in the states in which they practice. Furthermore, they must work for the necessary legislative amendments that would facilitate appropriate reforms so as to fulfill the dictum *primum nil nocere,* we must minimize harm.

Clients' rights

A right is the enjoyment of a privilege secured by law to a person. Persons with a mental illness who are hospitalized may experience a double limitation on their rights, one created by the organization of the hospital system and the other created by their illness. Although clients' illness may limit them to some extent, prejudging their competency by the staff may be a greater obstacle to clients exercising their rights. For example, a simple request to make a telephone call to home is subject to interpretation, evaluation, and possible denial if it is not deemed to be in the best interest of the client and the hospital organization. Thus a tension can exist in all psychiatric institutions between the client's need to exercise civil rights and the hospital's need to provide care in an effective, efficient manner. When the hospital's organizational needs take precedence over the client's treatment needs or civil rights, dehumanization, frustration, resignation, and despair can occur.

If it is proved that the individual is incapable of conducting his or her affairs, a **guardian** may be appointed by the court or by state authorities to protect the individual's rights and property. In some states this property guardian is called a conservator. If the amount of the client's property warrants the expense of guardianship or if business involving such property must be transacted, the guardian's responsibilities are not trivial. A guardian has direct responsibility for the individual's personal welfare and is generally a close relative. The guardian cannot confine the individual in an institution without permission or approval of the court, but this person can dictate, within certain limits, the nature of the treatment and can sign a permit for major surgery. The guardian may also have custody of the individual's minor children if the other parent is absent or incapable of accepting this responsibility.

A client's wife or husband rather than the parents is regarded as the natural guardian. All guardians must give bond for the proper performance of their duties. At regular intervals the guardian is required to make an accounting of expenses and income. The first consideration must be the comfort of the client. The guardian is required to protect the client's welfare judiciously.

The law has defined certain rules for the control of human conduct, including protection from injury-producing situations. These rules have been developed from rights that pertain to each individual and may not be violated without legal repercussion, unless the individual consents to their invasion. The first 10 amendments in the U.S. Constitution, adopted in 1791, deal with human rights. Some rights included in these amendments are the freedom of speech, the right of protection from unreasonable search and seizure, the right to a speedy trial, and the right to due process of law before being denied life, liberty, or property.

A serious loss of civil rights was often the consequence of involuntary commitment to a psychiatric hospital. As a result, in many states the committed person was not able to make valid contracts, vote, marry, or divorce. However, in almost all legal jurisdictions, legally committed individuals presently retain their constitutional and human rights, particularly those pertaining to their person, property, and civil liberties. Various rights have been listed in recent legislation, such as the following:

1. The right to keep clothing and personal effects
2. The right to communicate by telephone, to correspond, and to visit with persons outside the institution
3. The right to vote
4. The right to religious freedom
5. The right to enter contractual relationships
6. The right to make purchases
7. The right to make wills
8. The right to education
9. The right to habeas corpus
10. The right to be employed
11. The right to independent psychiatric examinations
12. The right to civil service status
13. The right to marry
14. The right to sue and to be sued
15. The right to retain licenses or permits established by law
16. The right not to be subjected to unnecessary mechanical restraint

In 1977 the President's Commission on Mental Health recommended that each state have a bill of rights for all individuals who are being treated for mental illness. Furthermore, it urged that a copy of these rights be displayed in all psychiatric settings, be given to each client using the facilities, and be explained in an easily understandable manner. A model client's bill of rights for mental health care was included in the Mental Health Systems Act passed by the U.S. Congress in 1980. Although the Omnibus Budget Reconciliation Act of 1981 included the repeal of parts of the Mental Health Systems Act, it did retain the bill of rights except for the provisions and funding for protection and advocacy. A summary of the **Mental Health Systems Act Bill of Rights** is found in the box on p. 29.

Statements regarding clients' rights have been developed because of judicial disillusionment with the way mental health professionals have

MENTAL HEALTH SYSTEMS ACT BILL OF RIGHTS

1. The right to appropriate treatment in the least restrictive setting
2. The right to treatment based on a current, accurate, individualized, written treatment plan that includes a description of mental health services that may be needed after discharge
3. The right to ongoing participation in the planning of treatment, along with appropriate explanations of its objectives, potential adverse effects, and alternatives
4. The right to refuse treatment, except in an emergency or as provided by law
5. The right not to participate in experimentation. When consent is given, the client has the right to have a full explanation of the procedure, its anticipated benefits, potential discomforts and risks, and alternative treatments, along with the right to revoke such consent at any time
6. The right to freedom from restraint or seclusion, except in an emergency or when these are prescribed as a part of treatment
7. The right to a humane treatment environment
8. The right to confidentiality of the client's mental health care records
9. The right to access of the client's own mental health care records, except to that information provided by third parties and that information deemed by a mental health professional to be detrimental to the client's health
10. The right to converse with others privately, to have convenient and reasonable access to the telephone and mails, and to see visitors during regularly scheduled hours, except when denied access to a particular visitor as part of the written treatment plan
11. The right to be informed promptly about these rights
12. The right to assert grievances regarding infringement of these rights, including the right to have such grievances heard in a fair, timely, and impartial manner
13. The right to obtain assistance from designated or otherwise qualified advocates
14. The right to exercise these rights without reprisal, including the denial of any appropriate, available treatment
15. The right to referral to other providers of mental health services on discharge

traditionally dealt with individuals being treated for a mental illness. It is important to recognize that the mere enactment of legislation designed to protect clients' rights does not ensure enforcement. Nurses seeking employment in psychiatric settings must be certain that these facilities have the proper internal structure to protect the client's rights. Facilities with no internal structure to enforce clients' rights are in a vulnerable position because clients may be forced to go outside the institution, possibly to court, to see that their rights are protected.

The following sections discuss selected client rights that are not self-explanatory or that have particular relevance to psychiatric nursing.

The right to habeas corpus

The object of the right to habeas corpus is to ensure the speedy release of individuals who claim that they are being deprived of their liberty and being detained illegally. This fundamental right has not always been respected. Kenneth Donaldson, a client in a civil commitment case decided by the Supreme Court, was refused writs of habeas corpus 18 times during his 15 years of hospitalization before he finally won his chance to have a court hear his case.

The right to treatment

In 1960 Morton Birnbaum advocated the recognition and enforcement of the legal right of an individual hospitalized in a public psychiatric institution to adequate medical treatment for psychiatric illness. Adequate treatment for hospitalized individuals who are mentally retarded or who have a mental illness is a constitutional right. The U.S. Second Federal Appeals Court and the Alabama Federal District Court have elaborated the following legal doctrines: (1) persons in custody for mental illness have a right to treatment;

(2) they may not be held without treatment; and (3) treatment can be legally defined.

In 1971 the guardians of committed clients and some employees of Bryce State Mental Hospital filed a class action suit against the Commiss'oner of Mental Health, members of the Alabana Mental Health Board, and others *(Wyatt v. Stickney)*. The defendants were charged with providing inadequate treatment to approximately 5000 clients. The court based its decision on the constitutional guarantee of a right to treatment. In 1972 the court issued an order that detailed criteria for adequate treatment: (1) a humane psychological and physical environment, (2) qualified staff in sufficient numbers to administer adequate treatment, and (3) individualized treatment plans.

The right to informed consent

If clients consent to treatment, their consent must be informed by staff explanation. It is important to understand what **informed consent** means. For a consent to be valid, it must be based on adequate knowledge and information and must be given by a person who has the legal capacity to consent. Furthermore, it must be voluntarily given. A rapidly growing mental health doctrine requires that clients be given specific and adequate information about the proposed treatment procedure. This is to include the administration of the treatment, its probability of success or failure, its risks and side effects, alternative treatment procedures, and the probable consequences of not receiving treatment.

The mental health professional has the duty to provide the necessary information whether or not the client requests it. The precise information given depends on the nature, severity, and consequences of the proposed treatment. The mental health professional misleads the client when the beneficial effects of a treatment are exaggerated or if the dangers of the treatment are minimized or withheld. If the client is injured, the mental health professional could be held responsible through malpractice or negligence claims.

The right to confidentiality-privacy

Confidentiality and privacy of information about the client must be respected at all times. The frequent necessity to exchange information about the client between health care professionals and institutions does not alter the legal requirements to protect the client's privacy. The individual revealing information about the client's condition without authorization could be subject to legal difficulties. A lawsuit for invasion of privacy, liability, or slander is possible, depending on the facts of the situation and the type of information revealed.

Statutes that pertain to the confidentiality of psychiatric records vary greatly among the states. Some statutes only prohibit disclosure of information about the client's diagnosis and treatment, whereas others prohibit disclosure of the fact of hospitalization. Most statutes permit disclosure to private physicians, welfare officials, police, and insurance companies. Some may permit disclosure to prospective employers. Other statutes prohibit disclosure to almost everyone unless the person consents to disclosure.

Clients should be told of the need to share information with other persons and agencies. They should be asked to sign the appropriate consent form.

Some states consider mental health professional–client communication, including nurse-client communication, privileged. Four criteria are used for judging whether communication is privileged:

1. The communication is given with confidence in its nondisclosure.
2. Confidentiality is essential to the maintenance of the relationship.
3. In the community's opinion the relationship should be zealously fostered.
4. The injury that would result to the relationship by disclosure of the communication is greater than the benefit gained in winning litigation.

The unnecessary disclosure of confidential information is considered improper by law. A breach of confidence is defined as the discussion of the client's confidential information with a third party. This type of unlawful disclosure may provide the client with a cause for action against the party revealing such information.

The right to an independent psychiatric examination

Fairness or due process requires that clients have an opportunity to secure a psychiatric examination by a physician of their choice. The provision of this independent judgment in commitment proceedings is designed to protect the client from the judgment of mental health professionals appointed by the court who may have motivations other than the client's interests. If the state is allowed to use such testimony, the client should have the same right. Furthermore, the constitutional right to present witnesses may also necessitate that clients be allowed to choose expert witnesses. Some authorities believe that the state should provide the client with sufficient funds to retain at least one expert witness.

The right to refuse treatment

An important basis of the right to refuse treatment is the constitutional right to privacy and personal autonomy. As long as public health, safety, or morals remained unharmed, the courts will respect a client's decision to refuse treatment.

In 1976 the Third Circuit Court of Appeals found at least three constitutional deprivations that may accompany the involuntary administration of medication (*Scott v. Plante*). The first involves the nature of psychotropic drugs, which affect mental processes and may interfere with a person's First Amendment rights to freedom of speech and association. The second deprivation occurs when medication administered against the client's will violates the right to consent to medical treatment. In the third the court considered that the involuntary administration of medication may raise an Eighth Amendment issue concerning cruel and unusual punishment. The nurse must be knowledgeable about these issues before forcefully administering medication that

the client refuses. Such an action by the nurse could result in a charge of assault.

The right to be free of restraints

During their hospital stay, clients may become violent, and the hospital is obliged to control them so that they do not harm others or themselves. If a delirious postoperative patient were left unattended by an open window and jumped from it, the hospital would be considered negligent.

However, the right to restrain a client is limited to the duration of real necessity. Although no one would dispute the right of hospital personnel to prevent a delirious individual from pulling out a catheter, in most situations hospital personnel cannot interfere with clients' actions. If, for example, clients shout obscenities but are not a threat to themselves or others, hospital personnel cannot tie them down or lock them up. To commit such acts invites a suit for false imprisonment.

Some state laws have specified the type of physical restraints that may be used, including the consistency of the material from which the restraint is made. Nurses must be mindful of such regulations. The restraint need not be physical; threats of force are sufficient cause for legal action. One who is physically restrained may have cause to file an action for battery. Alternatives for restraining clients must be considered, such as the provision of constant observation by nursing personnel. Nurses must also be aware that understaffing is not a suitable justification for the use of chemical or physical restraints. The issue of safety is the primary concern.

PSYCHIATRIC NURSING IN THE ACUTE CARE SETTING
On admission

Many say that a person has only one opportunity to make a first impression. The first impression of the person newly admitted to an acute care psychiatric setting and of the family lays a foundation for subsequent interactions and is likely to influence the nature and speed of the client's progress during hospitalization.

One of the nurse's goals during the admission procedure should be to establish a therapeutic alliance with both the client and the family. Persons admitted to an acute care psychiatric setting are likely to be experiencing at least two major fears. First, their symptoms are likely to be pronounced, or they would not require hospitalization. Clients may not have experienced these symptoms before and are likely to be frightened by them. Second, fear of the unknown is caused by an unfamiliarity with the staff and the setting. Nurses must remember that although they admit clients frequently, this procedure and the preceding events may be once-in-a-lifetime experiences for the client and family. Consequently the nurse and other personnel should assume that the person being admitted to the hospital is very frightened and should intervene on that basis. This means (1) behaving in a manner that expresses genuine concern for clients and treating them as important, worthwhile individuals; (2) conveying a sense of being in control of the situation and being able and willing to help; (3) explaining procedures in a simple, clear manner; and (4) responding to the concerns of the clients and of those who accompany them to the hospital.

For example, one client asked repeatedly about who would care for his dog while he was in the hospital. None of the staff answered him, probably causing him to wonder if he was being heard. As his voice grew louder and louder with the same question, the staff concluded he was on the brink of becoming violent and requested and received a physician's order for a tranquilizer, which they administered by force. This episode did little to establish a therapeutic alliance with the client.

A second goal to be achieved during the admission process is to learn clients' perceptions of why they are being hospitalized and what they hope to achieve as a result. Often a simple question such as, "What do you see as your problem?"

will elicit helpful information. Those who accompany the client to the hospital also should be asked for their perceptions of the problem. The responses to these questions provide goals toward which the treatment plan should be directed, since the client and family are likely to be most motivated to engage in activities related to issues they see as problems. For example, if the client is most distressed about hearing voices, it is useful to explain that the prescribed medication is designed to alleviate this symptom. This explanation may increase the client's willingness to take the medication because it clarifies the connection between the client's concern and the treatment. In contrast, the client who hears voices but expresses the most concern about lack of money can be helped to understand that the symptoms are likely to interfere with the client's ability to secure and retain a paying job. Therefore, taking the prescribed medication is a step toward this goal of obtaining more money. The client's presenting problem is referred to as the **target symptom.**

In addition to determining the client's target symptoms, questioning the client and accompanying persons about their perceptions of the problem can yield valuable information about the client's insight and the communication pattern between the client and these significant others. Most importantly, understanding what is most distressing to the client and accompanying persons forms the basis for the development of a treatment plan that is relevant to the client and the family.

A third goal is to orient the client and the family to the staff, the physical environment, and the routine. It is usually not wise to offer extensive information immediately on admission, but those who will be caring for the client must introduce themselves by name and role. In addition, such details as the location of the bedroom and the bathroom, the time of meals, and visiting hours are often major concerns. Many hospitals have a booklet about the facility and its procedures that is given to newly admitted clients and their families at admission. These booklets often have a section to write the names and telephone numbers of the client's physician, nurse, and other staff. People who are anxious often do not hear information correctly or at all, and written material provides a reference they can refer to later.

Many acute care units have locked doors, and the realization that they cannot leave at will may be frightening to some newly admitted clients. In contrast, some persons find the locked door reassuring. In either situation, another goal to achieve during the admission process and in the following days is to convey to clients that their safety and the safety of others of paramount importance to the staff. As with other people, clients new to the unit have learned the same stereo-

---

**ORIENTATION TO
HOSPITALIZATION FOR
PSYCHIATRIC TREATMENT**

Inform client of rights and responsibilities.
Explain treatment-planning process and client's participation in this process.
Provide guided tour of facility.
Explain unit rules and policies.
Introduce staff and other clients.
Describe staff's contribution to treatment process.
Provide information about schedule for next 24 hours.
Explain locked doors.
Explore client's thoughts and fears about being confined to hospital.
Facilitate client's verbalization of questions and provide information.
Explain treatment modalities and expectations of clients.
Provide information about rights, visiting hours, and process of increasing freedom.
Explain unit schedule, including meals, therapy, and free times.
Provide information about use of telephone, writing materials, and mailing procedure.
Provide rationales for restricted access to personal items and how they can be made available to client.

Modified from Haber J and others: *Comprehensive psychiatric nursing,* ed 4, St Louis, 1992, Mosby–Year Book.

---

types about persons with a mental illness. One of the most common stereotypes is that all persons with a mental illness are dangerous, so many clients are frightened of other clients. One of the quickest, most effective ways to help clients overcome this fear is to introduce them to one or two other clients, particularly those who are likely to be helpful. At the very least, the newly admitted client must be introduced to the roommate if a bedroom will be shared.

Another goal of the admission process is to establish a baseline assessment of the client. This means it is important to have an idea of what is normal or usual for this person in terms of physical parameters and daily routine. Therefore, if possible, a physical examination should be conducted and a history taken. If the client is upset, this should be postponed until the client is able to cooperate. Gathering information about a usual day for the client is often overlooked. Knowing preferred foods, usual sleeping patterns, and similar information can be invaluable in correctly understanding the client's response to the unit's standardized routine. For example, the client who has always worked from midnight to 8 AM initially may be unable to go to sleep at 10 PM.

The box at left outlines important components of the clients' orientation to hospitalization for psychiatric treatment.

During the treatment process

Information about treatment interventions specific to different types of clients is found in Section Four. However, it is important to understand that treatment should be as highly individualized as possible, which requires much thought, effort, and cooperation by all staff. Undoubtedly, it is easier to routinize procedures and insist that all clients comply with the same routine regardless of their needs or desires. Certainly, some basic rules that all must comply with are necessary in settings where groups of people live. However, the many rules that govern psychiatric units are often in place for the staff's

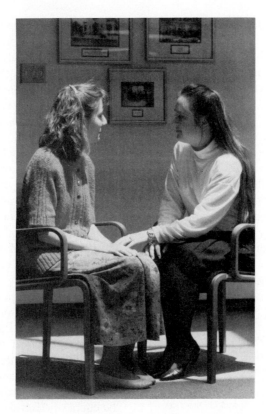

Figure 2-2
One-to-one relationship.

convenience and not for their therapeutic value. Also, the more individualized the treatment approach, the greater its help to the client.

Since clients are likely to feel secure when they can predict what will occur, individual staff members must agree on and support the unit's rules. Also, the staff must agree to be flexible in certain matters. An example of a rule that staff members could "agree to disagree on" is a somewhat arbitrarily determined bedtime. Although it is important that clients, especially those acutely ill, receive an optimum amount of sleep, the amount that is optimum varies among clients. The rule that all must be in bed no later than 10 PM, for example, is likely to be more a reflection of the staff's need to finish paperwork before the next shift's arrival than a desire to ensure the client has adequate sleep. It is also easier for staff to mandate that all go to bed at the same time than to explain to a client why it is important that he or she go to bed at 9 PM while others are staying up later.

Although many nurses practicing today have skill in the development and implementation of a one-to-one relationship (Figure 2-2), the short-term nature of hospitalization for treatment of an acute episode of a mental illness makes this intervention difficult to implement and sometimes inappropriate. Rather, the trend is for extended treatment to occur in group settings. The concept of the therapeutic community and the treatment modality of group therapy (Figure 2-3)

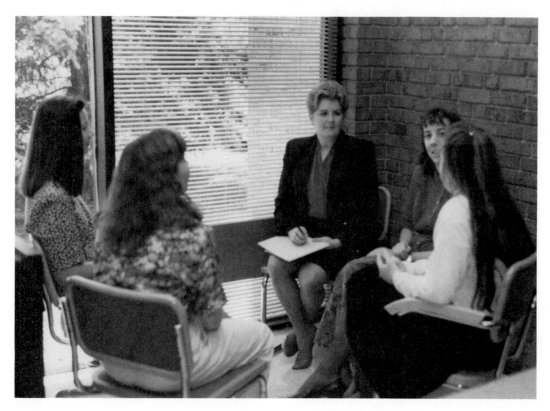

Figure 2-3
Group therapy in an acute care facility.

have been in existence for many decades, but only recently have group interventions been widely used. These interventions are likely to be educative in focus rather than psychotherapeutic, although any intervention that results in the client becoming more able to function satisfactorily is surely therapeutic. For example, it is imperative that clients understand the actions of their medications. Since teaching clients about their medications is a major function of nurses, nurses often conduct "medication groups." A frequent outcome of these groups is not only increased understanding of medications, but also increased social skills because clients have an opportunity to interact with and learn from each other as well as from the nurse.

The focus on group interventions is in apparent violation of the principle of individualized care. Reliance on group activities that are designed on the basis of the staff's interest and skills rather than the client's needs and interests does violate the principle of individualized care. However, when groups are formed because of clients' needs and interests and clients are assigned to groups on this basis, individualized care is truly achieved in a group setting.

Preparation for discharge

As is true with hospitalization for any reason, preparing for the discharge of the client who is hospitalized for the treatment of a mental illness should begin on admission. The client and family must be integral members of the team in the determination of what is to be achieved by hospitalization and when the client is ready to be discharged. The previously mentioned target symptoms determined at admission provide a useful reference in arriving at these decisions.

As clients become ready for discharge, they are often given "passes" to spend 1 or more days at home as a transition experience. On returning to the hospital from such a visit, the client is helped to evaluate the experience, including the aspects that went well and any unsuccessful areas. Treatment goals should be revised based on this evaluation.

A major function of the nurse in preparing the client and family for discharge is teaching. The following factors have been found to be most significant in the client's success in achieving a successful posthospitalization adjustment.

1. *An understanding of the illness.* This means not only a textbook understanding of the illness, but more importantly an awareness of factors likely to create stress with this particular client and how early symptoms of the illness are manifested in this person. These are called *premorbid symptoms* and are highly individualized. For example, one person with the medical diagnosis of schizophrenia may develop the belief that others are talking about him or her, whereas another person with the same medical diagnosis may have initial symptoms of being unable to bathe, arise in the morning, or otherwise fulfill activities of daily living. For all clients, however, the early identification of symptoms and prompt treatment may prevent the need for rehospitalization.

2. *An understanding of the nature of the prescribed medications and the importance of taking them.* Not long ago it was considered inappropriate, if not unprofessional, to teach the client and the family about the prescribed medication. Given the side effects of many of these medications, one should not be surprised to learn that many clients stopped taking their medications once they began to feel better. This prac-

tice, in turn, has been documented repeatedly as a major factor contributing to relapse and the need for rehospitalization. It is widely accepted practice today for the nurse to assume the primary responsibility for teaching the client and the family about the prescribed medication and what to do and whom to contact about questions and concerns.

3. *An ability to provide for the client's daily living needs.* Before discharge the treatment team must ensure that the client either is able to engage in activities of daily living or has available the supports necessary to enable the client to function on a daily basis. These activities include appropriate and adequate housing, food, clothing, work, and leisure activities. For example, the nurse would want to ensure that the client returning to an apartment had food available and that the electricity, heat, and telephone were operating. Although the social worker often has the responsibility for securing community support services, the nurse has a very important role in the discharge process because the nurse often has the most knowledge of the client's needs and how well the client is able to meet them.

Many clients are discharged to the homes of relatives, particularly parents. These relatives need to know what to expect and how to handle crises. They need to be helped to achieve a balance between treating the client as a child by reacting to every action and ignoring the client. They also need to learn what support groups are available to them in the community.

4. *An ability to handle questions about the client's absence and illness.* Many clients still face much discrimination about hospitalization for mental illness. The nurse should help clients prepare to answer questions about their absence and illness through role-playing anticipated situations. Even if these situations never occur, knowing they are prepared to respond appropriately is a comfort to many persons.

Many clients require continuing care after discharge. Usually the staff who treats the client in the community is a different group of people than the staff who treated the client in the hospital. This unfortunate practice contributes to the ineffectiveness of the mental health care delivery system. Nevertheless, as nurses work to effect change in the system, they can help ensure continuity of care of individual clients by completing referral forms in an accurate, timely manner. Some treatment settings have established linkages between hospital personnel and staff in the community whereby the two groups meet on a regular basis to discuss the care of clients about to be discharged.

PSYCHIATRIC NURSING IN THE LONG-TERM CARE SETTING

Government-supported hospitals for the care of those with a mental illness, particularly state-supported hospitals, are increasingly becoming long-term care facilities. At present, two major groups of clients reside in these settings. One group is persons whose illnesses have not been controlled by available treatments and who exhibit behaviors that interfere with living in the community. This group includes persons considered to be dangerous either to themselves or to others and who are likely to be in the hospital as a result of legal commitment.

The second major group is persons who have been hospitalized for decades, who consider the hospital their home, and who have few, if any, friends or relatives living outside the hospital. Even though these persons do not have an active mental illness, they have little incentive to leave the hospital, and few have the skills necessary to live successfully in the community.

Caring for these persons is one of the nurse's greatest challenges. Since change occurs slowly, if at all, with the first group described and treatment is not necessary with the second group, the staff often becomes discouraged and has low morale. The result is that institutions designed to provide long-term care of persons with a mental illness are at risk of becoming warehouses that do little more than provide custodial care. However, this does not need to be the case.

A frequently overlooked concept in the care of persons with a mental illness is the need for these persons to be rehabilitated. The need for rehabilitation of persons with a physical illness has long been recognized. Much effort and money are expended in helping those with residual physical illness adjust and adapt to the consequences of their illness. For example, an individual who is left paralyzed as a result of a cerebrovascular accident (stroke) is provided with the necessary physical supports, such as a motorized wheelchair and leg braces, and extensive training in the use of these devices so as to increase his or her independence. This has not been the case with individuals who have had a mental illness. The deinstitutionalization of these individuals and their inability to function in the community showed that persons with a severe mental illness have significant residual disability even if their illnesses have been successfully treated. The discipline of *psychiatric rehabilitation* was developed to address these disabilities.

The terms *impairment, disability,* and *disadvantage* are central to understanding psychiatric rehabilitation. Anthony, Cohen, and Farkas (1990) define *impairment* as any loss or abnormality of psychological, physiological, or anatomical structure or function; *disability* as resulting from an impairment and manifesting itself in any restriction or lack of ability to perform an activity and/or role in the manner or within the range considered normal for a human being; and *disadvantage* as resulting from an impairment and/or a disability and manifesting itself as a lack of opportunity for a given individual that limits or prevents the fulfillment of a role that is normal (depending on age, sex, social, or cultural factors) for that individual. These terms constitute the rehabilitation model (Table 2-1).

Clearly, many people with a severe mental illness who have been hospitalized for years have major disabilities and disadvantages, as a result

Table 2-1. Rehabilitation model for severe mental illness

STAGE	DEFINITION	EXAMPLES
Impairment	Any loss or abnormality of psychological, physiological, or anatomical structure or function	Hallucinations, delusions, depression
Disability	Any restriction or lack of ability to perform an activity and/or role in the manner or within the range considered normal for a human being (resulting from an impairment)	Lack of work adjustment skills, social skills, or ADL skills, which restricts one's residential, educational, vocational, and social roles
Disadvantage	A lack of opportunity for a given individual that limits or prevents the fulfillment of a role that is normal (depending on age, sex, social, or cultural factors) for that individual (resulting from an impairment and/or a disability)	Discrimination and poverty, which contribute to unemployment and homelessness

Modified from Anthony WA, Cohen MR, Farkas MD: *Psychiatric rehabilitation,* Boston, 1990, Boston University, Center for Psychiatric Rehabilitation.
ADL, Activity of daily living.

of the illness, their institutionalization, or both.

Psychiatric rehabilitation focuses on the consequences of the illness, not on the illness itself. It strives to help individuals to improve their functioning in a specific environment. The overall mission of psychiatric rehabilitation is to help persons with psychiatric disabilities become successful and satisfied in the environments of their choice with the least amount of ongoing professional intervention (Anthony, Cohen, and Cohen, 1983).

Psychiatric rehabilitation can be practiced by members of any of the mental health disciplines but is not routinely included in the educational programs that prepare these practitioners. What is taught is the treatment model, which focuses on impairment and is effective only with clients who have an active mental illness. Therefore, it is not surprising that nurses and other professionals who work with persons in long-term care settings are frustrated and demoralized, since their illness-oriented interventions do not address clients' rehabilitation needs.

It is beyond the scope of this chapter to discuss psychiatric rehabilitation in detail, and the student is referred to the many texts and articles on the subject. However, it is worth noting that the values and principles that undergird psychiatric rehabilitation are many of the same values and principles fundamental to the effective practice of psychiatric nursing. Examples include the emphasis on the client's strengths, the value of functioning, the emphasis on the here and now, and providing opportunities for client self-determination. Therefore, nursing is a particularly appropriate discipline in which to learn and implement the skills and techniques of psychiatric rehabilitation.

KEY POINTS

1. Individuals with a mental illness are now treated in a variety of settings, including acute care and long-term care hospitals.

2. Voluntary admission to a psychiatric hospital is characterized by the individual's admission and discharge via his or her own signature. Involuntary

admission is initiated by someone other than the client and results in a legal commitment to the hospital. It is important for nurses to know the laws of the state in which they practice.

3. The law has defined certain rights pertaining to persons hospitalized for the treatment of mental illness. It is vital that nurses know and understand these rights so that their practice reflects adherence to them.

4. When admitting a person to an acute care setting, the nurse should strive to achieve these goals:
   a. Establish a therapeutic alliance with both the client and the family.
   b. Learn clients' perceptions of why they are being hospitalized and what they hope to achieve as a result.
   c. Orient the person and the family to the staff, the physical environment, and the routine.
   d. Convey to clients that their safety and the safety of others are of paramount importance to the staff.
   e. Establish a baseline assessment of the person's physical parameters and usual daily routine.

5. Treatment interventions should be as highly individualized as possible. Group interventions based on clients' needs and interests serve as effective, efficient, and individualized interventions.

6. The client and the family must be integral members of the treatment team in the determination of what is to be achieved by hospitalization and when the client is ready to be discharged.

7. A major function of the nurse in preparing the client and the family for discharge is teaching them about the illness, the prescribed medications, how to provide for daily living needs, and how to answer others' questions about the hospitalization and illness.

8. A frequently overlooked concept in the long-term care of persons with a mental illness is their need for psychiatric rehabilitation. Psychiatric rehabilitation focuses on the consequences of the illness, not on the illness itself. Its overall mission is to help persons with psychiatric disabilities become successful and satisfied in the environments of their choice with the least amount of ongoing professional intervention.

SUGGESTED SOURCES OF ADDITIONAL INFORMATION

Andrews G: Private and public psychiatry: a comparison of two health care systems, *Am J Psychiatry* 146:881, July 1989.

Anthony WA: Psychiatric rehabilitation: key issues and future policy, *Health Aff (Millwood),* Fall 1992, p 164.

Anthony WA, Cohen MR, Cohen BF: Philosophy, treatment process, and principles of the psychiatric rehabilitation approach. In Bachrach LL, editor: *Deinstitutionalization,* New directions for mental health services, monograph 17, San Francisco, 1983, Jossey-Bass.

Anthony WA, Cohen MR, Farkas MD: *Psychiatric rehabilitation,* Boston, 1990, Boston University, Center for Psychiatric Rehabilitation.

Caverly S: Coordinating psychosocial nursing care across treatment settings, *J Psychosoc Nurs Ment Health Serv* 29(8):26, 1991.

Donner L and others: Increasing psychiatric inpatients' community adjustment through therapeutic passes, *Arch Psychiatr Nurs* 4:93, April 1990.

Farkas M: Utilizing the nursing process in the development of a medication group on an inpatient psychiatric unit, *Perspect Psychiatr Care* 26(3):12, 1990.

Feis C and others: Serving the chronic mentally ill in state and community hospitals, *Community Ment Health J* 26:221, June 1990.

Fetter M, Lowery B: Psychiatric rehospitalization of the severely mentally ill: patient and staff perspectives, *Nurs Res* 41:301, September/October 1992.

Freddolino P and others: Daily living needs at time of discharge: implications for advocacy, *Psychosoc Rehabil J* 11:33, April 1988.

Hunt A: The admission process, *Nurs Times* 87:30, 1991.

Kelly K and others: Fostering self-help on an inpatient unit, *Arch Psychiatr Nurs* 4:161, June 1990.

Koontz E and others: Implementing a short-term family support group, *J Psychosoc Nurs Ment Health Serv* 29(5):5, 1991.

Kurek-Ovshinshy C: Group psychotherapy in an acute inpatient setting: techniques that nourish self-esteem, *Issues Ment Health Nurs* 12:81, 1991.

Manderino M, Bzdek V: Social skill building with chronic patients, *J Psychosoc Nurs Ment Health Serv* 25(9):18, 1987.

McEvoy JP and others: Why must some schizophrenic patients be involuntarily committed? The role of insight, *Compr Psychiatry* 30:13, January/February 1989.

National Association of Mental Health Position Statement: Civil rights of mental patients, *Ment Hyg* 56:67, Spring 1972.

Osborne O and others: Forced relocation of hospitalized psychiatric patients, *Arch Psychiatr Nurs* 4:221, August 1990.

The revolution in psychiatric care, *US News & World Report,* Aug 5, 1991, p 49.

Robinson GM, Pinkney AA: Transition from the hospital to the community: small group program, *J Psychosoc Nurs Ment Health Serv* 30(5):33, 1992.

Rourke A: Self-care: chore or challenge? *J Adv Nurs* 16:233, 1991.

Sebastian L and others: Whose structure is it anyway? *Perspect Psychiatr Care* 26(1):25, 1990.

Smith J: Privileged communication: psychiatric/mental health nurses and the law, *Perspect Psychiatr Care* 26(4):26, 1990.

Stokes G, Keen I: Developing self-care skills and reducing institutionalized behaviour in a long-stay psychiatric population: the role of the nurse in behaviour modification, *J Adv Nurs* 12:35, 1987.

Wolpe P and others: Psychiatric inpatients' knowledge of their rights, *Hosp Community Psychiatry* 42:1168, November 1991.

Worley N, Lowery B: Linkages between community mental health centers and public mental hospitals, *Nurs Res* 40:298, September/October 1991.

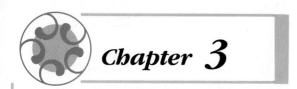

Chapter 3

Psychiatric Nursing in the Community

CHAPTER OUTLINE
Historical perspective
Living in the community with a long-term chronic mental illness
Community services
Components of an effective community support system
Community-based psychiatric nursing

LEARNING OBJECTIVES
After studying this chapter, the student will be able to:

* Discuss government initiatives to provide comprehensive community care for those with a long-term, chronic mental illness.

* Describe three categories of persons with a long-term, chronic mental illness who live in the community.

* Discuss the problems associated with securing appropriate housing for those with a long-term, chronic mental illness.

* Describe the types of community mental health services currently available.

* Discuss nine principles that should guide an effective community support system.

* List 10 component services, in addition to mental health treatment, considered necessary for an effective community support system.

* Discuss four characteristics of effective community-based nursing care of persons with a long-term, chronic mental illness.

An increasing proportion of persons who have a serious, persistent mental illness live in the community rather than in long-term, single-purpose psychiatric hospitals. With the increasing emphasis on community-based health care for all people, including those with a mental illness, this number is likely to increase. Therefore, growing opportunities will exist for nurses to practice psychiatric nursing in the community. The effective practice of psychiatric nursing in the community is different from traditional psychiatric nursing practice in the hospital not only because the needs of clients and their families may be different from their needs when the client is hospitalized, but also because the system for delivering mental health care in the community is still evolving. Therefore the student of psychiatric nursing must have an appreciation of the challenges of caring for persons with a mental illness in the community.

HISTORICAL PERSPECTIVE

As discussed in Chapters 1 and 2, treatment of those with a mental illness in the United States was generally limited to institutional care until the 1960s when the Joint Commission on Mental Illness issued its landmark report. Based on this report, President John F. Kennedy delivered a special message to the U.S. Congress in 1963. In this speech, the President called for a decrease in the number and size of state-supported psychiatric hospitals and a focus on providing community resources for the prevention of mental illness and the treatment of those who had a mental illness. The Community Mental Health Center Construction Act of 1963 resulted from this policy initiative. This act provided federal funding for the development of comprehensive community mental health centers designed to provide comprehensive mental health services to people in a delineated geographical region, referred to as a **catchment area.** Specific requirements for a fully developed, comprehensive community mental health center were identified in the law that made government funding available.

When fully developed, a comprehensive community mental health center was intended to include inpatient and outpatient services, day and night hospital units, crisis intervention centers, halfway houses, family therapy centers, rehabilitation centers, transitional facilities where individuals could receive board and care, and suicide prevention centers. In addition, the center was expected to offer services to the community that included consultation to community agencies and professional personnel, diagnostic services, and rehabilitative services, including vocational and educational programs. Finally, the comprehensive community mental health center was expected to provide training for professional and paraprofessional workers; to conduct research into the prevention, cause, and treatment of mental illness; and to evaluate the effectiveness of the programs offered.

Community mental health centers never fully achieved their goal of providing comprehensive mental health services. Some believe this failure resulted because the federal government did not use state mental health agencies to select and participate in the operation of community mental health centers (Shern and others, 1989). This was a problem because state governments in the 1960s and 1970s, as is true today, were committed to the ongoing deinstitutionalization of clients from state hospitals and to the restriction of admission to the hospital to only those individuals who had no other alternative. Since many community services were under the auspices of other agencies, it became difficult, if not impossible, to link deinstitutionalized clients appropriately with available community services. In addition, those services that were available often did not effectively address the needs of this particular population, since many centers focused on prevention and treatment of mental illness rather than on aftercare. As a result, many professionals and the public deemed deinstitutionalization a failure and became increasingly concerned about the number of people with a serious, persistent mental illness who lived on the streets of most large cities.

In an attempt to address the community care needs of these persons, the National Institute of Mental Health (NIMH) mounted the **Community Support Program** (CSP) in 1977. This program awarded federal money to the states for the purpose of coordinating the services offered by the variety of agencies attempting to serve individuals with a long-term mental illness.

In 1981 the **Omnibus Budget Reconciliation Act** drastically reduced federal funding for all health care services, including those for mental health. However, this act did allocate funds available for mental health to the states in the form of block grants. In turn, state governments awarded these monies to local governments in an attempt to refocus the community care system in a way that would meet the needs of those with a long-term, serious mental illness as well as the needs of the community for promotion of mental health and prevention of mental illness.

Despite these federal initiatives and the efforts of state and local governments, the mental health needs of the public are still unmet. The answer to what constitutes effective, efficient, comprehensive community mental health services is yet to be definitively defined. What is known, however, is that community care of those with a long-term mental illness is here to stay, and if these persons are to live and function in the community, they must have a range of coordinated basic community services and supports, referred to as a **community support system** (CSS). The challenge is to design and operate such a system in a clinically effective, cost-efficient manner and to educate mental health professionals with knowledge and skills relevant to practice within such a system.

LIVING IN THE COMMUNITY WITH A LONG-TERM CHRONIC MENTAL ILLNESS

Individuals with a long-term, chronic mental illness who live in the community fall into several categories, some of which overlap. One group is those who have been discharged from state-supported psychiatric hospitals, many of whom have lived in these settings for years. In addition to their individualized symptoms of dysfunction, these persons often have dysfunctions caused by prolonged hospitalization, such as lack of skills in activities of daily living because these needs were met by hospital staff. Many of these persons do not have families or friends in the community. Rather, their "family" was the hospital staff and other patients. Therefore they lack natural social support systems.

Another category of persons with a mental illness found in the community is young adults who have a chronic mental illness but who became ill after state hospitals stopped admitting anyone other than those who could not be treated elsewhere. As a result, this population does not have a history of long-term institutionalization but does have the expectation that their needs will be met by community services. Some of these persons live with their families. They tend not to take prescribed medications regularly but attempt to self-medicate by using alcohol and other substances. More importantly, they do not have appropriate, relevant, comprehensive treatment because of the current fragmentation of the community mental health system.

A third group of individuals in the community is elderly persons, who may or may not have a history of long-term psychiatric hospitalization. More than any other group, the number of elderly persons with a diagnosable mental illness is growing.

One of the tragedies resulting from inadequate community-based mental health care is that many jails are crowded with people who have a mental illness. In 1990 the Los Angeles County Jail was referred to as the largest mental institution in the United States, since it housed more persons with a mental illness than were found in any psychiatric hospital.

The most visible persons in the community who have a mental illness are those who are homeless (Figure 3-1). Because of the nature of homelessness, it is difficult to determine accurately the number of people who are homeless at any point in time. Estimates of homeless per-

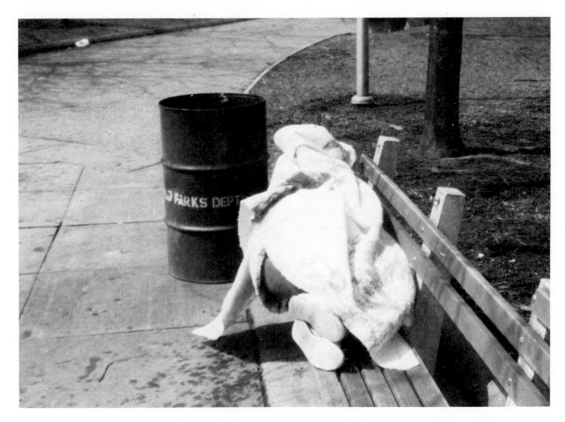

Figure 3-1
An estimated one third of people who are homeless suffer from a mental illness.
From Cookfair JM: *Nursing process and practice in the community,* St Louis, 1991, Mosby–Year Book.

sons in the United States range from 600,000 to several million. Most agree, however, that at least one third of those who are homeless have a diagnosable mental illness. Many of these persons have a history of prior long-term psychiatric hospitalization, but most are young adults with a chronic mental illness.

Housing is a fundamental need of all people. Housing not only provides shelter but also provides an address, which is necessary to establish eligibility for many entitlements. Securing appropriate housing for people with a mental illness is a major problem. A significant nationwide shortage of low-rent housing exists, and discrimination against those with a mental illness is

widespread and affects their ability to secure a share of the available low-rent housing.

A national survey in 1990 by the Robert Wood Johnson Foundation Program on Chronic Mental Illness found that group homes for people with chronic mental illness are among the types of facilities many people find unacceptable to have in their neighborhoods. Those who are most likely to object to such a facility are male, well educated, professionals, married, homeowners, and living in large cities or suburbs of large cities. This **NIMBY** ("not in my back yard") **phenomenon** reflects these people's stated belief that such facilities are necessary but should be in someone else's neighborhood. The most distressing fact about this finding is that this same group tends to be the opinion makers in U.S. society.

Many persons with a mental illness who have a residence live with their families. Young adults are likely to live with their parents; elderly persons often live with their adult children. Those who do not live with their families may live in congregate care facilities such as group homes, family care homes, and single-room occupancy (SRO) apartments. Some live alone or with friends in open-market apartments.

COMMUNITY SERVICES

Various types of community-based mental health services are currently available to those with a long-term, chronic mental illness. Among these are clinics, continuing care centers, and psychosocial clubs. However, these services are often inadequate, inappropriate, or inaccessible to those who need them. For example, homeless individuals may not know of these services or may not be eligible to use them. Furthermore, mental health clinics often operate by an appointment schedule to provide monitoring and treatment of only the person's mental illness. Continuing care centers are organized to provide daily activities for clients but are usually open only during the day, Monday through Friday. Although psychosocial clubs are operated by clients with minimum professional assistance and provide socialization opportunities and psychoeducational programs, they frequently do not meet reimbursement requirements.

A major problem with available services is their fragmentation. Often, clients must negotiate a very complex system if their needs are to be met. For example, the clinic that monitors the person's psychotropic medication is unlikely to provide physical health care, which the client must seek from another clinic or private community physician. The complexity of securing appointments, finding and using public transportation, explaining the problem, and arranging for payment is a challenge that most mentally healthy

adults would find daunting. Many with a mental illness are incapable of meeting this challenge, and therefore their needs remain unmet.

The existing system is an adaptation of institutional care in that clients usually are expected to go to the clinic or continuing care facility rather than the services being provided to clients in their area. In addition, services are often available only during the work week. These characteristics reflect the values of white, middle-class, healthy individuals and are not responsive to the needs of many persons with a mental illness whose ethnic, cultural, and health behaviors are different from those of the majority. Therefore, one should not be surprised to learn that many clients do not keep appointments or follow through on treatments, but rather make inordinate and inappropriate use of general hospital emergency rooms. The problem then becomes compounded because these persons are labeled uncooperative or noncompliant and deemed difficult to treat.

COMPONENTS OF AN EFFECTIVE COMMUNITY SUPPORT SYSTEM

An effective community support system for persons with long-term mental illness would be guided by the following principles (Stroul, 1989):

1. *Services are consumer oriented.* Services should be based on and responsive to the needs of the client rather than the needs of the system or of providers.
2. *Services empower clients.* Services should include self-help approaches and be provided in a manner that encourages clients to retain the greatest possible control over their own lives. This means actively involving clients in all aspects of policy making, planning, and delivering services.
3. *Services are racially and culturally appropriate.* Services should be available, accessible, and acceptable to members of racial and ethnic minority groups and to women.
4. *Services are flexible.* Services should be

EXAMPLES OF COMMUNITY SERVICES

Serving individuals

Rape crisis center
Churches and synagogues
Job-training agencies
Art shows
Recreation clubs (e.g., chess clubs, automobile clubs)
Adult education programs
Literacy programs
Employment agencies
Mediation groups
Renewal centers
Meals on Wheels
Colleges and universities
Mental health agencies

Serving families

Women, Infants, and Children (WIC)
Nutritional services
Community "welcome wagon"
Sex-counseling agencies
Family-planning agencies

Recreation centers
Children's groups (e.g., Camp Fire Girls)
Church groups
Day-care centers for children, disabled persons, and elderly persons
Family recreation centers and groups
Shelters for victims of domestic violence

Serving the community

Fresh Air Fund
Environmental groups
Education groups (e.g., American Lung Association, March of Dimes)
Utility companies
Community emergency shelters
Government agencies
Police department
Fire department
Fair-housing bureau or agency
Prisons
Performing arts centers
Public forests and parks

From Haber J and others: *Comprehensive psychiatric nursing,* ed 4, St Louis, 1992, Mosby–Year Book.

available whenever they are needed and for as long as they are needed. They should be provided in a variety of ways, with individuals able to move in and out of the system as their needs change.

5. *Services focus on client strengths.* Services should build on clients' assets and strengths to help them maintain a sense of identity, dignity, and self-esteem.

6. *Services are normalized and incorporate natural supports.* This implies that services are offered in the least restrictive, most natural setting possible. Clients should be encouraged to use the natural supports in the community and should be integrated into the normal living, working, learning, and leisure activities of the community.

7. *Services meet special needs.* Services should be adapted to meet the needs of various subgroups of persons with severe mental illness, such as elderly persons, young adults, individuals with substance abuse problems as well as mental illness, persons with a mental illness who are homeless, and persons with a mental illness who are inappropriately placed within the correctional system.

8. *Service systems are accountable.* Service providers should be accountable to the users of the services and monitored by the state to ensure quality of care and continued relevance to clients' needs. Primary consumers and their families should be involved in planning, implementing, monitoring, and evaluating services.

9. *Services are coordinated.* Coordination should occur between and among agencies providing services and between and among the various levels of government and the service agencies. At the very least, continuity of care between the hospital and community services should be ensured.

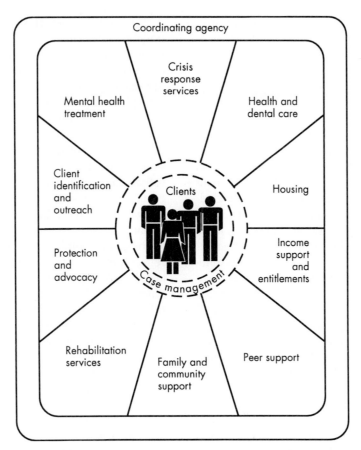

Figure 3-2
Community support system.
From Stroul BA: *Psychosoc Rehabil J* 12:14, January 1989.

Mental health treatment services alone are not sufficient to meet the needs of individuals with long-term, chronic mental illness who live in the community. Since these illnesses are all-pervasive, they are disabling in all aspects of the person's life. Consequently, effective community services must include an entire array of coordinated, accessible treatment, life support, and rehabilitation services (see box on p. 46). In addition to mental health treatment, components of such a coordinated system include client identification and outreach, crisis response services, health and dental care, housing, income support and entitlements, peer support, family and community support, rehabilitation services, protection and advocacy, and case management (Stroul, 1989). No one agency can or should provide all these services. Many agencies are already in existence but are not accessible to persons with a mental illness, especially if they must access them on their own initiative. What is needed, therefore, is an agency that is responsible for coordinating available services and developing unavailable services (Figure 3-2). Whether such an agency should be supported by state governments, local governments, or voluntary agencies is a subject of much current debate.

The box on p. 49 lists services and opportunities for persons with a long-term, chronic mental illness living in the community.

COMMUNITY-BASED PSYCHIATRIC NURSING

The nurse who provides community-based services to those with a mental illness is often required to exercise the greatest skill, creativity, diplomacy, and initiative. Not only are the consumers of the nurse's services likely to be challenging, but great ingenuity is required to surmount the limitations of the current system if the needs of clients and their families are to be met.

As described in Chapter 1, some nurses function as case managers and assume major responsibility for coordinating care and services for those persons who are most severely disabled by their mental illness. Other nurses work in the previously described clinics, continuing care centers, or psychosocial clubs. With increasing frequency, nurses employed by public health agencies are providing care to individuals with a mental illness and their families in homes. Regardless of their employing agency or their site of practice, nurses who care for people with a mental illness in the community should administer care that reflects the principles cited earlier. Specifically, nursing care is most helpful when it has the following characteristics:

1. *Care includes the client's family and significant others.* Families and significant others should not be viewed solely as sources of information about the client. Since their role as caretakers heavily impacts their own sense of well-being, the nurse has an opportunity to promote the mental health of these concerned persons and help them cope with the demands of the client's illness. Communities are increasingly making respite care available for clients who live with their families. The nurse can often be instrumental in making arrangements for such care, as well as encouraging families to use this service without guilt.

2. *Care is holistic.* This means that insofar as possible, the client should be assessed and treated as a whole person, not only for symptoms of mental illness. For example, it is well known that many persons who have a mental illness also have physical problems. These problems may or may not be related to their mental illness. Persons with a mental illness are often malnourished because of their inability to plan meals, shop for food, and cook meals. Homeless individuals frequently have impaired peripheral circulation, manifested by leg ulcers as a result of constantly being on their feet. Another example is many clients' understandable feelings of hopelessness and helplessness. These feelings may reflect spiritual distress and may be signs of emotional dysfunction. Finally, clients with a mental illness often are socially isolated and long for a relationship with other human beings. The nurse can and should be instrumental in identifying and addressing all these needs.

3. *Care is relevant and individualized to the client's needs, goals, and living situation.* This implies that nurses take the time to help clients explain their needs, goals, and living situations and that nurses involve clients in planning and evaluating their care. For example, making an appointment for a client with a physician whose office is inaccessible by public transportation is not helpful if the client does not have private transportation. On the other hand, the nurse displays interest in and concern for the client who has visual blurring as a side effect of psychotropic medication when the nurse provides large-print magazines so the client can participate in a reading group.

Flexibility is an important component of relevant, individualized care. Because nurses are not likely to see the client daily, they should not assume the client is necessarily the same person as when they last saw him or her. In other words, the client will have had many experiences in the day, week, or month since the nurse last saw him or her. Based on these experiences, the client's needs or interests might be different than when

COMPREHENSIVE ARRAY OF SERVICES AND OPPORTUNITIES FOR PERSONS WITH LONG-TERM, CHRONIC MENTAL ILLNESS

Basic needs/opportunities
Shelter

Protected (with health, rehabilitative, or social services provided on site)
Hospital
Nursing home
Intermediate-care facility
Crisis facility
Semi-independent (linked to services)
Family home
Group home
Cooperative apartment
Foster care home
Emergency housing facility
Other board and care home
Independent apartment/home (access to services)

Food, Clothing, and Household Management

Fully provided meals
Food purchase/preparation assistance
Access to food stamps
Homemaker service

Income/Financial Support

Access to entitlements
Employment

Meaningful Activities

Work opportunities
Recreation
Education
Religious/spiritual
Human/social interaction

Mobility/Transportation

Special needs/opportunities
General Medical Services

Physician assessment and care
Nursing assessment and care
Dentist assessment and care
Physical/occupational therapy
Speech/hearing therapy
Nutrition counseling
Medication counseling
Home health services

Mental Health Services

Acute treatment services
Crisis stabilization
Diagnosis and assessment
Medication monitoring (psychoactive)
Self-medication training
Psychotherapies
Hospitalization: acute and long-term care

Habilitation and Rehabilitation

Social/recreational skills development
Life skills development
Leisure activities

Vocational

Prevocational assessment counseling
Sheltered work opportunities
Transitional employment
Job development and placement

Social Services

Family support
Community support assistance
Housing and milieu management
Legal services
Entitlement assistance

Integrative Services

Client identification and outreach
Individual assessment and service planning
Case service and resource management
Advocacy and community organization
Community information
Education and support

From Department of Health and Human Services Steering Committee on the Chronically Mentally Ill: *Toward a national plan for the chronically mentally ill,* Pub No (ADM)81-1077, Washington, DC, 1981, US Government Printing Office.

the nurse last met with the client. Therefore, the nurse's plan for intervention must be flexible if it is to remain relevant to the client.

4. *Care includes repeated opportunities for the client and the family to learn about the illness and the prescribed medications and to develop self-care skills.* This involves not only knowledge acquisition but also skill development. Teaching must be in a form and manner that are meaningful to the client. For example, medication teaching should begin with issues the client is most concerned about, which may be such factors as the medication's effect on sexual potency or body weight. Any written material given to the client, perhaps about the prescribed medication, should be laminated so that it will remain useful for a longer time.

Research studies have documented that persons with a severe, long-term mental illness, particularly the schizophrenias, have difficulty in transferring and adapting skills learned in one setting to other settings where the environment is different. Therefore, it is most helpful when skills are practiced in the setting in which they are going to be used. One nurse spent hours over several weeks helping a client successfully learn to use a commerical washing machine in the continuing care center but was dismayed to learn he was still unable to use the machine in his local laundromat. Only after accompanying him to the laundromat did the nurse realize the problem was that the machine in the center was front loading, whereas the laundromat's machines were top loading!

The preceding four areas merely include examples of characteristics of nursing care that have been found to be helpful when working with clients in the community. Nurses in this role find fewer pre-established rules and procedures to guide their care than exist in hospitals. This fact can be viewed as an opportunity and a challenge to devise and deliver nursing care that is truly holistic, individualized, relevant, and therefore effective.

KEY POINTS

1. The Community Mental Health Center Construction Act of 1963 provided federal funding for the development of comprehensive community mental health centers. The goal of these centers, to provide comprehensive mental health services, was never fully achieved.

2. Despite federal initiatives and the efforts of state and local governments, the mental health needs of the public are still unmet.

3. Individuals with a long-term chronic mental illness who live in the community include those who have been discharged from state-supported psychiatric hospitals, young adults who became ill after state hospitals stopped admitting anyone other than those who could not be treated elsewhere, and elderly persons.

4. The most visible of those in the community who have a mental illness are homeless persons. Most authorities agree that this group constitutes one third of the total population of homeless people.

5. The fundamental need of all people for housing is difficult to meet for those with a mental illness because of the nationwide shortage of low-rent housing and the negative attitudes of many about group homes in their neighborhoods.

6. Community-based mental health services currently available are clinics, continuing care centers, and psychosocial clubs. However, these services are often inadequate, inappropriate, or inaccessible to those who need them.

7. Principles that should guide an effective community support system include:
   a. Services are consumer oriented.
   b. Services empower clients.
   c. Services are racially and culturally appropriate.
   d. Services are flexible.
   e. Services focus on client strengths.
   f. Services are normalized and incorporate natural supports.
   g. Services meet special needs.
   h. Service systems are accountable.
   i. Services are coordinated.

8. Components of an effective community support system include mental health treatment, client

identification and outreach, crisis response services, health and dental care, housing, income support and entitlements, peer support, family and community support, rehabilitation services, protection and advocacy, and case management.

9. To be effective, community-based nursing care of persons with a long-term, chronic mental illness must include the client's family and significant others; be holistic, individualized, and relevant; and include repeated opportunities for the client and family to acquire knowledge and develop skills.

SUGGESTED SOURCES OF ADDITIONAL INFORMATION

Anthony WA, Blanch A: Research on community support services: what we have learned, *Psychosoc Rehabil J* 12:55, January 1989.

Bachrach L and others: Homeless mentally ill patients in the community: results of a general hospital emergency room study, *Community Ment Health J* 26:415, October 1990.

Bawden EL: Reaching out to the chronically mentally ill homeless, *J Psychosoc Nurs Ment Health Serv* 28(3):6, 1990.

Brooker C: The health education needs of families caring for a schizophrenic relative and the potential role for community psychiatric nurses, *J Adv Nurs* 15:1092, 1990.

Connolly PM: Services for the underserved: a nurse-managed center for the chronically mentally ill, *J Psychosoc Nurs Ment Health Serv* 29(1):15, 1991.

Davidson RE and others: Brief report: psychiatric nursing roles in a community mental health center, *Community Ment Health J* 24:83, 1988.

Drew N: Combating the social isolation of chronic mental illness, *J Psychosoc Nurs Ment Health Serv* 29(6):14, 1991.

Ferguson MA: Psych nursing in a shelter, *Am J Nurs* 89:1060, August 1989.

Geiser R and others: Respite care for mentally ill patients and their families, *Hosp Community Psychiatry* 39:291, March 1988.

Gonzales-Osler E: The homeless chronically mentally ill: coping with transition, *J Psychosoc Nurs Ment Health Serv* 27(6):29, 1989.

Grella CE, Grusky O: Families of the seriously mentally ill and their satisfaction with services, *Hosp Community Psychiatry* 40:831, August 1989.

Gullberg P: The homeless chronically mentally ill: a psychiatric nurse's role, *J Psychosoc Nurs Ment Health Serv* 27(6):9, 1989.

Holmstrom C: Community living for the chronically mentally ill, *Can J Psychiatr Nurs* 30:6, December 1989.

Huddleston J: Family and group psychoeducational approaches in the management of schizophrenia, *Clin Nurse Specialist* 6(2):118, 1992.

Kozlak J, Thobaben M: Treating the elderly mentally ill at home, *Perspect Psychiatr Care* 28:31, April-June 1992.

Lamb HR: Perspectives on effective advocacy for homeless mentally ill persons, *Hosp Community Psychiatry* 43:1209, December 1992.

Lindsey AM: Health care for the homeless, *Nurs Outlook* 37:78, March/April 1989.

MacGilp D: A quality of life study of discharged long-term psychiatric patients, *J Adv Nurs* 16:1206, 1991.

Malone J: Concepts for the rehabilitation of the long-term mentally ill in the community, *Issues Ment Health Nurs* 10:121, 1989.

McNiel DE and others: Family attitudes that predict home placement of hospitalized psychiatric patients, *Hosp Community Psychiatry* 43:1035, October 1992.

Public attitudes toward people with chronic mental illness: executive summary, Prepared for The Robert Wood Johnson Foundation Program on Chronic Mental Illness, April 1990.

Report says confinement of mentally ill persons in U.S. jails reflects lack of community services, *Hosp Community Psychiatry* 43:1253, December 1992.

Riesdorph-Ostrow W: The homeless chronically mentally ill: deinstitutionalization: a public policy perspective, *J Psychosoc Nurs Ment Health Serv* 27(6):4, 1989.

Shern DL and others: Designing community treatment systems for the most seriously mentally ill: a state administrative perspective, *J Soc Issues* 45(3):105, 1989.

Stroul B: Community support systems for persons with long-term mental illness: a conceptual framework, *Psychosoc Rehabil J* 12:9, January 1989.

Struening EL, Padgett DK: Physical health status, substance use and abuse, and mental disorders among homeless adults, *J Soc Issues* 46(4):65, 1990.

Susser E and others: Some clinical approaches to the homeless mentally ill, *Community Ment Health J* 26:463, October 1990.

Wells DA: Management of early postdischarge adjustment reactions following psychiatric hospitalization, *Hosp Community Psychiatry* 43:1000, October 1992.

Wilkinson L: A collaborative model: ambulatory pharmacotherapy for chronic psychiatric patients, *J Psychosoc Nurs Ment Health Serv* 29(12):26, 1991.

Worley NK, Albanese N: Independent living for the chronically mentally ill, *J Psychosoc Nurs Ment Health Serv* 27(9):18, 1989.

Chapter 4

Issues in Psychiatric Nursing

LEARNING OBJECTIVES

After studying this chapter, the student will be able to:

* Identify one issue affecting psychiatric nursing from each of the following categories: economic, social, professional, clinical, delivery system, and educational.

* Discuss how each identified issue is likely to affect the future of psychiatric nursing.

KEY TERMS
Self-help trend
Role blurring
"Revolving door" syndrome

The final years of the twentieth century are times of challenge for psychiatric nursing. The very existence of this health care specialty is in question, while simultaneously the potential for it to make a valuable, unique contribution to the welfare of society has never been so great. Today's students of nursing will be practicing well into the twenty-first century and will be the nursing leaders of tomorrow. Since their nursing practice will be affected by how current issues are resolved, it is imperative that nursing students become aware of those factors that will shape the nature and scope of psychiatric nursing in the future.

This chapter highlights some of the major issues that confront psychiatric nursing. The nature of any issue is that solutions are not obvious. If they were, issues would not be present. Another characteristic of issues is the many factors that interrelate to create them. However, whenever a discussion of issues is attempted, it becomes necessary to separate artificially each factor to facilitate discussion. Consequently, this chapter presents my view of those issues facing psychiatric nursing but does not claim to supply solutions. It is hoped that the reader's awareness of these issues will be increased whether or not the reader agrees with my analysis. As a result of an increased awareness, it is further hoped that the reader will be motivated to formulate his or her own concerns and develop a plan to address them.

ECONOMIC ISSUES

Not since the Great Depression of the 1930s has the U.S. economy been as influential a factor in shaping daily events as it is today. Many economists agree that the current economic situation is unique in U.S. history. For example, for the first time, unemployment, traditionally limited primarily to those without education or skills, has affected all socioeconomic groups, from unskilled hourly workers to salaried corporate executives. In the past, high unemployment rates have dropped when people were rehired to fill the positions from which they had been laid off. Because businesses and governments are restructuring and permanently downsizing, this historical resolution to the unemployment problem is unlikely to occur in the future.

In addition to the economic problems caused by unemployment, many employed persons find themselves in a position where they have more income than ever before but also have expenses greater than their income. Unfortunately, this applies to all levels of government as well as to individuals and families and has resulted in deficit spending, with money borrowed to cover expenses. This practice, in turn, has resulted in a level of individual, familial, and governmental indebtedness unprecedented in U.S. history. A complete restructuring of the U.S. economy is being demanded.

The federal deficit is at an all-time high, and many state and local governments are unable to balance their budgets. Therefore, all expenditures are being scrutinized as never before. Since health care accounts for a major segment of all governmental budgets, it is being examined for cost-effectiveness and clinical efficacy. Although the United States is in the midst of a movement for total health care reform, mental health care is particularly vulnerable to cutbacks, since mental health care costs are believed to be the fastest rising segment of health care costs. Furthermore, treatment protocols are not as well established as are intervention measures for physical illnesses. Therefore, besides being expensive, mental health care is also suspect.

Some authorities believe that an outcome of health care reform might be rationing of services. This means that the government and/or insurance companies would set limits not only on the amount paid for certain procedures, but also on the procedures themselves. If this were to occur on a nationwide basis as it has in some states, only those with sufficient private funds would have access to health care measures that third-party payers considered too expensive or too ineffective. How will health care rationing affect people with long-term, chronic illnesses such as mental illness who do not have money to pay for their care? The concept of rationing health care services is an ethical dilemma with which every citizen, but particularly every health care professional, must grapple.

The effect of the economy is all-pervasive. It is a direct or indirect factor that influences all other issues in psychiatric nursing. For example, consumers faced with expenses equal to or greater than their income must establish priorities for the expenditure of the available funds. Often, health care takes a low priority, particularly health care designed to promote health and prevent illness. Furthermore, health care providers are being called to ever-increasing accountability for the expenditure of their time. Unfortunately, it is not usually possible to demonstrate that time spent in crisis intervention with an individual or family has prevented costly mental illness. This expenditure of time cannot be compared with the administration of a parenteral diuretic, for example, the results of which are quickly visible in the patient's improved cardiopulmonary function.

Nurses who care for persons with a mental illness, by their very function, are highly vulnerable to the economic issue. For example, the nurse and client may interact through such activities as walking together, playing cards, or sitting silently with each other. Understandably the casual observer of these activities would raise questions as to their value. Nurses must assume the initiative and responsibility for engaging in research that documents the efficacy of such interactions.

Economic constraints that result in demands for increased accountability also inevitably result in increased paperwork. Unfortunately the persons required to do this paperwork are often those who least wish to do so, that is, people prepared to function as clinicians. In addition, events that can be quantified, or reduced to numbers, are more easily accounted for than events that are not quantifiable. For example, consider the difference between health counseling, which may take 30 minutes, and changing a Foley catheter, which may take 15 minutes. The latter intervention can be easily documented as to need, action taken, and results achieved, whereas counseling may prove difficult to justify when the same criteria are applied. Therefore the necessity for accountability has increased the value of activities that can be quantified and has devalued activities that cannot be easily translated into numerical values.

A nationwide movement exists to treat persons with a mental illness in the least restrictive environment. This is resulting in a dramatic reduction in the number and size of state-supported psychiatric hospitals. Although this is a laudable goal, when it is combined with the economic constraints currently existing in most states, it results in some clients being discharged from the hospital before adequate community-based care is available. The consequence is an unprecedented number of persons with an active mental illness in the community. While many of these persons receive care through community-based services, some have no access to the mental health system because they are among the homeless. Equally tragic, others are in jails and nursing homes where they do not receive the care they require.

Since only physicians and nurses are licensed to administer medication, the many persons with an acute mental illness in the community have led many community-based psychiatric nurses to focus much of their time administering the necessary psychotropic medications and monitoring their effects. Although these functions are certainly within the scope of nursing practice, it is feared that they will become the nurse's primary function to the neglect of other equally necessary functions such as counseling, teaching, and socializing.

It is also feared that hospitals will cope with decreased budgets by eliminating or curtailing in-service education programs for nurses. Al-

though this would be a serious development for any area of nursing, it is potentially lethal for psychiatric nursing because limited time is spent studying this subject in formal educational programs and the discipline is rapidly changing. These issues are discussed further in this chapter under "Educational Issues" and "Professional Issues."

In this time of economic distress, some believe that nursing is pricing itself out of existence. Should nurses be willing to accept less pay than is equitable to prevent being replaced by less expensive (and less well-prepared) health care workers? Are nurses willing and able to make outcomes research a major priority to demonstrate the clinical and economic effectiveness of their interventions? Are they willing to publicize the results of such research to educate the public about the value of their services? The answers to these and other questions are likely to play a major role in determining the position nursing will have in the health care delivery system of the twenty-first century.

SOCIAL ISSUES

A major social trend that has had a direct impact on psychiatric nursing is the continued, organized effort of women to achieve social and economic equality. Since nursing is primarily a women's profession, changes in the status of women are closely intertwined with changes in the profession. No longer are women content to be dependent on men; no longer are nurses willing to be handmaidens to physicians. Women are demanding more education; nurses are becoming increasingly better educated. Women are demanding wages appropriate to their preparation and responsibilities; nurses are organizing and striking to receive salaries that more closely reflect their preparation and responsibilities.

An unfortunate but, it is hoped, temporary result of the women's movement is the tendency of young women to choose careers other than those traditionally associated with women, namely, teaching and nursing. Although all young people, both men and women, should have the opportunity to pursue careers for which they are best suited, it is unfortunate that many young women are dismissing nursing as a career merely because it has been historically associated with women. To compound this problem the number of persons, both male and female, in the 18- to 24-year-old age group is dropping steadily and will continue to do so well into the twenty-first century. Consequently, the pool of persons from which students of nursing are traditionally recruited is smaller than ever before and subject to the increased recruitment efforts of other occupational groups.

A positive trend is the increasing number of nontraditional students who are choosing nursing as a career (Figure 4-1). These individuals include housewives and holders of degrees in other fields. The presence of these persons with their varied life experiences and educational backgrounds enriches nursing in both the classroom and the health care delivery system.

An unprecedented social phenomenon is the **self-help trend.** Consumers no longer believe that professionals necessarily know best. Popular magazines regularly feature articles about health issues, ranging from diet to human behavior. Self-help books on a wide range of subjects are readily available, and some that deal with human emotions have been best-sellers. The result of this phenomenon is people who are well educated about health matters and who consequently demand quality care at reasonable cost. The field of psychiatry, which less than a century ago was scorned, has now become demystified. The implication of this trend is that all mental health care professionals, including nurses, are increasingly held accountable by consumers and cannot hide behind professional jargon and unexplained actions.

A social issue specific to psychiatric nursing is the stigma associated with mental illness. As the number of persons with a mental illness liv-

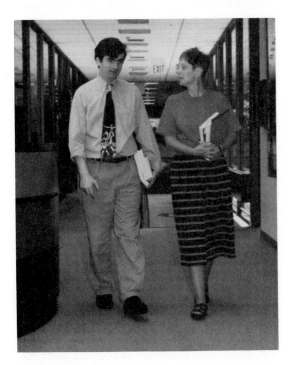

Figure 4-1

Nontraditional students are choosing nursing as a career.

OF SPECIAL INTEREST

Dr. Morton Kramer, noted epidemiologist from Johns Hopkins University, projects that in the year 2005 the population of the United States will be 267,603,300. If 10% of the population, or 26,760,300 people, require only 6 hours of psychiatric nursing care that year, Dr. Kramer estimates that 107,041 psychiatric nurses will be needed.

Did you know that there are only about 52,000 RNs practicing psychiatric nursing in the United States today?

From Kramer K: Target-populations for psychiatric-mental health nursing 1980-2005. In *Psychiatric-mental health nursing: proceedings of two conferences on future directions,* US Department of Health and Human Services, Washington, DC, 1986, US Government Printing Office.

ing in the community increases, the societal stigma against them seems to be growing, as evidenced by the NIMBY ("not in my back yard") phenomenon discussed in Chapter 3. Those who provide care to a stigmatized group, whether to persons with acquired immunodeficiency syndrome (AIDS) or those with mental illness, find themselves stigmatized as well. Therefore, stigma against those with a mental illness results not only in direct discrimination against this group, but also in barriers to the recruitment of an adequate number of nurses and other health care personnel to provide the necessary care.

PROFESSIONAL ISSUES

Advances in neuroscientific understanding of the interrelationships among the brain, behavior, emotion, and cognition have been phenomenal over the last decade. Many say that more has been learned about how the brain functions in the last 10 years than in all previous human history. These astounding revelations have been made possible by the development of such technologies as positron emission tomography (PET), which allows study of the brain while the person is alive. It is now believed that at least the most severe mental illnesses, such as schizophrenia and bipolar disorder, are diseases of the brain in the same way that diabetes is a disease of the pancreas. Therefore, such a state as "mental" illness may not exist.

Many health care professionals currently providing care to those with a mental illness were educated in the era when most mental illnesses were thought to result from interpersonal, social, or environmental dysfunctions, not physical malfunctions. The recent research findings that implicate brain dysfunction in the most severe mental illnesses have resulted in the development of two professional camps. The first is the group that wants to "medicalize" the practice of psychiatry. This simply means that this group sees all the knowledge gained from decades of research in the social and behavioral sciences as irrelevant to understanding human behavior and that only physiological functioning should be considered. The opposing group clings to traditional interpretations of human behavior and attempts to ignore current research findings and their implications for treatment.

In my opinion, neither of these extreme views will prove correct. Humans are holistic beings; the whole of the person is greater than the sum of the parts. Therefore, health care directed only to the body or only to the behavior will be ineffective and at worst harmful. All health care professionals must have an in depth knowledge of both the biophysical and the psychosocial sciences to practice effectively. This includes psychiatric nurses.

The question arises whether the nurse who cares for clients who have a mental illness is similar to any other nurse or whether she identifies more with other mental health disciplines. Traditionally, psychiatric nurses have participated in their alienation from the mainstream of health care professionals, as have psychiatrists. These groups have tended to define their practice as fundamentally different from the practice of their colleagues in other areas of nursing and medicine. This posture has had several benefits, including a separate source of federal funding for education and research through the National Institute of Mental Health (NIMH). This stance also has had its drawbacks, including inaccessibility to the political strength of mainstream nursing and medical organizations. Now that the NIMH has become a part of the National Institutes of Health, I believe that the drawbacks outweigh the benefits. However, whether this separatist view will continue is yet to be determined.

Another professional issue facing psychiatric nursing is role blurring. Before the advent of the phenothiazine derivatives, the roles of mental health professionals were more cleary defined. The nurse was primarily concerned with the client's activities of daily living, the psychiatrist focused on diagnosing and prescribing, the psychologist focused on testing and research, and the social worker concentrated on the client's family. Very little treatment occurred. When psychotropic drugs made clients more accessible to therapeutic interventions, all mental health disciplines began to claim these interventions within their scope of practice. The result was **role blurring,** in which members of all disciplines engage in individual, family, and group therapy. The question then arises as to what, if anything, differentiates the nurse from the physician, psychologist, or social worker. Psychiatric nursing must convincingly answer this question or be at risk of extinction.

Documentation is increasing concerning the inadequate number of professionals available to provide the mental health care needed by the public. This is particularly true in rural and inner-city areas. This personnel shortage, combined with economic constraints, has led to the question of whether the available professionals are being used in the most efficient, effective manner. Specifically, a movement exists for psychologists and nurses with master's degree preparation in psychiatric nursing to be prepared and certified to prescribe medications specific to their area of expertise. Some believe that advanced-practice psychiatric nurses would be easier to attract and retain in underserved geographical areas than psychiatrists. Not all nurses are supportive of this movement, partially because of the role-blurring issue just described. Other nursing groups see authority to prescribe as an opportunity to enhance more fully their psychiatric nursing role.

CLINICAL ISSUES

The incidence of mental illness in our society is clearly increasing. Factors such as economic pressures, changing moral values, and an increase in violent crimes all result from and contribute to a stress-laden lifestyle to which individuals and families must adapt. Intervention measures designed to promote mental health and to prevent mental illness are needed in addition to measures designed to treat those who already have a mental illness. Meeting the mental health needs of its citizens presents an enormous challenge to the United States.

Most authorities acknowledge that the most cost-effective and best way to meet many of these needs is through programs geared to prevention. These programs are designed to alter the environment in a way that is conducive to better mental health or to helping individuals, families, and communities to increase and diversify their coping mechanisms. An example of the former is efforts directed toward decreasing violence on the streets; examples of the latter are Head Start programs, victim assistance programs, and self-help groups such as Recovery, Inc.

Although almost universal agreement exists that prevention of mental illness and promotion of mental health are the best routes in terms of long-term goals, it is exceedingly difficult to document the effects of such programs in the short term. With a scarcity of resources, government and private agencies are less likely to allocate funds to such programs, feeling a need to concentrate limited resources on short-term, obvious problems, that is, the treatment of those who already have a mental illness.

As previously stated, the most severe, disabling forms of mental illness are now known to have a biophysiological basis. Despite this knowledge and protestations to the contrary, health care professionals still practice in a manner that perpetuates a dichotomy between the brain and the rest of the body. Some have called this a "brainless" practice. Based on this knowledge, major changes need to occur in the mental health care delivery system that take into account the biopsychosocial nature of the illness. Because of the enormity and severity of the problem of mental illness in our society, a need also exists for the development of appropriate treatment modalities and intervention techniques that address large population groups.

Traditional one-to-one, family, and group psychodynamically based treatment modalities are no longer viable as the main forms of intervention, particularly in short-term, acute care settings. These techniques have proved costly and, at worst, not necessarily therapeutically effective. In addition, these modalities clearly benefit only those who value feelings and thoughts, are verbally fluent, have financial resources, are highly motivated, and have the intelligence necessary to deal with the abstractions inherent in these treatment modalities. These criteria rule out many individuals and certain population groups, such as cultural minorities, children, elderly persons, and poor persons. These groups have the greatest incidence of mental illness, and for them we have the least understanding of effective means of treatment. Although the need for change is well accepted by most mental health disciplines, few ideas seem to exist as to what changes can and should occur. Consequently, mental health professionals are still being educationally and experientially prepared in the traditional modes of treatment while being told that in most instances their developing skills will be to no avail in solving the larger issues of the day.

What then is required? First and foremost, research must be conducted to find reliable answers to these problems. Although neuroscientific research into the causes and prevention of mental illness certainly needs to continue, a great need also exists for more behavioral research that focuses on appropriate treatment of those already ill. This is easier said than done. Research regarding human behavior is by its nature different from pure laboratory research in a variety of ways. First, many variables are difficult, if not impossible, to control. In a laboratory, chemical elements can be isolated and then systematically combined with other elements one by one and the effects clearly observed. When dealing with human beings, it is impossible to isolate a subject's personality from intelligence or from culture. Second, many laboratory experiments yield results in a relatively short period, at least within

the researcher's lifetime. In contrast, much behavioral research is longitudinal, requiring the observation and study of the subjects over a generation or two. In addition to the time and money involved, longitudinal research also runs the risk of incurring environmental changes that may affect the outcome such as an economic depression.

A prime concern in behavioral research and perhaps the core issue is the necessity in a democratic society to protect the rights of each individual. Therefore, procedures involved in research and treatment are subjected to vigorous scrutiny and are not approved if there is any potential for harm to the persons involved. Consequently the best that behavioral research can show is a relationship between and among variables after the fact. Despite these obstacles, however, it is essential that society continue to support behavioral research directed toward both understanding the cause of mental illness and developing effective treatment modalities.

DELIVERY SYSTEM ISSUES

The philosophical basis of the community health movement was and still is seen as a desired goal. Not only is it more humane, but it is also believed to be more cost-effective to maintain persons outside institutions. Although society and the health care professions endorse the result, it appears that little thought has been given to the changes that would be required in treatment methods and therefore in educational preparation of health care professionals. Unfortunately, in too many instances the community mental health movement has meant little more than a change of setting; the same treatment philosophy and methods have been moved from the institution to a decentralized center in the community.

Rather than solving any problems, this shortsighted approach often has compounded existing problems and created new ones. Major problems include the community disorganization and increased stigma resulting from scores of persons with a mental illness and with few or no resources being thrust into the community. Also, when adequate or appropriate community-based treatment and rehabilitation services are absent, the costly **"revolving door" syndrome** occurs. This syndrome is a phenomenon in which persons receive intensive care through hospitalization, are discharged to the community where they may or may not continue to receive care, and shortly require hospitalization again, repeating the cycle.

Another major delivery system issue is the geographical maldistribution of mental health care professionals and treatment centers, which tend to be clustered in large urban areas, particularly on the East and West coasts of the United States. In these areas, professionals can receive not only appropriate salaries but also the intellectual, cultural, and social stimulation they desire. As a result, large groups of consumers do not have geographical access to continuous mental health care.

As previously stated, mental health professionals continue to be educationally prepared in the traditional treatment modalities, so it is understandable that they choose to work with clients who can benefit from these techniques. Therefore, in addition to geographical maldistribution, disproportionately few mental health care professionals choose to work with poor persons, including the inner-city poor, educationally disadvantaged people, minority groups, children, and elderly persons. Since these groups represent the largest number of persons with a mental illness, the mental health needs of the United States clearly are not being met.

EDUCATIONAL ISSUES

The cost of higher education in the United States is skyrocketing and therefore placing college education out of the reach of more and more people at a time when scientific and technological advances require increasingly more educational preparation for most occupations. This situation is particularly problematic for women and members of cultural minorities who are attempting to achieve equality, in part, through education. Consequently a smaller proportion of black and Hispanic people and women are able to afford the cost of higher education, which in turn results in fewer health care professionals from those populations who require the most health care.

A great concern is that fewer and fewer nurses are choosing to work in psychiatric settings or to pursue graduate education in this field. The reasons for this are multiple and complex. Many psychiatric nurse educators, however, believe that a major contributing factor is the trend in undergraduate nursing programs to integrate content. This trend is a result of nursing's attempt to teach in a way that helps the student view the client holistically and to move away from the medical model that tends to segment clients according to their disease or illness. These goals are commendable, but one unexpected effect has been that some nursing students do not have a specific learning experience with clients who have a mental illness. Consequently, it is understandable that graduates of these programs are unlikely to choose psychiatric nursing as a field in which to work, and therefore the pool of persons interested in and qualified to pursue graduate education in psychiatric nursing is diminished. As with all other issues, the cyclical nature of this problem is evident because as fewer nurses become prepared at the graduate level, fewer psychiatric nurses will be prepared to teach, which in turn results in poorer preparation of beginning practitioners in psychiatric nursing, ending with fewer choosing to work in this area. Thus the cycle is complete and is set to repeat itself. Unless efforts to recruit qualified persons into psychiatric nursing are successful, this health care specialty will die a natural death and need not fear extinction from external forces.

KEY POINTS

1. The final years of the twentieth century are times of challenge for psychiatric nursing.

2. Psychiatric nursing is highly vulnerable to the current constraints on the U.S. economy. The apparent simplicity of traditional psychiatric nursing interventions, the demand for increased accountability and its resultant paperwork, and the need for nurses to focus on administration of medications to the exclusion of other important functions contribute to this vulnerability.

3. Major social issues impacting psychiatric nursing include the women's movement, the self-help trend, and the stigma associated with mental illness.

4. Professional issues include the need to incorporate into practice the latest research, which implicates brain dysfunction as a basis for the major mental illnesses. This means that all health care professionals, including psychiatric nurses, must have an in depth knowledge of both the biophysical and the psychosocial sciences if they are to practice effectively.

5. Professional issues also include the need for psychiatric nurses to resolve the question of whether they identify with the profession of nursing or with other mental health disciplines and whether they support authority to prescribe medications for psychiatric nurses prepared at the master's degree level.

6. Because of the enormity and severity of the problem of mental illness in our society, a need exists for the development of appropriate treatment modalities and intervention techniques that address large population groups.

7. Although neuroscientific research into the causes and prevention of mental illness needs to continue, need also exists for more behavioral research that focuses on appropriate treatment of those already ill.

8. Delivery system issues include the need for the development of an effective, efficient community-based mental health delivery system and the resolution of geographical maldistribution of mental health care professionals and treatment centers.

9. Educational issues include the need to recruit more nurses to the specialty of psychiatric nursing, especially members of cultural and ethnic minorities.

10. Unless efforts are made to recruit qualified persons into psychiatric nursing, this health care specialty will die a natural death and need not fear extinction from external forces.

SUGGESTED SOURCES OF ADDITIONAL INFORMATION

Abraham IL and others: Integrating the bio into the biopsychosocial: understanding and treating biological phenomena in psychiatric–mental health nursing, *Arch Psychiatr Nurs* 6:296, October 1992.

Chamberlain J, Marshall S: Recruitment problems from the psychiatric nursing education perspective. In *Proceedings: Psychiatric Mental Health Nursing Recruitment to the Specialty,* Rockville, Md, 1982, Department of Health and Human Services.

Custer W: *Issues in Mental Health Care,* February 1990.

Fagin C: Concepts for the future: competition and substitution, *J Psychosoc Nurs Ment Health Serv* 21:21, 1983.

Griffith H: Nursing practice: substitute or complement according to economic theory, *Nurs Economics* 2:105, 1984.

Kelly LS: Another look at the future of health care, *Nurs Outlook* 39:150, July/August 1991.

Lamb HR: Deinstitutionalization and the homeless mentally ill, *Hosp Community Psychiatry* 35:899, September 1984.

Lamb HR, Peele R: The need for continuing asylum and sanctuary, *Hosp Community Psychiatry* 33:798, August 1984.

Lapierre ED, Padgett J, editors: Answers professionally speaking: what is biological psychiatry? How will the trend toward biological psychiatry affect the future role of the psychiatric mental health nurse? *J Psychosoc Nurs Ment Health Serv* 30:33, 1992.

Lowery BJ: Psychiatric nursing in the 1990s & beyond, *J Psychosoc Nurs Ment Health Serv* 30:7, 1992.

Malone JA: The DSM-III-R versus nursing diagnosis: a dilemma in interdisciplinary practice, *Issues Ment Health Nurs* 12:219, 1991.

Martin EJ: A specialty in decline? Psychiatric–mental health nursing, past, present and future, *J Prof Nurs* 1:48, January/February 1985.

McBride AB: Psychiatric nursing in the 1990s, *Arch Psychiatr Nurs* 4:21, February 1990.

Pearlmutter DR: Recent trends and issues in psychiatric–mental nursing, *Hosp Community Psychiatry* 36:56, January 1985.

Peplau H: Tomorrow's world, *Nurs Times* 83:29, January 1987.

Peplau HE: Future directions in psychiatric nursing from the perspective of history, *J Psychosoc Nurs Ment Health Serv* 27(2):18, 1989.

Robinson L: The future of psychiatric/mental health nursing, *Nurs Clin North Am* 21:537, September 1986.

Slavinsky A: Psychiatric nursing in the year 2000: from a non-system of care to a caring system, *Image: J Nurs Scholarship* 16:17, Winter 1984.

Talley S, Brooke PS: Prescriptive authority for psychiatric clinical specialists: framing the issues, *Arch Psychiatr Nurs* 6:71, April 1992.

Trends to watch for in '92: health highest on American agenda, *Executive Wire,* National League for Nursing, January/February 1992.

Walgrove NJ: Mental health aftercare: where is nursing? *Nurs Clin North Am* 21:473, September 1986.

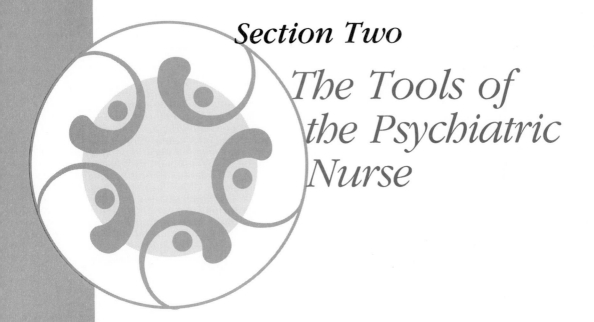

Section Two

The Tools of the Psychiatric Nurse

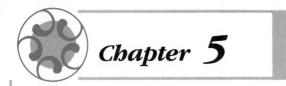

Chapter 5

Self-Awareness

LEARNING OBJECTIVES

After studying this chapter, the student will be able to:

* Explain the significance of self-awareness in the effective practice of psychiatric nursing.

* Differentiate between self-awareness and self-understanding.

* Discuss the nature of self-awareness.

* Describe four frequently used methods to increase self-awareness.

KEY TERMS

Unconscious mind
Beliefs
Feelings
Johari window
Introspection
Discussion
Enlarging experience
Role playing

Persons with a mental illness can be the most challenging group of individuals with whom the nurse has an opportunity to work. The relationship the nurse and the client develop can be one of the most important factors in the client's therapeutic experience. Whether the nurse can be a force for developing a truly therapeutic situation for the client depends on the nurse's ability to provide the client with new and more positive experiences in living with other people. To accomplish this, the nurse continuously strives to understand the client's behavior and the emotional needs expressed by that behavior. However, since the relationship between the nurse and the client has the potential for becoming a therapeutic experience for the client, it is not sufficient for the nurse to understand only the client; in addition, the nurse must develop self-awareness.

To practice psychiatric nursing effectively, the nurse's approaches to clients must be constantly adjusted and readjusted. Effective psychiatric nurses give much thought and consideration to their behavior as it influences the behavior of others. In other words, nurses need to be prepared to make positive use of their personality, a primary tool, as they work therapeutically with clients. Many nurses successfully make therapeutic use of their personality without recognizing their interpersonal effectiveness or being able to analyze how they succeed. However, nurses who work with persons with a mental illness cannot trust in luck in the hope of developing the self-awareness fundamental to being therapeutically effective. Although the effective practice of psychiatric nursing probably does not require particular personality attributes or attitudes, it does require a consistent, thoughtful effort directed toward developing awareness of self and others.

HISTORICAL PERSPECTIVE

The importance of self-awareness when working with persons who have a mental illness was not recognized until Freud's revolutionary discovery of the **unconscious mind** and its role in influencing behavior. Freud demonstrated how the origins of present behavior often lay in repressed emotions and earlier experiences. He logically concluded that what was true of his patients was also true of all human beings, namely, that much behavior is determined by **beliefs** and **feelings** that are beyond awareness. He also believed that if one is to help others, one must have an in-depth understanding of one's own beliefs and feelings so as not to interfere inadvertently with the patient's progress. The practice of psychoanalysis, the treatment procedure developed by Freud, therefore required the analyst to undergo much the same rigorous process of self-examination before being qualified to treat others.

Although Freud emphasized the importance of self-understanding, it soon became apparent that most mental health professionals could not or would not avail themselves of such a lengthy, costly, and emotionally disruptive process. Nevertheless, it became evident that increasing one's self-awareness had value to all persons, not just those involved in providing human services. During the 1960s and 1970s, sensitivity training and encounter groups became popular, and groups designed to enhance self-awareness abounded. The **Johari window,** described in this chapter, is a tool that became popular at that time. It was named for its developers, Joseph Luft and Harry Lipton.

Although the popularity of these self-awareness groups has diminished, it is now well accepted that increased self-awareness is desired for all persons but is mandatory for those, such as nurses, who work to assist others in achieving emotional growth (Figure 5-1).

SIGNIFICANCE OF SELF-AWARENESS

The major therapeutic tool of the nurse who works with persons with a mental illness is use of self in an interpersonal context. Since behavior is largely determined by one's beliefs and feelings, the nurse's ability to use the self as a therapeutic tool depends on adopting beliefs and feelings conducive to the effective practice of psychiatric nursing.

Beliefs are thoughts held to be true but not proved to be so. Beliefs differ from facts in that facts are truths that have been documented. Some beliefs stem from ignorance of the facts. Other beliefs have their source in the individual's prior experience or society's cultural norms. Some beliefs ultimately will be tested and proved to be either facts or falsehoods. Others are not amenable to testing because of their very nature. For example, a belief that stems from a value, such as the belief that human beings are basically good, does not lend itself to known methods of documentation.

Feelings are affective states or emotions. Recent research has demonstrated that feelings often arise from beliefs, rather than beliefs stemming from feelings, as is typically thought. For example, the mother of a teenage driver who is 2 hours late in arriving home often will think of all the negative events that could account for her child's delay. The belief that only a tragedy could cause her child to be late can result in the mother feeling great anxiety. On the other hand, if the same mother thought her child was delayed because of a positive event, or because he merely had overlooked the time, her resultant feeling likely would be pleasure or annoyance, not anxiety.

It is important to understand that beliefs and feelings are inextricably related and affect each other in a cyclical fashion. It is also important to understand and appreciate that the behavior of human beings, including nurses, is greatly influenced by their combined beliefs and feelings.

Many people in our society hold false beliefs about mental illness and those who have a mental illness. A recent survey conducted by the National Alliance for the Mentally Ill (NAMI) found that 71% of respondents believe mental illness is caused by some emotional weakness; 65% said

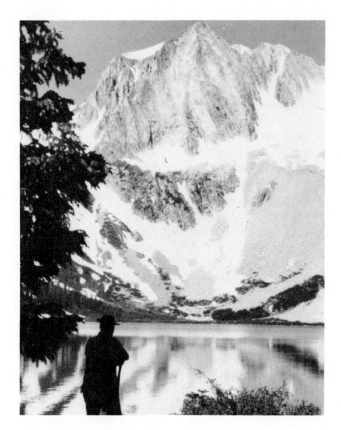

Figure 5-1
An individual's self-awareness is enhanced by enjoying a favorite activity.
From Rawlins RP, Heacock PE: *Clinical manual of psychiatric nursing,* St Louis, 1988, Mosby–Year Book.

poor parenting is at fault; 35% pointed to sinful behavior as a cause of mental illness; and 45% believed that those with a mental illness can bring on or turn off their illness at will. As a result of these and other erroneous beliefs, those with a mental illness are still stigmatized by society. Nurses, as with all members of society, have been influenced by these views. Therefore, it is likely nurses also have some of these beliefs, which, in turn, negatively affect the quality of their nursing care.

In addition to learned beliefs about those with a mental illness, nurses may have individually determined negative beliefs and feelings about clients who are overweight or underweight, young or old, wealthy or poor, or male or female or who reflect any of many characteristics. These prejudices inevitably interfere with the effective practice of psychiatric nursing.

Nurses whose beliefs and feelings are not conducive to the effective practice of psychiatric nursing cannot hope to alter them unless they can become aware of them. Furthermore, even if nurses have the beliefs and feelings necessary for the effective practice of psychiatric nursing, these cannot be used purposefully unless they are brought to a level of awareness. Although all nurses should learn to examine their beliefs and feelings, it is imperative for psychiatric nurses to do so.

The reader will note that the desired goal is self-awareness, not self-understanding. *Self-understanding* implies a knowledge of why one believes and feels as one does; this often requires a lengthy, in-depth process of self-examination guided by a qualified professional. Few nurses have the opportunity to engage in this process, and it is not necessary for most. However, all nurses can become *aware* of what they believe and feel without necessarily having to understand why they believe and feel as they do. Heightened self-awareness is within the grasp of all persons if they are willing to work at achieving it.

NATURE OF SELF-AWARENESS

A helpful model for understanding the nature of self-awareness is the Johari window (Figure 5-2). The window's upper left quadrant represents a person's beliefs and feelings that are known to the person and to others. This quadrant is termed "open." For example, nurses may believe that acutely psychotic persons are very amenable to therapeutic intervention. Furthermore, nurses may be aware that they are the type of person who is gratified by relatively rapid changes in a client's behavior. Consequently the nurse often volunteers to assume the nursing care of acutely psychotic clients, allowing others to infer this particular belief and feeling from the nurse's behavior.

The upper right quadrant, the "blind" quadrant, represents those beliefs and feelings hidden from a person's awareness, usually because of their anxiety-producing nature. The person defends against awareness of such beliefs and feelings by using mental mechanisms. However, the person's behavior reveals these beliefs and feelings to others. For example, the nurse may believe that clients who abuse alcohol are morally degenerate, and any contact with them makes the nurse angry. This belief and feeling may be unacceptable to the nurse and so do not exist at a level of awareness. However, the nurse's comments about these clients and behavior when around them reveal the nurse's negative feelings to others, including the clients.

The lower left quadrant of the Johari window represents beliefs and feelings known to the person but purposefully and consciously concealed from others. This quadrant is termed "private" and usually exists because the individual fears rejection if his or her beliefs and feelings were known. For example, the nurse may believe that clients who seek readmission to the hospital at the end of the month when they have run out of money are really malingerers, and therefore the nurse feels they are undeserving of care.

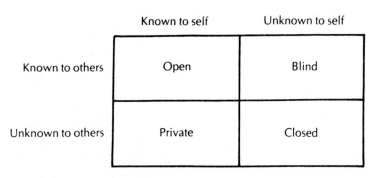

Figure 5-2
Johari window.

Being aware of this belief and consequent feeling but fearing criticism by peers if they were known, nurses extend themselves to provide care for these clients in an effort to conceal their attitude.

Finally, the lower right quadrant (the "closed" quadrant) represents beliefs and feelings so deeply buried in the person's unconscious mind that they are unknown both to the person and to others. This does not imply that these beliefs and feelings do not affect the person's behavior, but rather that behavioral manifestations are likely to be indirect and therefore not easily understood by either the person or others.

When the Johari window is used as a model, the goal of self-awareness can be understood to be the decrease of the size of the blind and private quadrants, thereby enlarging the size of the open quadrant. In this way, more beliefs and feelings will become known to the person and to others. Working toward this goal has major advantages. Because it requires energy to conceal beliefs and feelings from oneself or from others, an increase in self-awareness and self-disclosure can free energy that can then be used more profitably. An increase in self-awareness and self-disclosure also gives persons more control over their behavior as well as a better understanding of others' response to them.

Finally, one outcome of increased self-awareness often is an increase in acceptance of self and others. As one becomes more self-accepting, one values oneself more and therefore is more able to value others. As one becomes more self-aware, it becomes possible to judge oneself and others less harshly and to develop skill in affirming oneself and others. This skill is important in maintaining one's own mental health and becoming an effective psychiatric nurse.

Under usual circumstances, it is unlikely that the size of the closed quadrant will be reduced, but as is true of self-understanding, the effective practice of psychiatric nursing does not require complete self-awareness.

INCREASING SELF-AWARENESS

For nurses to increase self-awareness, they must examine their beliefs and feelings. Several methods can be employed to achieve this. However, all require a willingness to explore one's own behavior as a means of uncovering one's beliefs and feelings, much as the nurse who is learning a new psychomotor skill is willing to practice the technique until it is mastered. Unfortunately, this is more easily said than done because we are conditioned from birth to view our behavior and that of others judgmentally. In other words, we are prone to evaluate observed behavior as either good or bad and understandably to avoid recognition of our own behavior that we deem "bad." Nevertheless, when attempting to heighten self-awareness, we need to reserve such judgment in an effort to allow the underlying beliefs and feelings to surface.

OF SPECIAL INTEREST

The pursuit of self-awareness is not recent and is not limited to health professionals. Perhaps the earliest and best known reference to self-awareness is the statement, "The life which is unexamined is not worth living." This phrase is found in Plato's *Apology* and is thought by many to have been said by Socrates, Plato's mentor.

More recently, a moving tribute to the value of self-understanding was written by Katherine Mansfield, a New Zealand short-story writer. The end of her *Journal,* written in 1922, states: "I want, by understanding myself, to understand others. I want to be all I am capable of becoming.... This all sounds very strenuous and serious. But now that I have wrestled with it, it's no longer so. I feel happy—deep down. *All is well."*

Ms. Mansfield died of tuberculosis in January 1923 at the age of 34.

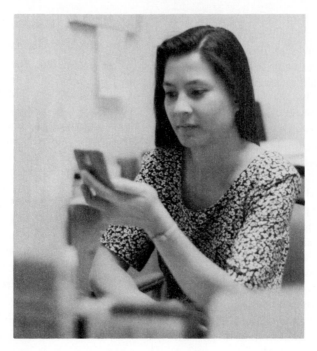

Figure 5-3
Increased self-awareness gives the individual more control over own behavior.

Four methods often used to increase self-awareness are described here.

Introspection

Introspection is the process of observing one's own behavior in various situations and identifying its themes and patterns. In a sense, introspection requires stepping out of oneself to watch oneself in interaction with others. This practice is aided by the use of a process recording, journal, or diary in which everything remembered from an interaction is written as soon as possible after it occurs. This includes thoughts and feelings as well as overt behaviors. Once behaviors are identified, the nurse can ask, "What beliefs and feelings underlie what I did?" This process of discovery is aided immeasurably by a state of relaxation, as is often achieved through meditation or yoga, when the mind is cleared of focused thoughts and allowed to roam freely. In

a sense, this is similar to free association, when one thought leads to another.

The advantage of introspection is that it can be engaged in at any time and place and does not depend on the presence of another person. The disadvantage of introspection is that its success depends on the individual's ability to overcome defenses and experience the potential emotional discomfort that may result from an unexpected discovery about oneself. As a result, introspection alone is a technique used most successfully by individuals who have already achieved some degree of self-awareness.

Discussion

Discussion is the process of having a focused conversation about one's behavior and can occur either in a group or with one other person, a dyad. Although both contexts can be helpful, most persons find themselves more comfortable in one or the other situation. In either instance, it is important that the participants have developed a degree of mutual trust and respect. Discussion directed toward increasing self-awareness often involves the nurse and the instructor or supervisor or a small group of nurse colleagues led by an experienced nurse. As with introspection, the discussion focuses on the nurse's behavior and attempts to discover that individual's underlying beliefs and feelings. In either dyadic or group situations, each person recounts observations and shares conjectures about what the behavior might indicate.

The advantages of discussion are that the insights of more than one person are brought to bear on the situation and that each participant is able to learn and be stimulated by hearing the perspectives of others. The disadvantage of discussion is that the observations made about another's behavior may be more reflective of what the speaker is thinking and feeling than what the subject is thinking and feeling. In addition, a skillful leader is necessary to help ensure that remarks remain nonjudgmental and that confidentiality is maintained.

Enlarging one's experience

Enlarging one's **experience** is the act of purposefully choosing to engage in unfamiliar activities and carefully noting one's reactions to them. This is a useful technique because one way human beings maintain their belief system is to limit their experiences to those familiar and known. For example, the nurse may believe that all persons with a mental illness are assaultive and therefore may fear contact with anyone diagnosed as mentally ill. However, when the nurse seeks contact with several persons with a mental illness, the nurse soon discovers that most of these individuals are fearful, withdrawn persons. This realization may lead to a re-examination of beliefs and an alteration of feelings. The nurse who is committed to increasing self-awareness will seek new experiences to test beliefs and feelings in light of reality.

The advantage of enlarging experience as a means of increasing self-awareness is that it increases one's ability and therefore one's self-confidence and almost forces becoming aware of and examining one's beliefs and feelings. The disadvantage of this method is that some preparation is required to benefit from the new experience. For example, nurses who are not prepared for an experience in psychiatric nursing may have their worst fears confirmed because their anxiety elicits assaultive behavior from the clients.

Role playing

Role playing is an exercise in which participants enact the parts of the persons involved in a real or anticipated interaction. It is seldom necessary to play out the entire interaction; often, one participant acts as timekeeper and stops the interaction at a predetermined time. To be useful, role playing must be followed by discussion (Figure 5-4). However, unlike discussion, in which interaction is limited to verbal and nonverbal exchanges about recent events, role playing allows the participants to behaviorally experience situations in the present. Role playing can occur between two people but is more effective when enacted in a small group.

The advantage of role playing is that the participants' reactions are likely to be spontaneous and less subject to unintentional censoring. In addition, this method is useful in developing empathy for the person whose role is enacted. The disadvantages are that many people feel uncomfortable role playing and are hesitant to try it and that a skilled, experienced leader is necessary for optimum benefits.

Nurses who are new to the practice of psychiatric nursing and who are just embarking on enhancing self-awareness may find themselves consciously preoccupied with analyzing their behavior and that of others. This is a perfectly normal occurrence, indicative of attempts to master the practice of self-awareness before it becomes automatic. This process is similar to the preoc-

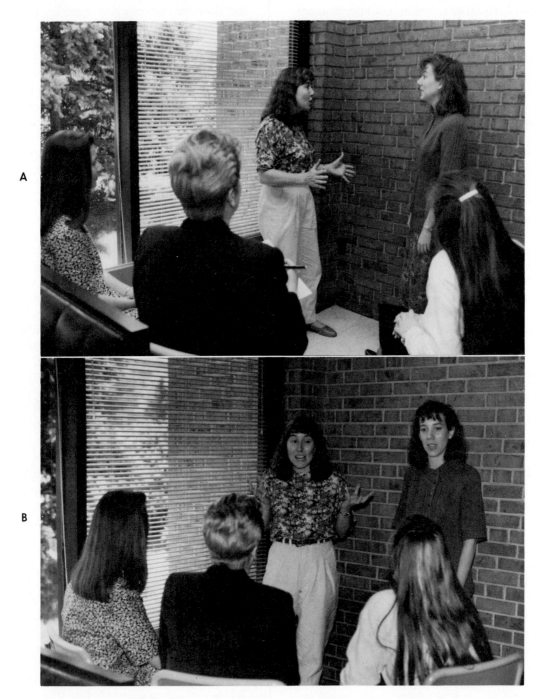

Figure 5-4
A, Role playing. **B,** Group discussion following role playing.

cupation nurses may have had with their physical health when they first studied pathophysiology. Concerns they may have about this preoccupation are appropriate topics to discuss with colleagues and experienced psychiatric nurses.

KEY POINTS

1. The major therapeutic tool of the psychiatric nurse is the use of self in an interpersonal context.

2. Nurses' beliefs and feelings about those who have a mental illness have been influenced by society's erroneous beliefs about mental illness. In addition, nurses may have individually determined negative beliefs and feelings about any number of human characteristics. Inevitably, prejudicial beliefs and feelings negatively affect the quality of nursing care.

3. The effective practice of psychiatric nursing requires that nurses learn to examine their beliefs and feelings.

4. Self-awareness differs from self-understanding in that self-awareness does not require a knowledge of why one believes and feels as one does.

5. Increased self-awareness frees energy, makes more control over one's own behavior possible, increases acceptance of self and others, and makes it possible to judge oneself and others less harshly, thereby enabling one to develop skill in affirming oneself and others.

6. When attempting to heighten self-awareness, nurses need to explore their behavior as a means of uncovering beliefs and feelings.

7. Four methods typically used to increase self-awareness are introspection, discussion, role playing, and enlarging one's experience.

SUGGESTED SOURCES OF ADDITIONAL INFORMATION

Brillhart B, Jay H, Wyers M: Attitudes toward people with disabilities, *Rehabil Nurs* 15:80, March/April 1990.

Bunkers S: A strategy for staff development: self-care and self-esteem as necessary partners, *Clin Nurs Specialist* 6(3):154, 1990.

Burnard P: Developing self-awareness, *Nurs Mirror* 158:30, May 1984.

Haber L: The role of the therapist's critical parent, *Issues Ment Health Nurs* 10:89, 1989.

Jerome A, Ferraro-McDuffie A: Nurse self-awareness in therapeutic relationships, *Pediatr Nurs* 18:153, March/April 1992.

Knowles R: Dealing with feelings: coping with lethargy, *Am J Nurs* 81:1465, August 1981.

Knowles R: Dealing with feelings: overcoming guilt and worry, *Am J Nurs* 81:1663, September 1981.

Knowles R: Dealing with feelings: managing guilt, *Am J Nurs* 81:1850, October 1981.

Knowles R: Dealing with feelings: handling anger: responding vs reacting, *Am J Nurs* 81:2196, December 1981.

Krikovian D, Paulanka B: Self-awareness—the key to a successful nurse-patient relationship, *J Psychosoc Nurs Ment Health Serv* 20:19, June 1982.

Landeen J, Byrne C, Brown B: Journal keeping as an educational strategy in teaching psychiatric nursing, *J Adv Nurs* 17:347, 1992.

Luft J, Ingham H: The Johari window: a graphic model of awareness in interpersonal relations. In Luft J, editor: *Group processes: an introduction to group dynamics,* Palo Alto, Calif, 1963, National Press Books.

Minot S, Adamski J: Elements of effective clinical supervision, *Perspect Psychiat Care* 25(2):23, 1989.

National Advisory Mental Health Council: *Mental illness in America: a series of public hearings—a report to the Congress of the United States,* Arlington, Va, 1992, National Alliance for the Mentally Ill.

Perez L: Safe and sound: orienting nurses to psychiatry, *Perspect Psychiatr Care* 26(3):7, 1990.

Peternelj-Taylor C: The effects of patient weight and sex on nurses' perceptions: a proposed model of nurse withdrawal, *J Adv Nurs* 14:744, 1989.

Rawlinson J: Self-awareness: conceptual influences, contribution to nursing, and approaches to attainment, *Nurs Educ Today* 10:111, 1990.

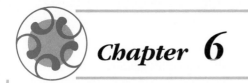

Chapter 6

Principles of Psychiatric Nursing

LEARNING OBJECTIVES
After studying this chapter, the student will be able to:
- State seven principles of psychiatric nursing, discussing the beliefs and feelings on which each principle is based.
- Define psychiatric nursing.
- Discuss each phase of the nursing process as it is used in psychiatric nursing.
- Describe the characteristics of an effective interview.
- Discuss observation as a means of client assessment.

KEY TERMS
Psychiatric nursing
Philosophy
Principles
Holistic
Adaptation
Homeokinesis
Assessment phase
Observation
Diagnostic phase
DSM
NANDA
Planning phase
Implementation phase
Evaluation phase

The current state of knowledge about human behavior is at best imprecise. It consists mostly of beliefs, and many of these beliefs are incompatible. For example, the medical model of health care holds the belief that aberrant behavior reflects an individual illness hypothetically amenable to treatment by somatic means. In contrast, a sociological model of health care dictates the belief that aberrant behavior is a sign of deviance rather than illness and must be assessed and treated within the larger context of the society. These examples illustrate the diversity of currently held beliefs about human behavior and the necessity for all health professionals to develop an awareness of the beliefs that guide their professional practice.

Being aware of one's beliefs and feelings is necessary but not sufficient for the effective practice of **psychiatric nursing.** To be useful, the nurse's beliefs and feelings must be organized into an internally consistent statement about the nature of human beings and their behavior. When combined with the nurse's knowledge of the scope and nature of nursing practice, these statements constitute a **philosophy** that, in turn, provides direction for developing principles of psychiatric nursing. **Principles** are rules or laws that have proved applicable in most, if not all, situations. Identifying principles of psychiatric nursing allows nurses to operationalize their beliefs and feelings as they provide nursing care.

HISTORICAL PERSPECTIVE

The principles that have guided the care of persons with a mental illness over the centuries have been largely determined, by definition, by the prevailing societal beliefs about the nature of mental illness. As discussed in depth in Chapter 1, these have ranged from the belief that those with a mental illness were possessed by the devil or other evil spirits or that the phases of the moon influenced behavior to the belief that mental illness is caused by biochemical imbalance. When it was believed that persons with a mental illness were possessed by demons, it was un-

derstandable, although not acceptable in today's views, that the principles guiding their treatment reflected the necessity to exorcise the evil spirits. When biochemical imbalance is believed to be the major determinant of mental illness, it follows that principles of care would emphasize somatic treatments, especially psychopharmacology.

In addition to principles of care being influenced by beliefs about the nature of mental illness, the society's economic status strongly influences the principles underlying the treatment of persons with a mental illness. For example, in prehistoric times, people had no means of accumulating or storing food beyond their daily needs and therefore did not have the ability to sustain members who were not able to care for themselves. Therefore the "principle" that guided the treatment of those whose behavior was aberrant was simply "each person for oneself." An affluent society, such as existed in the United States after World War II, could literally afford to believe that every human being has a right to the best possible treatment, regardless of the contribution that person makes to society.

Finally, the society's cultural heritage is a major determinant of its beliefs and therefore the principles underlying how its members are viewed and treated. The Western world is greatly influenced by its Judeo-Christian heritage, which dictates that each individual has worth and value. This belief has also helped to focus treatment efforts on the individual as opposed to the family or community. In contrast, Eastern cultures, which value the family unit above the individual's worth, tend to view the family as the focus of treatment concern.

BELIEFS, FEELINGS, AND PRINCIPLES OF PSYCHIATRIC NURSING

This chapter discusses my beliefs about the nature of human beings and their behavior, feelings conducive to the effective practice of psychiatric nursing, and the resultant principles of psychiatric nursing to which I adhere. Included is a definition of psychiatric nursing derived from my philosophy. Students are encouraged to examine their own beliefs and feelings about human beings and their behavior so that they may state a philosophy and definition of psychiatric nursing to guide their nursing care.

Viewing the client as a holistic being

Human beings are viewed as complex systems of interrelated parts, the whole of which is greater than the sum of the parts. This belief represents a **holistic** perspective, a stance that acknowledges the interdependence and interrelatedness of the parts to each other, to the person, and to the environment. Therefore, alterations in any aspect of the system require responsive alterations in other aspects of the system.

Nurses new to psychiatric nursing sometimes believe that the slightest change in the environment of a person with a mental illness will precipitate an untoward emotional response. It is also not unusual for such a nurse to believe that individuals with a mental illness are so emotionally fragile that they can be traumatized by an inexpertly phrased statement. These beliefs may cause some nurses to fear that they may injure clients emotionally, and as a result nurses may avoid contact with clients.

This fear and its resultant behavior are particularly unfortunate and unwarranted if the nurse views the client as a system. It is important to remember that persons with a mental illness are not defenseless and that they withstand the inappropriate approach of new staff remarkably well. It may be helpful to note that if clients were defenseless, it would be relatively easy to interact with them in a manner that would result in emotionally corrective experiences. Rather, clients, as with all human beings, are complex organisms who are usually able to sense the basic friendliness behind the nurse's approach even if it is not skillfully executed. Furthermore, the nurse who is new to psychiatric nursing has developed expertise in many other areas of nursing practice that can be brought to bear on the interaction. Consequently, nurses can develop the *feeling*

that they have the potential to be helpful to the client, even though they may not have yet developed expertise in the care specific to individuals with a mental illness.

A major principle of psychiatric nursing that stems from this belief and feeling is that *the nurse views the client as a holistic being with many interrelated and interdependent needs.* The implications of this principle are numerous. First, the nurse caring for the individual with a mental illness must be skilled in understanding the interrelatedness of all the client's subsystems. For example, mental illness does not provide immunity to physical illness; persons with a mental illness are prone to the development of physical illness just like other members of the population. Therefore the nurse needs to be constantly alert to the possibility that a client may develop a physical illness and thereby avoid the pitfall of assuming that all symptoms are simply manifestations of emotional stress. The individual must also be viewed as an integral part of the social system, simultaneously affecting the system and being affected by it. Therefore the person cannot be assessed accurately in isolation from the family, community, and the reference groups to which the person belongs. As a result, the well-prepared psychiatric nurse must have not only effective interpersonal skills but also current knowledge about pathophysiology and about the beliefs, norms, and practices of various subcultures and religions. This principle is often cited as the rationale for employing a nurse whose educational background includes preparation in the biophysical and psychosocial realms, instead of a nursing assistant whose on-the-job training focuses only on the psychosocial realm.

Focusing on the client's strengths and assets

Each individual has some strengths and a potential for growth, that is, a potential for developing increasingly effective adaptations to stress. I do not mean to suggest that all individuals have an equal number or the same type of strengths or the same potential for growth, but rather that each individual has some strengths and some potential for growth, no matter how small or great.

Sometimes nurses who are new to working with persons who have a mental illness feel despair at the slow progress some clients are able to make. Some nurses even feel hopeless about effecting any improvement. This feeling often emanates from inexperience in working with persons who have a chronic illness and for whom no specific treatment may exist. However, as the nurse gains experience and adopts the belief that each individual has potential for growth, despair will be replaced by hope. Interestingly, *the feeling of hope is therapeutic* in and of itself, since it conveys to the client the feeling that change is possible.

The principle of psychiatric nursing derived from this belief and from the feeling of hope is that *the nurse focuses on the client's strengths and assets, not on weaknesses and liabilities.* All clients have some strengths, no matter how few or insignificant they may seem. These strengths should be built on to encourage the individual's emotional growth. For example, the client who dresses without undue difficulty can build on this behavior by being encouraged to choose clothing appropriate to the occasion and weather. As the client learns to make these choices, an increasing sense of autonomy may develop, which in turn may carry over to other areas of daily living. This example is overly simplistic, but it is given to illustrate how this principle can be used in frequently encountered situations.

When mental health care was limited to institutional care, an illness orientation was all-pervasive. A client who was cooperative was too often seen as being overly submissive; if the same client became assertive, he or she ran the risk of being labeled rebellious. The focus on illness not only tended to reinforce the condition and therefore stifle the client's growth but also may have contributed to the development of illness. A positive outcome of the community mental health movement has been the necessity to focus on clients' healthy aspects in an effort to enable them to maintain themselves in the community and outside the institution. In many instances, this orientation has been even more successful than had been originally anticipated. Some authorities believe this may result because when an individual is helped to identify and accept strengths, the person is less threatened and therefore more open to exploring and altering dysfunctional behaviors. It should be noted, however, that a focus on the individual's strengths and growth potential does not mean that limitations should not be taken into account when assessing the person's behavior. Failure to do so and subsequent misjudgments have accounted for many failures that have also accompanied the community mental health movement.

Accepting the client as a unique human being

I endorse the belief that *each individual, although sharing much with other persons, is unique and has inherent value.* This belief is consistent with the view of human beings as complex systems that transform energy and matter in a unique way. The belief that each individual has inherent value is a product of the Judeo-Christian heritage of our society and is manifested in numerous ways through societal practices.

In contrast, American culture also places great value on an individual's capacity to contribute to the society and thus covertly devalues those persons who are unable or who choose not to do so. Certainly, many persons with a mental illness are not able to make an identifiable contribution to society's welfare, and therefore some nurses have the feeling that these persons have less inherent value than other more productive members of the population. It is important for the nurse to recognize this feeling if it exists and attempt to overcome it by focusing on the humanness of the client, regardless of level of productivity. Valuing the client may also be difficult because of appearance or behavior. Once the nurse is able to view these factors as indicators of the client's ineffective **adaptations,** the nurse is more likely to be able to *appreciate the uniqueness and inherent value of each human being.*

The principle of psychiatric nursing that stems from the belief in and feeling about the uniqueness and inherent value of each human being is that *the nurse accepts the client as a unique human being who has value and worth exactly as he or she is.* Most authorities agree that this principle is the most basic to the effective practice of psychiatric nursing.

The conviction that each individual is unique implies that the nurse has a responsibility to observe and listen carefully to each person as if he or she were the only one to whom care has ever been given. The nurse must not "tune the person out," even though the client's story has been told 100 times before. Psychological experiments have demonstrated that each person's perceptions of and reactions to the same situation are always different, depending on many variables, such as previous experience and present state of being.

This principle guides the nurse in respecting the worth and dignity of persons at all times, without regard to the acceptability of their behavior. Thus the effective nurse treats clients with respect even though their behavior may be unacceptable. Inherent in this principle is the attitude that information about clients is treated with appropriate professional confidentiality and that client problems must not become topics for social chatter. This principle also implies that the treatment methods in which health professionals engage must not in themselves be dehumanizing, even though such methods may have desired outcomes. In other words, if all human beings have inherent worth and value, treatment modalities that are dehumanizing do not justify even desired ends.

Although the nurse needs to convey to the client a belief in the potential to change and grow, acceptance of the client must not depend on reaching these goals. That would be conditional acceptance and may convey, "I value you only because of what you could become." Most clients have a long history of being rejected in social relationships because their behavior did not measure up to usual societal expectations. Therefore, such individuals enter treatment situations understandably expecting the responses with which they are so familiar. If they do receive these negative responses, they might just as well not have sought treatment because they will be receiving very little constructive help. Since nurses spend more time with the client than other professionals, they have the greatest opportunity to convey a feeling of acceptance. Calling clients by their surnames, such as Mr. Smith, unless requested otherwise is an example of how acceptance and respect can be conveyed.

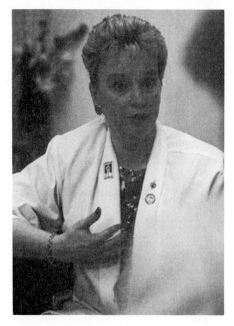

Figure 6-1

The nurse should convey a feeling of acceptance to the client.

From Potter PA, Perry AG: *Basic nursing: theory and practice,* St Louis, 1991, Mosby–Year Book.

Potential for establishing a relationship with most clients

In apparent contradiction to the belief that each individual is unique is the belief that *all human beings are sufficiently similar that a basis exists, no matter how small, for understanding and communicating with one another*. Harry Stack Sullivan, the developer of the interpersonal theory of psychiatry, has said that we are all more human than otherwise. I ascribe to this belief of similarity among human beings and further believe that differences in feelings and behavior are more likely to be differences in quantity rather than in quality. For example, all persons have experienced anxiety, although most individuals have not adapted to anxiety by withdrawing from reality. Almost everyone knows what it means to feel sad, or happy, or excited. Those who have a mental illness experience these same emotions, but to an exaggerated or diminished degree.

The very nature of this belief may elicit in nurses a fear that they may become mentally ill. Not too many decades ago, it was believed by lay people that if a person worked too long with persons who had a mental illness, that person also would become mentally ill. This belief had its origins in the lack of understanding of the causes of mental illness and in the observation that many who did work with persons who had a mental illness were emotionally disturbed themselves. This latter phenomenon resulted from the care of these people being seen as such an undesired job that only socially deviant persons who could not find employment elsewhere were willing to work in the asylums.

The nurse today brings into the mental health setting all the biases and prejudices of the society at large. When the nurse realizes that the behavior of most clients is not as bizarre as expected, another fear may be elicited—the fear that the nurse has more problems than the clients appear to have. Consequently, some nurses initially believe that they require psychiatric treatment or hospitalization. Although this may be true in a

very few instances, the nurse will learn that most persons enter a treatment situation because of an increasing inability to perform the usual activities of daily living in regard to both work and family life. In contrast, the nurse who is functioning despite possible emotional problems learns that the ability to function productively is an important criterion of mental health.

Beginning students of psychiatric nursing frequently experience anxiety about their state of mental health as they learn more about the dynamics underlying mental illness. This probably results from the student more easily identifying with the person who has a mental illness than with the person who has a physical illness. All human beings have experienced emotional trauma, anxiety, guilt, anger, and other emotions, but not all have experienced appendicitis, myocardial infarction, or other forms of major physical illnesses.

Once again, it is important for the nurse to remember that none of the feelings and few of the experiences of persons with a mental illness are different from those the nurse has personally known. In fact, the nurse will learn *to use her familiarity with the various emotions as a tool through which to develop empathy with the client's feelings*.

The principle of psychiatric nursing based on belief in the similarity of all human beings and the nurse's empathy with the client's feelings is that *the nurse has the potential for establishing a relationship with most, if not all, clients*. This principle implies that nurses who interact with clients who have a mental illness must continuously strive to discover the area of similarity between the person and themselves that can serve as a means of establishing communication. Nurses cannot hide behind the belief that it is useless to try to help others because their background, experience, and behavior are different from anything with which nurses are familiar. This does not suggest that a common cultural or experiential background between a client and a nurse may not be helpful in establishing communication, but rather that nurses must continue to strive to communicate with clients if their frame of reference is not immediately understood. Furthermore, in some situations when the nurse and the client have much in common, the nurse may fail to recognize the client's uniqueness and inappropriately attribute to the person the nurse's own feelings and reactions. This principle does not mean, however, that any one nurse should or could have a therapeutic relationship with all clients. The student will learn that to engage effectively in a therapeutic relationship with a client is very time-consuming and an emotionally and intellectually draining activity. Therefore, such interventions should be undertaken with clients who are most likely to benefit from the nurse's personality and style of interaction. However, the nurse can interact with every client in a helpful way if the nurse continuously looks for areas of similarities between them to use as a basis for increasing an understanding of the client.

Exploring client behavior for its need or message

A belief central to the effective practice of psychiatric nursing is that *all behavior is purposeful and designed to meet a need or to communicate a message.* No behavior is accidental or occurs by chance.

Some nurses fear the clinical practice of psychiatric nursing not only because it is a new experience but also because of many preconceived ideas about the behavior of persons who have a mental illness. Nurses may have heard discussions about unusual and frightening behavior of such individuals. These discussions often exaggerate the behavior being described and tend to arouse fear in the listener. A few nurses may have had an experience with a person with a mental illness that they found frightening.

The nurse with these feelings can cope more readily with the situation by acknowledging any concerns about personal safety, by facing them frankly, and by examining these fears to discover

what they involve. It is usually helpful to discuss such feelings in situations in which students and teacher can help each other in examining, understanding, and coping with these feelings. This method is particularly effective when the discussion focuses on a specific individual whose behavior is causing concern.

Much fear of persons with a mental illness grows out of cultural attitudes and beliefs handed down from one generation to another. Despite attempts to educate the public about mental illness, many persons still believe that all individuals with a mental illness are dangerous and require drastic measures to control their behavior. Nurses being introduced to a mental health setting will be surprised at the many clients whose behavior is socially acceptable. They will be surprised to find that many clients seem content to be inactive. Instead of requiring controls, these clients require stimulation and need to be helped to develop an interest in the available activities. Once the nurse has become familiar with the clients in the mental health setting and has gained more knowledge about human behavior, the nurse can replace fear of client behavior with a *feeling of curiosity about its meaning.*

The principle of psychiatric nursing that stems from the belief that all behavior is purposeful and from the accompanying curiosity about its meaning is that *the nurse explores the client's behavior for the need it is designed to meet or the message it is communicating.* This principle does not imply that all behavior must be accepted or condoned as it is expressed. On the contrary, tolerance of all behavior, no matter how antisocial, can convey to clients the idea that they are not important enough for the nurse to explore their behavior with them. Helpful nurses attempt to convey to the client their understanding that the client's behavior has meaning and their willingness to help the client meet the need or communicate the message in a socially acceptable way. Some clients have never become aware that socially acceptable means exist through which their needs can be met. When the nurse helps the client to evaluate the consequences of present behavior and test new patterns of behavior, the nurse does much in furthering the client's feeling of being a worthwhile human being. By treating the client's socially unacceptable behavior in this manner, nurses communicate that they are not being punitive or judgmental but are primarily concerned about the client's welfare.

Assisting the client to learn effective adaptations

Another belief regarding the nature of human behavior is that *it was learned as an adaptation to earlier stressors,* especially those experienced during the influential years of infancy and childhood, when the foundation of the personality is laid. Therefore *the individual's present behavior is believed to represent the best possible adaptation the person is capable of making at the time.* All behavioral adaptations were effective in maintaining **homeokinesis** (system stability) at the time they were learned. If, however, the interpersonal environment in which the behavioral adaptation was learned was unique or unhealthy, the behavior that was effective in the original situation becomes ineffective and dysfunctional when the person moves to a subsequent developmental stage or into the larger social system that functions in a more usual or healthy manner.

Even when they are seeking help, persons with a mental illness may be shy, suspicious, withdrawn, and preoccupied with their own thoughts and problems. Nurses may interpret these behaviors as a dislike of them and react with the socially familiar response of disliking the client. As the nurse develops an understanding of mental illness, she or he will realize that some clients behave in this manner, even when they want very much to become acquainted with the nurse, because they fear that they will not be accepted by her or him. The nurse cannot expect to like all clients thoroughly and cannot expect all clients genuinely to like her or him. However,

it is realistic to expect that the nurse will develop some understanding and acceptance of all clients and learn not to view all their behavior as a reflection of their feelings toward the nurse. The nurse will also be able to develop *the ability to care about clients even though they may not reciprocate this feeling* if the nurse works at developing a support group among peers rather than looking to clients for approval and gratitude.

The principle of psychiatric nursing based on these beliefs and feelings is that *the nurse views the client's behavior nonjudgmentally while assisting the client to learn more effective adaptations.* This principle is central to the effective practice of psychiatric nursing because it implies that the client can unlearn previous adaptations and relearn new, more effective adaptations if provided with an environment that facilitates and supports this goal. Further, this principle also implies that the nurse is likely to accept the client's behavior, withholding judgment. For example, adherence to this principle makes it inappropriate for the nurse to say that the client refuses to participate in group therapy; rather, the nurse is more likely to understand that at this time the client is not able to participate. In addition, this principle helps to dispel the aura of hopelessness that often surrounds the care of persons with a mental illness. Although it is important to be realistic about the changes any one individual can make, it is inappropriate to believe that a person's behavior cannot change or that overall adaptation to the stresses of life cannot become more effective.

Quality of the nurse-client interaction

A final belief basic to the effective practice of psychiatric nursing is the understanding that *an individual learns behavioral adaptations primarily in interaction with significant people in the environment.* Human beings do not exist in a vacuum; their survival depends on interaction with other human beings. However, an individual cannot be expected to learn new behavioral adaptations if not given an opportunity to interact with others who provide experiences that are more positive than those the person has known previously.

Nurses beginning an experience in psychiatric nursing sometimes find they have a strong desire to be helpful but simultaneously believe they are not skillful enough to assume a significant role in the client's treatment. These feelings present nurses with an uncomfortable personal dilemma from which they may seek to escape by becoming indifferent. To allow this feeling to develop would be unfortunate because indifference is one of the reactions that most persons with a mental illness have already experienced much too often in their relations with family and friends. Without such involvement, the nurse can be of little therapeutic help. However, it is essential to understand the meaning of involvement. *Involvement* implies that nurses are genuinely and sincerely interested in the client, that they give their time and themselves without expecting anything in return, and that they interact in a way that meets the client's needs instead of

their own. Although initially nurses may think that their interpersonal skills are not developed to a level that makes them feel adequate in the situation, with guidance, practice, and persistent study of self, the early feelings of inadequacy will be replaced with *feelings of competency in their ability to interact therapeutically* with persons who have a mental illness.

The principle of psychiatric nursing derived from the belief and feeling just discussed is that *the quality of the interaction in which the nurse engages with the client is a major determinant of the degree to which the client will be able to alter behavioral adaptations in the direction of more satisfying, satisfactory interpersonal relationships* (Figure 6-2). When individuals seek help from a treatment setting, they have little impetus to alter adaptive mechanisms if their characteristic behavior is met with the same negative, judgmental attitudes they have experienced from society. On the other hand, if, despite their behavior, individuals become involved with an interested, concerned nurse who values their

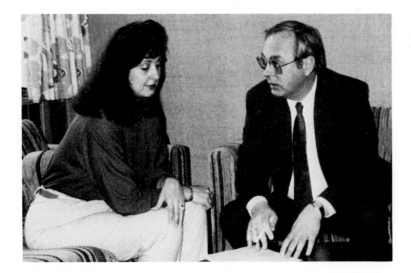

Figure 6-2

Therapeutic nurse-client interactions are important in helping the client develop more satisfying, satisfactory relationships.

From Cookfair JM: *Nursing process and practice in the community,* St Louis, 1991, Mosby–Year Book.

worth and dignity, positive satisfactory behavioral adaptations are likely to be elicited. This principle is particularly germane to the practice of psychiatric nursing because the nurse is the professional person who is likely to spend the greatest amount of time with the client and therefore is the person who has the greatest opportunity to create the environment in which the client can unlearn previous ineffective adaptations and learn new, more effective adaptations.

Table 6-1 outlines beliefs, feelings, and principles conducive to psychiatric nursing.

Table 6-1. Beliefs, feelings, and principles conducive to the effective practice of psychiatric nursing

BELIEF	FEELING	PRINCIPLE
Human beings are complex systems of interrelated parts, the whole of which is greater than the sum of the parts.	The nurse feels she can be helpful to the client, since she has expertise in many areas of nursing.	The nurse views the client as a holistic being with many interrelated and interdependent needs.
Each individual has some strengths and a potential for growth.	The nurse is hopeful about the client's ability to grow.	The nurse focuses on the client's strengths and assets, not on weaknesses and liabilities.
Each individual is unique and has inherent value.	The nurse appreciates the client's uniqueness and inherent value.	The nurse accepts the client as a unique human being who has value and worth exactly as he or she is.
All human beings are sufficiently similar that a basis exists for understanding and communicating with one another.	The nurse feels empathy with the client's feelings.	The nurse has the potential for establishing a relationship with most, if not all, clients.
All behavior is purposeful and is designed to meet a need or to communicate a message.	The nurse feels curious about the meaning of the client's behavior.	The nurse explores the client's behavior for the need it is designed to meet or the message it is communicating.
Behavior is learned as an adaptation to an earlier stressor and is the best possible adaptation the individual is capable of making at the time.	The nurse cares about clients even though they may not reciprocate this feeling.	The nurse views the client's behavior nonjudgmentally while assisting the client to learn more effective adaptations.
An individual learns behavioral adaptations primarily in interaction with significant people in the environment.	The nurse feels competent in her or his ability to interact therapeutically with persons who have a mental illness.	The quality of the interaction in which the nurse engages with the client is a major determinant of the degree to which the client will be able to alter behavioral adaptations in the direction of more satisfying, satisfactory interpersonal relationships.

DEFINITION OF PSYCHIATRIC NURSING

The nurse's philosophy of psychiatric nursing and the resultant principles provide direction for stating a definition of psychiatric nursing. The philosophy and principles just discussed lead me to define psychiatric nursing as a process whereby the nurse collaborates with others, as individuals or in groups, in the development of a more positive self-concept, a more satisfying pattern of interpersonal relationships, and a more satisfactory role in society.

THE NURSING PROCESS

Too often the same nurse who systematically plans, implements, and evaluates care for persons who have a physical illness relies on intuitive judgment of the moment in administering care to those persons who have a mental illness. This practice is likely to result in therapeutic interactions that occur more by chance than design and as a result decrease the probability of the client attaining a more satisfactory level of adaptation. Therefore, it is important to understand how the nursing process is used in the care of those who have a mental illness. The following discussion is not intended to be a comprehensive review of each phase of the nursing process. Rather, it is designed to highlight factors specific to the care of those with a mental illness.

Throughout each phase of the nursing process, it is important for nurses to validate their findings with the client to ensure their relevancy. For example, the nurse may develop a goal that has no meaning to the client and then wonder why the interventions do not elicit the desired behavioral change.

Assessment phase

Although psychiatric nursing is concerned primarily with the client's emotional, behavioral, and interpersonal responses, the nurse must remember that the human being is a unified, in-tegrated whole. Consequently, the nurse must assess the client comprehensively, considering all client responses, if accurate information is to be available to plan nursing care.

What to assess

To assess the client comprehensively and therefore accurately, the nurse needs to adopt an organizing schema to direct the **assessment phase.** Furthermore, for the assessment data to provide direction for planning nursing care, they must be not only comprehensive but also relevant to nursing practice. In other words, the assessment data must lead to the formulation of nursing diagnoses. Although the nursing profession agrees little about the nature of the appropriate organizing schema, consensus exists about its necessity. Several nursing models are available that meet the criteria of comprehensiveness and relevancy.

How to assess

It is important to collect data about the client from all appropriate sources. These include the client's chart, other health care workers, relevant texts and journals, and the client's family and friends. Although all sources of information about the client should be used, the client is the most important and significant source of information. To obtain data from the client, the nurse needs to perfect the skills of interviewing and observing.

An interview is conducted to obtain specific information. As such, it is not designed to be therapeutic or to convey information, although indirectly it may be helpful or informative to the client. An interview is guided by goals, and an effective interview requires that the nurse organize goals and approaches before meeting with the client. Because an interview is structured, it is likely that the nurse will be more directive and ask more questions than in an interaction designed to be therapeutic. Thus the nurse should plan sample questions, the answers to which will provide the data sought. Questions likely to be most effective in eliciting information are simple, concrete, and direct. For example, "What do you usually eat for breakfast?" is preferable to "Tell me about your usual diet."

On initiating an interview, the nurse should tell the client the purpose of the interaction and approximately how long it will last. As with all interactions, the nurse should introduce herself or himself to the client if they have not already met and take a position at eye level with the client. Ideally, both the nurse and the client should sit in comfortable chairs. However, sitting down is not always possible if the client is too anxious. In that case the nurse may wish to remain standing as well. If the nurse intends to take notes during the interview, its purpose should be explained at the onset. By orienting the client in this manner, the nurse establishes a foundation on which a future trusting relationship with the client can be built, either by the nurse or by another nurse.

One of the most important goals of an initial interview is to ascertain the clients' perception of their problems. Although it is generally advisable to avoid using "why" questions, they are sometimes useful when interviewing persons who are psychotic because "why" questions are concrete and direct. For example, a psychotic, hallucinating individual who is asked, "What brought you to the hospital?" might very well respond by answering, "A car brought me." In contrast, the same client might respond to "Why did you come to the hospital?" by answering, "To get out of the cold" or "Because I see my grandmother all the time, and I know she is dead." Either of these responses answers the nurse's question, which is not the case when use of a "why" question is avoided.

Having ascertained the client's perception of the problem, the nurse's next goal is to determine the duration of the problem, what circumstances led to the problem, who else is involved, and in what way the client expects the hospital or clinic to help. A determination of these variables is essential to an accurate, comprehensive assessment and allows the nurse to compare the client's perception of the problem with the perceptions of others. Then the nurse can design a plan of care that will be of the greatest help to the client.

Another major goal of the interview is to obtain information about such factual data as the client's daily activities, previous health history, educational level, and occupation. It is important, however, that the client not be bombarded with questions that can be answered by other sources. For example, if the nurse has access to a chart from the client's previous admission, the nurse should not ask for such information as the client's date of birth unless the nurse questions the reliability of the available information or is using the question to assess the client's memory.

The interview should be concluded as close to the time specified as possible. It is helpful to the client for the nurse to repeat what she or he said earlier about how the information the client shared will be used. It is also important that the nurse inform the client what will happen next, such as that the nurse will take the client back to the unit or that the client should schedule another appointment with the receptionist.

The other skill integral to the assessment phase of the nursing process is **observation.** Observation is a frequently used term for an active goal-directed process that uses all appropriate senses. While talking or otherwise interacting with the client, the nurse looks, hears, feels, and smells. In general, the goal of observation is to determine the appropriateness and congruence of the client's appearance, behavior, and verbalizations with each other and with the situation. This implies, then, that observations are planned. This should not imply, however, that the nurse should not observe unanticipated phenomena. It is important for the nurse to follow intuitive feelings about a situation. Experience has shown that, more often than not, these intuitive feelings are manifestations of the nurse's unconscious perceptions based on reality. The nurse needs to be alert to the client's facial expression, voice quality, neatness and appropriateness of dress and grooming, participation in activities, response to other clients and staff, and many other aspects of behavior while the nurse is interviewing and during the time the client spends in the treatment setting, whether 1, 8, or 24 hours.

To validate the information gained from observations and to determine their significance, observations of the same or similar events must be made repeatedly. For example, the nurse may observe that on one occasion a client who was unable to purchase his or her brand of cigarettes swore at the clerk and stalked out of the store. Many people occasionally feel this degree of frustration and sometimes act on it. If the client does not have a similar reaction in future situations, this incident probably is relatively insignificant. On the other hand, if the nurse observes that on subsequent days the same client yells and walks away because he or she must wait for the elevator and then later displays the same behavior because a meal contains food the client does not like, the nurse would be correct in determining that a theme or pattern has been identified in this client's behavior likely to be most indicative of a problem. With some clients, however, behavior that is strikingly uncharacteristic of the client may be highly significant and should be recorded and communicated to other members of the professional team. As the nurse learns to understand more about the meaning of human behavior and learns to know the client as an individual, the nurse will become more skillful in recognizing significant behavior.

Concluding the assessment

The final step in the assessment phase of the nursing process is to determine the meaning of the assessment data by sorting and organizing the data according to themes. Themes are recurring patterns that may have different manifestations but that stem from the same source.

For example, the nurse may observe that the client has an unkempt appearance, speaks deprecatingly of self, and refuses to join in group activities that are new. Even though these behaviors superficially may seem to have little or no relationship, with study the nurse will learn they all may be manifestations of the same pattern. Identifying themes of the client's responses is a precursor to the **diagnostic phase** of the nursing process.

Diagnostic phase

The second phase of the nursing process is the diagnostic phase, in which the nurse makes a nursing diagnosis. This phase is based on a synthesis of all available assessment data and provides direction for developing a plan for nursing care.

A classification of diagnoses of mental disorders has been available for many years. However, in 1980 the American Psychiatric Association published the *Diagnostic and Statistical Manual of Mental Disorders, third edition* (**DSM**-III), which for the first time not only defined and described mental disorders but also included physical disorders and conditions and categorized the severity of the client's psychosocial stressors and his or her highest level of adaptive functioning during the past year. This major revision of the psychiatric diagnostic taxonomy was a major step in viewing the client holistically. The DSM-III was revised in 1987 and is known as the DSM-III-R. The latest revision of this taxonomy is the DSM-IV, which is currently in press. Since the health care delivery system remains organized around the medical model of disease and illness, the psychiatric nurse must be conversant with the terminology and diagnoses used by psychiatrists. The DSM-III-R and proposed DSM-IV classifications appear in Appendixes A and B.

In recent years, efforts have been made to develop a classification system of nursing diagnoses that reflects characteristic responses of persons to common health problems. One of the most recent systems, and perhaps the one most widely used, is that developed by the North American Nursing Diagnosis Association **(NANDA).** No one claims this system is complete, and work on its development continues. The 1992 NANDA-approved nursing diagnostic categories are found in Appendix B.

The client's response to the health problem is often referred to as the nursing diagnosis. However, to be most useful in providing direction for nursing care, a nursing diagnosis must be a statement that identifies the client's response along with a phrase indicating its probable etiology or antecedent factor. Some nursing authorities reject this format because of our limited knowledge about definitive etiologies, especially in regard to psychosocial responses. Although this argument has validity, a nursing diagnosis that states only the client's response is of limited use in planning care. For example, the nursing diagnosis of "altered family role" is much less useful than the nursing diagnosis of "altered family role, related to marriage of youngest child." The reader will note that this example connects the human response with its postulated etiology by the phrase "related to." This format implies a relationship between the two phenomena but does not rule out other factors, indirectly acknowledging the imprecise state of knowledge about human behavior.

Most clients have more than one nursing diagnosis. However, if numerous diagnoses are identified for the same client, the nurse should question whether a unifying theme has been missed. In other words, as the nurse gains knowledge and experience, she or he will learn that the various client responses are usually interrelated. The nurse will attempt to identify those that provide direction for planning nursing care but omit those that result in an unnecessarily repetitive plan of care.

Planning phase

The third phase of the nursing process, the **planning phase,** is developing a plan for nursing intervention. The plan for nursing intervention is derived from the nursing diagnoses and contains statements including the goal of the care *(objective),* how the objective will be achieved *(nursing interventions),* and the anticipated results *(outcome criteria).*

Once stated, objectives need to be prioritized as short-term or long-term goals. Criteria for prioritization include the urgency of the situation, the time required to achieve the objective, and the anticipated length of contact with the client. Unless objectives are realistically prioritized, both the nurse and the client risk being continuously frustrated by failing to achieve the desired outcomes of nursing care. This is currently the case in many psychiatric hospitals where clients are discharged to aftercare clinics as soon as their behavior has stabilized. As a result, the nurses in the hospital may have contact with the client for only a few weeks, since a different nursing staff is at the clinic. In these instances the hospital nursing staff should limit objectives to those that can be achieved in a short time.

To be effective, nursing interventions must be related to the objectives of the care. In addition, they must be realistic in light of the resources available.

Outcome criteria are statements phrased in behavioral terms that enable the nurse to assess whether the goal has been achieved. Unlike objectives, outcome criteria are always stated in terms of client behavior and are most useful when they specify the conditions under which they will occur, their frequency, and the time in which they are anticipated.

The plan for nursing intervention is highly individualized for each client. However, all plans for nursing intervention should reflect the principles of psychiatric nursing discussed earlier in this chapter. See Table 6-2 for an example of a plan for nursing intervention.

Implementation phase

The fourth phase of the nursing process is the implementation of the plan of care. In the **implementation phase** the nurse employs a variety of roles. These roles are discussed in detail in Chapter 8.

Evaluation phase

The final phase of the nursing process is the **evaluation phase.** The phases of the nursing process previously cited have been described as if they are discrete entities, and the phase of evaluation is frequently seen as the last step in this process. In reality, however, all phases of the nursing process may occur simultaneously, and some form of evaluation must occur continuously. Therefore, it is imperative that the nurse review the assessment of the client, the nursing diagnoses, and the plan for nursing intervention, as well as the outcome of the nursing intervention. The results of the nursing care should be evaluated against the outcome criteria the nurse established in the plan for care. As previously mentioned, outcome criteria need to be stated in behavioral terms and as specifically as possible.

Inherent in all aspects of evaluation is the necessity for the nurse to evaluate personal behavior and to determine the degree to which it does or does not facilitate achievement of the objectives of the plan for intervention. Evaluation also frequently serves the purpose of identifying aspects of care that are helpful to the client and therefore should be continued. See Table 6-3 for a summary outline of the nursing process as used in psychiatric nursing.

Table 6-2.   Example of a plan for nursing intervention

Nursing diagnosis

Self-esteem disturbance, related to developmental stressors of adolescence and increased familial responsibility

OBJECTIVE	NURSING INTERVENTIONS	OUTCOME CRITERIA
The client will exhibit a sense of worth	Praise accomplishments, no matter how small. When client verbally derogates self, disagree if appropriate without arguing.	Within 1 month client: Makes statements reflecting self-worth (e.g., "Yes, I did do that well.") Makes few or no self-derogating remarks Exhibits well-groomed personal appearance and appropriate dress

Table 6-3.   Nursing process

PHASE	PURPOSE	EXAMPLES OF NURSING INTERVENTIONS
Assessment	To collect data	Observe client's present behavior, using all appropriate senses. Read client's chart and relevant texts and journals. Interview client, family, and other staff.
	To validate data collected from observation	Make repeated observations; discuss perceptions with others.

Continued.

Table 6-3.   Nursing process—cont'd

PHASE	PURPOSE	EXAMPLES OF NURSING INTERVENTIONS
Assessment—cont'd	To validate data collected from observation—cont'd	Read relevant texts and journals to confirm observations.
	To analyze data	Sort and organize data according to themes.
Diagnostic	To establish a nursing diagnosis	Synthesize all available assessment data.
		State client response and probable etiology.
Planning	To plan for nursing intervention, using nursing diagnosis as a basis	Individualize a plan for intervention and identify nursing goal, nursing interventions, and outcome criteria.
		Use principles of psychiatric nursing:
		1. Nurse views client as a holistic being with many interrelated and interdependent needs.
		2. Nurse focuses on client's strengths and assets, not on weaknesses and liabilities.
		3. Nurse accepts client as a human being who has value and worth, exactly as he or she is.
		4. Nurse has potential for establishing a relationship with most, if not all, clients.
		5. Nurse explores client's behavior for need it is designed to meet or message it is communicating.
		6. Nurse views client's behavior nonjudgmentally while assisting client to learn more effective adaptations.
		7. Quality of interaction in which nurse engages with client is a major determinant of degree to which client will be able to alter behavior in direction of more satisfying, satisfactory interpersonal relationships.
Implementation	To implement plan for nursing intervention	Function in a variety of roles while using principles of psychiatric nursing.
Evaluation	To make planned, critical assessment of care	Review assessment data for accuracy and currency.
		Review nursing diagnoses for accuracy and currency.
	To revise or confirm plan of care	Review plan for nursing interaction.
		Compare client's response to intervention with outcome criteria.
	To make self-assessment	Evaluate own behavior.
		Revise or confirm plan for nursing intervention based on overall evaluation.

KEY POINTS

1. To be useful, the nurse's beliefs and feelings must be organized into a philosophy that provides direction for the development of principles of psychiatric nursing.

2. The belief that human beings are complex systems of interrelated parts, the whole of which is greater than the sum of its parts, combined with the nurse's feeling of being potentially helpful to the client, is the basis of the principle that the nurse views the client as a holistic being with many interrelated and interdependent needs.

3. The belief that each individual has strengths and a potential for growth, combined with the nurse's feeling of hope about the client's ability to grow, is the basis of the principle that the nurse focuses on the client's strengths and assets, not on weaknesses and liabilities.

4. The belief that each individual is unique and has inherent value, combined with the nurse's appreciation of the client's uniqueness and inherent value, is the basis of the principle that the nurse accepts the client as a unique human being who has value and worth exactly as he or she is.

5. The belief that all human beings are sufficiently similar that a foundation exists for understanding and communicating with one another, combined with the nurse's feeling of empathy with the client's feelings, is the basis of the principle that the nurse has the potential for establishing a relationship with most, if not all, clients.

6. The belief that all behavior is purposeful and designed to meet a need or to communicate a message, combined with the nurse's feeling of curiosity about the meaning of the client's behavior, is the basis of the principle that the nurse explores the client's behavior for the need it is designed to meet or the message it is communicating.

7. The belief that behavior is learned and is the best possible adaptation the individual is capable of making at the time, combined with the nurse's caring about the client, is the basis of the principle that the nurse views the client's behavior nonjudgmentally while assisting the client to learn more effective adaptations.

8. The belief that an individual learns behavioral adaptations in interaction with significant others, combined with the nurse's feeling of competency in her or his ability to interact therapeutically, is the basis of the principle that the quality of the nurse-client interaction is a major determinant of the degree to which the client will be able to alter behavioral adaptation.

9. The nursing process includes the phases of assessment, diagnosis, planning, implementation, and evaluation.

10. Throughout each phase of the nursing process, it is important for the nurse to validate findings with the client to ensure their relevancy.

11. Although psychiatric nursing is concerned primarily with the client's emotional, behavioral, and interpersonal responses, the client must be assessed comprehensively.

12. The client is the most important and significant source of information.

13. An effective interview obtains specific information; is guided by goals; requires the use of simple, concrete, and direct questions; and occurs during a specified time.

14. Ascertaining the client's perception of the problem and obtaining factual information about the client are major goals of the initial interview.

15. While observing the client, the nurse's goal is to determine the appropriateness and harmony of the client's appearance, behavior, and speech patterns with each other and with the situation.

16. To be useful in providing direction for nursing care, a nursing diagnosis must be a statement that identifies the client's response along with a phrase indicating its probable etiology or antecedent factor.

17. All plans for nursing intervention should reflect the principles of psychiatric nursing.

18. In implementing the plan of care, the nurse uses a variety of roles.

19. Evaluating the plan of care includes reviewing the assessment data, the nursing diagnoses, the plan for nursing intervention, and the results of the nursing intervention in light of the outcome criteria.

SUGGESTED SOURCES OF ADDITIONAL
INFORMATION

Aidroos N: Use and effectiveness of psychiatric nursing care plans, *J Adv Nurs* 16:177, 1991.

Barker P: The conceptual basis of mental health nursing, *Nurse Educ Today* 10:339, 1980.

Davis CM: What is empathy, and can empathy be taught? *Phys Ther* 70:32, November 1990.

Glasso D: Guidelines for developing multidisciplinary treatment plans, *Hosp Community Psychiatry* 38:394, April 1987.

Holden RJ: Empathy: the art of emotional knowing in holistic nursing care, *Holistic Nurs Pract* 5(1):70, 1990.

Kerr NJ: Ego competency: a framework for formulating the nursing care plan, *Perspect Psychiatr Care* 26(4):30, 1990.

Milne D: "The more things change the more they stay the same": factors affecting the implementation of the nursing process, *J Adv Nurs* 10:39, 1985.

Morrison EF: Nursing adaptation evaluation: a method for evaluating nursing care, *Perspect Psychiatr Care* 26(4):11, 1990.

Morrison P, Burnard P: Students' and trained nurses' perceptions of their own interpersonal skills: a report and comparison, *J Adv Nurs* 14:321, 1989.

Mulhearn S: The nursing process: improving psychiatric admission assessment? *J Adv Nurs* 14:808, 1989.

Olsen D: Empathy as an ethical and philosophical basis for nursing, *Adv Nurs Sci* 14(1):62, 1991.

Parsons PJ: Building better treatment plans, *J Psychosoc Nurs Ment Health Serv* 24:8, 1986.

Peplau H: *Interpersonal relations in nursing,* New York, 1952, GP Putnam's Sons.

Reed PG: Constructing a conceptual framework for psychosocial nursing, *J Psychosoc Nurs Ment Health Serv* 25:24, 1987.

Rolfe G: The assessment of therapeutic attitudes in the psychiatric setting, *J Adv Nurs* 15:564, 1990.

Savage P: Patient assessment in psychiatric nursing, *J Adv Nurs* 16:311, 1991.

Chapter 7

Effective Communication

LEARNING OBJECTIVES

After studying this chapter, the student will be able to:

* Define the communication process.

* Discuss the four modes of communication.

* Give examples of effective verbal and nonverbal communication.

* Identify special problems and their solutions in communicating with persons who have a mental illness.

KEY TERMS

Communication
Verbal communication
Nonverbal communication
Body language
Therapeutic listening
Rapport
Reassurance
Double-bind communication

Communication refers to the reciprocal exchange of information, ideas, beliefs, feelings, and attitudes between two persons or among a group of persons. As such, it is a dynamic process requiring continual adaptations by those involved. Communication is effective when it accurately and clearly conveys the intended messages.

The communication process is basic to all nursing practice and, when effective, greatly contributes to the development of all therapeutic relationships. Knowledge of and skill in effective communication are essential for the nurse who works with clients with a mental illness because the quality of the nurse's communication skills is influential in determining the effectiveness of other interventions. Most important, effective communication has been demonstrated to be a powerful intervention with those who have a mental illness.

HISTORICAL PERSPECTIVE

Communication is not unique to human beings. Other species of animals communicate with each other. Only humans, however, have the ability to engage in the complex interaction evidenced by the use of language. The ability to use language is seen by many as an essential characteristic of being human. Effective communication is a major means by which people express many of their needs and subsequently have them met, thereby experiencing satisfying, satisfactory relationships with others.

The needs of primitive human beings most certainly centered around issues of physical survival. Therefore, their ability to listen for and respond appropriately to sounds that warned of danger or ensured safety was essential. Effective communication was achieved when verbal and nonverbal forms of communication were accurately transmitted and interpreted. Feedback about the effectiveness of communication was likely to be immediate. During this period of human development, communication was limited to face-to-face interaction between individuals and among small groups.

Although the alphabet was developed around 2000 BC, major changes in the communication process did not occur until the invention of the printing press in the fifteenth century. This invention made possible the mass production of the written word and essentially changed the culture of communication from a speaking-listening orientation to a visual orientation.

This change in orientation coincided with and contributed to a change in the standard of living in which the peoples of the Western world could afford to be less concerned about survival issues and more concerned about higher-level needs related to interpersonal relationships. Paradoxically, as concern with these needs intensified, people increasingly depended on the written word, which by definition is devoid of human contact. Some authorities believe that this dependence on the written word and consequently on a visual orientation to communication has diminished the ability of many contemporary persons to engage in the effective verbal and nonverbal communication that characterizes satisfying interpersonal relationships. Whether this is the case or not, it is well documented that ineffective communication patterns are a predominant symptom of many forms of mental illness and that engaging in effective communication with clients can have therapeutic results.

Because of the complexity of the communication process and its important role in interpersonal relationships, effective and disturbed communication patterns have been the subject of much study by contemporary theorists. One of the best known, psychiatrist Jurgen Ruesch, has written that communication is therapeutic when it is helpful. The following discussion of communication is designed to provide the nurse with guidelines for the development of helpful and therefore therapeutic communication patterns.

MODES OF COMMUNICATION

Everyone is familiar with communication through the written word. When written material is read, the reciprocal aspects of communication are limited to the reader's ability to understand and react to the ideas and concepts that the author is attempting to convey. If the reader does not receive the intended message, effective communication has not been achieved.

Another mode of communication with which everyone is familiar is the spoken word, or **verbal communication.** If persons who are speaking together understand the same language, a major reciprocal element is present as they exchange, question, challenge, clarify, and enlarge on statements.

A mode of communication that people are not always aware of is **nonverbal communication,** which is closely related to verbal communication and is usually an integral part of it. Nonverbal communication refers to the messages sent and received through such means as facial expression, voice quality, physical posture, and gestures. Thus a person's behavior conveys much to the astute observer. Nonverbal communication is often referred to as **body language.** Because nonverbal communication, or body language, is always present when people interact, it has been said that a person cannot *not* communicate.

Inner feelings are expressed by the manner in which individuals conduct themselves in even such simple activities as walking, opening and closing doors, reclining in an easy chair, speaking to other people, and asking questions. The nonverbal aspects of communication sometimes convey general attitudes, feelings, and reactions more clearly and more accurately than do spoken words. An understanding of the implications of nonverbal communication is important for all nurses, especially those who work with persons who have a mental illness. Not only must nurses be aware of the client's nonverbal communica-

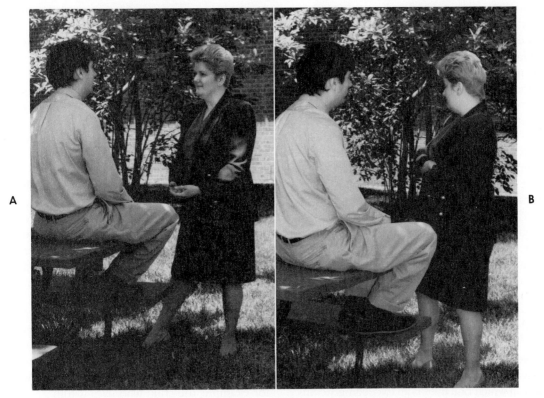

Figure 7-1

A, Nonverbal communication congruent with verbal communication. **B,** Nonverbal communication incongruent with verbal communication.

tion, but they must also be aware of their own nonverbal communication. Persons with a mental illness are more aware of nurses' nonverbal behavior than many nurses realize. Nurses who walk briskly, close doors emphatically, and answer questions sharply are likely to be seen as angry, unapproachable persons. Nurses who walk in an unhurried manner, smile, and speak in a warm, friendly manner convey an acceptance that may prompt clients to turn to them for help.

Another mode of communication, rarely recognized on a conscious level, is *metacommunication*. Metacommunication refers to the role expectation individuals have of each other in the context in which verbal and nonverbal communication occur. These role expectations strongly influence the nature of the verbal and nonverbal communication. For example, when a salesperson says to a customer, "May I help you?" both individuals understand that the salesperson is asking whether he or she can be of assistance in helping the customer to make a purchase. On the other hand, when the nurse in a treatment setting asks the same question of a client, both understand that the client is being asked if the nurse might do something, such as listening or helping the client with activities of daily living. Metacommunication and nonverbal communication are present in all situations when two or more persons are present, although verbal communication may be absent at times.

Communication is most effective when the three previously mentioned modes of communication—verbal, nonverbal, and metacommunication—are congruent. Imagine the reaction of the previously mentioned salesperson if the customer responded: "Yes, you can help me. My child is ill, and I am very worried about her." In this situation the customer's reply indicates a response only to the salesperson's verbal communication and ignores the metacommunication. Therefore the customer's reply illustrates incongruency between verbal communication and metacommunication, which is likely to result in an increase in the anxiety levels of both persons involved.

DEVELOPING EFFECTIVE MODES OF COMMUNICATION

Developing modes of communication that are effective within the family, the culture, and the society in which one lives is an exceedingly complex learning process that begins at birth and comprises a large part of subsequent developmental stages. Although some of this learning takes place in a formal way through such societal agencies as the school, the foundation of the communication process is laid within the family long before the child is ready to attend school. In this respect the family acts as the representative of the society at large.

Much teaching and learning about communication within the family structure are achieved indirectly. For example, the child learns certain words by hearing them used in the home and without anyone overtly teaching the child to associate the word with the object. This is illustrated by the 4-year-old child of two college professors who was asked by his nursery school teacher to identify pictures of objects. His classmates identified one as a "suitcase" or "bag," but he identified the same object as an "attaché case."

Furthermore, he was unable to identify the object called "apron" by the rest of his classmates. The strong academic influence and lack of domestic interest in this child's home were clearly demonstrated by the nature of his vocabulary.

In the same way the meaning of nonverbal communication is learned. In some cultures a loud tone of voice signifies anger. In other cultures the opposite is true; that is, silence signifies anger, whereas loud, animated talking is indicative of nothing more than enthusiasm. To survive, children must learn the meaning of both the verbal and the nonverbal communications of their family members, since they depend greatly on these persons for having their needs met. It is a comment on the great intellectual potential of human beings to note how quickly the child does learn the meaning of highly complex messages.

It is not sufficient, however, for the child merely to learn the meaning of the messages received. The child must also learn ways of responding that are acceptable within the family structure, and this is no simple task. Consider, for example, the child who lives within a family in which the verbal response to situations that are frustrating or anger producing is to swear. Not infrequently the first time the child responds to anger or frustration by repeating a swear word, the child is told by the adults that he is using a bad word that is forbidden and that if he continues to use it, he will be punished.

Despite the complexity of learning the communication process, most children are capable of doing so in a relatively short period and quickly become able to adapt that which they have learned in the home to the demands of a larger society. The previously mentioned 4-year-old child quickly learned what an apron was and how it was used and that an attaché case is only one type of bag. In some instances, however, effective adaptation is not possible or becomes possible only after experiencing much stress. The stress of adapting to the communication in a different culture can be observed when adults travel rapidly between countries by jet airplane. Many travel agencies give their customers brochures describing the customs and frequently used words of the countries to be visited to lessen the communication shock experienced by the traveler.

The preceding examples illustrate communication problems that are normal from the standpoint of mental health. At times, however, the learning of the communication process is accompanied by such a high level of stress that it produces a pattern of communication that is ineffective within either the family itself or society at large. *For our purposes, we can consider any communication to be ineffective if it does not accurately and clearly convey the message intended.* All persons occasionally experience ineffective communication. However, when this becomes a pattern (the rule rather than the exception), it frequently is a manifestation of mental illness and also a factor in perpetuating the illness.

USING EFFECTIVE COMMUNICATION IN THE CARE OF PERSONS WITH A MENTAL ILLNESS

Individuals with a mental illness need the opportunity to communicate with others who are sincerely interested in their problems and who care about them as people. It is important for nurses to learn to communicate in such a way that their conversations will become a part of the total therapeutic endeavor. The ability to communicate therapeutically with clients requires that the nurse have an attitude of acceptance and genuine interest in them.

A climate of mutual trust and respect must be developed before persons with a mental illness can feel safe enough to communicate with a nurse. This is not an easy climate to establish; it requires time, patience, knowledge, and skill. However, nurses are rewarded for their efforts by the knowledge that when a client is helped to converse effectively with a professional per-

son, an emotionally supportive experience often results.

Integral to establishing a climate of trust and respect is the skill of **therapeutic listening.** Listening therapeutically involves much more than merely hearing the client's words. It also involves focusing on the client to the exclusion of all other distractions, including the common tendency to think about one's next response.

Listening implies using silence at times, but it does not imply passivity. Listeners can and should be active, alert, and interested participants, even though they may make very few verbal contributions. The nurse gives evidence of interest by being genuinely interested in clients and what they are saying. This interest cannot be feigned. Evidence of genuine, sincere interest is shown by the expression on the listener's face, by the way the listener looks at the speaker, and by the verbal encouragement given to the speaker. Nodding the head to suggest that one understands or agrees is one way of giving encouragement. Comments such as, "That must

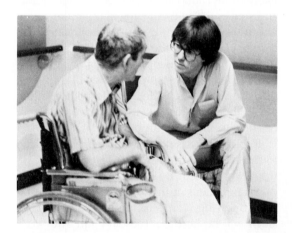

Figure 7-2

Effective communication requires the nurse to be an active listener.

From Burnside I: *Nursing and the aged,* ed 3, St Louis, 1988, Mosby–Year Book.

have been difficult for you" or "I see, go on," are encouraging when said at an appropriate time with a friendly, interested tone. If the listener cannot follow the logic of the client or the sequence of the related incidents, it is best to ask the client to review that part of the story again. The nurse might say, "Could you explain that last statement again for me? I do not believe I understood it clearly." Or the nurse might say, "I'm sorry, I didn't understand what you said a minute ago. Could you go over the last point again?" If the nurse fails to ask for clarification when it is needed, the client will soon discover that the nurse does not understand the conversation but is trying to act as if she or he does. The client may interpret this as a lack of interest. In contrast, when nurses ask for needed clarification, they convey a sincerity of interest that helps the client to develop trust in them.

Initiating a conversation

When the nurse meets the client, they are strangers. They must become acquainted before therapeutic communication can occur. Although some clients may be eager to talk, others are likely to be cautious in approaching the nurse, and some may be totally unwilling to engage in a conversation. In any event, it is not realistic for the nurse to expect the client, as with any other stranger, to be willing to share his or her most intimate feelings. Sensitive nurses will use some of the same skills in interacting with a client whom they have just met as they have used successfully to interact with other strangers.

If the nurse has not already been introduced to the client, she begins the conversation by introducing herself. It will be helpful if she explains her status at the same time. This can be done by saying, "I am Miss Jones, a student nurse, and I will be here on Tuesdays and Thursdays for the next 4 weeks." Or she might say, "I am Miss Smith, a graduate nurse, and I have come to work here." If the nurse does not know the name of the person to whom she has introduced herself, she might say, "Will you please help me

learn your name? I am sorry that I do not know it." With this invitation, most persons will introduce themselves. Having learned the client's name, the nurse uses it when speaking to the client. This simple but important technique helps to individualize the conversation and encourages the client to focus attention.

After the nurse and the client have been introduced, it is appropriate for the nurse to initiate a conversation. A conversation is one of the most common of the shared activities in which people engage. Just as one initiates the conversational topics with other strangers, the nurse may find it helpful with clients to introduce a neutral conversational topic appropriate for the time and place. Sports may be an appropriate topic. If the client seems interested in sports, the nurse may choose to initiate a conversation with a question about a recent game. For example, the nurse may begin by saying, "I did not have a chance to follow the game yesterday. What was the final score?" Other neutral topics that may be used include the headlines in the newspaper, the weather, or an approaching event. If a person is holding a newspaper, the nurse may begin a conversation by inquiring, "What interesting happenings are in the headlines today?"

Having introduced a topic, the sensitive nurse will wait for a response and will not feel compelled to avoid silences by immediately adding comments or opinions. After ample opportunity has been given for a response, the nurse should introduce a second conversational idea that logically follows the first.

Certainly the nurse should avoid approaching anyone with a barrage of words. In their desire to communicate effectively, nurses sometimes resort to asking a series of questions. Unfortunately, this is too often the type of conversation that is reported when nurses are asked to tell about a recent conversation with a client. "How are you today?" is one of the usual questions with which many nurses begin a conversation. Such an opening sentence usually does little to develop a conversation.

Developing effective verbal communication

To be effective, the nurse's verbal communication must be guided by goals. The nurse's therapeutic potential is greatly increased if a conscious effort is made to establish a goal for each conversation. The identified purpose for the conversation provides a guide to the appropriate approach used, the approximate duration of the conversation, and how it is terminated.

Obtaining specific information

Frequently the nurse talks with the client to obtain specific information. When initiating this type of conversation, the nurse should explain its purpose and that questions will be asked. Although in this instance it is appropriate that direct questions be asked, the nurse needs to understand that many persons with a mental illness may feel threatened by direct questions. Therefore the nurse should begin with questions designed to elicit answers that are factual and therefore likely to be seen as neutral, rather than questions that require responses that reveal feelings or opinions. Some examples are "What is your name?" and "Tell me your address." As a result of the exchange of factual information, the client may relax sufficiently to be able to provide more sensitive information, such as a response to the question, "What events brought you to the hospital?" Questions beginning with the word "why" usually are ineffective in soliciting an informative response.

A conversation with the goal of obtaining specific information is usually brief and is terminated with an expression of thanks for the client's cooperation.

Establishing rapport with the client

The nurse often approaches the client with the goal of establishing a beginning **rapport** that can serve as a basis for developing a meaningful future relationship. With such a goal, attention is focused on the client in a manner that conveys sincere interest and a willingness to listen. The focus of the conversation is on becoming acquainted and establishing a feeling of mutual trust. In such a situation, direct questions are rarely necessary or useful. Rather, statements that reflect observations are most productive. The comment, "The blue dress you are wearing looks nice with your blue eyes," is an example of such an observation, assuming this is the case.

The duration of a conversation with the goal of establishing rapport with the client is likely to be determined by its context. Thus, it may be a brief exchange when passing each other in the hall, or it may be quite long if, for example, the nurse and client are on a shopping trip. A conversation with this goal is most usefully terminated with a statement about when the interaction will resume. For example, the nurse might say, "I will be able to spend more time with you tomorrow at 10 AM and will meet you here. Is that time and place all right with you?" It is imperative that nurses make only those promises they are reasonably certain they can keep if the ultimate goal of establishing a feeling of mutual trust is to be achieved.

Encouraging expression of thoughts and feelings

If the conversation's purpose is to encourage the client to express thoughts and feelings, a nondirective approach would undoubtedly achieve the most positive results. In such a situation the client would be encouraged to initiate the conversation. Responding to the client's comments by reflecting thoughts and feelings back to the client might be helpful in encouraging him or her to continue expressing feelings without introducing new or unrelated ideas. For example, if the client speaks of an unhappy home life, the nurse might respond by saying, "It sounds to me as if you are saying that your home life is unhappy." This type of response conveys to the client that the nurse is listening and gives the client an opportunity to either accept or reject the nurse's impression of the communication.

Once having encouraged the client to express thoughts and feelings, the nurse may not be prepared to hear what the client has to say and may respond judgmentally. Such an attitude is reflected in statements such as, "Don't be silly!" or "How could you possibly think that?" Responses such as these discourage the client from further divulging thoughts and feelings. To be helpful, the nurse must withhold personal opinions about what the client is saying and avoid the use of words that convey a judgment.

The duration of conversations with the goal of encouraging the client to express thoughts and feelings should be determined by the client's response. In other words, the conversation should be continued for as long as it remains productive; it should be terminated if the client becomes unduly anxious or is unable to continue. The nurse should summarize the content of the discussion as a means of ending the conversation.

Arriving at a decision

When the client is in a situation that requires arriving at a decision, the nurse can be effective by helping the client explore possible alternatives and their consequences. This often involves assisting the client to gather additional information or to validate available information. However, this process is not the same as giving advice. Even though the nurse may have strong feelings about what would be the best decision, sharing these feelings should be avoided. The nurse is not the client and cannot know the choices that are best for the client in most situations. The nurse does not know all the past experiences that influence the client's present thinking and feeling and therefore is not qualified to give advice about what the client should do. Giving advice suggests that the client is not capable of making choices among the available alternatives. Furthermore, although giving advice may result in a temporary positive response because it relieves the client of the responsibility for making

a decision, in the long term it is likely to encourage the client to remain dependent on some other person to make future decisions. Instead of offering advice, it is more helpful for the nurse and client together to explore the positive and negative aspects of the possible decisions.

Most decisions have a time frame within which an action must be taken. The nurse can be helpful by assisting the client in determining that time frame and helping him or her to become aware that not making a decision within the necessary time frame is, in effect, making a decision.

The duration of conversations with the goal of arriving at a decision is determined by when the decision needs to be made and by the client's response to the problem-solving activity. Therefore, only one brief conversation may be required, or several conversations about the same subject may be held over time. This type of conversation is most effectively terminated by the nurse's encouraging the client to summarize the advantages and disadvantages of each identified alternative and the rationale for the choice made.

Providing reassurance

Almost all persons with a mental illness have low self-esteem and have had many negative experiences. Consequently, they are likely to need **reassurance** about their value and worth as human beings as well as about the outcome of stressful events. Nurses make many comments that they hope will provide reassurance but that actually fall short of this goal. Even though the nurse intends to be helpful, it is rarely helpful to make comments such as, "Don't worry," "Your doctor says this medicine will help you," "There are many people worse off than you are," and "Don't cry; you don't want people to see you crying." Such comments are unhelpful and are likely to convince clients that the nurse is not able to understand their problems. Reassurance is never achieved by use of meaningless clichés. Instead, it is reassuring to the client if the nurse considers the problem thoughtfully and asks intelligent, reality-oriented questions about the situation. It is reassuring to the client when the nurse accepts tears without comment or assures the client that crying is a reasonable reaction under the circumstances, provided the circumstances warrant such expression. It is reassuring to the client when the nurse listens to personal problems without showing surprise or disapproval when the client talks about past social behavior that is unusual or unacceptable to the nurse. It is reassuring when the nurse agrees that the client has a problem and works in trying to problem solve. It is reassuring to the client if the nurse sits with him or her even when the client does not feel like talking, thereby conveying a genuine interest in the problem and acceptance of the client. Finally, it is reassuring to the client when the nurse reflects back the tone of the feeling the client is expressing. For the nurse to say, "It sounds to me as if you are really upset," conveys that the feelings and the content of what the client is saying are being understood. Once again, the nurse is not imposing a feeling on the client by such a statement but rather is expressing a response.

The duration of conversations with the goal of providing reassurance tends to be longer than many other types of conversations. If the topic or the client's emotional state warrants reassurance, a brief conversation probably will not be effective. When approached by a distraught client, nurses often employ meaningless clichés, as just discussed, because they sense the conversation will be long and they believe they do not have the time to spend. If the nurse truly does not have sufficient time to spend with the client, the nurse should say so and then arrange for another time to talk.

A conversation with the goal of providing reassurance is terminated by the client indicating that he or she has exhausted the topic, at least for the moment. At this point, the nurse is often tempted to ask, "Do you feel better?" This question is rarely appropriate because it is designed to elicit an affirmative answer to reassure the nurse, not the client. Furthermore, if clients do feel better, they often will say so spontaneously; if they do not feel reassured, the nurse's question may lead them to believe they should and therefore add to their concern.

Stimulating client interest

Many persons with a mental illness avoid activities that involve other people as a means of protecting themselves from interpersonal interactions with which they believe they cannot cope. Others have so little energy and/or such low self-esteem that they do not attend to even the basic activities of daily living, such as bathing and grooming themselves. Much can be done to stimulate interest in activities and to help individuals alter social attitudes by using skillfully phrased suggestions. For instance, encouraging a client to participate in the activities offered by the occupational therapist may be accomplished by telling the client about the activities available and by using suggestions such as, "You might enjoy the finger-painting class." At another time a second comment about this activity might be, "Many clients seem to have an interesting time when they go to occupational therapy; I think you might, too." A male client who refused to wash his hair for several weeks may do so if several people with whom he is acquainted comment about his attractive appearance when his hair was clean a few weeks before. One suggestion is usually not sufficient to alter an attitude or help a person accept a new idea. Suggestion must be used frequently and skillfully by persons whose opinion the client respects.

The duration of conversations with the goal of stimulating client interest is almost always brief, although such conversations may occur frequently. If the goal is to be achieved, however, the nurse needs to resist the temptation to pressure the client, as would be the case if the nurse approached the client frequently to talk of nothing other than the desired activity. This type of conversation is terminated when the client indicates an interest in the desired activity.

Table 7-1 summarizes the goal, nurse's approach, usual duration, and termination of common conversations with clients.

Developing effective nonverbal communication

One of the first steps the nurse can take in developing effective nonverbal communication is to examine feelings toward clients and, if possible, to focus efforts on those for whom the nurse feels genuine interest and acceptance. If the nurse attempts to work closely with clients about whom she or he has many negative feelings, the nurse will surely communicate these feelings nonverbally. The nurse needs to recognize the importance of personal feelings in developing positive interactions with clients. It is also essential to recognize the role of nonverbal communication and to understand that it is impossible for every nurse to develop a meaningful and helpful relationship with every client. Equipped with this knowledge and understanding, the nurse can feel comfortable in admitting that she or he is not the appropriate person to provide care to a specific individual about whom the nurse has negative feelings.

After examining personal feelings toward clients, the nurse can take several specific steps to engage in effective nonverbal communication. One of the most important steps is to sit near a client when talking. Some nurses hesitate to sit beside clients even when they are trying to converse with them. This hesitancy probably comes from experience in previous nursing situations in which sitting was viewed as resting rather than working.

When nurses stand during a conversation, they convey that they are in a hurry, expect the conversation to be short, and are prepared to remain for only a few minutes. In such a hurried atmosphere, no one can expect clients to feel that sufficient interest or time exists for them to talk about anything important. Conversely, when sitting with a person who has a mental illness, it is important not to sit in such a way that the person feels trapped or in danger of attack. Astute observation of the client's nonverbal behavior quickly reveals if the nurse is sitting in a position that produces the best climate for conversation. Examples of behaviors likely to indicate that the client feels uncomfortable are the movement of the body or chair away from the nurse, focusing the eyes elsewhere, and physical signs of anxiety such as restlessness and agitation. The nurse should not hesitate to alter position if this seems appropriate from observations of the client's behavior. When the nurse conveys sincere interest in the client through position and through the warmth of the nurse's voice and facial expression, the first step has been taken toward the establishment of a helpful interaction.

Concluding a conversation

The conclusion of a conversation is as important as is its initiation. The conclusion often sets the tone for subsequent conversations between the nurse and the client. When needing to leave, the nurse should break off the conversation so that it can be resumed at another time. Thus the nurse might say, "I have been interested in what you have been telling me, and I hope we can continue this discussion later on." Of course, such a statement must be true. If the nurse has promised to talk with the client at another time, the nurse must find time for resuming the conversation. The nurse might begin by saying, "I have been thinking about our conversation of yesterday, and I am wondering if we could talk some more about the last point that you were making." The nurse would use this statement only if it were true. If such a statement were not true, the nurse would choose another that would be appropriate for the conversation.

CHALLENGES TO EFFECTIVE COMMUNICATION WITH PERSONS WHO HAVE A MENTAL ILLNESS

Although establishing and maintaining effective communication are integral to the effective

Table 7-1. Goal, nurse's approach, usual duration, and termination of common conversations with clients

GOAL	NURSE'S APPROACH	USUAL DURATION	TERMINATED BY
Obtaining specific information	Explain purposes. Begin with questions designed to elicit factual responses.	Brief	Thanking client for co-operation
Establishing rapport	Focus on client. Convey interest and willingness to listen.	Variable, depending on context	Planning for next conversation
Encouraging expression of thoughts and feelings	Be nondirective. Reflect back client's thoughts and feelings.	Determined by client's response	Nurse summarizing content discussed
Arriving at a decision	Assist client to explore possible alternatives and their consequences. Assist client to gather additional information or to validate available information. Assist client to determine time frame within which a decision must be made.	Determined by time frame of decision and client's response to problem solving	Client summarizing advantages and disadvantages of each alternative and rationale for choice
Providing reassurance	Ask intelligent, reality-oriented questions. Listen nonjudgmentally. Convey interest and acceptance.	Lengthy	Client indicating he or she has exhausted topic for now
Stimulating interest	Use skillfully phrased suggestions.	Brief but frequent	Client indicating interest in desired activity

care of persons with a mental illness, such communication is not always easy to achieve because dysfunctional communication is frequently a symptom of the illness itself. Therefore, some characteristic challenges exist when attempting to communicate effectively with persons who have a mental illness.

The first challenge is to communicate in a *congruent* manner. Although this is important when communicating with any person, it is essential when communicating with a person who has a mental illness. Individuals with a mental illness, particularly one of the schizophrenias, are very sensitive to communication in which the nonverbal message contradicts the verbal message. The consequence of this communication is that the receiver must decide to which message he or she will respond, being aware that either choice is incorrect. When this type of communication is routine rather than the exception, it may result in the receiver becoming unable to respond at all because of being immobilized by anxiety. The technical term for this type of disturbed interaction is **double-bind communication.** Some theorists believe that this pattern of communication is characteristic of dysfunctional families.

As the professional person spending the most time with the client in the treatment setting, the nurse has the greatest opportunity to create an environment in which the client can experience congruent communication.

To express congruent messages, nurses must be aware of themselves and personal feelings, a concept discussed in Chapter 5. A helpful suggestion is for nurses to make clear to the client what they are feeling, that is, to bring into verbal communication their nonverbal messages rather than letting the client guess the meaning. An example might be the nurse who says, after being purposely tripped, "Your behavior irritates me." It is important to note that this statement conveys a very different message than if the nurse were to say, "You irritate me." In the former statement the nurse is expressing and owning personal

feelings and not rejecting the client, whereas in the latter statement the nurse is blaming and rejecting the client, which is likely to end the possibility of any further communication.

Since nonverbal aspects of communication usually convey the intended message most clearly, persons with a mental illness, as with all others, usually accurately sense the staff's sincerity and kindness. Thus, it has been observed that a staff member who is gruff and outspoken with clients may be respected and loved by them because this person nonverbally communicates a basic attitude of kindness and a sincere interest in their welfare. A nurse who has adopted an unusually saccharine approach may be deeply resented by clients because this nurse nonverbally conveys a feeling of rejection.

Another challenge to effective communication with persons who have a mental illness is to avoid the use of cultural and professional jargon. Although the use of such jargon is not desired in any interaction with people from a different culture or those not in the same profession, people who are mentally healthy are often able to ask for clarification if they do not understand the meaning of what is said. In contrast, people who have a mental illness, particularly those who have thought disorders, may concretize, personalize, distort, or otherwise misinterpret the meaning if the nurse uses jargon unfamiliar to them. Therefore the nurse's verbal communication should be as free from jargon as possible. In addition, the nurse must be vigilant in validating the meaning of the client's words, especially if the client has a different cultural background. This is a particular problem in large urban areas, where nurses and clients are often from different ethnic and cultural backgrounds. A classic example of misinterpretation caused by cultural differences occurred when the nurse wrote on the client's chart that he was delusional because he believed he was a tree. The nurse received this impression because the client responded to her question about his sleeping habits by saying he "slept like a log."

Clients often ask nurses personal questions such as, "Are you married?" "What nursing school are you from?" or "Where do you live?" The natural curiosity of clients about the personal life of the professional staff is understandable. However, if the conversation is allowed to be focused on the nurse's personal life, it quickly loses its original goal: to achieve communication that is therapeutic for the client. If the nurse wants to do so, it is appropriate to respond to factual questions such as, "Are you married?" with a simple "Yes" or "No." If the client continues to ask personal questions, the nurse might state, "It seems you are very interested in me," or ask, "I wonder if we could find a topic other than my personal life to discuss?" Frequent personal questions directed to nurses should alert them to the need for focusing future conversation more carefully. It may suggest that clients hope to direct attention away from themselves.

Many persons with a mental illness struggle with the problem of not being able to trust other people. One way nurses can help such a person is to demonstrate that they can be trusted. If a client can begin to trust one person, trust may eventually be extended to other people. When attempting to help a client learn to trust them, nurses sometimes find themselves in a dilemma. A client with whom the nurse is interacting may confide information that puts the nurse in an untenable position. On the one hand, the nurse wants to respect the client's confidences, while at the same time the nurse hopes to carry out her responsibilities as a member of the professional staff. The following situation precipitated such a dilemma.

A client confided he was planning to leave the city during the next weekend, ostensibly to visit his family. He told the nurse he had stolen enough money to purchase a train ticket to a distant city where he was unknown and where he hoped to make a fresh start. The client cautioned the nurse not to tell anyone about these plans until after he was gone. The nurse had reason to be concerned about the client's safety and now was in conflict about keeping the confidence while still fulfilling her role as a member of the professional staff. She was understandably distressed about the situation.

It is important for the nurse to inform the client at the beginning of their interaction that the nurse will share information essential to the client's treatment or safety with other members of the treatment team. When the client begins to confide information to the nurse that should be shared with other members of the professional staff, the nurse has a responsibility to remind the client that the conversation must be reported to the appropriate people. The nurse might say to the client, "You know it will be necessary for me to share what you are telling me with the treatment team." Given this reminder, the client must then decide whether to continue the discussion. A reasonable guide to follow is that the nurse has a responsibility to tell the client's therapist and the nurse in charge if the client tells of plans that are dangerous to self or others or that interfere with the treatment plan.

OF SPECIAL INTEREST

Incongruency among the verbal, nonverbal, and metacommunication modes of communication is not the only source of ineffective, nontherapeutic communication. Within the mode of verbal communication alone, confusion can reign when speakers do not say what they mean or mean what they say. Knowledge of this communication problem is not limited to health care professionals, as illustrated in the following excerpt from Lewis Carroll's *Alice's Adventures in Wonderland.*

"Then you should say what you mean," the March Hare went on.

"I do," Alice hastily replied; "at least—at least I mean what I say—that's the same thing, you know."

"Not the same thing a bit!" said the Hatter. "Why, you might just as well say that 'I see what I eat' is the same thing as 'I eat what I see'!"

When the nurse has established a relationship with the client that allows the client to express thoughts and feelings freely, the nurse has a responsibility to listen with acceptance and understanding. The client confiding in the nurse indicates that an atmosphere of trust has been established. However, at times a client confides feelings and thoughts to the nurse that may be more appropriately discussed with another member of the treatment team. In this instance the nurse can suggest that this information be shared with the other team member and that the nurse could assist the client in doing so, if he or she desires.

Efforts to develop effective communication with persons with a mental illness require perseverance and a willingness to engage in a continuous examination of one's own communication. However, if the nurse truly appreciates the significance of effective communication as both a therapeutic intervention and a means to enhance other therapeutic interventions with persons who have a mental illness, the nurse should be as willing to work on developing this skill as on developing skills necessary for physical interventions (see the box below).

THERAPEUTIC COMMUNICATION TECHNIQUES

Technique: **Listening**
Definition: Active process of receiving information and examining one's reaction to messages received
Example: Maintaining eye contact and receptive nonverbal communication
Therapeutic value: Nonverbally communicates nurse's interest and acceptance to client
Nontherapeutic threat: Failure to listen

Technique: **Broad openings**
Definition: Encouraging client to select topics for discussion
Example: "What are you thinking about?"
Therapeutic value: Indicates acceptance by nurse and value of client's initiative
Nontherapeutic threat: Domination of interaction by nurse; rejecting responses

Technique: **Restating**
Definition: Repeating main thought client has expressed
Example: "You say that your mother left you when you were 5 years old."
Therapeutic value: Indicates nurse is listening and validates, reinforces, or calls attention to something important that has been said
Nontherapeutic threat: Lack of validation of nurse's interpretation of message; being judgmental; defending

Technique: **Clarification**
Definition: Attempting to put into words vague ideas or unclear thoughts of client to enhance nurse's understanding or asking client to explain what he or she means
Example: "I'm not sure what you mean. Could you tell me about that again?"
Therapeutic value: Helps to clarify client's feelings, ideas, and perceptions and to provide an explicit correlation between them and client's actions
Nontherapeutic threat: Failure to probe; assumed understanding

Technique: **Reflection**
Definition: Directing back to client his or her ideas, feelings, questions, and content
Example: "You're feeling tense and anxious, and it's related to a conversation you had with your husband last night?"
Therapeutic value: Validates nurse's understanding of what client is saying and signifies empathy, interest, and respect for client
Nontherapeutic threat: Stereotyping client's responses; inappropriate timing of reflections; inappropriate depth of feeling of reflections; inappropriate to client's cultural experience and educational level

Technique: **Focusing**
Definition: Questions or statements that help client expand on a topic of importance
Example: "I think that we should talk more about your relationship with your father."
Therapeutic value: Allows client to discuss central issues related to problem and keeps communication process goal directed
Nontherapeutic threat: Allowing abstractions and generalizations; changing topics

Technique: **Sharing perceptions**
Definition: Asking client to verify nurse's understanding of what client is thinking or feeling
Example: "You're smiling, but I sense that you are really very angry with me."

THERAPEUTIC COMMUNICATION TECHNIQUES—cont'd

Therapeutic value: Conveys nurse's understanding to client and has potential for clarifying confusing communication

Nontherapeutic threat: Challenging client; accepting literal responses; reassuring; testing; defending

Technique: **Theme identification**

Definition: Underlying issues or problems experienced by client that emerge repeatedly during nurse-client relationship

Example: "I've noticed that in all the relationships that you have described, you've been hurt or rejected by the man. Do you think this is an underlying issue?"

Therapeutic value: Allows nurse to best promote client's exploration and understanding of important problems

Nontherapeutic threat: Giving advice; reassuring; disapproving

Technique: **Silence**

Definition: Lack of verbal communication for a therapeutic reason

Example: Sitting with client and nonverbally communicating interest and involvement

Therapeutic value: Allows client time to think and gain insights, slows the pace of the interaction, and encourages client to initiate conversation, while conveying nurse's support, understanding, and acceptance

Nontherapeutic threat: Questioning client; asking for "why" responses; failure to break a nontherapeutic silence

Technique: **Humor**

Definition: Discharge of energy through comic enjoyment of the imperfect

Example: "That gives a whole new meaning to the word 'nervous,'" said with shared kidding between nurse and client

Therapeutic value: Can promote insight by making repressed material conscious, resolve paradoxes, temper aggression, reveal new options, and is socially acceptable form of sublimation

Nontherapeutic threat: Indiscriminate use; belittling client; screen to avoid therapeutic intimacy

Technique: **Informing**

Definition: Skill of information giving

Example: "I think you need to know more about how your medication works."

Therapeutic value: Helpful in health teaching or client education about relevant aspects of client's well-being and self-care

Nontherapeutic threat: Giving advice

Technique: **Suggesting**

Definition: Presentation of alternative ideas for client's consideration relative to problem solving

Example: "Have you thought about responding to your boss in a different way when he raises that issue with you? For example, you could ask him if a specific problem has occurred."

Therapeutic value: Increases client's perceived options or choices

Nontherapeutic threat: Giving advice; inappropriate timing; being judgmental

Modified from Stuart GW, Sundeen SJ: *Principles and practice of psychiatric nursing,* ed 4, St Louis, 1991, Mosby–Year Book.

KEY POINTS

1. Communication refers to the reciprocal exchange of information, ideas, beliefs, feelings, and attitudes between two persons or among a group of persons. Communication is effective when it accurately and clearly conveys the intended messages.

2. Written communication limits the reciprocal aspects of communication to the reader's ability to understand and react to what the author has written. Verbal communication is an exchange of words. Nonverbal communication refers to the messages sent and received through such means as facial expression, voice quality, physical posture, and gestures. It is always present when people interact and has led to the saying that one cannot *not* communicate. Metacommunication refers to the context within which verbal and nonverbal communication takes place.

3. Communication is most effective when the verbal, nonverbal, and metacommunication modes are congruent.

4. Communication is ineffective when it does not accurately and clearly convey the message intended.

5. Therapeutic listening is integral to establishing a climate of trust and respect with persons who have a mental illness. This climate is foundational to effective communication.

6. When the goal of the conversation is to obtain specific information, the nurse may appropriately ask questions that are more direct than those usually employed.

7. When the goal of the interaction is to establish a beginning rapport with the client, attention should be focused on the client in an attempt to convey a willingness to listen.

8. When the goal of the interaction is to encourage the client to express thoughts and feelings, a nondirective approach is most appropriate.

9. When the goal of the interaction is to arrive at a decision, the nurse can be effective by helping the client to explore possible alternatives and their consequences.

10. When the goal of the interaction is to provide reassurance, the nurse should listen in an accepting manner. Statements that represent meaningless clichés are never helpful.

11. When the goal of the interaction is to stimulate client interest, skillfully phrased suggestions are useful.

12. Sitting with clients is a nonverbal behavior indicative of acceptance.

13. Challenges characteristic to effective communication with persons who have a mental illness include communicating congruently, avoiding the use of cultural and professional jargon, focusing conversation on the client's needs, and knowing when to share communications with other members of the treatment team.

SUGGESTED SOURCES OF ADDITIONAL INFORMATION

Cochrane DA and others: Do they really understand us? *Am J Nurs* 92:19, July 1992.

Dunn B: Communication interaction skills, *Senior Nurse* 11:4, July/August 1991.

Gluck M: Learning a therapeutic verbal response to anger, *J Psychosoc Nurs Ment Health Serv* 19:9, March 1981.

Harden S, Halaris A: Nonverbal communication of patients and high and low empathy nurses, *J Psychosoc Nurs Ment Health Serv* 21:14, January 1983.

Impey L: Art media: a means to therapeutic communication with families, *Perspect Psychiatr Care* 19:70, March/April 1981.

Kasch C: Interpersonal competence and communication in the delivery of nursing care, *Adv Nurs Sci* 6(2):71, 1984.

Kemper BJ: Therapeutic listening: developing the concept, *J Psychosoc Nurs Ment Health Serv* 30(7):21, 1992.

Knowles RD: Building rapport through neurolinguistic programming, *Am J Nurs* 83:1010, July 1983.

Koshy KT: I only have ears for you, *Nurs Times* 85:26, July 1989.

Miller LE: Modeling awareness of feelings: a needed tool in the therapeutic communication workbox, *Perspect Psychiatr Care* 25(2):27, 1989.

Reusch J: *Disturbed communication,* New York, 1957, WW Norton.

Reusch J: *Therapeutic communication,* New York, 1961, WW Norton.

Stewart CJ, Cash WB: *Interviewing principles and practices,* ed 4, New York, 1985, William C Brown.

Tobiason SJB: Touching is for everyone, *Am J Nurs* 81:728, April 1981.

Watzlawick P, Beavin J, Jackson D: *The pragmatics of human communication,* New York, 1967, WW Norton.

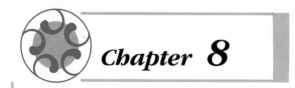

Chapter 8

Nurse-Client Interactions

LEARNING OBJECTIVES
After studying this chapter, the student will be able to:
- Discuss the concepts of acceptance and consistency as they relate to all nurse-client interactions.
- Discuss three types of nurse-client interactions in terms of their goals and degree of nurse-client involvement.
- Discuss the developmental phases of the nurse-client relationship.
- Describe the roles and functions the nurse may fulfill while engaging in nurse-client interactions.

KEY TERMS
Acceptance
Nonjudgmental
Consistent
Orientation or becoming acquainted phase
Working phase (maintenance)
Limit setting
Concluding phase (termination)
Target symptoms

Although therapeutic nurse-client interactions possess common elements, they are established and maintained differently based on the unique combination of characteristics of the individuals involved. If an interaction is to become therapeutic, the nurse must recognize the client as an important human being who experiences hopes, fears, joys, and sorrows as do all other people. The nurse also must recognize that the client's constellation of problems and reactions to life is unique. At the same time, the nurse must recognize that self-awareness is fundamental to the development of therapeutic nurse-client interactions. These recognitions can result in nurse-client interactions that are different from interactions with which the client is accustomed. Many persons with a mental illness have a long history of having failed at establishing and maintaining satisfying interpersonal relationships. To the degree that the nurse's interactions with the client focus on the client and reflect acceptance and consistency, they are likely to be therapeutic and may provide experiences that correct earlier, less helpful interpersonal experiences.

HISTORICAL PERSPECTIVE

In 1947 McGraw-Hill Book Company published *Nurse Patient Relationships in Psychiatry* by Helena Willis Render. She was the first author to introduce the idea that the relationship the nurse establishes with the client has a significant therapeutic potential. This book stimulated much attention from nurses concerning the potential therapeutic possibilities inherent in their interactions with persons who have a mental illness. In 1952 G.P. Putnam's Sons published the book *Interpersonal Relations in Nursing* by Dr. Hildegard E. Peplau, an active nurse clinician and educator. In many ways this book revolutionized the teaching and practice of psychiatric nursing in the United States. Peplau's text focused on the therapeutic potential of the one-to-one relationship. Not until the widespread use of the psy-chotropic drugs rendered clients amenable to interpersonally based treatment modalities, however, did psychiatric nursing begin to take its present form, making use of the concepts originally proposed by Render and Peplau.

Currently, it is acknowledged that how nurses use their personalities can be a great therapeutic influence in the experience of clients. The nurse's personality is the only tool that is unique and that the nurse alone directs. Although nurses may give dozens of daily medications and may assist with other somatic therapies, the major way in which they directly influence the care of clients is through the use they make of their personalities as they interact with clients.

DEVELOPING THERAPEUTIC NURSE-CLIENT INTERACTIONS

The foundation of all therapeutic interactions is **acceptance.** This is a frequently used word among nurses, although it is not universally understood or operationalized by them. Other equally important behaviors are expressed by the adjectives **nonjudgmental** and **consistent.** All these concepts are basic in developing therapeutic interactions with any client. They are discussed here in the hope of helping nurses to make effective use of them in caring for persons with a mental illness.

Acceptance of the client is demonstrated by using the client's name and by acting in a manner that reflects the nurse's belief that the client has the same basic personal rights as the nurse. Acceptance implies that the nurse tries to understand the meaning of the client's behavior. An accepting nurse recognizes that the client's behavior represents the best the client is capable of at a given time. The accepting nurse listens to the client's feelings, realizing that their expression is often a means of relieving tension. The nurse does not censor the client for statements and feelings that may not be conventionally acceptable but realizes that the client's comments may be a symptom of the illness.

The word *nonjudgmental* is usually used in conjunction with the word *attitude* and is closely related to the concept of acceptance. One cannot be achieved without the other. A nonjudgmental attitude is neither condemning nor approving. Through tone of voice and manner, the nurse conveys to clients a helpful attitude without morally judging their behavior. A nonjudgmental attitude toward the behavior of a person with a mental illness implies that the nurse recognizes that behavior, as with physical symptoms, is neither good nor bad or right nor wrong but rather a learned adaptation to stress. As such, the nurse also realizes that the client has the potential to change the behavior by learning new adaptations to stress.

Acceptance of persons with a mental illness and their behavior is often difficult to achieve, and almost everyone occasionally falls short of the ideal. Some clients' behavior is offensive at times. This is true, for example, of the behavior of clients who are so confused that they soil themselves. It may be impossible for the nurse to avoid feeling repelled by the sight of a person grossly soiled, but the nurse can avoid making that person feel offensive. Joking in front of clients about their behavior or describing their shortcomings to others within clients' hearing is neither respecting nor accepting them.

Consistency is another important characteristic of therapeutic interactions. The consistent nurse maintains the same basic attitude toward clients so that they derive security from being able to predict the nurse's behavior. Not only should the client be able to expect the same positive attitudes and approaches from an individual nurse, but also the entire nursing staff should interact with consistency regarding basic attitudes and overall policies. Consistency helps lessen the client's anxiety by simplifying decision making and by avoiding uncertainties.

All persons with a mental illness have some loss of self-esteem and self-confidence. If an interaction is to be helpful to clients, it must assist them in reestablishing self-confidence and restoring self-esteem. This is a slow process that requires consistent work over time. Recognizing clients as important human beings, expressing genuine interest in them, spending time with them, conversing with them, and listening with understanding to their expressions of feeling are all ways of helping clients feel worthwhile, important, and wanted. On the other hand, indifference, insincerity, and an impersonal attitude toward clients reinforce their sense of unimportance and further convince clients of what they may already believe, that they are lacking in value as persons.

A nurse cannot interact in a way that has the same therapeutic potential and the same meaning for each client. However, the nurse can learn to know the names and something of the needs of all clients with whom the nurse comes in close contact. The nurse can expect to develop a positive relationship with many of these persons. With a few clients, the nurse will be able to interact in a way that will lay the foundation for the development of a therapeutic relationship. With these individuals, the nurse will be able to carry on discussions that have therapeutic potential because she or he will know the clients well and will have developed a genuine interest in them as people.

TYPES AND CHARACTERISTICS OF THERAPEUTIC INTERACTIONS

The nurse is often involved in at least three types of one-to-one situations. These situations are differentiated on the basis of the degree of nurse-client involvement and whether the goal of the interaction is immediate, short term, or long term.

In the first situation the nurse and client do not know each other, and the client is in immediate, severe difficulty that requires the nurse to intervene. In other words, an emergency exists. The nature of the emergency can range from a life-threatening situation, such as a suicidal attempt, to the client being overwhelmed by a particular emotion, such as grief, and expressing this behaviorally. Ideally the person who intervenes in such situations should know the client and understand the plan of treatment. However, this is not always possible because of the necessity for immediate action or the unavailability of the appropriate staff member or because the client is new to the treatment setting. When such situations arise, nurses must not avoid intervening merely because they do not know the client. Rather, nurses must bring to the situation their knowledge of the dynamics of human behavior and their skill in psychiatric nursing. In these emergency situations, nurses should employ the principles of psychiatric nursing and good common sense. Clients have a right to be protected from harming themselves, either physically or emotionally, and from harming others.

Once the emergency situation is resolved, immediate efforts should be made to contact the mental health personnel involved with the client's treatment or to establish a treatment plan and begin its implementation if one has not already been developed.

In the second one-to-one situation the nurse and client have an association. Although they know each other, the nurse does not have major responsibility for the client's treatment. Unfortunately, some nurses believe that if they are not directly involved in the care of a particular client, they have little or no responsibility to behave in a thoughtful, goal-directed manner when interacting with the client. This is not the case, and the value of the interventions of other staff can be lessened by a nurse's thoughtless, offhand behavior. Although every nurse cannot have in-depth knowledge of all the clients in any treatment setting, every nurse can and must be aware of the treatment goals for all clients with whom they are likely to come in contact, no matter how superficially. With this awareness, on-the-spot interactions with clients can be designed to support and enhance the treatment being implemented by other personnel.

Spontaneous, seemingly casual nurse-client interactions are particularly common in psychiatric nursing, since, unlike many persons with a physical illness, persons with a mental illness usually are mobile and are able to approach the nurse whenever they choose. Sometimes a client seeks out one nurse to validate statements of another nurse or otherwise to engage the two nurses in a power struggle. The client's motivation may or may not be conscious and may be a manifestation of the stage of the relationship in which the client and nurse are engaged. In any event, how the nurse responds is frequently an important factor in enhancing or impeding the therapeutic endeavors of others. These on-the-spot, seemingly casual interactions should have support of the client's overall treatment as their goal.

In the third one-to-one situation the nurse seeks to develop a therapeutic relationship with a client in an effort to provide corrective interpersonal experiences. Because such a relationship requires an in-depth knowledge of the client and much of the nurse's time and energy, the nurse can have only a few such relationships in progress at any point in time. An understanding of the process of these relationships clarifies that it is inappropriate to use the term *nurse-client relationship* to describe all interactions between the nurse and all clients with whom she or he comes in contact. This is not to say that all nurse-client interactions should not be therapeutic, but rather that in only a few will the nurse be intensely involved in an ongoing relationship with the client that is designed to provide corrective interpersonal experiences. Since the nurse can be involved in only a few nurse-client relationships at any one time, the nurse must make the best use of time, energy, and skills by devoting them to those clients whose nursing diagnosis indicates a potential for benefiting from this type of nursing intervention. Not all nurses work equally effectively with all clients, since the nurse's personality is the major tool available for intervention. Therefore, when the nursing care plan indicates that a nurse-client relationship would be helpful, the nurse who develops such a relationship should have self-awareness indicating that the nurse would likely be effective with the particular client. Since both nurses and clients have the same wide variety of personalities, it is unlikely that a suitable nurse would not be available for any client.

Sometimes it is difficult for nurses to differentiate between social and therapeutic relationships when dealing with persons who have a mental illness. In a social relationship the needs of both individuals involved are considered. The needs of both must be met in a satisfying way if the relationship is to continue. A social relationship usually develops spontaneously without a conscious plan. The goal of such a relationship is usually shared by the participants and is frequently limited to personal pleasure. The participants in a social relationship share mutual concern regarding reciprocal approval. This may develop more or less satisfactorily without conscious awareness of the relationship's emotional significance.

In contrast, the therapeutic relationship focuses on the client's personal and emotional needs. Such a relationship is therapeutically oriented and is planned after consideration has been given to the client's needs and the nurse's therapeutic ability. There is always a therapeutic

goal toward which the nurse directs interventions. When accepting this role, the nurse must strive to be consciously aware of the developing relationship and its meaning. The nurse should seek help in reflecting objectively on the meaning of the interaction between self and client so that the nurse will be prepared to guide the client in developing more appropriate behavior. In a therapeutic relationship the nurse does not necessarily seek the client's approval. The nurse reevaluates the situation constantly so that she or he can distinguish between the client's needs and demands. As the time for the relationship to be terminated approaches, the nurse releases the client emotionally and strives to help this person move forward to more appropriate relationships.

Table 8-1 outlines the types of nurse-client interactions and their characteristics.

DEVELOPMENTAL PHASES OF THE NURSE-CLIENT RELATIONSHIP

Every therapeutic relationship developed by a nurse and a client has an initial phase, referred to as the **orientation** or the **becoming acquainted phase.** During this phase the nurse and client agree on a mutually acceptable contract that serves to establish the relationship's parameters. The goals of this phase are the development of trust and the establishment of the nurse as a significant other to the client.

Table 8-1. Types and characteristics of nurse-client interactions

TYPE OF INTERACTION	DEGREE OF NURSE-CLIENT INVOLVEMENT	GOAL OF INTERACTION
Emergency	Minimal	Immediate: resolve severe difficulty.
Association	Nurse and client know each other; nurse does not have major responsibility for client's treatment.	Short term: support and enhance treatment efforts of others.
Relationship	Great	Long term: provide corrective interpersonal experiences for client.

Although in some instances the client initiates the relationship, more frequently the nurse first approaches the client. Nurses do so by introducing themselves by name and position and suggesting that they would like to work with the client on the problems by meeting for a specific period and at a specified time and place. It is also important for nurses to ask how the client would prefer to be addressed. Most clients respond positively to this approach, ironically because the nurse is not yet an important part of their life and the idea of developing a relationship with the nurse is not threatening. Once the time and place of their conversations are agreed on, it is imperative that the nurse adhere strictly to this schedule. The nurse should also suggest a duration for each conversation, for example, 15 minutes. This period must be adhered to, even though the client sometimes may attempt to entice the nurse to stay longer by bringing up highly charged emotional issues 5 minutes before the end of the session. The nurse can handle this by acknowledging that the issues at hand sound important and by suggesting that the client reintroduce them at the beginning of their next meeting. This approach is therapeutic because it demonstrates that the nurse will follow through on what has been promised, in this instance, sessions of a 15-minute length, and therefore can be trusted to do what she or he says. It is important to understand that clients sometimes unconsciously introduce highly significant issues shortly before the end of planned sessions as a means of letting the nurse know what is disturbing them without running the risk of having to discuss these issues at length because they know that the session will soon be over. If the nurse succumbs to the temptation to continue the discussion beyond the agreed time, clients will learn that they have to be more guarded with the nurse in the future.

Some clients, rather than attempting to lengthen the sessions, try to shorten them by overt means such as walking away or covert means such as falling asleep. The nurse can ef-fectively deal with such situations by remembering that this period is set aside solely for interaction with this client and by stating this to the client. If the client still walks away or falls asleep, the nurse should remain in the designated meeting place for the remainder of the agreed time. This behavior also indicates to the client that the nurse can be trusted to do what has been promised, despite the client's behavior.

As the nurse becomes more meaningful to the client, the client's behavior toward the nurse often appears increasingly negative. Clients may not appear for the scheduled sessions, their language may become profane, or they may resist talking about themselves and state a preference for discussing the nurse's personal life. At this point, many nurses become discouraged and disappointed, since the earlier sessions had proceeded smoothly. In contrast, the nurse has reason to feel encouraged, since at this point in the relationship, the client's behavior most likely indicates that the nurse is becoming a significant other to the client. Persons with a mental illness have had much previous experience in familial and social relationships with persons who have initially accepted them but subsequently rejected them when their behavior became inappropriate. Therefore, clients have a need to test the nurse's reliability before allowing themselves to trust the nurse. If the nurse does not view this change in behavior as a test to determine just how much the client can rely on the nurse to be accepting and nonjudgmental, the nurse might feel discouraged and decide to end the relationship. To act on this feeling would be a mistake, since it would confirm the client's view of the nurse as being no different than others who have disappointed the client. More important, it would also confirm the client's view of being unworthy and unacceptable. Rather than discontinuing the relationship, the nurse must respond to the client's behavior with meticulous consistency. For example, if the nurse has agreed to meet with the client at a specified time and place, the nurse must be there even if the client does not appear. If the nurse continues in this manner, the client will soon have less need to test the nurse, and the first phase of the relationship will be concluded.

The second phase in a therapeutic relationship between a nurse and a client is called the **maintenance** or **working phase.** The goal of this phase is to identify and address the client's problem. Therefore the characteristics of this phase are highly individualized to the nature of the client's problems. Because each individual is unique and because the working phase of a relationship is so highly individualized to the particular client and nurse, few specific parameters can be given to guide the progress of this phase. An exception, however, is the necessity for **limit setting,** which often arises during this phase.

Limit setting is required when the client is threatening physical harm to self or others, when the client is destroying property or threatening to do so, and when the client's verbal hostility is upsetting and causing other clients or personnel to become tense and upset. If clients who require limit setting are willing to discuss their behavior, it may be sufficient for the nurse to point out that they are causing a dangerous, disturbing situation and to request that they stop. For some persons, such a request will be sufficient. However, others will require a more direct approach. In such an instance the nurse must speak firmly and explain that unless the disruptive behavior stops, the client will have to be segregated from the group and placed in a room alone or will be given a medication to assist him or her to gain control of the behavior.

If the nurse initiates and enforces limit setting in an empathic and nonpunitive manner, clients will often feel a sense of relief from anxiety because another person has assumed the responsibility for identifying and enforcing the boundaries of their behavior. Rather than damaging the relationship, limit setting often serves to further convince clients that the nurse cares about them as worthwhile individuals.

In summary, the maintenance, or working, phase of the nurse-client relationship is the time to identify and address the client's problems. Unless both the nurse and the client are actively involved in this process, the relationship cannot be effective. In maintaining a therapeutic relationship with clients, the nurse encourages them to express their concerns, fears, hopes, and problems. Sometimes the nurse will be able to achieve this by asking direct, specific leading questions. The nurse needs to recognize when she or he is able to intervene in the client's expressed concerns and when it is necessary to refer the client to other members of the treatment team who are prepared to address the specific problem. Therefore it is important for the nurse to understand how all members of the team share responsibility for the client's therapy.

The third phase of the therapeutic relationship is referred to as the **termination** or **concluding phase.** It is unrealistic to expect a relationship to continue indefinitely. This fact should be recognized and planned for in the orientation phase of the nurse-client relationship.

When the nurse learns that it will be necessary for the relationship to end, because either the nurse or the client is leaving the setting, the nurse should discuss this with the client as soon as possible. If the nurse knows at the outset of the relationship that it will be terminated at a specific time, the plans for the work of the nurse and the client should always include this fact. Terminating a relationship can be a traumatic experience for both the nurse and the client because they have shared much that is personal and important. At such a time, many clients express the feeling that the nurse is forsaking them. The loss of a trusted nurse is an especially difficult problem for a client who has been unable to trust other people. It is not unusual for clients to act out their frustration at the news of the impending loss of a trusted nurse.

In view of the possible traumatic difficulties that the nurse's departure presents to clients, the nurse must seek to understand their sense of loss and to help them express feelings and cope with them. The goal of this phase of the relationship is to help clients to review what they have learned through the process of the relationship and to transfer these learnings to their interactions with other persons.

If it is the nurse who is leaving the setting, the entire group of clients with whom the nurse has been working will respond in a variety of ways to the nurse's expected loss. Ideally, clients in a psychiatric setting should experience a relatively constant professional staff with whom they can establish meaningful relationships and work on emotional problems. Clients, as with all people, react to an anticipated loss in a variety of ways, depending on the characteristic way in which they respond to loss, their unique emotional needs, and the relationship they have developed with the departing staff member. Some clients may become depressed and unconsciously believe that they have been personally responsible for the nurse's loss. Other clients may not be able to accept the loss of this valued person and may repress the knowledge. They may report that no one told them the nurse was leaving. Other clients may respond with anger and may insist that the administrator take steps to see that the nurse does not leave.

When the nursing staff members are prepared for a variety of client responses, they can understand, accept, and cope with clients' behavior. This means that staff need to spend time talking with and listening to clients. Staff members must make themselves more available than usual to deal with the clients' many feelings about the situation and to reassure clients that they are not being abandoned. Sometimes it is helpful to encourage the clients to channel their feelings into some constructive activity. One way to redirect clients' concerns is to help them organize and carry out a party to honor the departing nurse.

It is unfortunate when clients are not given an opportunity to express their feelings about such a situation or not helped to handle their feelings. When this happens, as when a valued staff member simply disappears without any explanation, the feelings are not avoided but appear in many unusual behavioral reactions.

The client is not the only person who must cope with feelings of loss when the nurse-client relationship is terminated. By virtue of having established and maintained a relationship with the client, the nurse has invested much time, energy, thought, and emotion in the client. As a result, the nurse also experiences a sense of loss when the relationship is terminated. If nurses do not allow themselves to recognize these feelings, they might express them indirectly by showing undue concern for the client's future welfare, by encouraging the client to stay for a few more sessions, or by otherwise encouraging dependence on them. As with clients, nurses' previous experiences with and responses to loss are major determinants of their ability to cope effectively with their sense of loss when a nurse-client relationship is terminated. Most nurses find it helpful at this time to seek the guidance of the professional who is supervising the relationship. The nurse must remember that if the termination phase is not handled skillfully by encouraging the client to assume the independence he or she is ready for, the nurse can negate the value of the work that has been done in the preceding phase.

Table 8-2 summarizes the goals of and nurse behaviors in the nurse-client relationship.

ROLES AND FUNCTIONS OF THE NURSE

The three types of nurse-client interactions previously discussed provide the context within which the nurse assumes a variety of roles and functions. These shift frequently as the nurse strives to make contacts with clients therapeutic. The nurse is the creator of a therapeutic environment when providing opportunities for clients to experience acceptance in the environment. Frequently the nurse assumes the role of socializing agent when helping individuals or

Table 8-2.   Goals of and nurse behaviors in each phase of the nurse-client relationship

PHASE OF NURSE-CLIENT RELATIONSHIP	GOAL	NURSE BEHAVIORS
Orientation	Develop mutual trust. Establish nurse as a significant other to client.	Establishes mutually acceptable contract Responds to testing behavior of client by adhering strictly to terms of contract
Maintenance	Identify and address client's problems.	Highly individualized to the nature of client's problems Empathic, nonpunitive limit setting
Termination	Assist client to review what was learned and to transfer this learning to interactions with others.	Understands client's sense of loss Helps client express and cope with feelings Encourages client to channel feelings into constructive activity such as farewell party Recognizes own feelings of loss

groups to plan and participate in social events. The nurse finds that she or he must assume the role of counselor when clients need someone to listen with understanding and empathy while they talk about troublesome problems. The nurse is sometimes a teacher, especially when helping clients learn to understand their illness and its treatment. Frequently the nurse fills the role of parent surrogate when giving emotional support and understanding or when performing a nurturing activity such as feeding a client. Sometimes the nurse functions in the familiar technical role of nurse when performing such nursing duties as administering medications or treatments. Some nurses who have advanced educational preparation function in the therapist role by meeting with individuals, families, or groups at specified times and engaging them in a process designed to help them make fundamental system changes.

The nurse probably never functions in any single role at any given time; usually the nurse fulfills all or several of them at once. For the sake of clarity, however, these roles are discussed separately.

The nurse as creator of a therapeutic environment

One of the major therapeutic contributions the nurse can make is to develop a warm, accepting atmosphere. Although this atmosphere is related superficially to the environment's furnishings and decor, these attributes are no substitute for genuine human warmth, which springs solely from other human beings. If the situation is to be therapeutic for clients, it is essential that the nursing staff in close daily contact with the clients be honest, sincere, friendly people who really care about others. If the nurse is able to establish a warm, accepting atmosphere, the contributions of all members of the treatment team can be of maximum effectiveness.

A feeling of security is an essential element in developing a therapeutic climate. When clients are provided with an emotionally secure climate, feelings of acceptance, friendliness, warmth, safety, and relaxation are present. Many people who require psychiatric treatment are fearful, anxiety ridden, and insecure in their relationships with other people. A therapeutic climate should make it possible for such individuals to

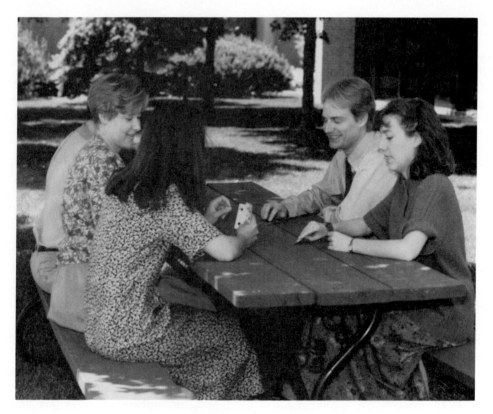

Figure 8-1
Group of patients enjoying a social activity.

behave as they need to behave because of their illness, secure in the knowledge that they will not be rejected and that they do not need to fear retaliation.

Another essential element in creating a therapeutic climate is an attitude that anticipates positive change and growth. If the climate is to be therapeutic, everyone working with clients must project an attitude that encourages improvement and positive change in behavior.

The nurse as socializing agent

Another important role is that of socializing agent. In fulfilling this role, the nurse helps clients participate successfully in group activities.

Physical facilities in many mental health settings are ideal for organizing and directing group activities. In a residential setting, group activities are particularly needed during that period in the day after the evening meal. Many scheduled activities stop before supper, and clients are frequently faced with long, unoccupied evenings. The nurse who cares for clients during the evening hours has a significant opportunity to contribute to these persons' mental health. Such a simple activity as an evening snack period can be the focus for group singing, group games, or group conversation. Activities organized by the clients themselves uncover and use hidden talent. In this way the group has an opportunity to recognize and encourage its own members and to contribute to developing the strengths of individuals. A dining room situation may lend itself to group activity. In such a situation the nurse has an opportunity to create an experience from which a feeling of belonging can develop. Mealtime is too often viewed solely from the standpoint of nutrition. Sometimes clients are hurried so that the staff can move to some other activity. Conversation is sometimes discouraged because it slows eating. The nurse who is with clients during mealtime may view this task solely from the standpoint of feeding the clients as efficiently and quickly as possible. When ascribing to these views, the nurse misses a valuable opportunity to facilitate positive learning experiences for clients.

In a nonresidential treatment setting, the nurse can assist clients to improve their social skills by introducing them to each other and then encouraging conversation by bringing up a neutral topic such as the weather. The community-based nurse who sits in an office waiting for clients to keep appointments misses an important opportunity to assist clients to develop social skills in the common social setting of the waiting room.

The nurse makes a contribution to improving clients' social skills by encouraging and developing the healthy aspects of their personalities. Many persons with a mental illness have learned to withdraw because of their extreme sensitivity and anxiety in relation to other people. The treatment setting provides opportunities for the nurse to design experiences in which clients can learn to achieve success in social situations, thereby developing feelings of security with other people.

The nurse as counselor

Empathic listening is another important aspect of psychiatric nursing. Probably no more important task exists than listening to a client in a positive, dynamic, empathic way without si-multaneously giving advice, stating opinions, or making suggestions. This type of active listening encourages clients to think through their problems and arrive at a helpful decision. Empathic listening helps clients to discharge anxiety and tension and tells them the nurse really cares.

Empathic listening demands much from the nurse in both time and emotional energy. It demands that the nurse be skillful in reflecting back the client's comments in such a manner that the client realizes the nurse is interested in the discussion and wants to hear as much as the client needs to tell. Some nurses may not understand the vital importance of this type of listening and may think they should stop the client's outpouring of problems. Unfortunately, this is easily done by a comment such as, "You can tell all that to your therapist tomorrow. He's the one who needs to know these things." The nurse also may respond with the even less helpful comment, "Things will be better tomorrow. Just keep a stiff upper lip." Clients often share their problems more freely with the nurse than with anyone else. The nurse and the other members of the mental health team need to agree on their roles with the client so the nurse and client can assess which concerns may appropriately be channeled to which team member.

The nurse's role is to help the client with problems of reality that deal with the here and now. Clients often discuss problems with the nurse that do relate to the areas that are the nurse's special concern, and in these situations the role as counselor is most frequently helpful.

Among the nurse's therapeutic responsibilities as a counselor is giving reassurance. Many situations in a client's life require that someone give some reassurance. Sometimes the nurse may suggest that reassurance should more logically be provided by the psychiatrist, chaplain, or social worker. The nurse needs to learn what services are available and how to obtain the assistance the client needs. However, more often than not, it is the nurse who must provide the needed reassurance. Such needs appear in every area of the client's life. There is the client who cannot sleep because he fears the treatment scheduled for the morning; the client who is upset because her husband did not visit as he had promised and she is now sure that he does not love her; the client who believes he is doomed forever because he has committed an unpardonable sin; and the client who is afraid of everything. The list is endless, and the needs for reassurance frequently appear at 11 PM or at 3 AM when no help may be readily available. This is why many day-care centers provide staff members who are available by phone during the entire 24-hour period. Often the staff members are nurses or trained mental health aides whose prompt intervention can prevent the need for hospitalization.

No set of rules or suggestions serves as a solution in each of these many situations. Probably the most effective reassurance for fearful, upset clients is a nursing staff whose members do not change frequently and are consistently kind and accepting. Merely sitting beside a client may be reassuring. This may help the client feel that someone on whom he or she can depend is there, ready to help in whatever way possible. Listening is one of the better ways of offering reassurance. Although logical, reasonable answers are frequently not helpful, they may be reassuring for some clients. Effective reassurance depends on the situation, the nurse, the relationship with the client, and the client's personality. A client who is suspicious requires a different form of help than one who is depressed.

Another aspect of the nurse's counseling role is in helping clients find acceptable outlets for anxiety. The client who is found sobbing hopelessly may be helped by a simple suggestion that he or she walk up and down the hallway with the nurse. Another client who is tense or excited may respond to the nurse's suggestion that the client take a warm tub bath before going to bed. Other ways in which the nurse may help clients find outlets for anxieties include assisting clients to participate in simple tasks, to become involved in some group activity, or to talk about their feelings.

The nurse as teacher

If purposeful therapeutic interventions can provide the individual with opportunities to learn to live a more satisfactory and satisfying life, they will make a significant contribution to the client's well-being. If the client is merely treated for the purpose of safeguarding family, community, or self, and if the client relies entirely on the judgment of professional personnel, the benefit of the experience is questionable. The nurse's role as teacher is in helping the client learn to cope in a more mature way.

The nurse's role as teacher has assumed critical importance as clients are increasingly likely to live in the community and become consumers of health care who demand and are expected to assume a major role in the determination and implementation of their care. To do so satisfactorily requires knowledge of the illness and the proposed treatment.

The nurse is in a pivotal position to teach clients (as individuals or groups), their families, and communities about mental illness and its treatments. Numerous surveys indicate that most people feel more comfortable confiding in nurses than in any other professional group and that they trust nurses' advice. Opportunities range from teaching the simple tasks of daily living, such as how to eat in socially prescribed ways, to how to deal with questions about the client's mental illness at large family gatherings during holidays. Usual concerns of clients and their families include the intended effects, side effects, and adverse reactions from prescribed medications; early symptoms of the reemergence of the illness; and how best to cope with the inevitable stressors of daily living. In other words, the nurse's teaching role includes educating clients and families about whatever is relevant to their situation.

Many persons with a severe mental illness

have cognitive and psychomotor disabilities. Therefore, not only must the *topic* of the teaching activity be relevant to the client and family, but the *method* of teaching also must be designed to consider these disabilities. Teaching techniques found to be successful with many persons with a mental illness include learning activities that require the active participation of the client and/or family, discussion and repetition of content, accompanying verbal instruction with culturally relevant written materials, and practicing skills in the location where the client is likely to use them in the future. Much success has been achieved in helping persons with a long-term, chronic mental illness retain employment by training them in the necessary skills in the place they will be working.

In addition to teaching clients and their families, nurses spend much time teaching each other about the latest developments in the care of those with a mental illness. Although this practice is highly desired, most nurses usually have access to a variety of other resources to gather this information. Meanwhile, the lay public remains ignorant of information that could change their negative attitude about those with a mental illness. Many nurses have invaluable information about mental illness and the care of persons with a mental illness that would be of interest and benefit to the general public. Since, as previously stated, nurses have much credibility among the public, they have a great opportunity to teach people about the facts regarding mental illness and the realities of living with a mental illness. Such opportunities frequently present themselves through church and civic groups. Psychiatric nurses fulfill their responsibilities as citizens and as professionals when they identify and use these opportunities.

The nurse as parent surrogate

Traditionally in this culture, the nurse has been a trusted person who performs personal services for sick people. Many of these services are similar to those a parent performs for chil-

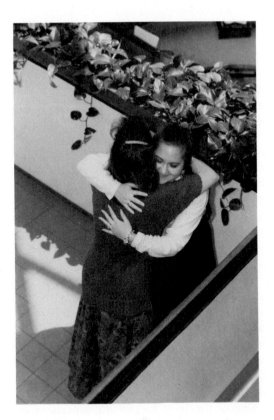

Figure 8-2
One of the roles of the nurse is parent surrogate.

dren. Nurses who work in mental health settings almost invariably become parent surrogates for some clients with whom they are closely associated. The role of parent surrogate is part of the nurse's traditional role, and although it does not imply becoming the client's parent, it includes many nurturing activities that may be required for some persons who have a mental illness. Although most clients are able to bathe, dress, and feed themselves, a few are too ill to perform these simple tasks. For some of these persons, the nurse may need to assume the traditional protective, supportive, parental role by giving physical care.

The nurse, as with an effective parent, realizes that it is important for clients to assume responsibility for their own physical care as soon as possible. Thus the nurse gives physical care to persons with a mental illness in an empathic, understanding way but looks for and seizes every opportunity to encourage them to assume responsibility for their own care as soon as possible. The effective nurse withdraws from the task of feeding or bathing clients as soon as they are able to take over the responsibility for themselves. In this way the nurse supports the client's increasing autonomy.

Besides assuming the parental role in relation to the client's physical needs, the nurse also does so in relation to managing the treatment setting. The nurse develops many policies concerning the environment that profoundly affect clients' lives. The nurse is indirectly responsible for almost every aspect of the treatment setting, from housekeeping to securing emergency medical care. The nurse sets the tone of the treatment situation, much as parents set the tone of the family.

One of the most therapeutic aspects of the nurse's traditional role as parent surrogate is in assisting individuals and groups of clients to set limits for their behavior. This aspect of the nurse's role probably overlaps the teacher role.

Clients who interact with each other over time may react toward each other as if they were members of the same family. These reactions are usually unconscious but are nonetheless real and may serve as a basis for much emotional and social unlearning and relearning. Therefore the nurse's role as parent surrogate offers an opportunity to provide clients with healthy experiences in the area of emotional relationships.

While serving as the object of many angry, hostile feelings that some clients cannot otherwise admit or express, the nurse may be able to supply the warm, accepting, nurturing relationship that some persons require to move toward more mature behavior. In conjunction with other members of the mental health team, the nurse is able to provide experiences that may prove to be corrective of the client's earlier unsatisfactory interpersonal experiences.

The technical nursing role

The nurse's traditional role includes those technical aspects involved in pouring and administering medications, monitoring vital signs, carrying out physical treatments, and observing and recording client behavior. Many nurses have become skilled in performing routine physical examinations. This activity, once limited to physicians, is important for nurses to master as the inextricable relationship between the mind and body is increasingly documented. Occasionally a client can accept a nurse as a helpful counselor or teacher only after the ability to perform the technical aspects of the nursing role has been demonstrated. Therefore the nurse must realize that such procedures as administering medications and taking vital signs provide an opportunity to enhance the therapeutic relationship with the client as well as to achieve the procedure's primary goal.

The nurse's responsibilities regarding medications and charting are discussed here because they are two technical functions common to all psychiatric nurses. Most important, the way in which these functions are carried out has the potential for having a great impact on the client's well-being.

Responsibilities in regard to medications

Because of the widespread use of psychotropic agents in the treatment of persons with a mental illness, it is not unusual for nurses to spend a large part of their time preparing and administering medications. Unfortunately, some nurses believe that their responsibility has been fulfilled once these tasks are completed. However, many other responsibilities are involved when nurses administer psychotropic agents to clients.

Before the client receives any medication, it

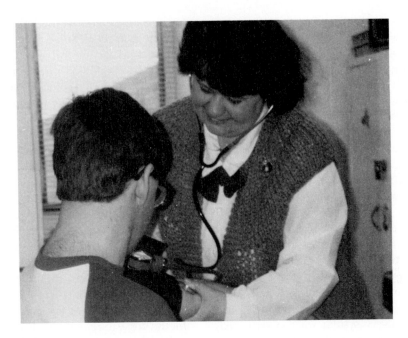

Figure 8-3
The technical nursing role.
From Cookfair JM: *Nursing process and practice in the community,* St Louis, 1991, Mosby–Year Book.

is essential for the nurse to make several assessments. Initially the nurse must obtain the client's medical history, especially in regard to seizure disorder; pregnancy; cardiac, hepatic, or renal disease; and substance abuse. In addition, the nurse should determine physiological baseline data about the client. These include blood pressure, both sitting and standing; pulse, both quality and rate; weight; sleep pattern; gait and movement; and blood chemistry. Many psychotropic agents affect these physiological processes, and the nurse cannot make an accurate assessment of their effect unless baseline data are available to which a comparison can be made. In addition, the choice of drug and dosage is influenced by these factors.

As the nurse works with clients before they receive a medication, the nurse often is in the best position to ascertain their attitude toward taking medications. Clients vary widely in their response to drug therapy, depending on such variables as their past experiences with psychotropic agents or other mind-altering drugs and their current state of orientation. Some clients are eager to receive medication and see it as the answer to all their problems. Others, particularly those who are suspicious, fear medication because of their feelings of loss of control. In most instances, both these extreme views are not reality based. The client needs to be helped to develop a realistic picture of what a psychotropic agent can and cannot do.

Once having ascertained the client's medical history, physiological baseline data, and attitude toward taking medication, the nurse is in a position to collaborate with the physician in determining the most effective medication, dosage, frequency, and route of administration. Although the physician usually has the responsibility for prescribing psychotropic medications, the assessments of a knowledgeable nurse are often relied on, especially in regard to dosage, frequency, and route of administration. If indicated by the assessment data, the nurse should suggest the medication be ordered by alternate routes.

The specific actions of the prescribed drug should address those symptoms of the client's illness that are most distressing to the client or to others. These symptoms are called **target symptoms,** and the degree to which they are ameliorated increases the likelihood of the client's continuing to cooperate with the treatment regimen. For example, a newly admitted client who is distressed by auditory hallucinations and for whom an antipsychotic drug is prescribed will often be relieved by the diminution of this disturbing symptom. If the client had been previously counseled by the nurse to expect this result, the client's trust in the nurse and in the health care delivery system will be increased. However, it is important that the nurse make clear that it often takes as long as 6 or 8 weeks before improvement in target symptoms is seen.

After a drug has been ordered for the client, the nurse is responsible for accurately preparing, administering, and recording the medication and its effects. As previously stated, some nurses unfortunately see this phase of the treatment as the only aspect of their role or, if not the only aspect, the most important one. In reality the nurse's success with this phase of the process depends greatly on the quality of the client assessment previously obtained and the degree of physician-nurse collaboration the nurse has been able to establish.

Most nurses have much experience in preparing medications, and doing so in a psychiatric setting does not differ from executing this task in other settings. On the other hand, administering medications to persons with a mental illness may be dramatically different than what the nurse is accustomed to. First, most clients with a mental illness are ambulatory, and the nurse must use caution that the medications intended for a group of clients not be accessible while the

nurse is occupied with administering medications to one client. Some clients will try to steal medications for use as barter for items such as cigarettes. In addition, clients may take medications to save until a sufficient amount has been accumulated so they may attempt suicide. Finally, clients may accidentally knock the medications over, resulting in the potential loss of medication and the actual loss of the nurse's valuable time. Therefore the nurse should keep the medications inaccessible to the client group and administer them to one client at a time.

While administering medication, the nurse has a valuable opportunity to observe the client for side effects and adverse reactions as well as for changes in behavior. Of equal importance, the nurse has the opportunity to interact in such a way as to gain the client's acceptance of the medication. In this regard, it is most often helpful for the nurse to refer to the drug as "medication" rather than using the word "drug" to prevent confusion with mind-altering street drugs. Nurses sometimes feel so rushed when administering medications that they resent the client asking questions about medications or otherwise lengthening the process. As a result, it is not unusual for the nurse to be drawn into a power struggle with the client around the issue of whether or not and when the client will take the medication. This common situation is unfortunate not only because it usually takes much time but, more important, because it sets a negative tone associated with taking medications. Rather than engaging in a power struggle with the client, the effective nurse takes the time to answer the client's questions and otherwise gives the client as much control of the situation as possible. Clients have the right and the need to know the name, dosage, actions, side effects, and adverse effects of the medicine they are taking.

Clients who refuse medication present a particular challenge to the nurse. Before deciding to omit the dose or to administer it parenterally, the nurse should make an assessment of why the client is refusing. Once again, this takes time, but time might be saved in the long run. One chronically ill client was readmitted to the hospital because of an exacerbation of visual and auditory hallucinations probably precipitated by having stopped his antipsychotic medication a month previously because of lack of money. Even though this client was known to the nursing staff as being cooperative, he refused to take his oral medication. Every time the nurse would extend her hand with the medication cup, the client would become visibly distressed, perspire profusely, and wrap his arms tightly around himself. Although the staff agreed that what this client needed most was the prescribed antipsychotic medication, they disagreed about how it should be administered. Some maintained that the client should be restrained and given the medication by injection. The nurse who knew him best, however, was struck by his uncharacteristic refusal of the medication and by the consistency of his behavior when offered it. She hypothesized that the client was perceiving the nurse's extended arm as an attack and consequently was experiencing massive anxiety when efforts were made to give him medication. Based on this assessment, this nurse approached the client from the side, laid the medication and water cups on the counter, slowly explained what they were, and gently directed the client to take the medication. Within a very short time the client complied. This thoughtful intervention by the nurse allowed the client to maintain control of the situation, accomplished the nurse's goal, and avoided the difficult and potentially traumatic situation of having to administer an injection forcibly .

It is important that the nurse document and otherwise communicate to other staff interpersonal interventions that have proved useful in working with clients who resist taking medications. The use of the same approaches will help to ensure consistency in treatment and increase the client's trust in the staff.

Once the client has begun a regimen of psychotropic medications, it is the nurse's responsibility to monitor physiological responses to the medication. To do so effectively, the nurse must be knowledgeable about the intended effects, side effects, and adverse effects of the drugs the client is receiving. The nurse must observe the client carefully and listen to reports with concern. When side effects appear, the nurse can reassure the client that these are anticipated and make suggestions for reducing the discomfort. For example, the dry mouth associated with the phenothiazines can be diminished by the client chewing sugarless gum or sucking on hard candy. If adverse effects occur, the nurse must notify the physician immediately and usually withhold the medication.

The ultimate goal of treatment with psychotropic medications is to enable the client to function at the highest level possible with the least amount of medication. To achieve this goal, the nurse is most helpful when working with the client on developing nonchemical adaptations to the symptoms, such as increasing interpersonal resources and skills. For clients who must continue taking maintenance doses of medication, the nurse has the responsibility to help clients learn as much as they are able about the medication and also to learn how to administer it to themselves correctly.

Responsibilities in regard to charting

One of the nurse's most significant responsibilities is the accurate, perceptive observation and recording of the client's behavior. In carrying out this function skillfully and meaningfully, the nurse contributes to the understanding that all members of the mental health team have about the client's problems. Nurses are the professional persons who are with clients for the longest time; as such, they have a unique opportunity to help other professionals understand clients' needs through effective recording of samples of conversation, sleep patterns, interpersonal relationships, socialization activities, and descriptions of personal habits.

It is recommended that the client's behavior be described rather than labeled. Not only do labels have stereotypical meanings, but they may also convey different messages to different readers. Instead of recording that a client is hallucinating, it is more meaningful to record exactly what was observed. The following is an example of this type of recording: "Stood near the ventilator for 10 minutes with hand cupped around ear as if trying to hear better. Carried on an animated conversation. Although no other person was present, the client could be heard saying, 'How dare you call me those names! You are a liar.'"

Instead of recording that the client is disoriented and misidentifies people, it would be more meaningful to record the following: "Mr. J. greeted the nurse by saying, 'Good morning, Mary. Have you cooked breakfast yet?' In the afternoon he asked, 'When are we going to have breakfast?' Client believes that this nurse is his wife, and he is not able to differentiate between morning and afternoon."

By recording observations in this manner, the nurse permits readers to make their own interpretation of the meaning of the client's behavior.

The nurse as therapist

For many years some nurses who have had the benefit of a master's degree in psychiatric nursing have functioned in the role of the nurse therapist. When nurses assume this role, they use the principles developed through the practice of psychotherapy.

Nursing therapy has developed differently in each situation, but basically it follows the same general guidelines. The nurse collaborates with other mental health professionals in the situation and confers regularly with those responsible for developing the treatment plans for the clients with whom the nurse is working. The nurse's intervention becomes a part of the total treatment plan for the client.

As with all therapists, it is essential that the nurse identify a skilled professional therapist to function on a regular basis as preceptor or supervisor while the nurse is working as a nurse

therapist. By doing so, the nurse therapist enhances the effectiveness of interactions with the client and increases personal knowledge and skill.

The nurse therapist should record each therapy session so that it can be used to (1) review the dynamics of the relationship, (2) analyze the problems that have been presented, and (3) evaluate client progress against the established treatment goals.

The following situation depicts the way a nurse fulfilled a variety of roles in an unanticipated clinical situation.

"Please take me back to the ward, Miss S., I feel sick." Tall, dark-haired 17-year-old Sam G. had walked across the dance floor and was pleading with the nurse to be allowed to leave the regular Wednesday evening dance. The dance was part of the recreational program for clients. Both Sam and the nurse knew that clients were usually encouraged to remain at the dance until it was over. She also knew that Sam had not made such a request before, and intuitively she felt that something at the dance had been upsetting to him.

Miss S. quietly made the necessary arrangements with the staff member in charge of the dance and took Sam back to the unit. Then she took his pulse, temperature, and respirations to be certain that he was not physically ill. When she found that these physical signs were within the normal range, she suggested that he help her make some sandwiches. Together they went into the kitchen, where they prepared a snack for the other clients who would soon be returning from the dance. Sam seemed happy to help. He and the nurse chatted and joked together. He spoke at length about his mother's illness and his family's financial problems, but he did not mention feeling ill.

After finishing the sandwiches and cleaning the kitchen, the nurse thanked Sam for his help, remarking on the speed with which he accomplished the task. They then went together into the living room and sat down on the couch. "Do you think that my face is changing?" he asked. "I just looked in the bathroom mirror, and it seems to me that my nose is getting a lot longer and uglier."

The nurse looked carefully at his face and said, "It looks just the same to me. It seems to you that your nose is getting longer?"

Soon the other clients arrived from the dance. The unit was filled with the busy noise of 25 people discussing the dance and eating the evening snack. Sam took part in all this activity but sought the nurse several times to ask questions: "Do you think you ought to call my doctor?" "Will I be able to sleep tonight?" "You think that I am going to be all right, don't you?"

Each time Sam came to ask a question, the nurse took time to listen carefully to his questions and to answer truthfully and sincerely. She did call the physician on duty that evening and told him about Sam's behavior. He agreed to come to see Sam. Because the physician was not well acquainted with Sam, the nurse spent several minutes telling him briefly about Sam's family problems. She pointed out that he had been anxious and tense during the evening and had seemed to cling to her and to be asking for reassurance. The physician talked with Sam. He believed that by allowing Sam to leave the dance, the nurse had been able to help him avoid an anxiety attack. The physician told the nurse that her empathic listening and her efforts at reassuring Sam had been partially successful. The next day, Sam's regular therapist was able to help him look more objectively at the problem that had been so upsetting to him. As a result of the nurse's intervention and the physician's help, Sam was able to attend the dance the following week without experiencing undue anxiety.

This example is typical of situations that nurses who work in inpatient psychiatric settings frequently encounter. In her interaction with Sam, the nurse used the technical nursing role by taking and evaluating his vital signs. She simultaneously engaged in the role of parent surrogate and socializing agent when she worked with Sam to prepare and serve snacks for the other clients. The therapeutic effectiveness of this activity became apparent when Sam spoke about his family's problems and then became able to communicate his concern about his physical appearance. The nurse's response to this concern reflects the role of counselor, since she listened attentively and responded in a truthful, reassuring way. The nurse displayed an understanding of the necessity for professional collaboration by calling the physician and carefully sharing with

him her assessment of the client. In summary, the nurse saw this clinical situation as an opportunity to use a variety of nursing roles, which proved to be very helpful to the client. Without an awareness of the therapeutic potential of these activities, the nurse might have insisted that Sam remain at the dance and thereby could have contributed to the exacerbation of an acute anxiety attack.

KEY POINTS

1. The major way in which nurses directly influence the care of clients is through how they interact with clients in face-to-face situations.

2. Acceptance of the client as an important human being with worth and value is foundational to effective nurse-client interactions. Nurse behaviors that reflect acceptance include calling the client by name, trying to understand the meaning of the client's behavior and believing that it represents the best the client is capable of at the time, and listening attentively to the client's expressions of feelings and concerns.

3. Consistency is an important characteristic of therapeutic interactions. The consistent nurse maintains the same basic attitude toward the client, enabling the client to predict the nurse's behavior.

4. Nurses may be in situations where they must interact with clients whom they do not know but who are experiencing an emergency. The goal of these immediate interactions is to resolve the emergency and ensure ongoing care.

5. The most frequent type of nurse-client interaction occurs in situations where the nurse and client are associated but the nurse does not have major responsibility for the client's treatment. In these short-term situations the goal of the interaction is to support and enhance the treatment efforts of others.

6. The third type of nurse-client interaction is in situations where the nurse seeks to develop a therapeutic relationship with a client in an effort to provide corrective interpersonal experiences. This long-term type of interaction is called a nurse-client relationship.

7. The goals of the orientation, or becoming acquainted, phase of the nurse-client relationship are the development of mutual trust and the establishment of the nurse as a significant other to the client.

8. The goal of the maintenance, or working, phase of the nurse-client relationship is to help the client identify and address problems. It is often necessary for the nurse to set limits during this phase.

9. The goal of the termination, or concluding, phase of the nurse-client relationship is to assist the client to review what was learned from the relationship and to transfer these learnings to interactions with others.

10. Roles of the nurse in nurse-client interactions include those of (1) creator of a therapeutic environment, (2) socializing agent, (3) counselor, (4) teacher, (5) parent surrogate, (6) technician, and (7) therapist. These roles shift frequently as the nurse strives to make interactions with clients therapeutic.

SUGGESTED SOURCES OF ADDITIONAL INFORMATION

Barrass D: The nurse as patient educator. *Br J Nurs* 1(5):241, 1992.

Bayer M: Saying goodbye through graffiti: it all began when we were about to discharge Hilda, *Am J Nurs* 80:271, February 1980.

Beeber L and others: Peplau's theory in practice, *Nurs Sci Q* 3:6, Spring 1990.

Bowditch B: Brief encounter, *Nurs Times* 87:41, Oct 2, 1991.

Burnard P, Morrison P: Nurses' interpersonal skills: a study of nurses' perceptions, *Nurs Educ Today* 11:24, 1991.

Chalmers H: Peplau's development model, *Nurs Times* 86:38, Jan 10, 1990.

Clarke AC: Nurses as role models and health educators, *J Adv Nurs* 16:1178, 1991.

Forchuk C, Brown B: Special feature: Hildegard Peplau: establishing a nurse-client relationship, *J Psychosoc Nurs Ment Health Serv* 27(2):30, 1989.

Kasch CR: Toward a theory of nursing action: skills and competency in nurse-patient interaction, *Nurs Res* 35:226, July/August 1986.

Lego SM: The one-to-one nurse-patient relationship, *Perspect Psychiatr Care* 18:67, March/April 1980.

Loomis ME: Levels of contracting, *J Psychosoc Nurs Ment Health Serv* 23(3):8, 1985.

Olson JK, Iwasiw CL: Nurses' verbal empathy in four types of client situations, *Can J Nurs Res* 21:39, Summer 1989.

Payton R: Truth is essential for trust between nurse, patient, *Am Nurse* 16(6):11, 1984.

Reed RC, Lewkowitz S: The interactive model of psychotherapy, *Perspect Psychiatr Care* 25(3/4):27, 1989.

Schroder PJ: Recognizing transference and countertransference, *J Psychosoc Nurs Ment Health Serv* 23:21, February 1985.

Tommasini NR: The use of touch with the hospitalized psychiatric patient, *Arch Psychiatr Nurs* 4:213, August 1990.

Topf M, Dambacher B: Teaching interpersonal skills: a model for facilitating optimal interpersonal relations, *J Psychosoc Nurs Ment Health Serv* 19:29, December 1981.

Trotter CMF: I never promised you a rose garden but I must remember to tell you about the thorns, *J Psychosoc Nurs Ment Health Serv* 23:15, March 1985.

Tudor GE: A sociopsychiatric nursing approach to intervention in a problem of mutual withdrawal on a mental hospital ward, *J Psychiatry* 15:193, 1952.

Yuen FKH: The nurse-client relationship: a mutual learning experience, *J Adv Nurs* 11:529, 1986.

Chapter 9

The Therapeutic Environment

LEARNING OBJECTIVES

After studying this chapter, the student will be able to:

* State the goals of a therapeutic environment in an inpatient treatment setting.

* Discuss the characteristics of a therapeutic environment in an inpatient treatment setting.

* Explain the necessity for setting limits in a therapeutic environment.

* Discuss the influence of the physical environment on the therapeutic environment.

* State the significant aspects of a therapeutic community.

* Discuss the implications of the therapeutic environment for the role of the nurse.

KEY TERMS

Therapeutic community
Ward Atmosphere Scale (WAS)

Research has documented that the environment in which persons with a mental illness are treated is a major factor in enhancing or impeding the therapeutic effects of other treatment modalities. When the environment itself becomes a treatment modality, it is referred to as a therapeutic community, a specialized form of the therapeutic environment.

It is well accepted that an environment that is therapeutic is necessary regardless of the type of setting in which a client is treated. Because an increasing number of persons with acute mental illnesses are being treated in short-term, general hospital units, and because many with long-term chronic illnesses are being treated in the community and in long-term care facilities, it becomes necessary to design environments differently based on the clients' needs and the setting's characteristics. For example, research has documented that clients who are acutely ill respond best to an environment that is structured, consistent, and nonstimulating. In contrast, individuals living in the community often benefit from treatment environments that they have an active part in creating and maintaining.

Because the nurse is with the client in the treatment setting for a longer time than any other professional, and because both the nurse and the client are directly affected by the environment, it is well accepted that the major responsibility to create and maintain a therapeutic environment lies with the nursing staff. The following is a discussion of the principles of a therapeutic environment in an inpatient treatment setting. In other treatment settings the nurse can and should adapt these principles based on the clients' needs and the setting's characteristics.

HISTORICAL PERSPECTIVE

The archives of American psychiatry include records of early successful attempts to develop a homelike atmosphere for persons hospitalized for mental illness, including provision for social and recreational activities. Physicians and their families joined other staff members in initiating and directing some of these activities. Early in the nineteenth century, emphasis on a homelike environment, recreational activities, and a sympathetic approach to clients was referred to as *moral treatment.* In 1842 Boston State Hospital was reported to have placed emphasis on moral treatment for its clients. The superintendent of one psychiatric hospital in Massachusetts is reported to have invited "inmates" to his home for Sunday dinner. Intimate discussions of personal problems and difficulties were part of the therapy offered in those institutions at that time.

Some authorities believe that the era of moral treatment ended because of the large numbers of immigrants who arrived in the United States after the Civil War. Many of these people could not cope with the problems of adjustment presented by the radically different environment they found and were therefore deemed mentally ill. Large numbers of inmates with differing cultural backgrounds and languages swelled the wards of mental institutions and made it difficult, if not impossible, to provide a homelike environment. Thus the era of moral treatment passed.

By 1940 large public hospitals were filled to overflowing. Because of the ever-increasing patient population, the task of the hospital personnel was staggering. They were able to do little more than keep the inmates bathed, dressed, and fed.

An unprecedented national concern for the welfare of persons with a mental illness after World War II and the introduction of the first of the antipsychotic drugs in the early 1950s fostered a resurgence of interest in the therapeutic potential of the hospital environment. It was within this context that *Social Psychiatry,* a small book by Dr. Maxwell Jones, was published in England in 1953.

When published in the United States, Dr. Jones's book was titled *The Therapeutic Community,* and it soon became one of the motivating factors in the movement to use the hospital environment therapeutically in the treatment regimen of persons with a mental illness. This influential book was a report of efforts at Belmont Hospital in England during and after World War II to rehabilitate patients with neuroses through group methods. That experience in group living at Belmont Hospital came to be known as the **therapeutic community,** a specialized form of therapeutic environment. In the therapeutic community, particular attention was paid to the development of the hospital's social structure and to communication between patients and the hospital staff. Dr. Jones dedicated his book to "The Nursing Staff who have formed a framework around which our therapeutic communities have been built." Although the nurses to whom he referred were not registered nurses, they were intelligent, capable, mature women who used the interpersonal skill and understanding required in psychiatric nursing. The dedication is appropriate. Without a nursing staff with insight, understanding, personal warmth, and skill in directing groups, the concept of a therapeutic community could not have developed into a reality.

GOALS AND CHARACTERISTICS OF A THERAPEUTIC ENVIRONMENT IN AN INPATIENT TREATMENT SETTING

As with any treatment regimen, a therapeutic environment is most likely to be successful if its implementation is consistent with the professional staff's philosophy and if it is guided by goals derived from that philosophy. Based on the philosophy stated in Chapter 6, the goals of a therapeutic environment are to help individuals increase their self-esteem and feelings of personal worth, to improve their ability to relate to others, and to enable them to work and live more effectively in the community. The probability of these goals being achieved is increased in a treatment setting that has the following characteristics:

1. The client's physical needs are met.
2. The client is respected as an individual with

rights, needs, and opinions and is encouraged to express these.

3. Decision-making authority is clearly defined and distributed appropriately among clients and staff.

4. The client is protected from injury from self and others, but only those restrictions necessary to afford such protection are imposed.

5. The client is afforded increasing opportunities for freedom of choice, commensurate with ability to make decisions.

6. All personnel, but particularly nursing staff, remain constant; for example, unit and shift assignments remain stable.

7. The environment provides a testing ground for the establishment of new patterns of behavior.

8. Emphasis is placed on social interaction between and among clients and staff, and the environment's physical structure and appearance facilitate this interaction.

9. Programming is structured but flexible.

Providing for the client's physical needs

Although most characteristics of a therapeutic environment focus on its socioeconomic climate and physical structure, the nurse must understand that no environment can be therapeutic if it does not provide for meeting the client's physical needs. Great effort has been expended to improve the care of persons with a mental illness by altering long-term treatment settings from custodial to therapeutic environments. In the process, however, some benefits of "custodial" care have been discarded. For example, ensuring that clients have adequate diet and rest and appropriate clothing and are monitored for signs of illness may be sacrificed in the service of socioemotional interventions. The probability of focusing solely on the client's physical or emotional needs is enhanced by the dualistic manner in which the health care delivery system continues to function. The reality is that humans are holistic beings and therefore respond holistically. For example, clients sometimes have nu-

tritional deficits because they eat more food with empty calories than nourishing meals. Furthermore, many psychotropic drugs typically used to treat persons with mental illness have very serious potential side effects. Therefore, in an environment that is truly therapeutic, the nursing staff continuously assesses and intervenes with each client in a comprehensive, holistic manner.

Socioemotional climate essential to a therapeutic environment

Once it is ensured that the environment is designed to address the client's physical needs, the socioeconomic climate of the treatment setting must be addressed. To be therapeutic, this climate must reflect respect for the client as a human being who has value and worth. As such, the nursing staff recognizes and respects the client's rights and opinions and sees the client as an indispensable ally in the formulation and implementation of the treatment plan. Although it is important that both the staff and the clients understand who is responsible for making which decisions, the nursing staff in a therapeutic environment frequently solicits the clients' opinions about matters that affect them. For example, rules regarding television viewing are often more productively made by the clients rather than by the staff.

An environment that is therapeutic provides for the protection of the client from injury from both self and others. Protecting the client from injury includes, but is not limited to, physical protection. It also includes safeguarding the client against making significant decisions when he or she is not well enough to do so. Thus the nursing staff may find it necessary to help the client avoid making decisions about such matters as a pending divorce or separation or the sale of property.

Some clients want and need reassurance that the staff will establish rules of conduct within which all clients will function. The process of establishing and enforcing such guidelines is referred to as limit setting. The establishment of limits is best done by all those affected by the rule, including the clients and the entire treatment team. The basis for rules should be an anticipated positive effect on clients' growth.

By involving all those affected by the rule in its establishment, the likelihood of imposing the personal standards of behavior of one person on all others is decreased. Before any rule that regulates client activity is established, all aspects of the results of such action should be considered, including enforcing the rule once it is established. Consistency in enforcing limits is necessary if the rule is to have its desired effect. However, a rule that cannot be enforced is less therapeutic than no rule at all, in that clients can become quite anxious about the staff's apparent lack of control of the situation.

The nurse can easily confuse limit setting with control of behavior. The nurse may rationalize that many imposed controls are limits placed on the situation for the safety and security of clients when in reality they exist because of tradition, personal idiosyncrasies of one or more staff members, or to facilitate ease of management of the setting. When groups of people live together, rules need to be established that may not be necessarily equally beneficial to all involved. Nevertheless, rules designed to make life easier for the nursing staff that have no benefit to the clients should be recognized as such and avoided.

Although appropriate limit setting is essential to the establishment and maintenance of an emotional climate conducive to a therapeutic environment, the nursing staff also strives to establish as few rules and regulations as possible for client behavior and restricts activity only when necessary. Opportunities for freedom of choice are provided. As clients demonstrate the ability to accept more responsibility for their behavior, opportunities for making choices are increased.

A nursing staff that is sensitive, friendly, and concerned about the welfare of every client is imperative if an environment is to be therapeutic. Although it is unlikely that every nurse will care deeply about every client, each client should be-

lieve that at least one nurse can be relied on as an advocate. To establish such a relationship requires that there be constancy among staff in the treatment setting. Unfortunately, the major determinants of staffing assignments are often the setting's managerial needs and the staff's personal preferences. Ironically, clients' relationship needs are the last factor to be considered, if they are considered at all.

As clients improve, they will experiment with different ways of viewing the world and the people in it. Thus, they will develop new ways of responding to others and of coping with stress. Some of these new methods of dealing with problems may not be appropriate. If the environment is truly therapeutic, these attempts at learning new patterns of behavior will be recognized as such and met with understanding by the nursing staff. Frequently, clients need encouragement to continue testing new patterns of behavior until they have achieved more satisfying and satisfactory patterns of behavior.

Finally, if the environment is to be therapeutic, the client needs to know what to expect there. Research has shown that persons with a mental illness respond most favorably in environments with structured activities. On the other hand, the activities should not be so structured that their implementation becomes the goal rather than meeting clients' needs. For example, it is usually useful to have a week's activities preplanned and made known to clients and staff alike. However, if an untoward event such as a client suicide occurs, or if an unanticipated opportunity such as a trip to the circus arises, the staff should be flexible enough to cancel the planned activity to deal with the event or to take advantage of the opportunity.

INFLUENCE OF PHYSICAL ENVIRONMENT ON THE THERAPEUTIC ENVIRONMENT

A therapeutic climate for persons with a mental illness depends on the staff's attitude toward mental illness and the clients' needs and does

OF SPECIAL INTEREST

One of the most widely used tools to measure ward atmosphere is the **Ward Atmosphere Scale (WAS)** (Moos RH: *Evaluating treatment environments: a social-ecological approach,* London, 1974, Wiley). This instrument consists of 10 subscales that both staff and clients complete in terms of their perception of ward atmosphere as it actually exists and what they believe should exist. The differences between the "real" and the "ideal" provide the basis for instituting change in the environment that is likely to be accepted by all concerned. The subscales and their definitions* are:

1. *Involvement.* Measures how active and energetic clients are in the day-to-day social functioning of the ward, both as members of the ward as a unit and as individuals interacting with other clients; also assesses attitudes such as pride in the ward, feelings of group spirit, and general enthusiasm
2. *Support.* Measures how helpful and supportive clients are toward other clients, how well the staff understand clients' needs and are willing to help and encourage clients, and how encouraging and considerate physicians are toward clients
3. *Spontaneity.* Measures the extent to which the environment encourages clients to act openly and to express freely their feelings toward other clients and staff
4. *Autonomy.* Assesses how self-sufficient and independent clients are encouraged to be in their personal affairs and in their relationships with staff; how much responsibility and self-direction clients are encouraged to exercise; and to what extent the staff are influenced by clients' suggestions, criticism, and other initiatives

5. *Practical orientation.* Assesses the extent to which the clients' environment orients them toward preparing themselves for release from the hospital and for the future; considers such factors as training for new jobs, looking to the future, and setting and working toward practical goals
6. *Personal problem orientation.* Measures the extent to which clients are encouraged to be concerned with their feelings and problems and to seek to understand them through openly talking to other clients and staff about themselves and their past
7. *Anger and aggression.* Measures the extent to which clients are allowed and encouraged to argue with other clients and staff, to become openly angry, and to display other expressions of anger
8. *Order and organization.* Measures how important order is on the ward, in terms of clients (how they look), staff (what they do to encourage order), and the ward itself (how well it is kept); also measures organization, again in terms of clients (do they follow a regular schedule, do they have carefully planned activities) and staff (do they keep appointments, do they help clients follow schedules)
9. *Program clarity.* Measures the extent to which clients know what to expect in the day-to-day routine of the ward and how explicit the ward rules and procedures are
10. *Staff control.* Measures the extent to which it is necessary for the staff to restrict clients, that is, in the strictness of rules and schedules, in the relationships between clients and staff, and in measures taken to keep clients under effective control

*Modified from Milne D: Planning and evaluating innovations in nursing practice by measuring the ward atmosphere, *J Adv Nurs* 11:206, 1986.

not develop because of any fixed type of architecture. A therapeutic climate can be developed in any type of setting if the staff focuses on meeting clients' needs. However, it is helpful if certain structural features are present. Clients' needs can be met more effectively if facilities for privacy, socialization, and planned activities are available. If such facilities are not already present, innovations must be introduced if a therapeutic environment is to be created.

If a person's self-esteem is to be raised, it is essential to provide an opportunity for privacy and a place where personal belongings can be kept. In most settings a substitute has been found for the barracklike dormitories and public showers once present in many large psychiatric hospitals. The mass approach to the care of human beings destroys self-esteem and the sense of individual worth. The key to a therapeutic environment is providing for the unique needs of individuals rather than dealing with clients as members of a crowd. In the past the idea that nothing should be arranged for one client unless it could be arranged for the group led many hospital staffs away from treating people as individuals. This attitude sometimes increased the client's difficulties rather than providing opportunities to solve problems.

If clients are to receive individualized care, and if the environment is to be therapeutic, living quarters must be attractive and inviting. In most instances, no more than two persons should share the same bedroom. If possible, single rooms should be provided for individuals who have strong feelings about sharing a room with another person. Clothes closets and dressers or satisfactory substitutes for this equipment must be available. It is important for clients to bring personal clothing and other equipment to the hospital so that they can be attractively and appropriately groomed. The use of hospital clothing may be necessary in rare instances, but in the past this dress helped to depersonalize the clients and reduced them to a group of human beings with a universal attitude of hopelessness. Because it is therapeutic for clients to assume responsibility for their personal cleanliness, laundry facilities should be available.

Furniture arrangement in communal areas such as day rooms is very important in facilitating social interaction between and among clients and staff. A variety of comfortable chairs and sofas should be organized in conversational groupings to encourage spontaneous discussion. Furthermore, the furniture should be light enough to be easily moved when a larger group needs to be accommodated. Although a television set is almost always present in a day room, it should not be the focal point of the room with all the furniture arranged to facilitate easy viewing. In such a setting, even the casual observer understands that the solitary activity of television viewing is more valued than social interaction.

Dining room facilities are important in developing a therapeutic environment. Mealtime should be a leisurely experience and a time for sharing ideas and reinforcing friendly relationships. It is not merely a time for the intake of food. Nurses can profitably assume a therapeutic role by serving as hostesses at small tables that seat groups of four to six clients. The role of hostess is more effective if the nurse shares the meal with the clients. This plan has been used successfully in some hospitals. As hostess the nurse can encourage conversation and can help make mealtime a happy, relaxed, and rewarding group experience. Such mealtime experiences cannot be initiated unless a dining room is attached to the unit itself. Serving meals in large, noisy dining rooms where hundreds of people are fed makes it impossible to achieve other therapeutic goals.

Bathrooms should provide privacy. Although locks on doors may not be advisable, it is possible to provide toilet doors that close and shower rooms equipped with screens. The past practice of showering 10 to 15 persons at a time helped to reduce the individual to a member of a crowd and negated other attempts to help the client feel like a respected human being. The therapeutic environment can develop most effectively when physical surroundings help clients to feel that they are respected and that their personal preferences are recognized, appreciated, and considered.

THE THERAPEUTIC COMMUNITY—A FORM OF THERAPEUTIC ENVIRONMENT

The therapeutic community is a treatment modality wherein the environment is used as a therapeutic intervention. The therapeutic community strives to involve clients in their therapy, to restore their self-confidence by providing many opportunities for decision making, to increase their self-awareness, and to focus their attention and concern away from self and toward the needs of others. It has been organized in various ways in different settings and has been most successful with groups of clients who are in contact with reality.

Significant aspects of a therapeutic community include the following:

1. The emphasis in a therapeutic community is placed on social and group interaction, with both individual clients and staff as important members of the community.
2. The goal of the therapeutic community is to provide a favorable climate in which clients can gain an awareness of their feelings, thoughts, impulses, and behavior; try new interpersonal skills in a relatively safe environment; increase personal self-esteem; and realistically appraise the potentially helpful and destructive aspects of their behavior.
3. The work of the therapeutic community and the maintenance of an open network of communication are achieved through a daily meeting attended by all staff members and all clients who work and live on the specific unit.
4. A successful therapeutic community requires that both staff and individual clients become fully aware of their roles, limitations, responsibilities, and authority.
5. Staff members in a therapeutic community make information openly available to clients with whom they share treatment responsibilities.
6. The treatment arena in the therapeutic community includes all relationships among the members of the community, with special attention being given to the network of communication among members.

An important feature of a therapeutic community is the establishment of a democratic environment in which those people affected by a decision are involved in making it. Historically, administrators and professional staffs have believed that persons who are ill enough to require hospitalization are incapable of making wise judgments and therefore must have all decisions made for them. Clients in most hospitals where this philosophy has been implemented have been reduced to a dependent state. There is a growing realization that forcing an adult person into such a dependent role is not usually necessary and is not therapeutic. Some completely dependent persons must have decisions made for them, such as acutely ill or unconscious patients. However, despite the reason for hospitalization, most adults are able to make valid decisions about many things involving their welfare. Forcing the dependent role on some persons with a mental illness may be particularly unfortunate. Some have spent a lifetime struggling with a desire to be dependent. When hospitalization forces this role on such an individual, he or she may never be able to relinquish it.

A therapeutic community requires that clients have an opportunity to participate in the formulation of rules and regulations that affect their personal liberties. Following through with such a plan means that clients would be involved in formulating policies that regulate bedtime; late night privileges; weekend passes; social activities; control of the radio, television, and piano; check-in time when returning to the hospital from a weekend; reporting for meals; and the many other aspects of personal life influenced by rules in the usual inpatient psychiatric setting. Also, it is thought to be therapeutic to involve clients in making decisions about behavior and relationships among the unit population. Thus, clients in a therapeutic community might be given responsibility for rendering a judgment about the infringement of unit rules, settling arguments between clients, judging the appropriateness of granting weekend privileges for certain members of the group, and many other decisions regarding the regulation of life on the unit.

Careful preparation of both the staff and the clients should be ensured before a therapeutic community is initiated. The staff may have difficulty accepting the activities and responsibilities granted to clients. Before a therapeutic community is initiated, a thorough exploration of the implications of such an undertaking should be carried on through group discussions. All levels of staff, including support staff such as secretaries and housekeepers, should be involved in these group discussions because all will be affected by the therapeutic community. All members of the staff must have a thorough understanding of the goals and limitations of the undertaking. Clients should also have an opportunity to explore its implications through group discussions. Both clients and staff must understand what responsibilities they can and cannot assume.

Active administrative sanction, acceptance, and interest are essential if the therapeutic community is to be successful. Involving clients in decision making represents a drastic change in the entire administrative philosophy of many hospitals. The therapeutic community cannot be expected to function smoothly at all times, and problems will undoubtedly arise. Decisions made by clients will not always be the most ap-

propriate. Unless the entire staff believes that involving clients in decision making is therapeutically valuable and worth the struggle, dissenting forces may destroy the undertaking.

Meetings of the therapeutic community should be held regularly and at specific times if they are to be effective. Meetings should not be allowed to deteriorate into complaint sessions or to focus entirely on what the hospital should do for clients. This can be avoided if the group has some real responsibility for solving problems relating to clients' needs.

In one instance the members of a therapeutic community in a small unit of a large psychiatric hospital held a meeting to consider the problem of three suicide attempts made in 1 week by a young woman on the unit. Their decision was to institute a buddy system so that she would be accompanied at all times by one of a group of clients, each of whom would be assigned to spend a specific amount of time with her daily. Several weeks after this decision was made, the system was working well, and the woman had made no further suicide attempts. At this same meeting, other problems considered were the late return of a client from a weekend holiday, a fight between two clients, and the request by a new client for a weekend pass.

It is much easier for the staff to make all decisions for clients, but this procedure has minimum therapeutic value. When clients have the opportunity to make decisions about their own and other people's behavior, they are presented with a realistic learning experience.

THE IMPLICATIONS OF THE THERAPEUTIC ENVIRONMENT FOR THE NURSE

It is not possible to develop a therapeutic environment without a nurse's strong, intelligent leadership. When many traditional rules and regulations of the psychiatric unit are discarded and it becomes a place that focuses on meeting the needs of the individual and the group, nurses are forced to accept a more active therapeutic role with clients. Nurses find it necessary to assign the clerical work, which formerly kept them confined to the nurse's station, to a secretary to free themselves to give leadership to the personnel as they participate with clients in all the planned activities. Persons with a mental illness require mature help and guidance in initiating and carrying out social activities.

When clients begin to experiment with new ways of behaving, they will make use of the nurse as an understanding person with whom they can discuss daily problems and emotional stressors. The nurse needs to be more alert than ever to changes in behavior. In a therapeutic environment, many traditional safeguards are removed, and therefore safety of clients depends more than ever on an alert nursing staff. Thus it becomes the nurse's responsibility to recognize changes in mood and behavior of clients and to intervene at appropriate times.

Skill in understanding group behavior and in directing groups is essential in the therapeutic environment. The nurse needs to work actively with the client government to solve many unit problems. Finally, active, functioning channels of communication are essential. The nurse's ability as a leader is reflected in the total effectiveness of the psychiatric team and ultimately in the therapeutic climate of the psychiatric unit. The effectiveness of the client's total hospital experience depends greatly on the level of professional leadership provided by the nurse.

KEY POINTS

1. Creating and maintaining a therapeutic environment are major responsibilities of the nursing staff. For an environment to be truly therapeutic, its design must be based on the clients' needs and the setting's characteristics.

2. The goals of a therapeutic environment in an inpatient treatment setting are to help increase the client's self-esteem and feelings of personal worth, to improve the client's ability to relate to others, and to enable the client to work and live more effectively in the community.

3. Meeting clients' physical needs is a fundamental characteristic of a therapeutic environment, although many other of its characteristics reflect socioemotional climate and physical structure.

4. Limit setting in a therapeutic environment means establishing rules of conduct involving all those affected by the rules. Rules should be kept to a minimum; those that exist should be both enforceable and beneficial to the clients.

5. A therapeutic environment can be developed in any setting. However, it is helpful if the physical environment is attractive and provides for privacy, informal socialization, and planned group activities.

6. Significant aspects of a therapeutic community include emphasis on social and group interaction; a growth-producing socioemotional climate; a daily meeting of all staff and clients; an awareness by all of roles, limitations, responsibilities, and authority of members; availability of information; and a focus on the network of communication among members.

7. The nurse must take an active leadership role in creating a therapeutic environment, delegating tasks that formerly kept the nurse confined to the nurses' station. It is also essential for the nurse to have skill in understanding group behavior and in directing groups.

SUGGESTED SOURCES OF ADDITIONAL INFORMATION

Baldwin LJ, Ramos NB: Role of the health care supervisor in management of a therapeutic milieu, *Health Care Supervisor* 4:12, July 1986.

Baldwin S: Effects of furniture rearrangement on the atmosphere of wards in a maximum security hospital, *Hosp Community Psychiatry* 36:525, July 1985.

Bell MD, Ryan ER: Where can therapeutic community ideals be realized? An examination of three treatment environments, *Hosp Community Psychiatry* 36:1286, December 1985.

Corey LJ and others: Psychiatric ward atmosphere, *J Psychosoc Nurs Ment Health Serv* 24:10, October 1986.

Devine B: Therapeutic milieu/milieu therapy: an overview, *J Psychosoc Nurs Ment Health Serv* 19:20, March 1981.

Emrich K: Helping or hurting? Interacting in the psychiatric milieu, *J Psychosoc Nurs Ment Health Serv* 27(12):26, 1989.

Greenblatt M, York RH, Brown IL: *From custodial to therapeutic patient care in mental hospitals,* New York, 1979, Arno Press.

Gutheil TG: The therapeutic milieu: changing themes and theories, *Hosp Community Psychiatry* 36:1279, December 1985.

Islam A, Turner D: The therapeutic community: a critical reappraisal, *Hosp Community Psychiatry* 33:651, August 1982.

James I: A systematic comparison of feedback and staff discussion in changing the ward atmosphere, *J Adv Nurs* 15:329, 1990.

Jones M: *Beyond the therapeutic community* New Haven, Conn, 1968, Yale University Press.

Jones M: *The therapeutic community: a new treatment method in psychiatry,* New York, 1953, Basic Books.

LeCuyer E: Milieu therapy for short stay units: a transformed practice theory, *Arch Psychiatr Nurs* 1(2):108, 1992.

Main S and others: Patient and staff perceptions of a psychiatric ward environment, *Issues Ment Health Nurs* 12:149, 1991.

Milne D: Planning and evaluating innovations in nursing practice by measuring the ward atmosphere, *J Adv Nurs* 11:203, 1986.

Mulvihill D: Therapeutic relationships in milieu therapy, *Can J Psychiatr Nurs* 30(1):21, 1989.

Raskinski K, Razinshy R, Pasulka P: Practical implications of a theory of the "therapeutic milieu" for psychiatric nursing practice, *J Psychosoc Nurs Ment Health Serv* 18:16, May 1980.

Tuck I, Keels M: Milieu therapy: a review of development of this concept and its implications for psychiatric nursing, *Issues Ment Health Nurs* 13:51, 1992.

Warner S: Humor and self-disclosure within the milieu, *J Psychosoc Nurs Ment Health Serv* 22:17, April 1984.

White J: Resistance within the therapeutic community, *Perspect Psychiatr Care* 25(1):28, 1989.

Yurkovich E: Patient and nurse roles in the therapeutic community, *Perspect Psychiatr Care* 25(3,4):18, 1989.

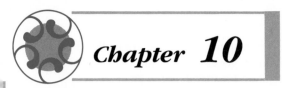

Chapter *10*

Psychopharmacology

Barbara L. MacDermott

LEARNING OBJECTIVES
After studying this chapter, the student will be able to:
* Identify frequently prescribed antipsychotic agents, antidepressants, antianxiety agents, and antimanic agents.
* Describe the mechanism of action of antipsychotic agents, antidepressants, antianxiety agents, and antimanic agents.

* List the common side effects and adverse reactions of antipsychotic agents, antidepressants, antianxiety agents, and antimanic agents.
* Identify frequently used medications that interact with antipsychotic agents, antidepressants, antianxiety agents, and antimanic agents.
* List the usual contraindications and precautions for antipsychotic agents, antidepressants, antianxiety agents, and antimanic agents.

KEY TERMS
Phenothiazines
Thioxanthenes
Butyrophenones
Dihydroindolones
Dibenzoxazepines
Extrapyramidal side effects (EPS)
Akathisia
Parkinsonism
Dyskinesias
Dystonias
Tardive dyskinesia
Neuroleptic malignant syndrome
Tyramine

Since psychotropic agents continue to increase as a major modality for persons with a mental illness, and since the nurse has the responsibility for administering these medications and monitoring their side effects, it is more important than ever that the nurse understand the actions of these medications. This chapter introduces the classifications of the major drugs typically used to treat mental illnesses: antipsychotic agents, antidepressants, antianxiety (anxiolytic) agents, and the antimanic agent lithium. Each classification is discussed in relation to its physiological actions and intended uses. Contraindications and precautions, side effects and adverse reactions, and interactions with other medications or substances are also presented.

Other drugs discussed in this chapter are those used as adjunctive agents: barbiturates, chloral hydrate, and diphenhydramine.

Because the focus of this chapter is limited to a discussion of the drugs typically used in the treatment of persons with a mental illness, nursing implications, including client teaching, are integrated throughout this text. For example, the importance of client assessment before the administration of these potent chemical agents is discussed in Chapter 8 as a major aspect of the nurse's technical role. Client teaching regarding each classification of drug is included in the chapter that discusses the disorder for which the drug is usually prescribed.

HISTORICAL PERSPECTIVE

For hundreds of years, persons with a mental illness were isolated from society, hidden in the cellars or attics of their homes, often poorly treated and ignored by family members except for meeting their most basic needs. During the first half of the twentieth century, the number of persons with a mental illness increased dramatically. By the early 1950s, more than half the hospital beds in the United States were in psychiatric wards. Most beds were in large psychiatric hospitals that were controlled by state or county governments and where patients remained for months or years.

Until the advent of antipsychotic drug therapy, treatment of persons with a mental illness consisted of physical restraints such as straitjackets, brain surgery (lobotomy), insulin or electrical shock therapy, and water or ice pack therapy. The few medications used were primarily sedatives: barbiturates, chloral hydrate, and paraldehyde.

The first of the antipsychotic agents, chlorpromazine (Thorazine), was introduced in 1956, beginning a revolution in the treatment of persons with a mental illness. Since then, many pharmacological agents have been marketed to treat the symptoms of schizophrenia. Other agents have been developed to treat depression, anxiety, and mania.

As research continues on the causes of mental illnesses, pharmaceutical research also continues in an effort to find even more effective medications to treat persons with these illnesses. In the past 30 years, evidence has increasingly indicated that substances in the nervous system called neurotransmitters, specifically a catecholamine called dopamine, may cause schizophrenia and that a lack of other catecholamines may cause depression. The history of drug therapy to treat persons with a mental illness continues to be written. All health care workers are responsible for keeping abreast of the latest developments in this treatment modality.

REVIEW OF THE NERVOUS SYSTEM

An understanding of the nervous system is foundational to an accurate understanding and appreciation of the effects of medications on the symptoms of mental illness.

The nervous system consists of two divisions: the *central nervous system* (CNS) and the *peripheral nervous system* (PNS). The CNS is composed of the brain and spinal cord and controls all body functions. It is responsible for behavior, consciousness, memory, learning, abstract reasoning, and creative thought. The CNS also regulates blood pressure, body temperature, gastric secretions, heart rate, muscular activity, and respirations.

The PNS transmits information to and from the CNS via a system of neurons (nerve fibers). The PNS has two divisions: the *somatic nervous system* (SNS) and the *autonomic nervous system* (ANS). The somatic nervous system controls voluntary or skeletal muscle.

The ANS is further divided into the *sympathetic* and *parasympathetic nervous systems*. The ANS acts on the cardiac muscle, smooth muscles,

and the glands. Figure 10-1 shows the divisions of the nervous system.

The following sections describe the central and autonomic nervous systems in more detail.

Central nervous system

The CNS consists of the brain and the spinal cord (Figure 10-2). The *cerebrum* is the largest part of the brain and is divided into two hemispheres, right and left, connected by a band of tissue called the *corpus callosum*. The outer surface of each hemisphere is composed of gray matter and is called the *cerebral cortex*. The cortex is believed to be the site of consciousness.

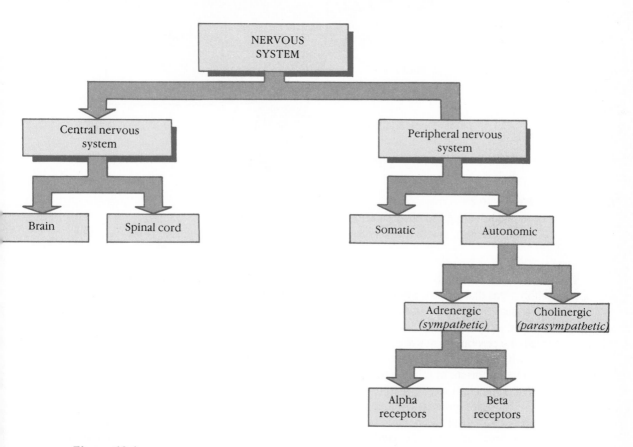

Figure 10-1

Overview of the nervous system.

From McKendry L, Salerno E: *Mosby's pharmacology in nursing,* ed 2, St Louis, 1992, Mosby–Year Book.

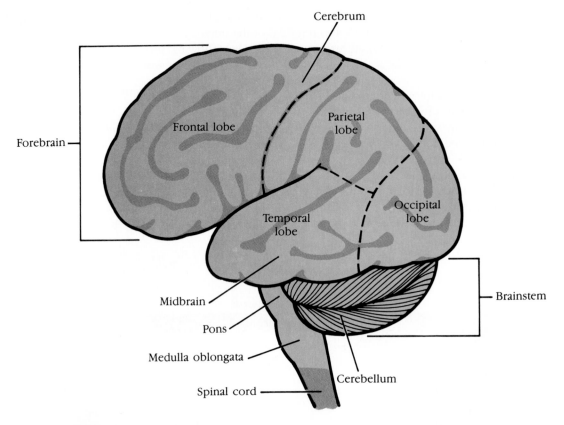

Figure 10-2
The human brain and other parts of the central nervous system.
From McKendry L, Salerno E: *Mosby's pharmacology in nursing,* ed 2, St Louis, 1992, Mosby–Year Book.

The cortex is divided into sensory, motor, and association areas that receive impulses from the sensory organs (eyes, ears, nose, mouth, skin) and from the joints, muscles, and tendons.

Beneath the cerebral cortex are structures and tracts of white matter, several of which are thought to be important in relation to the causes of mental illnesses and to the medications currently used in treating them. The thalamus, hypothalamus, and certain other tissue masses make up the area called the *diencephalon.* The *thalamus* is the major relay center for impulses to and from the cerebral cortex, including the sensory impulses of temperature, touch, and

pain. The *hypothalamus* is a major link between the mind and body in that it, as well as other areas of the brain, is involved with the control of emotions. The hypothalamus connects the nervous system to the endocrine gland processes. The adrenal cortex hormones, growth and thyroid hormones, and hormones affecting the sex glands or functions are under the control of the hypothalamus. Antipsychotic agents act on the hypothalamus and produce certain side effects: menstrual irregularities and amenorrhea in women, stimulation of the appetite with resulting weight gain, and changes in body temperature. Tricyclic antidepressants are thought to act on

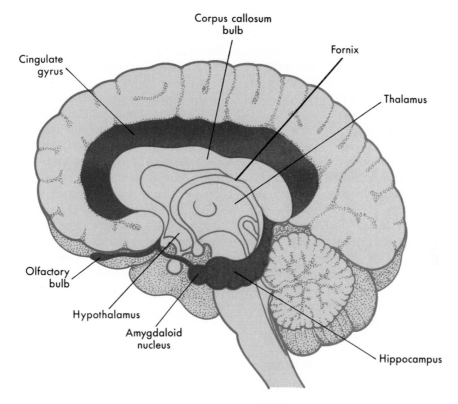

Cingulate gyrus

Corpus callosum bulb

Fornix

Thalamus

Olfactory bulb

Hypothalamus

Amygdaloid nucleus

Hippocampus

Figure 10-3

The limbic system.

Modified from McKendry L, Salerno E: *Mosby's pharmacology in nursing,* ed 2, St Louis, 1992, Mosby–Year Book.

the hypothalamus to reverse some symptoms of depression, including anorexia and weight loss, insomnia, and decreased libido.

The basal ganglia (corpus striatum, claustrum, amygdaloid nucleus) are located near the lateral ventricle of the cerebrum. The hippocampus, a mass of gray matter, is connected by a tract of fibers (fornix) to the hypothalamus. The hippocampus, fornix, amygdaloid nucleus, hippocampal gyrus, and uncus make up the *limbic system,* which is thought to be concerned with the conscious experience of emotion, especially those emotions associated with fear, pleasure, rage, and sexual behavior. The limbic system also plays

a role in the regulation of appetite, biological rhythms, and learning. Some antianxiety medications are thought to depress the limbic system, resulting in drowsiness and sleep. Figure 10-3 shows the location of the limbic system structures.

The *reticular activating system* (RAS) is a system of specific areas in the brainstem (medulla, pons, midbrain, diencephalon) that serves as a relay station for impulses between the spinal cord and the cerebral cortex. The RAS functions as the arousal or alerting system (consciousness) for the cerebral cortex and seems to play a role in filtering out extraneous stimuli, which in turn allows for concentration on a particular subject. It is thought that phenothiazine and antipsychotic agents may stimulate the RAS and strengthen the filtering process, leading to increased concentration. This may help reduce hallucinations in individuals who experience them as a symptom of their psychosis.

The reticular formation, part of the RAS, is a diffuse network of fibers and cells located throughout the medulla, pons, and midbrain. It has ascending and descending pathways that influence alertness, waking, sleeping, and some reflexes. Barbiturates depress the ascending reticular formation, which in turn decreases cortical stimuli and results in drowsiness or sleep.

The *extrapyramidal system* (EPS) is a motor pathway in the CNS associated with posture and movements of muscle groups. Antipsychotic agents that block dopamine receptors may produce side effects or adverse reactions related to the EPS.

Neurons and neuronal transmission

The neuron (nerve cell) is the basic structure of the nervous system. Neurons connect with each other but never touch each other. Between the end of one neuron and the cell body of another is a small gap called the *synapse.* Nerve transmission requires electrical conduction along the neuron and chemical transmission from neuron to neuron.

Neurotransmitters are chemicals produced and stored in the presynaptic neuron. When the neuron is stimulated and the electrical impulse reaches the end of the axon (the long "tail" of a neuron), it releases a neurotransmitter into the synapse. The neurotransmitter then diffuses across the synapse and reaches the postsynaptic site (or myoneural junction), which may be another neuron or a muscle cell.

Acetylcholine and the catecholamines (dopamine, norepinephrine, serotonin) are the major neurotransmitters in the CNS. *Acetylcholine* is found in high concentrations in the cerebral cortex. *Dopamine* is a precursor of norepinephrine

synthesis, and it is found in high concentrations in the corpus striatum and caudate nucleus (limbic system). High levels of *norepinephrine* are found in the hypothalamus, medulla, limbic system, and cranial nerve nuclei. *Serotonin* is found in the hypothalamus, midbrain, and spinal cord.

Medications such as the phenothiazine antipsychotic agents block the effects of dopamine, and this action is thought to be therapeutic in the treatment of psychoses. Dopamine blockade also accounts for the extrapyramidal side effects seen in clients taking these medications.

Changes in the levels of serotonin and norepinephrine in the nervous system are associated with behavioral changes and depression. Antidepressants inhibit the reuptake of serotonin and norepinephrine, enhancing the effects of these catecholamines and relieving depression.

Autonomic nervous system

The basic structure of the ANS consists of a preganglionic neuron, a ganglion, and a postganglionic neuron. Acetylcholine is the neurotransmitter released from the preganglionic nerve endings in both the sympathetic and the parasympathetic systems and from the postganglionic nerve endings in the parasympathetic system. Nerve fibers that release acetylcholine are called *cholinergic fibers.* Norepinephrine is the neurotransmitter released from the postganglionic nerve endings in the sympathetic nervous system. Nerve fibers that release norepinephrine are called *adrenergic fibers.* The antipsychotic and tricyclic antidepressant classifications of medication discussed later in this chapter have anticholinergic side effects. Antidepressants act on the mechanisms that usually destroy or inactivate norepinephrine and other catecholamines.

ANTIPSYCHOTIC AGENTS

The advent of antipsychotic agents (also called neuroleptic agents) in the 1950s led to extensive research to find additional medications useful in treating persons with mental illnesses. The spectrum now includes five groups of antipsychotic agents: **phenothiazines, thioxanthenes, butyrophenones, dihydroindolones,** and **dibenzoxazepines.** Table 10-1 lists these groups and individual agents with their dosage range and routes of administration.

Phenothiazines

About two thirds of the antipsychotic medications are phenothiazines. They are usually divided into three subgroups: aliphatics, piperidines, and piperazines. All phenothiazine derivatives have similar action but differ in potency and in the nature and severity of their side effects. The phenothiazines are described here as a group; the differences among the subgroups are noted at the end of this section.

Mechanism of action

Phenothiazine derivatives act primarily to block dopamine receptors in brain tissue. Do-

Table 10-1. Antipsychotic medications: dosage and administration

MEDICATION (TRADE NAME)	DOSAGE RANGE	ROUTE OF ADMINISTRATION
Phenothiazines		
Aliphatics		
Chlorpromazine (Thorazine)	50-2000 mg daily	Oral, parenteral, rectal
Triflupromazine (Vesprin)	30-150 mg daily	Oral, parenteral
Piperidines		
Mesoridazine (Serentil)	150-400 mg daily	Oral, parenteral
Thioridazine (Mellaril)	75-800 mg daily	Oral
Piperazines		
Fluphenazine (Permitil, Prolixin)	2-40 mg daily	Oral, parenteral
Fluphenazine decanoate (Prolixin Decanoate)	12.5-100 mg every 2-3 weeks	Parenteral
Perphenazine (Trilafon)	12-64 mg daily	Oral, parenteral
Prochlorperazine (Compazine)	15-150 mg daily	Oral, parenteral, rectal
Trifluoperazine (Stelazine)	4-40 mg daily	Oral, parenteral
Thioxanthenes		
Thiothixene (Navane)	5-60 mg daily	Oral, parenteral
Chlorprothixene (Taractan)	40-60 mg daily	Oral, parenteral
Butyrophenones		
Haloperidol (Haldol)	2-60 mg daily	Oral, parenteral
Haloperidol decanoate (Haldol Decanoate)	20-100 mg every 4 weeks	Parenteral
Dihydroindolones		
Molindone (Lidone, Moban)	15-225 mg daily	Oral
Dibenzoxazepines		
Loxapine (Daxolin, Loxitane)	15-250 mg daily	Oral, parenteral

pamine is a neurotransmitter in the subcortical area and in the basal ganglia in the brain. These areas are associated with emotions, motor functions, and cognitive functioning. Excessive dopamine activity is believed to be an important factor in the development of schizophrenia.

Phenothiazines also depress the release of most hormones from the hypothalamus and pituitary gland, produce blockade of alpha-adrenergic receptors in the sympathetic nervous system, and inhibit the action of dopamine within the medulla in the chemoreceptor trigger zone (CTZ). In addition, these agents depress the reticular system in the brainstem and block the effect of the vagus nerve in the gastrointestinal tract. Phenothiazines may increase the release of prolactin, a hormone produced by the pituitary gland.

Phenothiazines, especially the aliphatic subgroup, tend to lower the seizure threshold of the cerebral cortex and produce electroencephalographic (EEG) patterns associated with epileptic seizure disorders. Clients with a history of seizures who take anticonvulsants may need to have the dose of their anticonvulsant increased.

Indications for use

Although the major clinical indication for use of the phenothiazines is schizophrenia (see Chapter 15), they are also used to treat other psychiatric disorders, such as chronic brain syndrome, the manic phase of bipolar affective disorder, and alcohol withdrawal if the patient exhibits psychotic symptoms. Because of action on the CTZ and their antivagal effect, phenothiazines are effective in preventing nausea and vomiting (antiemetic effect). They are also used to treat intractable hiccups, although the mechanism of action is unknown. Phenothiazines potentiate the action of the narcotic analgesics (pain relievers) by an unknown mechanism. Administration of a phenothiazine concurrently with a narcotic allows a smaller dose of the narcotic to be effective, and tolerance to the narcotic does not build as rapidly.

Side effects and adverse reactions

Phenothiazines act in the ANS as well as in the CNS. These actions account not only for their therapeutic effects but also for many side effects and adverse reactions. ANS action causes anticholinergic and alpha-adrenergic blocking effects. Anticholinergic effects include dry mouth, tachycardia, blurred vision, increased intraocular pressure, urinary retention, and constipation. The major adrenergic-blocking effect is hypotension, especially orthostatic hypotension. Other antiadrenergic effects include dizziness, fainting, and tachycardia. Electrocardiographic (ECG) changes also occur because of abnormal impulse conduction through the ventricles of the heart. Because of these side effects, clients with cardiovascular disease, glaucoma, and urinary retention should be monitored carefully when antipsychotic agents are used.

CNS effects of the phenothiazines include excessive sedation, depressed respirations, endocrine changes, and changes in body temperature. The person exhibits drowsiness, fatigue, lethargy, and impaired mobility and mental processes. Breathing may become slow and shallow. Temperature changes result from action on the hypothalamus, with a decrease in body temperature (hypothermia) more common than an increase (hyperthermia). Endocrine changes are caused by a decrease in hormones from the pituitary gland and hypothalamus. Women experience menstrual irregularities and may be unable to become pregnant. Males have a decreased sex drive and may develop impotence. Endocrine changes also contribute to weight gain.

Extrapyramidal side effects are thought to be caused by an imbalance between the neurotransmitters dopamine and acetylcholine in the extrapyramidal tracts in the CNS. **Akathisia** (motor restlessness, inability to sit still, pacing) is the most common. **Parkinsonism** is another extrapyramidal effect, characterized by muscle rigidity and tremors, a shuffling gait, excessive salivation and drooling, a masklike facial expression, and loss of muscle movement. Other extrapyramidal effects include **dyskinesias** (involuntary rhythmic body movements) and **dystonias** (bizarre and uncoordinated movements of the extremities, eyes, face, neck, tongue, and trunk).

When extrapyramidal symptoms occur, medications are usually prescribed to relieve them. Table 10-2 lists these medications with their dosage and the forms available. The anticholinergic action of these medications helps correct the effects of acetylcholine in the CNS and restores the dopamine/acetylcholine balance in the basal ganglia of the brain, thereby relieving extrapyramidal symptoms.

Tardive dyskinesia, a potentially irreversible neurological disorder, may occur at any time during treatment with phenothiazines: within a few months, a few years, or even after treatment has been discontinued. Tardive dyskinesia is characterized by facial grimaces, blinking, spasms of the eyelids, lip smacking, sucking, puffing and chewing of the cheeks, lateral jaw movements, and tongue thrusting. Peripheral effects include foot tapping, rocking from side to side, and jerking and writhing motions of the extremities. No known treatment exists. Clients taking phenothiazines need to be monitored carefully for tardive dyskinesia. The Abnormal Involuntary Movement Scale (AIMS) (Appendix C) developed by the National Institute for Mental Health is a helpful tool nurses may use to assess clients receiving treatment with antipsychotic agents.

Hypersensitivity reactions to phenothiazines include cholestatic jaundice, blood dyscrasias (abnormalities), and skin reactions. The incidence of cholestatic jaundice (sometimes called cholestatic hepatitis) has decreased in recent years, probably because of the improved quality of the manufacturing process. It may occur, however, and any changes in the color of the sclera of the eye or skin or complaints of dry, itching skin should be reported to the physician.

Abnormalities in the blood may range from a slight decrease in the white blood count (WBC) to life-threatening agranulocytosis. The onset of agranulocytosis may be sudden, and the appearance of any symptoms of a flulike illness or upper respiratory infection in a person receiving antipsychotic medications indicates the need for a WBC immediately.

Several types of skin disorders may occur with antipsychotic medications, especially the phenothiazines. A hypersensitive reaction may occur, such as hives, macules (discolored spots or patches on the skin), papules (raised red areas), or edema in the extremities. Contact dermatitis may occur in personnel who handle medications, especially chlorpromazine. Photosensitivity, a reaction similar to a severe sunburn, is relatively common even with moderate doses. Clients taking these medications should be cautioned about

Table 10-2. Medications used to treat extrapyramidal side effects of antipsychotic agents

MEDICATION (TRADE NAME)	DOSAGE RANGE	FORMS AVAILABLE
Amantadine (Symmetrel)	200-400 mg daily	Capsules, syrup
Benztropine (Cogentin)	0.5-6.0 mg daily	Tablets, ampules
Biperiden (Akineton)	2-16 mg daily	Tablets, ampules
Diphenhydramine (Benadryl)	75-150 mg daily	Capsules, vials, ampules
Ethopropazine (Parsidol)	50-600 mg daily	Tablets
Procyclidine (Kemadrin)	8.5-20 mg daily	Tablets
Trihexyphenidyl (Artane)	1-15 mg daily	Tablets, elixir, sustained-release capsules

exposure to the sun and instructed to wear an effective sunscreen. Some of these side effects and adverse reactions are presented in Tables 10-3 and 10-4.

Contraindications and precautions

Phenothiazines are used cautiously in clients with glaucoma because mydriasis (dilated pupil) is a common anticholinergic effect. Clients with a family history of this disease should be monitored closely and have their intraocular pressure checked at regular intervals. Another anticholinergic effect is urinary retention, and men with prostatic hypertrophy (enlarged prostate gland) need to be monitored carefully. Phenothiazines can lower the seizure threshold. Clients with a seizure disorder may need a higher dose of anticonvulsant medications.

Because of the many actions on the cardiovascular system, phenothiazines are usually contraindicated in persons with any form of cardiovascular disease. If these agents are prescribed, clients should have their blood pressure monitored frequently and periodic ECGs taken.

Interactions

CNS depression may be enhanced when antipsychotic agents are given with other CNS depressants, including alcohol, antihistamines, narcotic analgesics, and sedatives and hypnotics. These interactions most often cause excessive sedation and severe respiratory depression.

Anticholinergic side effects from antipsychotic agents may be pronounced, and when these agents are given concurrently with other medi-

Table 10-3. Side effects of antipsychotic agents

SIDE EFFECT	COMMENTS
Dry mouth, blurred vision, constipation, urinary hesitancy, paralytic ileus	These effects result from drug's interference with acetylcholine. First three effects should be treated symptomatically and client reassured. In clients with urinary hesitancy and paralytic ileus, medication should be withheld until medical evaluation is obtained.
Orthostatic hypotension	Drug is used with great caution if cardiovascular disease is present and in elderly persons. Client should be warned about possible occurrences and taught to rise slowly and dangle legs before standing.
Photosensitivity	Occurs most frequently with chlorpromazine. Protect client from ultraviolet light. Use sunscreen. Examine skin frequently.
Endocrine changes	Weight gain, edema, lactation, and menstrual irregularities. Treat symptomatically. Reassure client.
Extrapyramidal system	Dose and duration related. Symptoms are managed by adjusting dose of drug or adding antiparkinsonian drug.
Pseudoparkinsonism	Typical shuffling gait, masklike facies, tremor, muscular rigidity, slowing of movements, drooling, and other symptoms mimicking those seen in Parkinson's disease
Akathisia	Continuous restlessness, fidgeting, and pacing; verbal complaints of "jitters"
Dystonias	Spasm of neck muscles, extensor rigidity of back muscles, carpopedal spasm, rolled-back eyes, and swallowing difficulties. Acute onset occurs, but condition is reversible with appropriate medication. Reassurance should be provided until symptoms subside.
Akinesia	Lethargy, feelings of fatigue, muscle weakness, and blunt affect; must be differentiated from withdrawal

cations that also cause these effects (e.g., anti-depressants, some antiparkinsonism agents), the anticholinergic effects may be excessive.

The risk of agranulocytosis is increased when phenothiazines are given with antithyroid medications. When antacids or antidiarrheal suspensions are taken at the same time as antipsychotic medications, the absorption of antipsychotic medications is blocked. Since antipsychotic agents may lower the seizure threshold, the dosage of anticonvulsants such as phenytoin (Dilantin) may need to be increased.

Phenothiazine subgroups

The *aliphatic* phenothiazines are especially effective in the control of psychotic symptoms, including hallucinations and delusions. Chlorpromazine, the first of the antipsychotic agents discovered, is still considered the prototype for this class of medication. Aliphatics produce strong sedative effects and moderate to strong extrapyramidal effects.

The *piperidine* phenothiazines have strong sedative effects and moderate to strong anticholinergic effects. They produce weak extrapyramidal effects.

The *piperazine* phenothiazines are the largest group of antipsychotic medications in current use. They have mild sedative effects but strong extrapyramidal effects. Piperazines cause fewer anticholinergic side effects and less hypotension than other phenothiazine subgroups.

Table 10-4. Possible adverse reactions to antipsychotic agents

ADVERSE REACTION	COMMENTS
Skin reactions	Urticarial, maculopapular, edematous, or petechial responses may occur 1 to 5 weeks after initiation of treatment. Withhold drug until after medical evaluation.
Jaundice	Develops in about 4% of clients and is a dangerous complication; drug should be discontinued.
Agranulocytosis, leukopenia	Chlorpromazine depresses production of leukocytes. Initial symptoms of sore throat, high temperature, and lesions in mouth indicate that drug should be stopped immediately. Outcome may be lethal, but this is rare.
Ocular changes	Corneal and lenticular changes and pigmentary retinopathy may occur with high dosages over long periods. Periodic ocular examinations are recommended.
Convulsions	Antipsychotic agents lower seizure threshold, making seizure-prone persons more likely to have seizures. Clients with a history of seizures or organic conditions associated with seizures require an increased dosage of anticonvulsant medication if antipsychotics are used.
Tardive dyskinesia	Insidious onset of fine vermicular movements of tongue occurs, which is reversible if drug is discontinued at this time. Can progress to rhythmical involuntary movements of the tongue, face, mouth, or jaw with protrusion of tongue, puffing of cheeks, and chewing movements. No known treatment; often irreversible. Prevention is imperative. Females over 50 years of age receiving prolonged doses are particularly at risk. Do *not* withhold drug until after medical evaluation; symptoms will increase.
Neuroleptic malignant syndrome	High fever, tachycardia, increased respirations and pulse, diaphoresis, muscular rigidity, stupor, tremor, and incontinence occur. *This condition is life-threatening.* Early recognition is critical. Discontinue medications, notify physician, and provide supportive care.

Thioxanthenes

Thiothixene and chlorprothixene are chemically different but pharmacologically similar to the phenothiazines in terms of antipsychotic and antiemetic action. They have weak anticholinergic, hypotensive, and sedative side effects, but the incidence of extrapyramidal symptoms is similar to that of the phenothiazines.

Butyrophenones

Haloperidol is the only drug in this group used for psychiatric disorders. A related drug, droperidol, is used in anesthesia and as an antiemetic. Haloperidol is chemically different from but pharmacologically similar to the phenothiazines. It is effective in the treatment of psychoses and may be useful in the manic phase of bipolar disorders (see Chapter 16).

Haloperidol is the drug of choice for clients with two neurological diseases, Tourette's syndrome and Huntington's disease (chorea). Huntington's disease is a genetic disorder involving progressive psychiatric symptoms and involuntary movements. Gilles de la Tourette's syndrome is a neurological disorder that begins in childhood and continues through the life span. It occurs more often in males than in females. Symptoms include facial and vocal tics (blinking and grimaces, barking, grunting, shouting, compulsive swearing) and involuntary purposeless movements. No cure exists for Tourette's syndrome, but haloperidol and pimozide often produce dramatic improvement. *Pimozide* is an antipsychotic agent approved only for the treatment of Tourette's syndrome in clients who do not respond to haloperidol.

Haloperidol has side effects and adverse reactions similar to those of the phenothiazines. However, the incidence of hypotension is lower, whereas extrapyramidal effects occur more frequently with haloperidol.

Neuroleptic malignant syndrome (NMS) is a serious, potentially fatal reaction. The occurrence of NMS is not limited to association with haloperidol or even with antipsychotic drugs; it can occur with any medication that alters dopamine mechanisms in the CNS. NMS is discussed here because haloperidol is a highly potent agent that causes extensive dopamine blockade in the brain.

NMS occurs in association with other extrapyramidal symptoms, including parkinsonism, akathisia, and dystonic reactions. Risk for NMS is dramatically increased by the use of two or more neuroleptic agents concurrently and by depot injections of antipsychotic agents. NMS can occur after only one dose or after years of treatment. Signs and symptoms of NMS often develop suddenly. The first symptom is usually rapid onset of muscular rigidity and akinesia, often with respiratory difficulty. Hyperthermia occurs in the range of 101° to 103° F, but the temperature may go much higher. An increased temperature is the cardinal sign of NMS; the client should be closely monitored. An elevated temperature should cause the nurse to suspect NMS if other symptoms are present. General physical decline is progressive over the next 48 to 72 hours and is accompanied by signs of autonomic dysfunction, including tachycardia, diaphoresis, rapid and labored breathing, fluctuations in blood pressure, and incontinence. NMS also produces CNS symptoms such as confusion, delirium, catatonic-like posturing, and combativeness.

At times the onset may be more gradual, and the person may develop less severe symptoms such as tachycardia, diaphoresis, and severely altered consciousness or delirium. These symptoms may be mistaken for an infection or an acute exacerbation of the mental illness, especially if they spontaneously remit.

Death from NMS occurs from an accumulation of secondary and tertiary complications, such as kidney failure or respiratory failure. Treatment is not specific but addresses the symptoms and may require the client's admission to an intensive care unit of a general hospital. Because of its life-threatening nature, any client receiving neuroleptic agents who has symptoms of NMS should be taken off these drugs immediately, even if this means an increase in combative behavior (Blair and Dauner, 1993). The physician should be notified as soon as NMS is suspected.

Dihydroindolones

Molindone is the only drug of this chemical class available for psychiatric use. It blocks dopamine receptors in the RAS and limbic system in the same way as do the phenothiazines. Molindone is not recommended for children under age 12 years. Because the oral tablets contain calcium citrate, molindone may reduce the absorption of the tetracyclines, a subgroup of anti-infectives, and phenytoin, an anticonvulsant. Dosages of these drugs may need to be increased if the client is also taking molindone.

Dibenzoxazepines

The dibenzoxazepine loxapine is currently recommended for use only in the treatment of clients with long-standing symptoms of schizophrenia who have not responded to other agents. Another medication in this class marketed in 1990 is clozapine, but the drug is currently available only under certain restrictive conditions. Clozapine does not cause extrapyramidal effects, but there is an increased risk of agranulocytosis, a blood disorder characterized by a significant, potentially life-threatening decrease in white blood cells. Weekly WBCs are ordered if a patient is receiving this medication.

ANTIDEPRESSANTS

Antidepressants are used in the treatment of clients with affective disorders, sometimes called mood or depressive disorders (see Chapter 16). The current classifications of major affective disorders are bipolar affective disorder and unipolar disorder. *Bipolar affective disorder* is characterized by periods of depression interspersed with periods of mania or hypomania. *Unipolar disorder* is characterized by periods of depression, without mania, interspersed with periods of normal mood. The cause of depression is un-

clear, but it seems to relate either to a deficiency of the neurotransmitters norepinephrine and serotonin in the postsynaptic adrenergic receptors in the brain or to an increased sensitivity of these receptors to the neurotransmitters. Medications used to treat depression include tricyclic and tetracyclic antidepressants and monoamine oxidase inhibitors. In recent years, several medications have been marketed that are chemically different from tricyclic antidepressants and whose action is specific to inhibition of serotonin reuptake. Another agent, bupropion, is the first in a new chemical class of antidepressants. Table 10-5 lists the antidepressants (as well as lithium, the antimanic agent), their dosages, and routes of administration.

Tricyclic/tetracyclic antidepressants

The tricyclic antidepressants (TCAs) are usually the first medications prescribed to treat clients with affective disorders. Tetracyclic antidepressants are also used, although rarely as the first course of therapy.

Mechanism of action

TCAs may block the reuptake of the catecholamines norepinephrine and serotonin in the sympathetic nervous system. When a catecholamine is released from the postganglionic neuron, some of it diffuses through the capillaries into the bloodstream, and some is deactivated by the enzymes monoamine oxidase (MAO) and catechol-O-methyltransferase (COMT). However, most of it is taken back into the postganglionic neuron and stored again for use later, a process called the *reuptake mechanism.* TCAs are thought to block this process, making norepinephrine and serotonin available in larger amounts and for a longer time. It requires up to 4 weeks to achieve maximum therapeutic response to TCAs.

Indications for use

TCAs have several uses other than for depression. Clomipramine is useful in treating obses-

Table 10-5. Antidepressants and antimanic agents: dosage and administration

MEDICATION (TRADE NAME)	DOSAGE RANGE	ROUTE OF ADMINISTRATION
Tricyclics		
Amitriptyline (Elavil, others)	50-300 mg daily	Oral, parenteral
Amoxapine (Asendin)	100-400 mg daily	Oral
Clomipramine (Anafranil)	25-250 mg daily	Oral
Desipramine (Norpramin, Pertofrane)	25-300 mg daily	Oral
Doxepin (Adapin, Sinequan)	25-300 mg daily	Oral
Imipramine (Tofranil, others)	30-300 mg daily	Oral, parenteral
Nortriptyline (Aventyl, Pamelor)	30-150 mg daily	Oral
Protriptyline (Vivactil)	15-16 mg daily	Oral
Trimipramine (Surmontil)	50-300 mg daily	Oral
Tetracyclics		
Maprotiline (Ludiomil)	50-225 mg daily	Oral
Serotonin reuptake inhibitors		
Fluoxetine (Prozac)	20-80 mg daily	Oral
Sertraline (Zoloft)	50-200 mg daily	Oral
Trazodone (Desyrel)	50-400 mg daily	Oral
Monoamine oxidase inhibitors		
Isocarboxazid (Marplan)	10-30 mg daily	Oral
Phenelzine (Nardil)	15-90 mg daily	Oral
Tranylcypromine (Parnate)	10-60 mg daily	Oral
Aminoketones		
Bupropion (Wellbutrin)	100-450 mg daily	Oral
Antimanic agents		
Lithium (Eskalith, Lithane)	900-1800 mg daily	Oral

sive-compulsive disorder (see Chapter 17). Imipramine is an effective medication used to treat childhood enuresis (nocturnal bedwetting) and phobic attacks, especially agoraphobia (fear of being alone in public or large open spaces). In recent years, low doses of TCAs have been found to be effective as adjuncts to analgesics (pain relievers), and in some persons, they have been effective in decreasing pain levels when given alone, especially in clients with intractable pain, peripheral neuritis, and neuralgia.

The use of a particular antidepressant is often based on its side effects. For example, TCAs that cause a high degree of sedation and block primarily the reuptake of serotonin (amitriptyline, doxepin, nontricyclic fluoxetine) may be prescribed for a client who is depressed and also agitated. Antidepressants that block norepinephrine uptake (desipramine, nortriptyline) are more often prescribed for the depressed client who is withdrawn.

Since the side effects of hypotension and tachycardia could be detrimental to clients with cardiac disease, medications that cause a lower degree of these effects may be chosen. Nortriptyline and desipramine cause less hypotension, and imipramine and desipramine cause less tachycardia than other TCAs.

Side effects and adverse reactions

Anticholinergic side effects seen with the tricyclic/tetracyclic antidepressants are dry mouth, constipation, tachycardia, blurred vision, and urinary retention. Drowsiness and sedation often occur, especially at the beginning of therapy. Although antidepressants usually correct the sleep dysfunction characteristic of depression, they may also cause insomnia. This probably relates to the increased activity of the sympathetic nervous system, as do the side effects of confusion, dizziness, hypotension, postural (orthostatic) hypotension, nervousness, and tremors.

Extrapyramidal side effects may be seen in some clients who take these medications; the incidence is highest with amoxapine.

Contraindications and precautions

TCAs are contraindicated in clients with narrow-angle glaucoma and benign prostatic hypertrophy or a history of urinary retention because the anticholinergic side effects exacerbate these conditions. TCAs may lower the seizure threshold, so they are usually contraindicated in clients with known seizure disorders. High-dose therapy may cause dysrhythmias, sinus tachycardia, and prolonged conduction time, and persons with severe cardiovascular disease need to be monitored very carefully if TCAs are prescribed. An exacerbation of psychotic symptoms may occur in clients with schizophrenia, and careful monitoring is required. Individuals who are depressed and have suicidal ideations also should

be carefully monitored, since they are more likely to have the energy and motivation to make a suicidal attempt as their depression lifts. If they should take an overdose of a TCA, death may result. Severe renal or hepatic disease is another contraindication to the use of these medications.

Interactions

TCAs used with alcohol and other CNS depressants (antihistamines, narcotics, sedative/hypnotics) may enhance CNS depression, especially lethargy and respiratory depression. Atropine and scopolamine, antihistamines, some antiparkinsonian medications, and the phenothiazines have anticholinergic effects, and when given concurrently with TCAs, these effects may be greatly enhanced. The use of TCAs and other medications that may cause extrapyramidal effects (e.g., antipsychotic agents) may enhance the risk and severity of these symptoms. Therefore, the nurse must carefully monitor the reactions of a client who is taking both TCAs and other medications that may cause extrapyramidal effects.

The risk of agranulocytosis increases when TCAs are used concurrently with antithyroid medications. The histamine$_2$ antagonists cimetidine and ranitidine may inhibit the metabolism of TCAs, with resultant increased serum levels and toxicity of the TCAs. Dosage reductions of the TCAs may become necessary.

TCAs may decrease the antihypertensive effects of the antihypertensive agents clonidine, guanadrel, and guanethidine. Blood pressure should be monitored carefully, and doses of the antihypertensive agent may need to be increased. For some clients, these particular antihypertensive agents are discontinued and others prescribed in their place.

Oral contraceptives may affect serum levels of TCAs, and clients receiving these medications concurrently should be monitored closely for either a decrease in the therapeutic response to TCAs or for symptoms of toxicity.

Concurrent use of TCAs and monoamine oxidase inhibitors is contraindicated because hypertensive crises, hyperthermia, convulsions, and death have been reported. If the client needs to be changed from one classification of antidepressant to another, a 2-week drug-free period is advised to enable the body to eliminate the medication completely.

TCAs used with sympathomimetic medications, many of which are found in over-the-counter (OTC) medications (phenylephrine, pseudoephrine, ephedrine), increase the incidence and severity of cardiac dysrhythmias, hypertension, and tachycardia.

Monoamine oxidase inhibitors

Monoamine oxidase inhibitors (MAOIs) are the second major classification of antidepressants. Iproniazid, the first MAOI used clinically, was originally used to treat tuberculosis. It caused marked hypotension and CNS stimulation but also improved these clients' mood. These effects led to further investigation of the use of MAOIs for treating depression and hypertension.

Mechanism of action

MAO is an enzyme that deactivates the catecholamine neurotransmitters norepinephrine, dopamine, and serotonin in the CNS and ANS. MAOIs block the action of this enzyme, resulting in an increased level of the neurotransmitter at the postsynaptic junction and a more intense response at the target cells. Since evidence indicates that a lack of catecholamines, especially norepinephrine and serotonin, may cause depression, these medications are believed to be effective because they cause a response that supplies the missing neurotransmitter.

Indications for use

MAOIs are used to treat hypertension and depression. In addition, one agent (procarbazine) is an antineoplastic agent, and another (furazolidone) is an antibiotic. MAOIs are now used chiefly for depressed clients who do not respond to the tricyclic antidepressants.

Side effects and adverse reactions

The most frequent side effects of the MAOIs are CNS stimulation, hypotension, and anticholinergic effects. Signs of CNS stimulation include acute anxiety, agitation, dizziness, drowsiness, euphoria, headache, muscle twitching, and weakness. The MAOIs may lower the seizure threshold in some clients, so the dosage of anticonvulsants may need to be increased. Hypotension is the most common cardiovascular side effect. Severe hypotension may reduce coronary blood flow, causing anginal pain.

The most common anticholinergic side effects are dry mouth, blurred vision, and constipation. Urinary retention and tachycardia are seen less often. Some side effects and adverse reactions are paradoxical and may relate to dosage levels or indiviual responses to the medication. Examples of paradoxical reactions are sedation and insomnia as well as constipation and diarrhea. The box at left on p. 155 lists some common side effects of and adverse reactions to MAOIs.

MAOIs interact with foods containing **tyramine** and many medications, causing a hypertensive crisis. Tyramine is a precursor to norepinephrine and has a similar effect on blood pressure. The box at right on p. 155 lists foods and beverages containing tyramine. Clients taking MAOIs and their family members should be taught the signs and symptoms of severe hypertension: severe headache, severe chest pain, nausea and vomiting, diarrhea, changes in pulse rate (tachycardia or bradycardia), and diaphoresis.

Leukopenia, skin rashes, and sexual disorders, especially impaired erection and ejaculation in males, may also occur.

Contraindications and precautions

MAOIs are usually contraindicated in clients with a seizure disorder because they can decrease the seizure threshold. Clients with a history of cardiovascular or cerebrovascular disease (angina, cerebrovascular accident, dysrhythmias) should not have these medications prescribed

---

COMMON SIDE EFFECTS OF AND ADVERSE REACTIONS TO MONOAMINE OXIDASE INHIBITORS (MAOIs)

Side effects

Blurred vision
Constipation
Diarrhea
Drowsiness
Dry mouth
Headache
Insomnia
Orthostatic hypotension
Sedation
Sexual dysfunction
Tremors
Urination difficulty
Vertigo
Weakness
Weight gain

Adverse reactions

Edema of lower extremities
Fainting spells
Hypertensive crisis
Nervousness
Severe orthostatic hypotension
Tachycardia

FOODS AND BEVERAGES CONTAINING TYRAMINE

Cheese* (aged, including blue, brie, Camembert, cheddar, Gruyère, mozzarella, parmesan, Romano, Roquefort)
Meat and fish that has been aged without refrigeration (caviar; dried, salted fish such as pickled herring; sausages such as bologna, salami, pepperoni)
Beef and chicken livers
Certain fruits and vegetables (overripe avocados, fava beans, raisins, figs)
Alcoholic beverages (beer; liquors; sherry; red wines, especially Chianti)

---

*Cottage cheese, cream cheese, sour cream, and yogurt are allowed when eaten in moderation and only when they are fresh. Small amounts of chocolate, coffee, cola, and tea (caffeine-containing foods) are considered safe.

---

because of the effects on blood pressure. MAOIs are not recommended for elderly persons who may have some degree of cerebral atherosclerosis. These agents are used very cautiously with diabetic clients, especially if these persons are insulin dependent, because MAOIs may potentiate hypoglycemia.

Interactions

A major interaction of MAOIs is with foods containing a moderate to high amount of tyramine, an intermediate product in the conversion of the amino acid tyrosine to epinephrine. MAOIs taken with such foods may cause a hypertensive crisis. Tyramine is found in most cheeses and in foods such as beer, broad bean pods, yeast, wine,

and chicken liver. The box at right above gives a more complete listing of foods to avoid when taking MAOIs.

MAOIs used with insulin or the oral hypoglycemic agents may cause severe hypoglycemia. Concurrent use with other medications that have anticholinergic effects (atropine-like medications, antihistamines, some antiparkinsonian agents, antipsychotic agents, many OTC cold and allergy preparations) exaggerate dry mouth, blurred vision, constipation, and urinary retention.

Using MAOIs with sympathomimetic medications may lead to a dangerous hypertensive crisis. Sympathomimetic medications include amphetamines, dopamine, and OTC cold, allergy, and weight loss preparations containing ephedrine, pseudoephedrine, phenylephrine, and phenylpropanolamine.

Other antidepressants

In recent years, several agents have been discovered that are chemically different from the cyclic antidepressants and the MAOIs. Bupropion (Wellbutrin), fluoxetine (Prozac), sertraline (Zoloft), and trazodone (Desyrel) inhibit primarily the reuptake mechanism for serotonin and affect the reuptake of norepinephrine only minimally or not at all.

Bupropion causes fewer anticholinergic and cardiovascular side effects than other antidepressants. It also causes CNS stimulation rather than depression, so it does not produce sedation. The incidence of seizures is especially high in clients taking bupropion.

Fluoxetine has a long half-life, which accounts for its effects being seen for some time after it has been discontinued. Serious side effects include skin rashes and urticaria (hives). Nausea and diarrhea are common gastrointestinal side effects. Anxiety, insomnia, and nervousness have occurred in a high percentage of clients. Fluoxetine should not be given concurrently with MAOIs because of a potentially fatal interaction. If fluoxetine therapy must be changed to MAOI therapy, fluoxetine must be discontinued for at least 5 weeks before MAOI therapy begins. Changing from MAOI to fluoxetine therapy also requires 5 weeks during which the MAOI is discontinued.

Sertraline has a long half-life, which allows for once-a-day dosage and accounts for reaching therapeutic levels as quickly as 7 days. It is a selective inhibitor of the serotonin uptake mechanism in that it does not have a strong effect on cholinergic receptors, thereby causing few anticholinergic side effects. Sertraline also has minimum effect on histamine$_1$ receptors and does not produce the sedation, weight gain, and hypotension typically seen with TCAs. The most common side effects are diarrhea, insomnia, and nausea.

Trazodone is used to treat depression. Males have a significant risk of priapism (persistent, abnormal, and painful erection of the penis); in some cases, surgical intervention has been necessary. Trazodone should be taken with food, since total drug absorption is up to 20% higher when the medication is taken with food rather than on an empty stomach. Trazodone has less anticholinergic activity than many other antidepressants.

ANTIANXIETY AGENTS

Anxiety is a state in which the person experiences feelings of apprehension, fearfulness, nervousness, and worry. It is a normal response to a stressful situation and may be beneficial if the anxiety state stimulates the person to take constructive action. However, when anxiety is severe or prolonged, the person becomes unable to cope with the situation, and the usual activities of daily living are affected, therapeutic interventions, including treatment with antianxiety (anxiolytic) agents, may become necessary. In addition to generalized anxiety disorder, the American Psychiatric Association delineates anxiety into several other categories: phobias and panic disorders, obsessive-compulsive disorders, post-traumatic stress syndrome, and atypical anxiety disorders (see Chapter 17).

Medications used to treat anxiety include sedatives and hypnotics, primarily the barbiturates, meprobamate, and the benzodiazepines. The barbiturates and meprobamate have been largely replaced by the benzodiazepines. Medications used to treat anxiety are listed in Table 10-6.

Benzodiazepines

Benzodiazepines are among the most widely prescribed medications used to treat anxiety. The prototype, diazepam (Valium), was the most frequently prescribed medication in the United States during most of the 1970s and early 1980s. Benzodiazepines produce an antianxiety effect at relatively low doses. Drowsiness and other symptoms of CNS depression occur less frequently than with comparable doses of meprobamate and barbiturates. The benzodiazepines have a high potential for drug abuse.

Mechanism of action

Benzodiazepines have a wide range of selective actions in the CNS, including antianxiety, anticonvulsant, skeletal muscle relaxant, and hypnotic effects. Although the exact mechanism of action is unknown, benzodiazepines appear to

Table 10-6. Antianxiety agents: dosage and administration

MEDICATION (TRADE NAME)	DOSAGE RANGE	ROUTE OF ADMINISTRATION
Benzodiazepines*		
Alprazolam (Xanax)	0.5-4 mg daily	Oral
Chlordiazepoxide (Librium)	15-300 mg daily	Oral, parenteral
Clorazepate (Tranxene)	7.5-60 mg daily	Oral
Diazepam (Valium)	4-50 mg daily	Oral, parenteral
Halazepam (Paxipam)	20-160 mg daily	Oral
Lorazepam (Ativan)	1-10 mg daily	Oral, parenteral
Oxazepam (Serax)	30-120 mg daily	Oral
Prazepam (Centrax)	10-60 mg daily	Oral
Nonbenzodiazepines		
Buspirone (BuSpar)	15-60 mg daily	Oral
Hydroxyzine (Atarax, Vistaril)	200-400 mg daily	Oral
Meprobamate (Equanil, Miltown)	1200-2400 mg daily	Oral

*Includes only those benzodiazepines used to treat anxiety.

work in the hypothalamic, thalamic, and limbic areas. The limbic system has a highly dense area of benzodiazepine receptors, and it is believed that by binding with these receptors, benzodiazepines increase the effects of gamma-aminobutyric acid (GABA) in the RAS. GABA is an inhibitory neurotransmitter, the overall effect of which is to decrease the stimulation and arousal of the limbic cortical areas in the brain, thereby relieving anxiety.

The dorsal spinal cord also has a concentration of benzodiazepine receptors. When the benzodiazepines bind with these receptors, spinal reflexes are blocked and skeletal muscles relax. Some direct action on motor neurons may occur as well, resulting in diminished muscular activity.

Indications for use

Table 10-7 lists the benzodiazepines and their usual indications. In general, they are used for anxiety disorders, in prevention of agitation and delirium tremens in acute alcohol withdrawal, for some neuromuscular diseases, as preoperative medication (adjunctive to general anesthesia and for sedation during invasive diagnostic tests such as angiography and endoscopy), for sleep disorders, and for seizure disorders.

Side effects and adverse reactions

Benzodiazepines may cause anticholinergic side effects, especially when higher doses are used or if the drug is given parenterally. CNS effects include drowsiness and sleep, ataxia, and loss of dexterity. Elderly or debilitated clients may have a paradoxical excitement, including apprehension, insomnia, and hallucinations. In some clients, pulse rate is slowed and blood pressure lowered. Additional adverse reactions include behavioral problems such as anger and decreased ability to concentrate (primarily in children), pruritus (itching) and skin rashes, muscle weakness, and mental depression.

Contraindications and precautions

Benzodiazepines are usually contraindicated in clients with severe respiratory disorders, se-

Table 10-7. Benzodiazepines and their usual indications

MEDICATION (TRADE NAME)	INDICATIONS
Alprazolam (Xanax)	Anxiety disorders, adjunct medication with associated depression
Chlordiazepoxide (Librium)	Anxiety disorders, alcohol withdrawal, preoperative medication
Clonazepam (Clonopin)	Seizure disorders
Clorazepate (Tranxene, Tranxene-SD)	Anxiety disorders, alcohol withdrawal
Diazepam (Valium)	Anxiety disorders, alcohol withdrawal, preoperative medication, seizure disorders, skeletal muscle spasms, other neuromuscular disorders
Flurazepam (Dalmane)	Sleep disorders
Halazepam (Paxipam)	Anxiety disorders
Lorazepam (Ativan)	Anxiety disorders, adjunct medication with associated depression, preoperative medication
Midazolam (Versed)	Preoperative medication
Oxazepam (Serax)	Anxiety disorders, adjunct medication with associated depression, alcohol withdrawal
Prazepam (Centrax)	Anxiety disorders
Temazepam (Restoril)	Sleep disorders
Triazolam (Halcion)	Sleep disorders

vere kidney or liver disease, and a history of hypersensitivity to any individual agent. Because benzodiazepines have a high potential for drug abuse, they should not be prescribed for those with a history of drug abuse to any substance. Other contraindications are related to anticholinergic effects: glaucoma, enlargement of the prostate gland, and a history of severe constipation or other gastrointestinal conditions involving decreased intestinal motility.

Interactions

When benzodiazepines are used concurrently with other CNS depressants, including alcohol, antidepressants, antihistamines, narcotic analgesics, and sedatives and hypnotics, there is increased risk of significant CNS depression, especially respiratory depression. Alcohol should be avoided and doses of analgesics reduced. When benzodiazepines are used concurrently with the antiviral agent zidovudine (azidothymidine, AZT) or the anticonvulsant/antiarrhythmic phenytoin (Dilantin), the metabolism of zidovudine or phenytoin may be inhibited, and therefore the risk of their toxicity is increased. The effectiveness of the antiparkinsonian agent levodopa may be decreased if used with the benzodiazepines.

Nonbenzodiazepine agents

Antianxiety agents that are not benzodiazepines include buspirone, hydroxyzine, and meprobamate.

Buspirone

Buspirone (BuSpar) is a nonbenzodiazepine agent used to treat anxiety disorders. It is as effective as the benzodiazepines with less sedation, and it does not cause skeletal muscle relaxation. The mechanism of action is unknown. Buspirone does not affect GABA and has no significant affinity for benzodiazepine receptors. It does have an affinity for serotonin and certain dopamine receptors.

Common side effects of buspirone are headache, increased nervousness, and nausea. Other side effects include abdominal distress, dry mouth, blurred vision, insomnia, nightmares, muscle spasm, and decreased ability to concentrate. Buspirone should not be given with MAOIs because a hypertensive crisis may occur. It is given cautiously with digoxin because it replaces digoxin from plasma protein binding sites. This increases digoxin serum levels and increases the risk of digoxin toxicity.

Hydroxyzine

Hydroxyzine (Atarax, Vistaril) has antianxiety, antihistaminic, antiemetic, and sedative effects. It competes with histamine at histamine₁ receptor sites, an action that may account for its sedative and antihistaminic effects. Hydroxyzine decreases vestibular stimulation and also acts on the labyrinth in the inner ear. It may also affect the chemoreceptor trigger zone in the medulla. These CNS actions account for its antiemetic effect.

The most common side effects are sedation and anticholinergic effects, especially dry mouth. Since hydroxyzine is a CNS depressant, when it is used concurrently with other agents with similar actions, CNS depression may be enhanced.

Meprobamate

Meprobamate (Equanil, Miltown) was introduced as an antianxiety agent before the benzodiazepines were marketed. Its approved use is only as an antianxiety agent, but it is sometimes prescribed as a sedative-hypnotic agent. Meprobamate has skeletal muscle relaxant properties, although it has been largely replaced by other agents for this purpose. Meprobamate enhances the analgesic effects of other medications.

Drowsiness and ataxia are the most common side effects of meprobamate. Hypotension may occur. Hypersensitivity is relatively frequent, and the incidence is greater in persons with a history of other allergies. Meprobamate may exacerbate porphyria, a rare hereditary metabolic disorder. Abruptly discontinuing the medication is likely to cause withdrawal symptoms.

ANTIMANIC AGENTS

Mania is a disorder characterized by flight of ideas, elation, speech and motor hyperactivity, reduced sleep requirements, poor judgment, and aggressiveness. A manic state may occur and recur with little or no depression, or it may be accompanied by alternating periods of depression (bipolar affective disorder) (see Chapter 16). One theory is that an increase in catecholamines (norepinephrine, dopamine) or an increased sensitivity of the catecholamine receptors may be responsible for manic symptoms.

Lithium

Lithium is the only antimanic agent in current use, although the calcium channel blocker verapamil shows promise of becoming another effective agent in the treatment of mania.

Mechanism of action

The mechanism of action is unknown, but lithium is thought to (1) accelerate the deactivation of catecholamines at the synapse, (2) inhibit the release of catecholamine neurotransmitters at the synapse, and (3) decrease postsynaptic receptor sensitivity. The cumulative result is a decrease in catecholamine response and improvement of the manic state.

Lithium is transported across cell membranes. Not all of it is removed by the sodium pump, leaving a small amount in the cell. This decrease in intracellular sodium accounts for some side effects and may be partly responsible for the decrease in manic symptoms.

Indications for use

Lithium is used to treat the manic phase of bipolar affective disorder or mania that occurs without cycles of depression. It decreases the severity and frequency of manic episodes and is effective in about 80% of clients. Clinical effectiveness is not immediate; it may require several weeks for symptoms to disappear. Lithium is also under investigation to prevent or treat cluster headaches, premenstrual syndrome, bulimia, and genital herpes. It has been used successfully to increase the neutrophil count in clients with chronic neutropenia and in those with neutropenia caused by some antineoplastic agents.

Side effects and adverse reactions

Common side effects of lithim include thirst and increased urination, nausea, diarrhea, tremors of the hands, and weight gain. Adverse reactions include dyspnea on exertion, increased weakness, and fainting. Early signs of toxicity are anorexia, diarrhea, drowsiness, nausea and vomiting, slurred speech, and muscle weakness. As toxicity worsens, the client has blurred vision, confusion, ataxia, severe trembling, and seizures.

Contraindications and precautions

Lithium is generally contraindicated in clients with significant renal or cardiovascular disease, dehydration, or severe hyponatremia (sodium depletion). It is used cautiously in clients with hypothyroidism, which may worsen with lithium treatment.

Interactions

Many drugs interact with lithium to cause decreased metabolism and excretion, leading to increased lithium serum levels and possible lithium toxicity. These include diuretics, salt substitutes, and nonsteroidal antiinflammatory agents. Other drugs increase lithium excretion and reduce serum levels, worsening manic symptoms: the diuretic acetazolamide, alcohol, the bronchodilator aminophylline, antacids, caffeine, corticosteroids, and sodium substances, including sodium bicarbonate and sodium chloride.

Concurrent use of lithium with antipsychotic agents may reduce serum levels of the antipsychotic, thereby causing psychotic symptoms to increase. In addition, the antiemetic effects of the phenothiazine antipsychotic agents may mask signs of lithim toxicity. The use of lithium with haloperidol may cause irreversible neurotoxicity.

Lithium acts synergistically with potassium iodide, and hypothyroidism may result. Clients taking lithium who require neuromuscular blocking agents should be monitored very closely, since respiratory depression may be prolonged and risk of respiratory arrest is increased. Mechanical respiratory support may be needed.

SEDATIVES AND HYPNOTICS

Sedatives and hypnotics are often used as adjunctive medications in the treatment of mental disorders, especially anxiety disorders. Sedatives produce relaxation and decrease anxiety. Hypnotics produce sleep. Sedatives and hypnotics cause varying degrees of CNS depression, ranging from drowsiness and mild sedation to sleep and anesthesia. Larger doses may cause respiratory depression, coma, and death. Some sedatives and hypnotics are used as antianxiety, anticonvulsant, and anesthetic agents.

Barbiturates are considered the prototype of this classification. Nonbarbiturates include the benzodiazepines (discussed under antianxiety agents), chloral hydrate, and the antihistamine diphenhydramine.

Barbiturates

Barbiturates are classified according to their duration of action: long-acting, intermediate-acting, short-acting, and ultra-short-acting agents. The onset of long-acting barbiturates is more than 60 minutes, with the peak action in 10 to 12 hours. The onset of intermediate-acting barbiturates is 45 to 60 minutes, with a peak in 6 to 8 hours. Short-acting agents have an onset of 10 to 15 minutes and a peak in 3 to 4 hours, whereas ultra-short-acting agents act within seconds and are used for intravenous anesthesia.

Mechanism of action

The barbiturates act at all CNS levels, producing effects that range from mild sedation to deep anesthesia. These effects depend on the medication given, the dose, and the method of administration. Although all barbiturates in current clinical use depress the motor cortex in large doses, only the long-acting agents (phenobarbital, mephobarbital, metharbital) exert a selective action on the motor cortex in small doses. This accounts for their use as anticonvulsants. Large doses of barbiturates, especially when given intravenously, depress the respiratory and vasomotor centers.

The barbiturates also act on the inhibitory neurotransmitter GABA in the RAS, decreasing the stimulation and arousal of the limbic and cortical areas of the brain, thereby relieving anxiety.

The barbiturates stimulate the microsomal liver enzyme system, causing some drugs (oral anticoagulants, some anticonvulsants, oral estrogen contraceptives, corticosteroids) to be metabolized in the liver at a faster rate, resulting in a decreased therapeutic effect and shorter duration of action of these agents.

Indications for use

The short-acting barbiturates are used as hypnotics to treat insomnia and as hypnotics or sedatives for preanesthetic relaxation. They may be ordered the night before surgery to ensure sleep and on the morning of surgery to reduce anxiety. If used as hypnotics, barbiturates should be ordered for only short periods because they tend to lose effectiveness after about 14 days. The benzodiazepines have largely replaced the barbiturates both as hypnotics and as preanesthetic agents.

Barbiturates in lower doses may be used to treat anxiety and nervousness because of their sedative effects. However, the benzodiazepines have largely replaced daytime use of barbiturates because they cause less drowsiness.

The long-acting barbiturates are used as anticonvulsants to control or prevent seizures associated with eclampsia, epilepsy, meningitis, and tetanus. Ultra-short-acting agents, thiopental and methohexital, are used for surgical procedures, especially those of short duration. They are sometimes used alone but are frequently combined with other agents for muscle relaxation and analgesia in balanced anesthesia.

Side effects and adverse reactions

The most frequent side effects of barbiturates are ataxia, drowsiness, dizziness, and a "hangover" effect. Other effects include nausea and vomiting, constipation, restlessness, insomnia, headache, and night terrors. The most common adverse reaction is hypersensitivity manifested by skin rash, exfoliative dermatitis, fever, sore throat, edema, and urticaria. Apnea, bronchospasms, and Stevens-Johnson syndrome are other hypersensitivity symptoms. Stevens-Johnson syndrome is a severe allergic reaction characterized by fever, bullae (large blisters) of the skin, and ulcers of mucous membranes (mouth, nose, genitalia).

Elderly and debilitated clients may exhibit confusion or disorientation as well as mental depression when taking barbiturates. Increased excitability, a paradoxical reaction, may occur in these same individuals and also in children.

Toxic effects of the barbiturates include severe confusion and profound irritability, laryngospasm, apnea, ataxia, extreme weakness, and visual disturbances. These signs and symptoms should be reported immediately to the physician for possible medical intervention.

Contraindications and precautions

Barbiturates are contraindicated in clients with severe respiratory, hepatic, or renal disorders, since these conditions predispose affected individuals to the respiratory depressant effects of these agents. Hepatic and renal dysfunction alters the rate of metabolism and excretion of the barbiturates and may lead to increased CNS depressant effects. A prior history of hypersensitivity or addiction to barbiturates is considered a contraindication. Barbiturates are also contraindicated in clients with acute intermittent porphyria. Porphyria is characterized by physical and neurological disturbances, including severe abominal pain and sensitivity to the light.

Interactions

Concurrent administration of barbiturates with other CNS depressants such as alcohol, antihistamines, narcotic analgesics, other sedatives or hypnotics, and antidepressants may enhance CNS depression, especially respiratory depression.

Because the barbiturates stimulate the microsomal liver enzyme system, they enhance the metabolism of oral anticoagulants, the hydantoin anticonvulsants, corticosteroids, and oral estrogen contraceptives. This decreases the serum levels and therefore the therapeutic effects of these agents. Prothrombin times should be done more frequently if a client is taking a coumarin or indanedione anticoagulant. The metabolic effect of barbiturates on the hydantoin anticonvulsants is unpredictable, so serum levels should be closely monitored. On the other hand, the metabolism of barbiturates may decrease if the client is also taking the anticonvulsant valproic acid. This may lead to elevated serum levels of the barbiturate and severe CNS depression. The half-life of valproic acid may also be reduced, so blood levels should be monitored. Dosage adjustments may be necessary to prevent seizures.

Nonbarbiturate agents

Nonbarbiturate sedatives and hypnotics include some benzodiazepines, chloral hydrate, and diphenhydramine. Among the benzodiazepines, those most frequently used as sedatives and hypnotics are chlordiazepoxide (Librium), chlorazepate (Tranxene), flurazepam (Dalmane), temazepam (Restoril), and triazolam (Halcion).

Chloral hydrate and derivatives

Chloral hydrate is the oldest sedative-hypnotic still in use. The exact mechanism of its action is unknown, but it is converted into a metabolite, trichloroethanol, in the liver. This metabolite produces the sedative and hypnotic effect. The oral and rectal forms of chloral hydrate are both rapidly absorbed. The onset of a hypnotic dose is within 30 minutes, and the half-life is 7 to 10 hours. Side effects include nausea and vomiting, abdominal distress, dizziness, and ataxia. Confusion, hallucinations, skin rash, and urticaria are possible adverse reactions. As with all sedatives and hypnotics, chloral hydrate enhances the effects of CNS depression when given with other CNS depressants. Clients taking both chloral hydrate and another CNS depressant must be monitored for respiratory depression and extreme lethargy. Chloral hydrate may displace the oral anticoagulants from their binding sites, leading to an increased therapeutic effect and excessive bleeding.

Chloral betaine (Beta-Chlor) and triclofos sodium (Triclos) are derivatives of chloral hydrate with the same onset and duration of action.

Diphenhydramine

Diphenhydramine (Benadryl) has antitussive, antihistaminic, and antiparkinsonian effects. However, because it causes drowsiness and sleep, it is frequently prescribed as a sedative or hypnotic, especially for elderly clients. Since elderly persons tend to be more sensitive to the effects of diphenhydramine, low doses should be prescribed initially, with close monitoring for side effects and adverse reactions.

KEY POINTS

1. The development of medications to treat persons with mental illnesses opened new ways to treat clients with psychoses, depression, and anxiety.

2. An imbalance of neurotransmitters, especially dopamine, norepinephrine, and serotonin, is thought to cause psychoses, depression, and anxiety. Antipsychotic agents, antidepressants, and antianxiety agents (anxiolytics) seem to correct these imbalances in the central nervous system (CNS).

3. Treatment with medications does not cure the disorder but rather alleviates symptoms of mental illness and allows the client to participate more readily in other forms of therapy.

4. Phenothiazines are the most frequently used class of medications for the treatment of psychoses. Their exact mechanism of action is unknown but is thought to involve dopamine blockade in specific areas of the CNS.

5. All phenothiazines have similar actions but vary in their potency and in the nature and severity of side effects.

6. Extrapyramidal side effects caused by the antipsychotic agents often occur. The Abnormal Involuntary Movement Scale (AIMS) is a valuable tool to determine the presence of these symptoms, especially in the early stages.

7. Anticholinergic side effects (dry mouth, blurred vision, urinary retention, constipation) and orthostatic hypotension are common side effects of both the phenothiazine antipsychotic agents and the tricyclic antidepressants (TCAs).

8. In addition to their usefulness in treating depression, TCAs are used for panic and phobic disorders and as analgesics, especially for neuralgias and neuritis.

9. Because TCAs have many cardiovascular side effects and adverse reactions, clients with cardiovascular diseases are at increased risk for dysrhythmias, tachycardia, congestive heart failure, and cerebrovascular accident.

10. Antipsychotic agents and antidepressants are more likely to cause side effects and adverse reactions in elderly clients. These individuals should be carefully evaluated throughout the course of therapy. A lower dose is usually recommended.

11. Monoamine oxidase inhibitors (MAOIs) are used to treat both depression and hypertension but are rarely the first choice in treating either condition.

12. Foods containing tyramine and over-the-counter preparations containing epinephrine-like medications (phenylephrine, pseudoephrine, ephedrine, phenylpropanolamine) taken concurrently with MAOIs may cause a hypertensive crisis. The client must be taught to avoid food and other substances containing tyramine.

13. Newer antidepressants seem as effective as TCAs and MAOIs in treating depression, without some of the side effects. These medications include bupropion, fluoxetine, and sertraline.

14. When clients with anxiety are treated with medication, they most likely will receive one of the benzodiazepines.

15. Benzodiazepines have a high potential for abuse. Clients taking these medications should be monitored closely, and the medications should be prescribed for as short a time as needed.

16. Lithium is the only antimanic agent currently on the market.

17. Persons taking lithium should not be on a low-sodium diet and should not concurrently be taking sodium-depleting drugs, such as the thiazide diuretics, because lithium toxicity may develop.

18. Sedatives and hypnotics, especially barbiturates, are used as adjunctive medication, especially in the treatment of anxiety.

19. Barbiturates have a high potential for abuse and should not be prescribed for clients with a history of abuse of any other substance.

20. Since sedatives and hypnotics depress the CNS, their use with other CNS depressants (e.g., alcohol, antihistamines, narcotic analgesics) should be monitored carefully because acute respiratory depression may result.

SUGGESTED SOURCES OF ADDITIONAL INFORMATION

Abrams A: *Clinical drug therapy: rationales for nursing practice,* ed 3, Philadelphia, 1991, Lippincott.

Antipsychotic agents. In *Information for the pharmacist,* St Louis, 1991, Facts and Comparisons.

Aslam M, Friedman T, Pollard A: Wonder drugs? *Nurs Times* 84(30):21, 1988.

Beeber L: Checking the effects, *Nurs Times* 84(30):28, 1988.

Beeber L: It's on the tip of the tongue: tardive dyskinesia, *J Psychosoc Nurs* 26(8):32, 1988.

Beeber L: Undesirable weight gain and psychotropic medications, *J Psychosoc Nurs Ment Health Serv* 26(10):38, 1988.

Black J: Antipsychotic agents: a clinical update, *Mayo Clin Proc* 60:777, November 1985.

Blair D, Dauner A: Dangerous consequences: neuroleptic-induced tardive akathisia, *J Psychosoc Nurs Ment Health Serv* 30(3):41, 1992.

Blair DT, Dauner A: Neuroleptic malignant syndrome: liability in nuring practice, *J Psychosoc Nurs Ment Health Serv* 31(2):5, 1993.

Boodhoo J: Anticholinergic antiparkinsonian drugs in psychiatry, *Br J Hosp Med* 46(3):167, 1991.

Butler F, Burgio L, Engel B: Neuroleptics and behavior: a comparative study, *J Gerontol Nurs* 13(6):15, 1987.

Chapman T: The nurse's role in neuroleptic medications, *J Psychosoc Nurs Ment Health Serv* 29(6):6, 1992.

Chutka D: Cardiovascular effects of the antidepressants: recognition and control, *Geriatrics* 45(1):55, 1990.

Cole J: The drug treatment of anxiety and depression, *Med Clin North Am* 72(4):815, 1988.

Cole J, Bodkin J: Antidepressant drug side effects, *J Clin Psychiatry* 41(suppl 1):21, January 1990.

Gilman A and others, editors: *Goodman and Gilman's the pharmacological basis of therapeutics,* ed 8, New York, 1990, Pergamon.

Gomez G, Gomez E: The special concerns of neuroleptic use in the elderly, *J Psychosoc Nurs Ment Health Serv* 28(1):7, 1990.

Harris B: Lithium: in a class by itself, *Am J Nurs* 89(2):190, 1989.

Harris E: The anti-psychotics, *Am J Nurs* 88(11):1508, 1988.

Hartman C, Knight M: Pharmacotherapy. In Cook JS, Fontaine KL, editors: *Essentials of mental health nursing,* ed 2, Redwood City, Calif, 1991, Addison-Wesley.

Hollister L: On the horizon: new psychotherapeutic drugs, *Pharmacol Toxicol,* March 1991, p 195.

Hooper J, Herren C, Goldwasser H: Neuroleptic malignant syndrome: recognizing an unrecognized killer, *J Psychosoc Nurs Ment Health Serv* 29(7):13, 1989.

Jones J, Barklage N: Nonpsychiatric uses of antidepressants, *Hosp Ther* 14(6)24, 1989.

McKendry L, Salerno E: *Mosby's pharmacology in nursing,* ed 18, St Louis, 1992, Mosby–Year Book.

Physician's desk reference, ed 45, Oradell, NJ, 1991, Medical Economics.

Product monograph: Zoloft (sertraline HCl), New York, 1992, Roerig, Division of Pfizer.

The safety of fluoxetine—an update, Indianapolis, 1990, Dista Products, Division of Eli Lilly.

Shlafer M, Marieb E: *The nurse, pharmacology, and drug therapy,* Redwood City, Calif, 1989, Addison-Wesley.

Strome T, Howell T: How antipsychotics affect the elderly, *Am J Nurs* 91(5):46, 1991.

Taft L, Barkin P: Drug abuse? Use and misuse of psychotropic drugs in Alzheimer's care, *J Gerontol Nurs* 16(8):4, 1990.

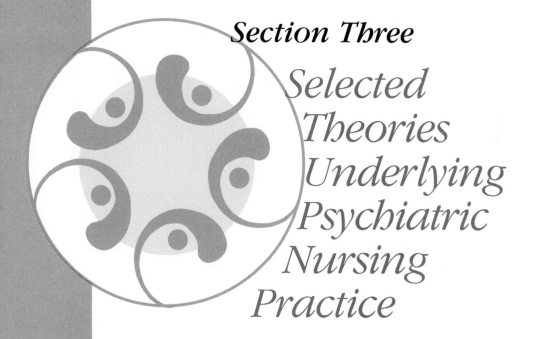

Section Three

Selected Theories Underlying Psychiatric Nursing Practice

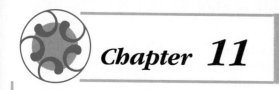

Chapter 11

General Systems Theory and Stress and Adaptation
one conceptual framework

LEARNING OBJECTIVES
After studying this chapter, the student will be able to:

• State the purpose of a conceptual framework.

• Discuss the concepts of general systems theory as applied to human systems.

• Discuss the concept of stress and adaptation as a process used by human systems.

• State an example of a nursing intervention using the conceptual framework of systems theory and stress and adaptation.

KEY TERMS
Conceptual framework
System
Subsystem
Environment
Input
Output
Matter
Energy
Potential energy
Kinetic energy
Nonsummativity
Wholeness
Throughput
Relatively closed system
Entropy
Relatively open system
Negentropy
Feedback
Stressor
Adaptation
General adaptation syndrome
Coping mechanism
Defense mechanism

For nurses to practice efficiently and effectively, they must do so within the context of a **conceptual framework.** The purpose of a conceptual framework is to provide a logical, coherent structure through which phenomena of concern can be understood and discussed. No conceptual framework is right or wrong. Rather, a conceptual framework is more or less appropriate; its appropriateness is determined by its applicability and usefulness. A conceptual framework appropriate for nursing must help explain the profession's phenomena of concern: the concepts of person, environment, and health and the interactions between and among these concepts. This framework must also be broad enough to be applicable to most, if not all, clinical situations but not so broad that it becomes meaningless.

The conceptual framework chosen for this text is general systems theory and the theory of stress and adaptation. This framework has been selected because of the applicability of its theories to psychiatric nursing and because several nursing theorists use these theories as a basis for their models of nursing practice.

HISTORICAL PERSPECTIVE

General systems theory, as reviewed in this chapter, was first discussed by Ludwig von Bertalanffy in 1968. However, other theorists, notably Kurt Lewin, had used its principles decades earlier to formulate their theories. General systems theory has been enthusiastically embraced by the helping professions because it is so useful in explaining relationships among apparently disparate entities. Nevertheless, some critics of this theory believe it is too mechanistic to apply to human systems.

In the 1930s Walter Cannon was the first theorist to mention the role of stress as a factor in causing disease. However, the foremost authority on the theory of stress and adaptation is probably Hans Selye, whose pioneering work on the subject was limited to a biochemical model of stress

and adaptation. Since that time, much research has demonstrated the same processes in the emotional and social realms.

GENERAL SYSTEMS THEORY

A **system** is usually defined as a complex of elements in interaction wherein a relationship between these elements and their properties can be theoretically demonstrated. Since all elements can be theorized to have ultimately a direct or indirect interactional relationship, the only true system is the universe. For example, it is often said that an individual's emotional problems are related to problems within the family. The family's problems in turn are attributed to problems within the community, whose problems in turn result from state, regional, and national concerns. These concerns in turn are closely related to international problems.

The study of the universe as the true system is not possible or desired because of the enormous amount of data that would have to be considered. Consequently, it is necessary to delin-

---

OF SPECIAL INTEREST

Although general systems theory was first addressed by scientists in the 1960s, many thoughtful persons were undoubtedly aware of the existence of an ordered, interrelated universe long before the twentieth century. A notable example of such an individual is Nathaniel Hawthorne (1804-1864), author of *The Scarlet Letter* and one of America's greatest writers of fiction. Hawthorne was deeply involved in the perennial debate concerning the nature of human beings and in 1835 wrote in the short story *Wakefield:* "Amid the seeming confusion of our mysterious world, individuals are so nicely adjusted to a system, and systems to one another and to a whole, that, by stepping aside for a moment, a man exposes himself to a fearful risk of losing his place forever."

eate a subsystem and define it as "the system" for the purposes of study.

Systems are delineated by the establishment of *boundaries,* which enclose those elements determined to have the greatest interactional qualities in terms of energy, matter, or both. The aggregate of elements that fall within the boundary is referred to as the "system"; each element becomes a component or a **subsystem** of the newly defined system. For example, mental health professionals often define the family as the system of concern and the individuals who make up the family as components or subsystems of the family system.

Each subsystem has its own elements, which are components or subsystems of that system. For example, the individual as a system is composed of a variety of subsystems, such as the physiological, psychological, and social subsystems. These subsystems, when viewed as systems themselves, consist of their own subsystems. For example, the physiological system consists of the cardiovascular and gastrointestinal subsystems, among others.

Elements that lie outside the boundary serve as the system's **environment,** which is in reality composed of other systems. Therefore the community system serves as an environment for the family system, the family system serves as an environment for the individual system, the physiological system serves as an environment for the psychological system, and so on.

It cannot be overemphasized that boundary delineation is an artifical demarcation of one aspect of the whole—artificial, but necessary, to limit the focus of concern to that which is relevant and thereby to increase the probability of comprehending the system. Because boundary delineation is artificial and is intended to enable the nurse to understand the system, boundaries can be enlarged or reduced as experience with the system dictates. For example, when the family is the system of concern, an initial assessment might indicate that the system should be limited to those members living under the same roof.

After working with this system, however, the nurse may discover that the grandparents who live in another state are integral components of this family system. The nurse would then enlarge the original system to include this subsystem, rather than viewing it as part of the environment.

The boundaries of a system have the necessary characteristic of permeability. This permeability may be greater or lesser when systems are compared; the degree of boundary permeability may also change at various times and places within any given system. The permeability of the system boundary regulates the exchange of matter and energy between the system and its environment. Matter and energy that move from the environment through the boundary into the system are referred to as **input.** Matter and energy that move from the system through the boundary into the environment are referred to as **output.**

In a system, matter and energy are integral parts of both the system and the system's environment. **Matter** is defined as anything that has mass and occupies space. **Energy** is defined as the ability to do work. Two types of energy exist: potential and kinetic. **Potential energy** is energy not currently engaged in work but available for use; it is stored energy. In contrast, **kinetic energy** is energy currently being used and therefore unavailable for additional work.

Energy can be neither created nor destroyed; it can only be converted from one form into another or transported from one place to another. When energy is used, it does not disappear but merely goes elsewhere or is changed to another form. The principle that energy can be neither created nor destroyed is the first law of thermodynamics; it is reminiscent of Freud's concept of psychic or libidinal energy, as explained in Chapter 12.

Systems are in a constant state of dynamic movement as they exchange matter and energy within themselves and between themselves and their environments. Any attempt to study a system is to suspend artificially this motion and therefore risk an inaccurate assessment. Nevertheless, it is necesssary to take this risk if systems are to be studied, but any conclusions should take this factor into account.

Systems are characterized by the concept of **nonsummativity,** which states that the whole of the system is greater than the sum of its parts. The parts of a system are that system's subsystems, and the system in its totality cannot be understood or appreciated by a mere summation of its subsystems. Perhaps the most familiar example of this concept is the Indian folk tale of the six blind men who each felt a part of an elephant's body. Each then described that part to the others, and as a group they attempted unsuccessfully to describe the whole. The primary reason that the whole is greater than the sum of its parts is that each subsystem interacts directly or indirectly with all other subsystems by exchanging matter and energy, a concept called **wholeness.** The uniqueness of the system results from the transformations of matter and energy that take place in this exchange, a process known as **throughput.**

Because of the interactional quality of the system's components, changes in any one component will automatically effect compensatory changes in all other components. These changes are compensatory because a system continuously strives to maintain itself as it is. In other words, the system continuously regulates itself to attain a steady state. When referring to living organisms, this process is known as *homeokinesis.*

Human beings are complex systems of interrelated and interdependent subsystems in constant interaction with each other and with their environments. Therefore, alterations in any aspect of the system require responsive alterations in other aspects of the system. For example, a person who has a physical illness, for whatever reason and to whatever degree, has concomitant emotional reactions to this lack of physical well-being. Conversely, there are physical side effects of emotional reactions, such as the stomach upsets, the lightheadedness, and the heart palpitations that accompany severe anxiety or fear.

This holistic view of human beings also provides direction for assessing the individual as an integral part of his or her social system, simultaneously affecting that system and being affected by it. This view implies that an individual cannot be assessed accurately in isolation from the family, community, and reference groups to which the person belongs. Nurses new to working with persons with a mental illness have had the experience of assisting an individual to achieve a higher level of emotional wellness only to be surprised by the observation that the behavior of another family member becomes increasingly disturbed. This common phenomenon reflects the family operating as a system and behavioral change in one member requiring a compensatory reaction by the family system, often manifested by altered behavior in other family members.

Those human systems who are most successful in achieving their goal of maintaining themselves as close to their original state as possible ironically are systems whose existence is in jeopardy. These systems are **relatively closed systems** and are likely to show signs of illness or dysfunction. The boundaries of relatively closed systems have little permeability, and relatively little exchange of matter or energy occurs with the environment. However, boundaries cannot be totally closed in a living system. Some permeability is necessary to exchange matter and energy, a process necessary for life. The bulk of energy in a relatively closed system is used in maintaining a steady state, leaving little potential energy available to respond to input. Because input into the system is minimal, energy is ultimately lost into the system's environment, leading to increased system disorganization. This situation is termed **entropy.**

The reader is probably familiar with a family that does not respond to notes from school about the children's poor academic performance, initially resulting in the family system being undisturbed by this news and thereby maintaining a steady state. Ultimately, however, this system's inability to recognize and process relevant input may lead to the children being left behind and perhaps eventually dropping out of school. This in turn means that the children are poorly prepared to leave home and to function as financially independent adults, resulting in the family's financial resources becoming increasingly depleted. In the long term, this fictional family does not change and grow but rather becomes increasingly ineffective in fulfilling its functions. This example, although oversimplified, illustrates the counterproductivity of a system attempting to achieve a steady state by maintaining relatively closed boundaries.

In contrast, a system that survives, grows, and develops is characterized by a semipermeable boundary that allows for exchange of matter and energy with its environment and by the availability of a sufficient amount of potential energy to use input in the service of system growth. This type of system is known as a **relatively open system** and is characterized by movement toward integration and growth, a situation referred to as **negentropy.**

A system in a state of negentropy is likely to manifest signs of health or to be considered functional. A discussion of the personality attributes of mentally healthy individuals is found in Chapter 12.

Finally, an understanding of systems theory must take into account the concept of **feedback,** a unique form of input derived from the system's output. In other words, system output is transformed by the environment (in reality another system) and in turn becomes that system's output. Part of that output is fed back as input to the original system. This process is often referred to as the *feedback loop.* Feedback is the message that the system receives about the degree to which it is successful in attaining a steady state and is therefore essential if the system is to adjust or regulate itself. A time lag always exists between the system's perception of the feedback and its ability to use it in the service of self-regulation.

Positive feedback reinforces the system, thereby encouraging the maintenance of a steady state and leading to entropy. *Negative feedback* is information that indicates change is necessary within the system for the system to grow. These concepts are often difficult for students to understand because of the belief that positive feedback is desired and negative feedback is to be avoided. Positive feedback does reinforce behavior, encouraging people to continue those behaviors that are rewarded. However, inadvertently perhaps, positive feedack discourages growth if altered behavior is necessary for growth. Negative feedback, on the other hand, is growth producing only if the system has the energy available to use the feedback and alter itself. For example, very intelligent students are not motivated to achieve their potential if minimal efforts are rewarded with high grades. On the other hand, students who are not as intellectually capable and who are working to capacity but receiving low grades will not be helped to do better merely through criticism of their work. They do not have the energy available to use the negative feedback, whereas their highly intelligent counterparts do.

This brief discussion of general systems theory demonstrates its applicability to nursing practice in regard to describing the structure of human systems. However, its language and concepts only hint at explaining the process. For example, we know that energy is exchanged between systems, but systems theory alone does not allow us to describe the nature of that energy. Therefore, to understand better the nature of the processes in which systems engage, we need to turn to another theory, stress and adaptation.

STRESS AND ADAPTATION THEORY

Human beings are continuously exposed to many and varied stimuli. These stimuli may be physical, emotional, physiological, social, or spiritual and may take the form of matter or energy.

These stimuli are input to the system and may emanate from within the system through the feedback loop or from external sources. The system's boundary screens and sorts input to protect the system from becoming overwhelmed while at the same time allowing sufficient input to transcend the boundary and ensure the system's viability.

In the terminology of stress and adaptation theory, system input is called a **stressor.** A stressor, in and of itself, is neither positive nor negative but rather has a positive or negative effect, depending on the way the system processes it. This concept helps to explain why different people respond differently to the same stressor. For example, the death of a spouse is considered a negative event in our society. After the initial grieving period, however, the surviving spouse may respond with more vigor and interest in life than before the spouse's death. Conversely, the birth of a baby is generally considered a positive event, but for some families an additional child may strain emotional and financial resources unbearably.

Stressors may be classified as *developmental* or *situational.* The significance of this classification is that developmental stressors can be anticipated but situational stressors cannot; situational stressors are untoward events. For example, the adolescent is assaulted with physiological, emotional, and social stressors. Because these are a normal, expected part of the maturation process, anticipatory guidance of the adolescent and the family can greatly strengthen the resources this system has available for dealing with these stressors. In contrast, the situational stressor of a middle-aged executive with two children in college who loses his job must be dealt with after it happens.

Regardless of whether a stressor is developmental or situational, the variables that determine a system's response to a stressor are multiple but always reflect the amount of potential energy available to deal with the stressor and the meaning of the stressor to the system. For ex-

ample, a mild laryngitis would not greatly distress a dock worker but would be a major stressor to the opera singer.

When a stressor transcends the system's boundary, it disturbs the system's steady state, automatically thrusting the system into a condition of stress. Therefore, *stress* is defined as a condition in which the human system responds to input that has disturbed its steady state. As such, stress is necessary to life and is neither positive nor negative, although it is capable of causing either positive or negative effects. This technical view of stress differs greatly from the way the term is used in everyday language. One often hears the word "stress" used only in a negative sense and often as descriptive of an event rather than the condition of being.

Stress in human beings is a subjective phenomenon that cannot be observed directly but rather must be inferred from the person's response to the stressor. This response is called an **adaptation.** Integral to the theory of stress is the concept that the human system adapts holistically to stress. Regardless of the nature of the stressor, the human being responds in all dimensions. A physiological stressor elicits not only a physiological adaptation, but also psychological and social adaptations. Similarly, a social stressor elicits social, physiological, and psychological adaptations. In other words, the human system is not able to respond selectively to stressors. This generalized, nonspecific response to stress is called the **general adaptation syndrome** and is consistent with the systems theory concept of wholism. For example, an adolescent experiencing the stress of her first date responds with fear about the appropriateness of her appearance and behavior. However, this response is not limited to the emotion of fear but also affects her physiological subsystem by raising her blood pressure and decreasing the blood supply to the digestive subsystem, rendering her unable to eat. This response is actually preparing her for "fight or flight" as if the stressor were life-threatening. This fight or flight response, if prolonged with no outlet, can result in the stress-related diseases that constitute major health problems in today's society.

In addition to the general adaptation syndrome, there may be a specific adaptation to the stressor. Although the general adaptation syndrome is involuntary and unconscious, adaptations specific to a stressor may be either voluntary or involuntary and conscious or unconscious. When adaptations are voluntary and conscious, they are called **coping mechanisms;** when they are involuntary and unconscious, they are called **defense mechanisms.** For example, a student in a state of stress because of an impending examination might adapt by voluntarily and consciously planning time to study and then adhering to the plan. Another student might respond to the same stressor by involuntarily using the unconscious defense mechanism of rationalization by believing the examination is less important than attending social events, and therefore this student might plan not to study. On the surface it would seem that the second student was more successful than the first in returning to the desired state of homeokinesis in that this second student, unlike the first, is no longer under stress. One should remember, however, that the second student must use some available energy to remain unaware of the reality of the situation; the student then has less energy available to deal with subsequent stressors. In either event, this example is not complete until the outcome of each adaptation is examined. When the time of the examination arrives, one can conjecture that the first student who studied would be prepared and therefore would do well on the test. The feedback this student would receive is positive, thereby reinforcing the behavior of studying before a test. The second student, however, would be unlikely to do well, and the feedback would be negative, thereby disrupting the system further and causing additional stress with less available energy to deal with it. If sufficient energy were available, however, the student could benefit from this negative feedback

by using it to alter his or her behavior and plan to study for examinations in the future.

Once again, this example is overly simplistic in that it implies a linear cause-and-effect relationship between the stressor and the adaptation. In reality, the human system is always being affected by multiple stressors, and its adaptations reflect the system's ability to test reality, its previous adaptations, and its amount of potential energy. Human systems that cannot regain homeokinesis because of an inability to test reality, or that have had no previous experience with the stressor, or that lack sufficient energy to adapt to the number and potency of the stressors encountered are in a state of crisis. This condition is discussed fully in Chapter 24.

The student of psychiatric nursing should be aware that Axis IV of the *Diagnostic and Statistical Manual of Mental Disorders (third edition, revised)* (DSM-III-R) (see Appendix A) provides for an assessment of the severity of the individual's psychosocial stressors in terms of both acute events (duration less than 6 months) and enduring circumstances (duration greater than 6 months). Although the scale used to assess psychosocial stressors may change in the DMS-IV, the inclusion of such an axis in this diagnostic taxonomy reflects a continuing recognition by the medical profession that psychosocial stressors may both contribute to and result from mental illness. On examination of the current axis, the student should note that suggested examples of stressors include both developmental and situational events that range from those encountered by many people to highly unusual situations likely to be experienced by only a few persons. The student should also note that the list of examples includes not only negative events but also those usually considered positive, such as graduation from school or marriage.

IMPLICATIONS FOR NURSING

The conceptual framework of systems theory and stress and adaptation provides nurses with organizing theories through which human behavior that seems arbitrary or inexplicable can be understood. It also provides a basis for conceptualizing the broad goals of all nursing interventions. Simply stated, the goal of all nursing interventions is to protect the system from noxious stressors or to increase the system's potential energy, thereby enhancing its ability to adapt to the stressor, or to diminish the stressor's potency. The following case history exemplifies how these goals can be achieved.

Mary Smith, a 16-year-old unmarried high school student, informed her parents that she was 2 months pregnant. Although this news was extremely upsetting to all, Mary's parents rallied around her, and after many family discussions, often late into the night, the family made several decisions. Mary would not marry the child's father because they had little in common other than a strong sexual attraction. She would carry the baby to term, and after the birth she would give the infant up for adoption so that she would be able to continue her education by going to college and perhaps fulfill her lifelong dream of becoming a lawyer. It was also decided that Mary would continue to attend the local high school. Mary's parents met with the school administrators, who agreed to this plan. They also contacted an adoption agency to initiate plans for the adoption of the unborn child. These decisions were congruent with the family's values, were agreeable to all, and seemed feasible to implement. Having adapted to the stressor of Mary's pregnancy, the Smith family regained its homeokinesis by devoting themselves to accomplishing the many household and business tasks left undone while its energy was focused on coping with this system change.

All things went well for the Smith family until the fifth month, at which time Mary was visibly pregnant. Her classmates began openly taunting her, her best friends no longer telephoned her or invited her to their homes, and the school board received a petition from irate parents demanding that Mary be suspended from school until the baby was born. Although the school board did not take this action and Mary's parents remained empathic and supportive, Mary became increasingly depressed, unable to eat or sleep. Mr. and Mrs. Smith became alarmed and made an appointment

at the mental health clinic. After several sessions at the clinic, the decision was that it would be best for Mary if she were to move to her grandparents' home in a different school district for the duration of her pregnancy. While she was there, she would continue to receive counseling focused on helping her to cope with the birth and subsequent adoption of her child, as well as exploring responses she might use when questioned about her pregnancy. Finally, the mental health counselors in Mary's town were concerned about the larger issue of the townspeople's attitudes, not only for Mary's sake, but also because of what this attitude of intolerance meant to the mental health of her classmates. Since part of the mission of the mental health clinic was community education, the personnel organized evening seminars under the school's auspices. These seminars were designed to assist interested students and parents to explore their interpersonal relationships and human values.

This case history depicts a family system thrust into a state of disequilibrium by changes in one of its subsystems caused by a situational stressor (Mary's pregnancy). The family system did not go into a state of massive disequilibrium on experiencing this change, which shows that it had potential energy available to bring to the situation. The family apparently used a problem-solving approach as the members engaged in many family discussions. The relative openness of this system's boundaries is attested to by the parents meeting with the school administrators and sharing their plans with them. The parents also were able to seek help from the mental health clinic when Mary's behavior alarmed them. A system with relatively closed boundaries would probably be unable to exchange information effectively with other systems in its environment.

The decision for Mary to move out of the school district to her grandparents' home is an example of an intervention that used available resources to protect Mary and her family from the noxious stressor of peer rejection, with which they were apparently unable to cope. Increasing Mary's potential energy, thereby enhancing her ability to adapt to future criticism, was accomplished by the reality-oriented counseling she continued to receive while at her grandparents' home. Finally, the action of the mental health clinic in conducting human relations seminars for the townspeople is an example of an intervention designed to diminish the stressor's potency.

Although this situation does not specifically refer to the nurse as the mental health professional involved, the interventions employed are well within the scope of practice of a nurse functioning in a community mental health clinic.

KEY POINTS

1. A conceptual framework provides a logical, coherent structure through which phenomena of concern can be understood and discussed. The conceptual framework of general systems theory and the theory of stress and adaptation is particularly applicable to the practice of psychiatric nursing.

2. Systems are delineated by artificially determined boundaries that enclose elements with the greatest interactional qualities.

3. Each element within a system is a subsystem.

4. Elements outside the system's boundaries form the system's environment.

5. Matter and energy that move from the environment through the boundary into the system are called input. Matter and energy that move from the system through the boundary into the environment are called output.

6. Mattter is anything that has mass and occupies space. Energy is the ability to do work and is either potential (or stored) or kinetic energy.

7. Systems are characterized by the concept of nonsummativity; that is, the whole is greater than the sum of its parts.

8. The uniqueness of each system results from the transformations of matter and energy between and among the subsystems, a process known as throughput.

9. Systems constantly regulate themselves to attain a steady state, a process known as homeokinesis.

Therefore, changes in one component of the system automatically effect changes in all other components.

10. Human beings are complex systems of interrelated and interdependent subsystems in constant interaction with each other and with their environments.

11. The boundaries of relatively closed systems have little permeability, and the bulk of the system's energy is bound in maintaining a steady state, leading to energy loss and increased system disorganization. This situation is called entropy.

12. The boundaries of relatively open systems allow for adequate exchange of matter and energy. A sufficient amount of potential energy to use input in the service of system growth and integration is available. This situation is called negentropy.

13. Feedback is a unique form of input that sends a message to the system about the degree to which it is successful in attaining a steady state. Positive feedback reinforces the system and encourages a steady state. Negative feedback disrupts the system, encouraging change and growth if the system has the potential energy available to use the input.

14. System input is called a stressor. A stressor is neither positive nor negative but has a positive or negative effect on the system.

15. Stressors may be developmental or situational.

16. Stress in human beings is a condition of being in which the human system responds to input that has disturbed its steady state. Stress is neither positive nor negative but is necessary to life.

17. The human system's response to stress is called an adaptation. Human systems respond holistically to stress. This generalized, nonspecific response to stress is termed the general adaptation syndrome.

18. There may be a specific adaptation to a stressor, which may be voluntary and conscious (coping mechanism) or involuntary and unconscious (defense mechanism).

19. The goal of all nursing interventions is to protect the system from noxious stressors, increase the system's potential energy, or diminish the stressor's potency.

SUGGESTED SOURCES OF ADDITIONAL INFORMATION

Blattner B: *Holistic nursing,* Englewood Cliffs, NJ, 1981, Prentice-Hall.

Botha ME: Theory development in perspective: the role of conceptual frameworks and models in theory development, *J Adv Nurs* 14:49, 1989.

Hazzard ME, editor: A systems approach to nursing, *Nurs Clin North Am* 6, September 1971.

Hill M: When the patient is the family, *Am J Nurs* 81:536, 1981.

Kinney CK, Erickson HC: Modeling the client's world: a way to holistic care, *Issues Ment Health Nurs* 11:93, 1990.

Leidy NK: A physiologic analysis of stress and chronic illness, *J Adv Nurs* 14:868, 1989.

Moore SL, Munro MF: The Neuman system model applied to mental health nursing of older adults, *J Adv Nurs* 15:293, 1990.

Murphy S: After Mt. St. Helen's: disaster stress research, *J Psychosoc Nurs Ment Health Serv* 22:8, July 1984.

Onega LL: A theoretical framework for psychiatric nursing practice, *J Adv Nurs* 16:68, 1991.

Selye H: *Stress without distress,* New York, 1974, Lippincott.

Spiegel J: *Transactions: the interplay between individual, family, and society,* New York, 1971, Science House.

von Bertalanffy L: *General systems theory: foundations, development, and applications,* New York, 1968, George Braziller.

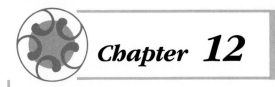

Chapter *12*

Psychosocial Theories of Personality Development

LEARNING OBJECTIVES
After studying this chapter, the student will be able to:
* Describe briefly the history of the study of personality development.

* Define the term *personality*.

* Discuss the personality attributes of a mentally healthy adult.

* Discuss the major concepts underlying the Piagetian theory of cognitive development and the Freudian, Eriksonian, and Sullivanian theories of personality development.

* Discuss each stage of cognitive and personality development in terms of its process and outcomes.

KEY TERMS
Personality
Psychosexual theory
Interpersonal theory
Maslow's "hierarchy of needs"
Intrapsychic
Libidinal energy
Conscious
Preconscious
Subconscious
Unconscious
Id
Ego
Superego
Pleasure principle
Conscience
Ego ideal
Developmental tasks
Dynamisms
Schema
Assimilation
Accommodation
Primary narcissism
Omnipotence
Empathic linkage
Self-concept
Security operations

Understanding mental health and mental illness depends greatly on understanding the processes through which human beings develop, emotionally and cognitively. Although it is imperative that the psychiatric nurse fully understand these theories, *all* nurses should be familiar with them, since nursing assessment and intervention for any client must be developmentally appropriate if they are to be accurate and effective.

HISTORICAL PERSPECTIVE

Before the beginning of the twentieth century, the physical, emotional, and cognitive development of human beings was poorly understood. Children were viewed as miniature adults and, as such, were treated with little or no understanding of their developmentally related needs. Furthermore, the attainment of physical maturity was thought to signal the achievement of emotional and cognitive maturity. If growth was complete, so was development! Not until the early twentieth century did the study of **personality** development of children begin in earnest. Major strides in understanding cognitive development were not made until the midtwentieth century. Interest in the personality development of adults has emerged only recently and is currently the subject of much study because the number of persons of middle and older age is rapidly increasing.

The theories proposed by Sigmund Freud (1856-1939) revolutionized the way in which clinicians and laypersons viewed human behavior. It was Freud's writing that first stressed the crucial importance of early chilhood experiences in the development of human personality and the relationship between some emotional problems in adult life and the negative influences that occurred during the individual's early years. Freud's theory of personality development is called the **psychosexual theory** of development.

During and after Freud's pioneering work, many other theorists addressed the study of personality development to better understand human behavior. Investigators such as Erik Erikson and Harry Stack Sullivan adapted, modified, and enlarged on Freud's basic theories; their work has resulted in theories seen as significantly different from those of Freud.

Erik Erikson was born in Frankfurt, Germany, in 1902 of Danish parents. His mother and father had separated before he was born, and when he was about 3 years old, his mother married a pediatrician who was a German Jew. With this mixed cultural heritage, Erikson had difficulty establishing his own sense of identity. His personal quest for identity was probably a major factor in the development of his theory of personality development, referred to as the *Eight Ages of Man*. At age 25 Erikson left Germany to go to Vienna, where he studied the new discipline of psychoanalysis. He immigrated to Boston in 1933.

Harry Stack Sullivan was born in Norwich, New York, in 1892 and died in 1949. Sullivan became a psychiatrist during the early years of Freud's profound influence on American psychiatry. However, unlike many of his colleagues, Sullivan studied only in the United States, working closely with a group of psychoanalysts and social psychologists who were pulling away from the classical psychoanalytical model established by Freud. Sullivan's theories postulate that the most critical factor in personality development is the individual's relationship with other significant people. His theories emphasize the nature and the quality of these relationships. This fact is best illustrated by his reference to the *mothering one* to distinguish between the roles of the biological mother and the person (male or female) who provides nurturing experiences for the infant. Although Sullivan viewed the relationship between the infant and the mothering one as fundamental to personality development, he also placed great emphasis on the importance of relationships with significant others such as peers, spouse, and offspring as the person progresses throughout life. Therefore, Sullivan's theory is called the **interpersonal theory** of psychiatry. Since the nurse's role with persons who have a mental illness is heavily focused on the relationship that is developed with them, Sullivan's theory seems to be particularly applicable to nursing practice.

The pioneering work on cognitive development was undertaken by Jean Piaget (1896-1980), a Swiss psychologist. Piaget was not alone in observing that children at various ages differ in their ability to think, remember, and problem solve. He was the first, however, to study systematically the processes by which these abilities develop. Piaget began his exploration of cognitive development by exhaustively observing his own three children; his resultant theory helps to clarify and augment what is known about the development of the personality.

DEFINITION OF PERSONALITY

Before a discussion of personality development can become meaningful, it is essential to understand the definition of the term *personality*. Unfortunately, this word has been used to convey many different meanings and ideas. In ordinary conversation, it usually refers to the personal response that the individual evokes from others. It is not unusual for someone to comment that an individual has a pleasing personality or that a certain person has a poor personality. When used technically, the term *personality* refers to *the aggregate of the individual's physical and mental qualities as these interact characteristically with the person's environment*. Thus, personality is expressed through behavior. The characteristic combinations of behavior distinguish one individual from another and endow individuals with their own unique identity.

This definition of personality includes the individual's biological and intellectual endowment, the attributes acquired through experience, and the person's conscious and unconscious reactions and feelings. Personality development is a complex, dynamic process. As such, the personality is constantly evolving from what it was to something different, but it always retains a certain identifiable consistency. It is important to remember that from birth to death, personality is ever changing and ever developing. This fact makes it possible for individuals of all ages to profit from corrective experiences and to modify behavior in a positive direction. This is the rationale underlying all psychotherapeutic endeavors.

PERSONALITY ATTRIBUTES OF THE MENTALLY HEALTHY ADULT

The first attempts to describe the personality attributes of the mentally healthy adult were based on inferences drawn from what was known about persons with a mental illness, often leading to erroneous conclusions. Consequently, mental health was initially described in negative terms, such as the absence of incapacitating anxiety. Not until the late 1950s did psychologist Marie Jahoda identify criteria of positive mental health. This work was done under the auspices of the Joint Commission on Mental Illness and Health, whose report was published in 1961.

It is important to understand that the personality attributes of the mentally healthy adult are not amenable to precise measurement, as are many indices of physical health. Rather, these attributes are inferred from behavior, including what the individual says about self and others. In general, socially acceptable behavior is considered indicative of mental health; socially unacceptable behavior is often considered a sign of mental illness. Consequently, mental health is culturally bound in the sense that the very same behavior acceptable in one culture may be deemed unacceptable in another. Furthermore, mental health is relative to time and place and situation. For example, individuals who would never consider harming another under usual circumstances but who are able to defend themselves by hitting an assailant when attacked are displaying the ability to assess reality accurately, a major criterion of mental health.

The individual's level of self-acceptance is usually mentioned as an important reflection of the degree of mental health. All human beings have strengths and limitations; a mentally healthy adult works at maximizing strengths and minimizing limitations but at the same time accepts strengths and limitations without inordinate pride or shame. In other words, the capacity to be comfortable with oneself is considered an important attribute of the mentally healthy adult.

The way a person perceives reality is another significant dimension of the degree of mental health. Mentally healthy individuals view their environment realistically, not as filtered through their unique need system. Therefore, mentally healthy adults are unlikely to view the world either as always hostile and threatening or as always friendly and accepting. Rather, they are able to evaluate each situation and validate their perceptions with others whom they trust.

Self-acceptance and a realistic perception of reality greatly influence the achievement of another attribute of mental health, environmental mastery. Environmental mastery suggests that the individual feels in control of self and the environment and has made an investment in living that has necessitated the high-level development of inherent abilities.

The mentally healthy or emotionally mature individual will have developed the capacity for independent thinking and action. This capacity is described by some as efficiency in problem solving and by others as autonomy or self-determination.

A final capacity usually included in a discussion of mental health is the individual's ability to synthesize all psychological functions and personal attributes, which in turn enables the person to achieve a unifying, integrated outlook on life and a sense of direction in relation to his or her role in it. The box on p. 181 outlines personality attributes of the mentally healthy adult.

These manifestations of mental health are consistent with those behaviors identified by another pioneer in the study of mental health, Abraham Maslow (1908-1970). Maslow believed that mental illness could be understood only within a framework of an understanding of mental health. He developed the widely used "**hierarchy of needs**" theory, often referred to as the *theory of self-actualization* (Table 12-1). This theory states that all human beings strive to develop, but all have inherent basic needs, which are ordered hierarchically and which emerge only when lower-level needs have been satisfied. Further, the individual's behavior is directed toward meeting the need that is operative at the time. This explains the oft-quoted observation that a child who is hungry cannot learn. A mentally healthy individual, according to Maslow, is a self-actualizing person whose energy is directed toward meeting his or her unique potential. Although the behavior of self-actualizing people differs because of their uniqueness, all share the ability and willingness to see reality as it is, a sense of humility integrated with creativity, an acceptance of self with little or no inner conflict, and importantly, a capacity for joy in themselves, others, and the world in which they live.

BASIC CONCEPTS OF PERSONALITY DEVELOPMENT

Although some psychiatrists believe it is important to adhere strictly and consistently to the tenets of one school of thought, psychiatric theories currently used in the United States are becoming increasingly eclectic. That is, concepts from various schools of thought are being used in combination to develop a useful theory of personality development. The necessity of an eclectic approach is particularly apparent in nursing practice; the role of the nurse in interaction with clients is probably more varied than in any other discipline. Consequently, the following discussion describes the basic concepts of Freud, Erikson, and Sullivan, with a subsequent discussion of each stage of personality development as described by these theorists. It is hoped that this approach enables the student to compare and contrast these theories and use what is applicable as she or he plans, implements, and evaluates nursing care.

Freudian concepts

Freud's theories are often referred to as **intrapsychic** because they emphasize the individual's internal emotional life as the most significant factor in personality development. Even though Freud deviated widely from the accepted medical theories and practices of his day, his theories are largely based on a biological model. For example, Freud believed that each individual is born with a genetically determined amount of **libidinal energy,** a form of psychic energy that seeks pleasure in an attempt to avoid tension or pain. In this sense, libidinal energy is viewed as sexual energy. This energy cannot increase or decrease in amount but must be shared among the various parts of the personality. Freud developed his conception of the stages of personality development largely around the concept of libidinal energy and delineated each stage of development according to the area of the body where he believed the energy was focused. For example, the first stage of development is characterized by the libidinal energy being concentrated on the mouth. Through the mouth the infant expresses tension and pain; through the mouth, pleasure is perceived. As the child matures physiologically, the libidinal energy shifts from the mouth to other parts of the body until adulthood, when the libidinal energy is focused on the genital area, enabling the individual to establish a mature heterosexual relationship, which Freud saw as the hallmark of the normal development of personality. Therefore, Freud delineated only five stages of personality development, seeing this process as being complete at adulthood, with major personality alterations

---

PERSONALITY ATTRIBUTES OF THE MENTALLY HEALTHY ADULT

Accepts strengths and limitations
Perceives reality accurately
Exhibits environmental mastery
Engages in independent thinking and action
Achieves a unifying, integrated outlook on life

Table 12-1. Maslow's hierarchy of needs

NEED	CHARACTERISTICS
Physiological	Satisfying needs for oxygen, water, food, shelter, sleep, relief of sexual tension
Safety	Avoiding harm and achieving security and physical safety
Love and belonging	Giving and receiving affection, developing companionship, and gaining acceptance by a group
Esteem and recognition	Achieving recognition by others, leading to self-esteem and feelings of prestige; achieving success in work
Self-actualization	Achieving one's own unique potential in all dimensions
Aesthetic and cognitive	Achieving an unbiased understanding and appreciation of the beauty and unity of the world and one's role in it

unlikely thereafter under usual circumstances. Because of the libidinal energy theory and its relationship to personality development, Freud's theory of personality development is called the *psychosexual theory.*

Freud's topographical descriptions of the psyche are important for the student to understand, since these concepts are used almost universally in the United States and contribute much to understanding human behavior.

Levels of consciousness

One way in which Freud described the mind topographically was from the standpoint of levels of consciousness. These levels are referred to as the conscious, the preconscious or subconscious, and the unconscious parts of the mind.

The **conscious** part of the mind is aware of the here and now as it relates to the individual and the environment. It functions only when the individual is awake. The conscious mind is concerned with thoughts, feelings, and sensations. It directs the individual as he or she behaves in a rational, thoughtful way.

In the **preconscious,** or **subconscious,** part of the mind, ideas and reactions are stored and partially forgotten. It is not economical for human beings to burden the conscious mind with many facts that are infrequently used and currently not in demand. The preconscious also acts as a watchman; it prevents certain unacceptable, disturbing unconscious memories from reaching the conscious mind. These two functions make the preconscious an extremely valuable device. Material relegated to this handy storehouse can usually be brought into conscious awareness if the individual concentrates on recall.

The **unconscious** is by far the largest part of the mind and is sometimes compared with the large hidden part of an iceberg that floats under the water. In this comparison the small part of the iceberg that appears above the water represents the conscious mind. The unconscious is the storehouse for all the memories, feelings,

and responses experienced during the individual's entire life. The unconscious is one of Freud's most important concepts. Freudian theorists believe that the human mind never actually forgets any experience but stores in the unconscious all knowledge, information, and feeling about all experiences. These memories cannot be recalled at will. The individual is rarely aware of the unconscious mind, except as it demonstrates its presence through such means as dreams, slips of the tongue, unexplained behavioral responses, jokes, and lapses of memory. Material stored in the unconscious has a powerful influence on behavior because the accompanying feelings continue to act as motivating, dynamic forces. The individual is unaware of the ideas themselves but may continue to experience an emotional reaction as if the material were in the conscious mind. This theory underlies the belief that all behavior has meaning. In other words, no behavior occurs by accident or chance; rather, all behavior is an expression of feelings or needs of which the individual frequently is not aware.

Structure of the personality

The second topographical description developed by Freud is frequently referred to as the structure of the personality. This structure includes the concepts of the **id,** the **ego,** and the **superego.**

The *id* is part of and derived from the unconscious. It is unlearned, primitive, selfish, and the source of all libidinal energy. It contains the instinctual drives, including the drive for self-preservation, the drive to reproduce, and the drive for group association. The id is without a sense of right and wrong and ruthlessly insists on immediate satisfaction of its impulses and desires.

When born, the individual is said to be a bundle of id, seeking only to satisfy needs and find release for physiological tensions. By crying, infants insist on receiving attention when tensions build up. Infants disregard all other factors in the environment as they demand that their needs be met.

During the individual's entire life, the id persists in pushing the organism toward the achievement of its primitive, instinctual goals. It is described as operating on the basis of the **pleasure principle.** That is to say, the id presses for avoidance of pain at all costs and seeks to maintain pleasure. *Pleasure* in this sense refers to release of tension and the establishment of emotional and physiological equilibrium. *Pain* refers to tensions that are present when the infant is cold, hungry, frightened, or anxious. As the child matures, the concept of pain encompasses additional aspects of body equilibrium, including sexual tension, tensions that result from cultural pressures, and tension from physiological needs. Throughout the individual's entire life, the id insists that the individual seek release of tension, regardless of the social outcome. It is the duty of other parts of the personality to censor the id and to keep it under control.

The development of the *ego* is a result of the individual's interaction with the environment. The ego is initiated when the infant recognizes the breast or the bottle as part of the environment rather than as part of his or her body. The ego promotes the individual's satisfactory adjustment in relation to the environment. Its main function is to establish an acceptable compromise between the crude, pleasure-seeking strivings of the id and the inhibitions of the superego. The means through which the ego achieves this goal is reality testing. The ego deals with the demands of reality as it strives to control and derive satisfaction from the environment. Thus, as the individual matures, the ego becomes the rational, reasonable, conscious part of the personality and strives to integrate the total personality into a smoothly functioning, unified, coherent whole. In the mature adult the ego represents the self to others and individualizes the person from other human beings.

Chronologically, the *superego* develops last. Its development is partially a result of the so-

cialization process that the child undergoes. The superego incorporates the taboos, prohibitions, ideals, and standards of the parents and other significant adults with whom the child associates. It operates mostly at the unconscious level and at this level is an inhibitor of the id. The superego is blindly rigid, strictly moralistic, and as unrelenting and ruthless as the id. Two aspects of the superergo exist: (1) the **conscience** punishes the individual through guilt and anxiety when behavior deviates from the strict standards of the superego; and (2) the **ego ideal** rewards the individual through feelings of euphoria and well-being when behavior emulates those standards believed by the superego to be desired. It is important to understand that neither the punishing nor the rewarding functions of the superego are based on the reality of the situation. Rather, they are based on the individual's internalized standards of right and wrong, good and bad, which were learned at an early age and which are stored primarily in the unconscious mind.

If the individual does not develop an ego strong enough to arbitrate effectively between the id and the superego, he or she will surely develop intrapersonal and interpersonal conflicts. When the id is not controlled effectively, the individual functions in antisocial, lawless ways because primitive impulses are expressed freely. If the superego is so strong that the individual's life is dominated by its restrictions on behavior, the person is likely to be inhibited, repressed, unhappy, and guilt ridden. Thus a mature, effective, stable adult life depends on the development of an ego powerful enough to test reality adequately and then to mediate successfully between the demands of the id and the superego.

Eriksonian concepts

Erikson's theories include and build on Freudian concepts. However, their emphasis is not on Freud's intrapsychic theories but rather on the ego's ability to develop in a healthy, adaptive manner given a facilitative environment.

Therefore, Erikson's theories are variously referred to as neo-Freudian, ego psychology, and cultural. Erikson has also extended the stages of personality development to include the totality of the life span, introducing the important idea that personality development does not cease at the achievement of adulthood. This belief helps to explain the fundamental changes in an individual's feelings and behavior that characteristically occur during adult life.

A major contribution Erikson has made to the understanding of personality development is his identification of **developmental tasks** for each developmental period. These developmental tasks are age-specific achievements that are largely culturally determined. Achievement of each task increases the individual's ego strength and enhances the probability of satisfactory achievement of subsequent tasks. Erikson sees the individual's ability to complete each developmental task satisfactorily as dependent not only on genetic endowment and intrapsychic development, but also primarily on the quality of interaction with the environment. It is important to understand that the developmental tasks identified by Erikson include both positive and negative outcomes. This means that the individual who has not satisfactorily achieved the developmental task for a specific stage of development will develop, as a result, an undesired, less healthy attribute instead. The most obvious example is the developmental task of the first developmental period, basic trust versus basic mistrust. The infant who is not successful, for whatever reason, in developing a sense of basic trust will not be left with an ego structure that demonstrates a mere lack of trust. The alternative is the development of an even more negative characteristic, a sense of basic mistrust. The significance of this paradigm is illustrated simply by the difference between the feelings of "I'm not sure that I can trust you" and "I'm sure that I cannot trust you." Therefore, to understand Erikson's theory of personality development fully, the student must understand the negative as well

as the positive outcomes of each developmental period.

Sullivanian concepts

Sullivan's theories are firmly based on the belief that human beings are more basically different from than similar to all other animals. The uniqueness of human beings, according to Sullivan, lies in their interdependence; as a result of interactions with others, not physiological endowment, the human personality is developed. As previously stated, Sullivan's theories are referred to as *interpersonal* because of their emphasis on human interaction. Sullivan believed that all human behavior is goal directed toward the fulfillment of two needs: the need for satisfaction and the need for security. The need for satisfaction represents the person's biological needs for air, food, sex, and so on. The need for security represents the individual's emotional needs for such feeling states as interpersonal intimacy, status, and self-esteem. When these needs are perceived, internal tension results, and the individual employs a variety of methods to meet them and thereby reduce the tension. Sullivan called these methods **dynamisms.** Partially around the dynamisms characteristic of each age group, Sullivan built his theory of personality development. For example, during the first stage of development the oral cavity is used almost exlusively by the infant as the method to meet needs for satisfaction (by crying to be fed) and needs for security (by crying to be held). Therefore the stage of infancy is characterized by the oral dynamism, and the oral cavity becomes important because it is the means through which the individual establishes interpersonal contact, which in turn is the means through which needs are met and tension is reduced. Not only does the individual have needs met through interpersonal contact, but also through this contact the person establishes the fact of his or her existence. Sullivan believed that an individual's self-concept is developed as a result of the quality of interpersonal relationships with significant others in the person's infancy and childhood. Sullivan defined the self-concept as the result of the reflected appraisals of significant others.

The concept of anxiety is central to Sullivan's theory of personality development. He postulated that anxiety is a response to feelings of disapproval from a significant adult. It is important to understand that these feelings may or may not be based in reality, and that the adult whose disapproval is feared may be real or a symbolic representation. According to Sullivan, therefore, the development of the personality consists of a series of interpersonally based learnings in which dynamisms are used as the individual attempts to gain approval and avoid the anxiety associated with disapproval.

BASIC CONCEPTS OF COGNITIVE DEVELOPMENT

Although cognitive development refers specifically to the individual's ability to think, to remember, and to problem solve, it is inextricably related to personality development and, as such, is included in this discussion. Piaget's theory of cognitive development places heavy emphasis on sequential interactions between the individual's genetically determined intellectual potential and the environment, with the goal of adjusting to the environment. Piaget believed that each individual has an innate knowledge structure, called **schema,** that initially allows the person to organize mentally ways to behave in the environment. Each new environmental experience demands *adaptation,* which entails the simultaneous processes of **assimilation** and **accommodation.** Assimilation refers to the adjustment of the experience so that knowledge of it can be incorporated into the child's existing body of knowledge; accommodation refers to the simultaneous modification of the body of knowledge based on the newly incorporated knowledge. In this way, schemata are built, refined, and organized within and among each other.

Piaget's theory describes four main, discrete stages of cognitive development: the sensorimotor stage, the preoperational stage, the stage of concrete operations, and the stage of formal operations.

STAGES OF PERSONALITY AND COGNITIVE DEVELOPMENT

It has been said that the first 6 years in a child's life contributes the most to personality development. When one considers that these years provide the foundation for future patterns of behavior, this statement appears to be true. However, the nurse must understand the influence of all stages of development on the personality to accurately assess the behavior of adults. The following sections describe and discuss each developmental stage according to the theories of Freud, Erikson, Sullivan, and Piaget.

Infancy

The period of infancy roughly extends over the first year and a half of life. Freud referred to this period as the *oral stage* because the child's libidinal energy is focused on the mouth and its functions to the exclusion of all other considerations. This singular focus on self is technically referred to as **primary narcissism,** which means self-love.

In the first months of life, infants are unable to differentiate between the self and the environment. They therefore feel that all that happens to them is caused by them. This feeling of being all powerful is termed **omnipotence.** Infants' awareness of themselves is in terms of comfort or discomfort, and their total being is focused on fulfilling the demands of the id, which insists on relief from hunger and cold, which are perceived as a diffused tension. They seek relief from this tension by using the mouth, lips and tongue to cry, suck, and swallow. These activities provide the infant with the greatest pleasure, since they reduce discomfort. In the earliest months the infant depends on a nurturing adult to supply the nipple that meets the need for sucking and through which the infant obtains milk to swallow, appeasing the tension caused by hunger. Accidentally, infants soon find the thumb and discover that they can meet their own needs for sucking. Although sucking the thumb provides pleasure, it is experienced as being different from sucking the nipple. Through this simple realization, the infant begins the complex, lengthy process of differentiating the self from the environment. In this way the ego, the recognition of the self, or the "me" begins to develop.

When weaning is initiated, the infant begins to receive fewer oral satisfactions from the environment. When the cup and solid food are substituted for the breast or bottle, the infant feels frustrated. With the adoption of more rigid schedules, the infant is denied the mother's complete attention. The infant may react to these frustrations orally in an aggressive, sometimes destructive way and may begin to bite and may seek symbolic oral gratification by sucking other objects.

Because food and love are given simultaneously during the oral period, oral needs become synonymous with protective love and security. These needs are universal and continue throughout life in one form or another. In adult life, release of tension through oral gratification is achieved through chewing gum, eating, and drinking. Freud believed that these activities are residuals of the oral stage of personality development.

Erikson's view of infancy is very similar to the Freudian view just described, although he terms it the *oral-sensory stage*. Unlike Freud, however, Erikson emphasizes the significance of the mother-child relationship in the achievement of the developmental task of the oral stage: *basic trust versus basic mistrust*. Erikson theorizes that if the infant's great need for love and attention is met consistently and unconditionally by a giving, loving mother, the infant will learn to trust her. Since the infant has no alternative but to view the mother as representing the world at large, this attitude of basic trust in her will strongly influence the infant's perceptions of other people and the environment. Therefore a healthy resolution of this stage of personality development, according to Erikson, results in the development of a basic sense of trust in the mother, which serves as the basis for the development of future trusting relationships. On the other hand, if the infant's experiences with the mother are characterized by inconsistencies and anxiety, the infant will learn to mistrust her and subsequently generalize this attitude to the world at large. One can quite easily appreciate the many great differences between the feelings and behaviors of adults who have achieved a sense of basic trust and those who have achieved a sense of basic mistrust.

Sullivan referred to the first year and a half of life as the stage of infancy rather than the oral stage because he believed that the oral cavity has significance only in that it is the vehicle through which the infant establishes interpersonal contact. Sullivan introduced several important concepts regarding the first stage of development. He coined the term *mothering one* to reflect the belief that the most important person in the infant's life is the individual who consistently nurtures the infant and that this person does not necessarily have to be the biological mother. Whether the mothering one is the biological mother or not, Sullivan believed that this person and the infant must establish an interpersonal relationship, through which they become highly significant to each other. This relationship is unique to the stage of infancy and is characterized by the **empathic linkage,** a symbolic emotional umbilical cord that makes the infant and the nurturing adult highly sensitive to each other's feeling states. Other theorists refer to this process as bonding. Through the empathic linkage, both positive feelings of love and acceptance and negative feelings of anxiety and rejection are conveyed. Sullivan also believed that the development of the **self-concept** begins in the stage of infancy and is closely related to the quality of the infant's feeding experiences. Since the self-concept develops as the result of the reflected appraisals of significant others, if infants frequently experience satisfaction and security from the mothering one during the feeding process, they begin to see themselves as being worthwhile individuals; that is, they begin to develop a "good me" self-concept. Conversely, if the experience with the mothering one is frequently fraught with tension and inconsistency, the foundation is laid for the development of a "bad me" self-concept, and the infant begins to see the self as being not worthwhile. If severely deprived during this stage, infants respond with great anxiety that threaten their life. To preserve life, infants defend themselves by disassociating the anxiety-generating experiences. As a result, they cannot develop a sense of self from reflected appraisals, so they develop a "not me" self-concept. This latter situation lays the foundation for the subsequent development of severe emotional problems.

Once the foundation is laid for its development, the self-concept tends to perpetuate itself. For example, children whose earlier reflected appraisals of significant others have led to the development of a "good me" self-concept sense that they are worthwhile, valued persons and tend to behave as such. This behavior, in turn, evokes further positive feedback from significant others and thereby reinforces the existing "good me" self-concept. However, as children grow, they inevitably encounter people who do not respond to them in the accustomed manner. This unfamiliar experience evokes anxiety and is dealt with by the use of what Sullivan termed **security operations,** enabling the child to ignore this differing input. This process is just as applicable to people who have developed "bad me" and "not me" self-concepts and helps to explain why some persons succeed against all odds and others fail despite all advantages.

Piaget's first stage of cognitive development is called the *sensorimotor stage* and is operative between birth and 24 months of age. During the initial phase of this stage, the infant responds to the environment in an undifferentiated way. For example, when the newborn is startled by a loud noise, the entire body reacts. The infant is also egocentric, viewing the self as fused with the environment and at its center. By the end of this stage, however, the child learns that he or she is separate from the environment. The child also learns that objects have permanence, that objects have not disappeared because they are out of sight. Mastering the concept of object permanence is the basis for the infant's pleasure in the game of peek-a-boo. Finally, by the end of the sensorimotor stage, the infant's behavior in familiar situations becomes goal directed. These cognitive outcomes are consistent with and related to the personality outcomes of the first stage of development as described by Freud and Sullivan.

Early childhood

All theorists agree that the successful resolution of the first stage of development greatly enhances the probability of a successful resolution of subsequent stages.

The period of early childhood is a phase of personality development that occurs roughly between the ages of 18 months and 3 years. Freud termed this time the *anal stage* because the libidinal energy shifts from the oral cavity to the anus and the urethra.

In the early part of this period, the child freely gratifies love of self with the pleasurable sensations involved in evacuating the bladder and bowels naturally and without restriction. Although the mouth remains an important zone of pleasure, the child derives greatest pleasure from the anus and the urethra during these early years.

Ego development continues in this period as the child continuously develops a better-defined concept of self. Superego development is initiated as the mother begins to insist that the child accept certain restrictions and controls regarding toileting. At this point the child experiences the first major frustration of id drives. The child is forced to confront the reality of the situation. To retain the mother's approval (love), the child must learn to postpone the immediate pleasure of urinating or evacuating until the appropriate time and place are available. The necessity for adapting to the mother's wishes regarding toileting places the child and the mother in conflict. As the mother makes demands in an attempt to force the child to accept her standards in relation to toileting, the child develops *ambivalence* toward her; that is, the child simultaneously loves and hates her.

Freud believed that if great stress is placed on remaining clean during this period, the child may grow up to be compulsively clean and meticulous. On the other hand, the child may unconsciously deal with anxiety by the use of reaction formation as a defense mechanism and become very untidy and unconcerned about cleanliness in adult life. Other adult attitudes thought to be traceable to rigid toilet training include stubbornness, hoarding and collecting, excessive concern with bowel function, and sadistic or masochistic tendencies.

Erikson refers to this stage of development as the *muscular-anal stage* and identifies *autonomy versus shame and doubt* as the developmental task to be addressed. Of great significance, according to Erikson, is the mother's response to the child's interest in assuming control over the self by controlling urine and feces. If the mother treats the child with respect as an individual who is separate from her, the child will begin to develop a sense of autonomy, or self-sufficiency. On the other hand, if efforts to do for themselves are ridiculed or interfered with, children will develop a sense of shame and doubt their capabilities.

Sullivan used the term *early childhood* to refer to this period of life. He acknowledged the shift in the child's interest from the mouth to the anus but emphasized the sense of power the child feels when attempting to control the self and others, particularly the mothering one. This feeling of power often puts the child and the mothering one in conflict as the mothering one attempts to toilet train the child. The process and outcome of this power struggle are believed to serve as the prototypical experience for similar interpersonal conflicts in later life. Of equal importance during this stage of development is Sullivan's belief that the child sees feces as an extension of the self, and therefore the mothering one's response to the child's pleasure in his or her feces is seen by the child as a reflection of the mother's view of him or her. In this way the self-concept established in the stage of infancy is reinforced or altered.

The developmental stages of early and later childhood encompass the second period of cognitive development, which Piaget calls *preoperational.* The preoperational stage is divided into two periods, the *preconceptual,* which occurs from ages 2 to 4 years, and the *intuitive,* which occurs from ages 4 to 7 years. During the preconceptual period the child begins to understand symbols and can think in terms of past, present, and future. Increasing language development provides a powerful tool for environmental exploration. By the end of the intuitive period the child is able to think in terms of classes; see relationships, especially if they involve the self; and handle number concepts. For example, the child can recognize a variety of seats as "chairs" even though they may look quite different, can understand that he or she will be punished if a rule is broken, and knows that eight of any object is more than two of the same object.

Later childhood

The period of later childhood is a phase of development that includes ages 3 to 6 years. Freud called this period the *phallic stage.* This descriptive term refers to the focus of pleasurable sensations having shifted from the mouth and the excretory organs to the genitalia. The child begins to identify with the parent of the same sex and unconsciously wishes to replace that parent in the family situation. Thus a girl in this age group might speak of "marrying Daddy" or a little boy might say, "Go away, Daddy, I will take care of Mommy."

From ages 3 to 6 years, children purposefully begin to examine their own bodies and the bodies of their playmates. They discover that pleasurable sensations can be aroused from manipulation of the penis or the clitoris. The difference between the genitalia of men and women is of great interest to them, and they wonder about the girl's lack of an obvious sexual organ. Children of this age may conclude that the penis can be lost in some way, since some people whose bodies they have observed have apparently lost this organ. Anxiety about the loss of the sex organ may develop among children in this age group. A little boy may express fears concerning the loss of his penis through punishment or an accident. These fears are referred to as *castration anxiety*. Unfortunately, some parents reinforce these fears by threatening to cut off the penis if the child is observed fondling it. A little girl notices that she has no penis and may conclude that she lost it or that it has been taken away. She naturally wants what she observes some other children possess. Freud referred to this little girl's attitude as *penis envy*.

Many contemporary theorists believe that any evidence of castration anxiety or penis envy in children of this age is a result of cultural conditioning and not an inherent element in personality development. A serious student of human behavior should keep an open mind, observing for behavioral changes in children as cultural changes occur.

During this period the little boy who has always had much attention and love from his mother begins to feel very possessive toward her. He wants her for himself, and he resents the close tie that exists between his mother and father. He develops competitive feelings toward his father and tries to become a rival with him for his mother's love. The father is such a large and formidable opponent that the little boy develops great resentment and fear of him. This situation is referred to as the *Oedipus complex*. It may precipitate castration anxiety because the little boy may begin to fear that the father will punish him for his resentment toward the father and his attempt to replace the father in his mother's life. Eventually the little boy concludes that being like his father is a more effective way of achieving his mother's love and attention. Thus he begins to take on his father's masculine behavior. This is referred to as *identification*. In this way the little boy begins to learn the male's role in the culture.

Similarly during this period, the little girl begins to identify with the feminine role. The process through which the girl passes in identifying with the parent of the same sex is not as clearly understood as is the process for little boys. The girl thinks that somehow her mother is responsible for her not having a penis. The girl also notices that she does not have breasts as her mother does. She may blame her mother for not having provided her with a complete body and may display much hostility and antagonism toward her. The little girl turns to her father for love and affection and frequently competes openly with the mother for his attention. She begins to imitate her mother because she believes that in this way she may be able to please her father. This is a difficult period for the little girl, who must keep her mother's love and approval because she still depends on her. It is essential that the child maintain a positive relationship with her mother if she is to accomplish the task of identifying with the feminine role.

The birth of a baby in the family at this time presents both boys and girls of this age with a particularly difficult adjustment problem. Children 3 to 6 years of age use almost all their energy in controlling their incestuous desires toward the parent of the opposite sex and their rage toward the parent of the same sex. The necessity to compete with a helpless infant for the parents' attention often results in overt sibling rivalry.

Superego development is also at its height at this time, since in most societies the issues being addressed are seen as moralistic ones. Therefore, unless this stage is successfully resolved, the potential exists for the child to develop long-lasting feelings of guilt because of the incestuous wishes for the parent of the opposite sex and the rage against the parent of the same sex.

Erikson refers to this stage of development as the *locomotor-genital stage* and describes it as having the developmental outcomes of *initiative versus guilt.* He agrees with Freud that children of this age desire to possess exclusively the parent of the opposite sex. To achieve this goal, the child makes the first move, that is, takes the initiative. In a healthy family environment the child inevitably fails to achieve this goal, but the child learns much about being assertive and is able to turn failure into the process of learning how to become a spouse and parent in the future. If, on the other hand, the child experiences great punitiveness and withdrawal of basic approval, the feelings of guilt already present are reinforced and persist in subsequent stages.

Sullivan designated this period of life as *later childhood.* Sullivan believed that the major significance of this stage of personality development is that the child becomes capable of giving up personal and private language and substitutes language that has universal meaning. The importance of the acquisition of the tool of language cannot be overemphasized, since it allows the child to begin to affirm perceptions and feelings with others. The term that describes this process is *consensual validation.* The ability to validate experiences consensually with others is a major factor in enabling the child to develop relationships with peers in the neighborhood or in the nursery school.

Latency

The stage of personality development that occurs roughly between ages 6 and 12 years was called *latency* by Freud. He chose this term because he believed that the child's libidinal energy was not focused on any one area of the body as it had been in the previous three stages. He believed that this energy was lying dormant, and therefore nothing of psychosexual significance occurred during this stage. The relatively stable behavior and even-tempered nature of most children of this stage attest to the temporary intrapsychic equilibrium achieved by the id, ego, and superego.

Erikson recognizes the very important role that school experiences play in the child's personality development during this period. Although he agrees with Freud that no specific area of the body is of particular interest to children during this stage, he believes that psychic energy is being actively used in pursuit of knowledge and skills. In other words, children are purposefully involved in acquiring tools through which they can deal with the environment both in the present and in the future. According to Erikson, if children are successful in this endeavor, they will have achieved the developmental task of *industry.* If unsuccessful, they will feel inadequate and develop a sense of *inferiority.*

Sullivan saw this period as being very critical to the development of a healthy adult personality. He divided Freud's and Erikson's 6-year span into two periods: the *juvenile era,* lasting roughly from ages 6 to 10; and *preadolescence,* lasting roughly from ages 11 to 12, or to the onset of puberty. During the juvenile era the child turns away from the parents as being the most significant people in life and looks to peers of the same sex to fill the functions of providing a sense of security and companionship. This is the period of gang formation and fierce gang loyalties. The gang requires strict adherence to the group's rules, and the child slavishly complies with them. During this period the child tries to find a place among peers. In so doing, the child acquires two very important interpersonal tools: the ability to compete and the ability to compromise. As the child tests these modes of behavior with peers, their responses help the child to learn to use both appropriately.

Another very important function of the peer group is the reinforcement or alteration of the self-concept. A child who enters this stage of development with a positive or "good me" self-concept is likely to behave in a manner that elicits responses from peers that confirm and reinforce the child's view of self. When the child enters this period with a negative or "bad me" self-concept, positive reflected appraisals from the peer group can do much to alter the child's view of self. This fact indicates the significant role the peer group plays in the child's life during this period.

During preadolescence the child maintains great interest in the group but simultaneously develops an intense love relationship with a particular person of the same sex whom the child perceives to be very similar to himself or herself. Sullivan called this special relationship a *chum relationship*. Until this time the child's love has been self-centered, but in the chum relationship the child experiences for the first time the capacity to put the needs of someone else ahead of his or her own. Sullivan saw this experience as a necessary prerequisite to the establishment of a satisfactory heterosexual relationship in subsequent stages of development. The emotional intimacy that the chums experience also helps them to explore and clarify their feelings in a way that builds self-esteem.

Sullivan also stressed the importance of the school experience in the development of the child's personality. At school, children meet significant adults who greatly influence the development of their self-concepts. In this culture, success at school is rewarded with much approval, whereas lack of success often begins a series of defeats that carry over into adult life. The self-concept of children who do poorly in school may be irreparably damaged by the reactions of teachers, the significant adults in that important environment. On the other hand, understanding, helpful teachers may provide the child with a positive basis for self-evaluation and in some instances may constitute an opportunity for corrective interpersonal experiences with adults. Teachers are extremely important in the lives of children and need to be aware of their potential for therapeutic experiences in their day-to-day contacts with children.

Sullivan's emphasis on the importance of the school experience for children in this developmental stage is validated by their stage of cognitive development. The third stage of cognitive development, according to Piaget, occurs between ages 7 and 12 years, is termed *concrete operations,* and is characterized by major intellectual and conceptual development. The enthusiasm and joy of learning exhibited by children of this age are well known by adults who have sustained contact with these children. During this stage, children develop the ability to handle more numbers in an increasingly complex way, to think logically, to relate external events to each other even if the events do not involve them, and to classify persons or objects along more than one dimension. For example, children learn to understand that chairs are also furniture and that their mother is also a nurse and a wife.

Puberty and adolescence

The stage of puberty and adolescence covers the years from age 12 to approximately age 18. Because all theorists agree that this stage of development is initiated by the active functioning of the sexual glands and because individuals mature physiologically at different rates, it is difficult to make a definite statement concerning the span of years included in adolescence.

Freud saw adolescence as the final stage of personality development, characterized by a reactivation of libidinal energy and the focusing of this energy on the genital area. As such, he designated this period the *genital stage.* Although Freud believed that this final stage lasted for the rest of the person's life, he emphasized that the intense work of this period was completed when the individual achieved a satisfactory heterosexual relationship with a mate and began the life cycle anew by establishing a family.

Adolescence can be a highly problematic stage of personality development. As adolescents mature physiologically, they are faced with the necessity of handling powerful sexual urges that threaten to put the influence of the id out of balance with the influences of the ego and superego. Because of this imbalance of psychic forces, unresolved conflicts and unsolved problems of earlier developmental periods often reemerge at this time. This is particularly true of the Oedipal conflict because of the similar sexual urges experienced at both stages. Therefore the adolescent is simultaneously drawn toward the parents and driven away from them. This ambivalence is manifested by much conflict between the adolescent and the parents as the adolescent vacillates between behaving in a dependent, immature, childlike way and in an independent, mature, adult manner.

Erikson builds on Freud's theory by elaborating on the conflictual nature of the parent-child relationship. Erikson sees the developmental task of puberty and adolescence as the development of a sense of *identity versus role diffusion*. During this time, adolescents must emancipate themselves from their parents, not only physically but also emotionally by establishing for themselves their own sense of identity. They must answer the most fundamental questions of "Who am I?" and "What am I?" This requires many decisions regarding familial, occupational, and social roles. Adolescents are strongly influenced by the family's norms and values as they struggle to make these decisions. However, if they are to master this developmental stage successfully, they must accept these norms and values as their own or reject them and establish new guidelines for themselves. In other words, the adolescent's primary task is to develop an ego that has integrated previous learnings and experiences so that the adolescent develops a sense of continuity and sameness in life. Unsuccessful mastery of this stage results in a diffuse, fragmented sense of self, the most problematic aspect of which is often the shifting between an adult and a child orientation.

Sullivan designated the period between 12 and 17 or 18 years of age as *early adolescence*. As the person experiences sexual urges (termed *lust* by Sullivan), he or she turns from the chum relationship to the task of establishing a relationship with a peer of the opposite sex. The peer group remains an important aspect of the adolescent's life during this stage because it serves the important function of providing security and consensual validation of the adolescent's feelings and behaviors. The influence of the peer group in regulating the adolescent's behavior is very strong.

Successful resolution of the stage of adolescence is greatly impeded when the child is seen as unacceptable by the peer group, perhaps because of physical handicaps or major cultural differences. The consequence of this nonacceptance may be a prolonged clinging to parents or parent figures to feel a sense of security and belongingness. Another pitfall of this stage occurs when the adolescent's peer group is composed of individuals who are antisocial and engage in delinquent behavior. Although adolescents will avoid the anxiety of isolation by identifying with this group, it is also likely that they will develop behaviors that are antagonistic to society and that will impede them in the successful achievement of subsequent developmental tasks.

The final stage of cognitive development begins during the stage of adolescence, approximately at age 12, and continues throughout adulthood. Piaget terms this last stage *formal operations* (Table 12-2). During this stage the individual develops abstract thinking and is able to see multiple, complex relationships among objects, categories, and events. This ability permits sophisticated use of problem solving, as in the scientific method. With use, this cognitive ability continues to develop and be refined throughout the remainder of the person's life.

Table 12-2. Piaget's stages of cognitive development

AGE	STAGE	CHARACTERISTICS
Birth to 2 years	Sensorimotor	Initial egocentrism and nondifferentiation from environment
		Learns object permanence and that he or she is separate from environment
2 to 4 years	Preoperational: preconceptual	Understands symbols
		Thinks in terms of past, present, and future
		Increased language development
4 to 7 years	Preoperational: intuitive	Thinks in classes
		Understands relationships that involve him or her
		Understands number concepts
7 to 12 years	Concrete operations	Handles more numbers in a complex way
		Thinks logically
		Understands relationships that do not involve him or her
		Classifies persons or objects along more than one dimension
12 years to adulthood	Formal operations	Thinks abstractly
		Sees multiple, complex relationships
		Engages in complex problem solving

Young adulthood

The period of young adulthood has its onset at the end of adolescence and continues until adulthood. It is almost impossible to state a chronological age range for this period with any degree of accuracy, although many authorities state that it usually begins sometime in the person's twenties and is concluded in the late thirties or early forties. As the life span increases and the entry into the adult work world is delayed by the need for increasingly advanced education, the age ranges of the later developmental periods will have to be re-evaluated.

As previously stated, Freud believed that the healthy young adult will have achieved psychosexual maturity. By this he meant that individuals will have integrated their libidinal drives in a manner that enables them to love a member of the opposite sex with whom they hope to establish a home and nurture a family. At the same time the healthy young adult retains enough self-love to seek satisfaction for personal needs without being destructive to others. In addition, the person is able to direct positive feelings toward other people in the environment, to work effectively, to achieve creatively, and to use fully the capacities with which he or she has been endowed without being hampered by crippling anxieties. The ability to achieve these mature capabilities depends greatly on the person's heredity and constitutional endowment. However, psychosexual development is powerfully influenced by the experiences that the person has had during early formative years.

Although Freud's theory of psychosexual development does not preclude the potential influence of events on personality in the individual's adult life, Freud postulated that the early developmental stages were critical and that the final stage begins in the late teens and lasts for the remainder of the person's life, with major alterations in personality development being unlikely during this time under usual circumstances.

Erikson, on the other hand, sees the personality as continuing to develop dynamically throughout the remainder of the life span.

Erikson sees the necessity for the individual in young adulthood to continue making decisions about significant aspects of life, such as choosing a mate with whom the individual can experience both physical and emotional intimacy. Erikson expresses this by stating that the task to be mastered during this period is the development of *intimacy versus isolation*. The ability to develop an intimate relationship with an adult of the opposite sex depends greatly on satisfactory mastery of previous developmental tasks and leads to the establishment of a safe, congenial family environment in which children can be reared. Accepting the role of parent and the responsibility for nurturing, safeguarding, and rearing children is essential if the culture is to be perpetuated. The individual's ability to be successful in these activities is determined largely by experiences as a child within a family. Erikson also emphasizes the significance of successfully building one's lifework during this state. Children cannot be effectively nurtured unless the family has a reasonable degree of social and financial security. Thus, acceptance of family responsibilities requires that the young adult be reasonably effective in performing some aspect of work.

If the developmental task of intimacy and its concomitant responsibilities are not achieved, young adults are likely to develop a sense of emotional isolation, having the sense that they "do not fit." Although young adults who retreat into isolation often do so to avoid the emotional pain risked by the vulnerability associated with intimacy, they ironically discover that the price of self-protection is not having their needs met, which increases the need to protect themselves.

Sullivan referred to young adulthood as the stage of *late adolescence*. He believed that the major task of this period is the incorporation of intimacy (which developed during preadolescence with a chum) with lust (which became the mode of relating during early adolescence) so that these are not experienced in isolation from each other. Sullivan viewed this mode of relating

as the hallmark of adult maturity and therefore did not identify any subsequent stages of development.

Adulthood

As previously stated, neither Freud nor Sullivan identified developmental dynamics beyond the achievement of adolescence or early adulthood. However, both these theorists implied that it may take the remainder of the individual's life to develop the maturity that theoretically should have been achieved by those periods. Erikson, however, continues to elaborate on developmental tasks specific to later life.

According to Erikson, the developmental task of adulthood is the development of *generativity versus stagnation*. Erikson believed that as emotionally healthy individuals grow older, it becomes increasingly important to them that they transmit their values to the next generation, thereby helping to ensure their own immortality through the perpetuation of their culture. Therefore the adult may become very involved in activities concerned with the community and society. On the other hand, the individual who developed a sense of isolation during the previous period becomes increasingly self-absorbed and is often acutely aware of "marking time." This person receives little fulfillment from interpersonal relationships or work and has few, if any, meaningful goals. Erikson refers to this state as *stagnation*.

Current literature about the stage of adulthood makes it clear that this period is one about which we still need to learn more. Several authorities believe that adults, because of physiological alterations, aging parents, an increasing awareness of community and societal needs, and grown children who lead lives independent of them, confront their own mortality for the first time. It is believed that this confrontation results in much uneasiness about the status quo and a subsequent reevaluation of one's goals and purposes in life. Persons who have previously led relatively unexamined lives often find themselves in a state of crisis, which they may attempt to hide from others, since to them their concerns do not seem to be reality based. Societal manifestations of this turmoil are a marked increase in the divorce rate and major shifts in career patterns. For example, the woman who has been relatively satisfied as a homemaker for the past 15 to 20 years senses that she has been left out of the mainstream of life and suddenly develops a need to become involved in a career outside the home. Likewise, a husband and father at this stage of life may have a feeling that the occupation in which he has been involved for the previous 20 years is unsatisfying, regardless of his monetary or social success.

Understandably, such a reaction on the part of either wife, husband, or both, causes much disequilibrium in the family system. Many middle-aged persons decide they have made a mistake, not only in choice of vocation, but also in marriage partner, geographical location, and hobbies. Unfortunately, many decisions are made precipitously, and these feelings are not recognized as being valid within the developmental context in which they occur.

Margaret Mead, world-famous anthropologist, eloquently pointed out that the needs and requirements of marital partners, as with those of their children, change as the relationship matures. Thus the maintenance of a happy, successful marriage relationship requires that the partners continuously seek to relate to each other as individuals whose needs are in a process of dynamic evolution.

Maturity

The role of aged individuals who have retired from an active social and economic life is unique in U.S. culture. Unfortunately the wisdom they have accumulated through the years is not considered of value as it is in some cultures. Aging persons find it necessary to adjust to a reduced income, waning physical strength, and deterio-

rating health. This may be an anxiety-producing experience, since it represents a loss of power and independence. Loneliness is another experience with which elderly people must cope. Frequently their friends and marital partners die, leaving them in social isolation. Such lonely individuals who are no longer able to cope efficiently with their physical requirements need to adjust to the establishment of living arrangements that are acceptable, while at the same time being faced with the need to accept a dependent role. Older persons need to establish social relationships with a group of interested, understanding peers. This need leads many older individuals to seek an affiliation with a "golden age" club or a similar organization.

The preceding statements about the stage of maturity are pessimistic in tone because of the current nature of the society in which we live and the ways in which elderly people are viewed. It should be clear that the older person must inevitably make many adjustments to altered physiological, social, and financial states. If previous developmental tasks have been satisfactorily achieved, however, it is possible for the elderly person to make the necessary adjustments with grace, dignity, and minimum undue anxiety.

The major dynamic of the stage of maturity is the acceptance of the inevitability of death. To develop this acceptance, individuals engage in a life review. If, on the whole, aged persons are able to feel satisfied with the uniqueness and achievements of their past life, Erikson believes they will develop a sense of *ego integrity,* which in turn enables them to view death as the ultimate conclusion of life. If, on the other hand, the life review finds individuals lacking, they will develop a sense of *despair* because time is too short for them to undo and redo their lives to achieve the sense of fulfillment they lack.

As with adulthood, maturity is a stage of life about which much more must be learned. Interest in and concern about this stage of devel-

Table 12-3. Interpersonal age-related experiences and behavioral outcomes based on Erikson's theory of personality development

AGES OF MAN	INTERPERSONAL AGE-RELATED EXPERIENCES	AGE-RELATED BEHAVIORAL OUTCOMES	EGO QUALITIES
Oral-sensory			
Positive	Infant is held lovingly and tenderly by mother; needs met with sensitivity and consistency.	Infant sleeps and feeds easily; is usually relaxed and snuggles closely when held.	Basic trust
Negative	Infant continuously experiences anxiety in contact with mother; needs met inconsistently.	Infant generally tense and crying; not comforted by holding; rages when left by mother.	Basic mistrust
Muscular-anal			
Positive	Toddler's efforts to stand on own feet are respected and encouraged; relaxed, unhurried toilet training.	Toddler takes pride in self-expression, whether making bowel movements or playing.	Autonomy
Negative	Toddler experiences rejection as efforts at self-sufficiency are ridiculed; cleanliness overemphasized.	Toddler is self-conscious, hiding face or self from others; is stubborn and has temper tantrums.	Shame and doubt
Locomotor-genital			
Positive	Child's need to explore body is accepted matter-of-factly; sexual curiosity handled without anxiety.	Child begins to imitate parent of the same sex; approaches tasks with enthusiasm.	Initiative
Negative	Child's masturbatory activities are condemned and punished; sexual curiosity ignored or rebuked.	Child experiences nightmares, often symbolic of castration; hides masturbatory activities.	Guilt
Latency			
Positive	Child's efforts at learning are supported; new interests and friendships encouraged.	Child is obedient, prefers order and limits; works on projects to completion with peers.	Industry
Negative	Child is ridiculed in front of peers; friends and interests criticized.	Child fears failure and gives up; does not try to perform or to learn.	Inferiority
Puberty and adolescence			
Positive	Youth's beginning emancipation from family is accepted; vocational choices supported.	Youth turns from parents to peer groups, joining cliques and clubs; develops "crushes" on other figures.	Identity
Negative	Youth's rapidly changing body, awkwardness, and interest in opposite sex are ridiculed; parents try to dominate.	Youth is unable to separate from parents; is embarrassed over physical changes; is unable to make job choice.	Role diffusion

Table 12-3. Interpersonal age-related experiences and behavioral outcomes based on Erikson's theory of personality development—cont'd

AGES OF MAN	INTERPERSONAL AGE-RELATED EXPERIENCES	AGE-RELATED BEHAVIORAL OUTCOMES	EGO QUALITIES
Young adulthood			
Positive	Young adult experiences support, interest, approval, and tenderness in love relationship; has job satisfaction.	Young adult is well rounded; has varied interests in family, job, friends, and hobbies.	Intimacy
Negative	Young adult's choice of partner is rejected by parents; parents try to hold and control offspring.	Young adult sacrifices relatedness for work and drive to succeed; is unable to give emotionally to others.	Isolation
Adulthood			
Positive	Adult experiences orgasm with loved, trusted, and respected partner; experiences love and respect from offspring.	Adult is productive and creative; bears and nurtures children; teaches and gives to others.	Generativity
Negative	Adult experiences rejection and hostility in adult relationships; takes no pleasure in community affairs.	Adult experiences impotence/frigidity; becomes bored and resentful with job.	Stagnation
Maturity			
Positive	Individual experiences love and respect from maturing offspring; has satisfying past recollections.	Individual looks forward to retirement as opportunity to try new things; recalls past with pleasure.	Ego integrity
Negative	Individual experiences alienation from family; loneliness occurs as friends, spouse, and others die.	Individual faces death with fear, preoccupied with reliving life because of dissatisfaction with the past.	Despair

Modified from Lofstedt CR: *Mereness' essentials of psychiatric nursing learning and activity guide,* ed 3, St Louis, 1990, Mosby–Year Book.

opment are increasing as the number of older persons in society increases.

Table 12-3 outlines the age-related interpersonal experiences and behavioral outcomes experienced by human beings as they traverse the eight ages of man identified by Erikson. They are outlined here because of their comprehensiveness and applicability to nursing practice.

KEY POINTS

1. Children were historically viewed as miniature adults who were thought to develop emotionally at the same rate that they developed physically. This view did not change until the early twentieth century. Interest in the personality development of adults has emerged only recently.

2. Personality is defined as the aggregate of the individual's physical and mental qualities as these

interact characteristically with the person's environment.

3. A mentally healthy adult accepts strengths and limitations, perceives reality accurately, exhibits environmental mastery, engages in independent thinking and action, and achieves a unifying, integrated outlook on life.

4. Major concepts underlying the Piagetian theory of cognitive development include schema, adaptation, and assimilation and accommodation.

5. Major concepts underlying the Freudian theory of personality development include libidinal energy, levels of consciousness (conscious, preconscious or subconscious, unconscious), the structure of the personality (id, ego, superego), the pleasure principle, and avoidance of pain.

6. A major concept unique to the Eriksonian theory of personality development is the process of ego development resulting from the person's struggle with developmental tasks specific to each period of the entire life span.

7. Major concepts underlying the Sullivanian theory of personality development include the uniqueness of human beings, their interpersonal interactions, their need to fulfill the need for satisfaction and the need for security, and the concept of anxiety.

8. Freud, Erikson, and Sullivan describe the process of personality development from infancy through adolescence. Erikson extends the description of personality development through maturity.

9. Each theorist views the development of the personality in a different way, although their views have much in common and have significance for the practice of psychiatric nursing.

10. Piaget defined five stages of cognitive development, from birth to adulthood: sensorimotor; preoperational, preconceptual; preoperational, intuitive; concrete operations; and formal operations.

11. Freud defined five stages of personality development: oral, anal, phallic, latency, and genital.

12. Erikson described eight developmental tasks, each specific to a stage of development: basic trust versus basic mistrust, autonomy versus shame and doubt, initiative versus guilt, industry versus inferiority, identity versus role diffusion, intimacy versus isolation, generativity versus stagnation, and ego integrity versus despair.

13. Sullivan defined five stages of personality development: infancy, early childhood, later childhood, early adolescence, and late adolescence.

SUGGESTED SOURCES OF ADDITIONAL INFORMATION

Arnold H: Snow White and the seven dwarfs: a symbolic account of human development, *Perspect Psychiatr Care* 117(5):218, 1979.

Bednar RL and others: Self-esteem: a concept of renewed clinical relevance, *Hosp Community Psychiatry* 42(2):123, 1991.

Bowlby J: *Maternal care and mental health,* series no 2, Geneva, 1952, World Health Organization.

Bowlby J: *Attachment,* New York, 1980, Basic Books.

Bowlby J: *Separation,* New York, 1980, Basic Books.

Bowlby J: Developmental psychiatry comes of age, *Am J Psychiatry* 145:1, January 1988.

Cumming E, Henry W: *Growing old: the process of disengagement,* New York, 1979, Arno Press.

Denehy JA: Interventions related to parent-infant attachment, *Nurs Clin North Am* 27(2):425, 1992.

Erikson EH: *Childhood and society,* ed 2, New York, 1964, Norton.

Freud S: *The ego and the id,* New York, 1962, Norton (edited by J Strachey).

Freud S: *A general introduction to psychoanalysis,* New York, 1972, Pocket Books.

Hemmelgarn B, Laing G: The relationship between situational factors and perceived role strain in employed mothers, *Fam Community Health* 14(1):8, 1991.

Howell E, Bayes M, editors: *Women and mental health,* New York, 1981, Basic Books.

Kerr NJ: The ego competency model of psychiatric nursing: theoretical overview and clinical application, *Perspect Psychiatr Care* 26(1):13, 1990.

Maslow A: *Toward a psychology of being,* Princeton, NJ, 1962, Van Nostrand.

Maslow A: *Motivation and personality,* ed 2, New York, 1970, Harper & Row.

May R: *Sex and fantasy: patterns of male and female development,* New York, 1980, Norton.

Muller ME: A critical review of prenatal attachment research, *Scholarly Inquiry Nurs Pract* 6(1):5, 1992.

Munroe R: *Schools of psychoanalytic thought,* New York, 1955, Dryden Press.

Piaget J: *The growth of logical thinking from childhood to adolescence,* New York, 1958, Basic Books.

Piaget J: The child's conception of the world, Ames, Iowa, 1963, Littlefield, Adams.

Powers M: Universal utility of psychoanalytic theory for nursing practice models, *J Psychosoc Nurs Ment Health Serv* 18:28, April 1980.

Sheehy G: *Passages—predictable crises of adult life,* New York, 1976, Dutton.

Sullivan HS: *Interpersonal theory of psychiatry,* New York, 1953, Norton.

Symonds B: Sociological issues in the conceptualization of mental illness, *J Adv Nurs* 16:1470, 1991.

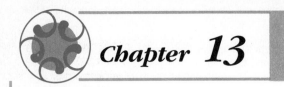

Chapter 13

Anxiety
one response to stress

CHAPTER OUTLINE
Historical perspective
Definition and characteristics of anxiety
Origin of anxiety
Adaptations to anxiety
   Ego defense mechanisms
   Security operations
   Coping mechanisms

LEARNING OBJECTIVES
After studying this chapter, the student will be able to:
• Define the concept of anxiety and list its characteristics.

• Discuss the process through which anxiety originates, as theorized by Freud and Sullivan.

• Discuss how ego defense mechanisms, security operations, and coping mechanisms serve as adaptations to anxiety.

KEY TERMS
Anxiety
Normal anxiety
Pathological anxiety
Mental mechanisms
Ego defense mechanisms
Security operations
Coping mechanisms
Compensation
Displacement
Denial
Fixation
Sublimation
Reaction formation
Identification
Introjection
Undoing
Isolation
Rationalization
Repression
Regression
Projection
Symbolization
Condensation
Conversion
Apathy
Somnolent detachment
Selective inattention
Preoccupation
Suppression

Anxiety is the most universal of human emotions and is experienced by all persons throughout their entire life span. Despite its all-pervasive nature, however, **anxiety** cannot be observed directly. Rather, its presence can be inferred only from behavior.

Anxiety is simultaneously an adaptation and a stressor. It functions as an adaptation in that it is a response to system disequilibrium and initially reduces the level of stress by obscuring the nature of the stressor. In the long term, anxiety is a nonproductive adaptation because it prevents the system from focusing on and directly dealing with the source of the stress. Nevertheless, its existence is a signal that the system is having difficulty maintaining homeokinesis, and in that sense it serves a valuable function.

Anxiety also serves as a stressor in that it, unlike any other emotion, is always perceived as negative. Thus its presence thrusts the system into a state of stress, sometimes compounding rather than relieving the original stress. Because anxiety is always perceived as being negative, the system deals with it by employing various mechanisms that are themselves adaptations.

Because anxiety is a basic factor in the development and manifestation of human behavior, it is necessary for the nurse to acquire an in-depth understanding of its characteristics, its origin, and the usual adaptations to it.

HISTORICAL PERSPECTIVE

It is reasonable to assume that people have experienced anxiety since the dawn of humanity. Until recently, however, human beings have had to struggle merely to survive. Consequently, it is likely they more frequently experienced fear than anxiety.

Fear and anxiety are indistinguishable to the person experiencing them. Fear is a response to a real stressor that threatens the system's existence. Because the stressor can be identified, it becomes possible to deal with it directly by fighting it or fleeing it. These adaptations provide a direct outlet for the physiological and psychological tension resulting from fear.

Such is not the case when the adaptation to a stressor is anxiety. In this instance the feeling perceived is the same as that experienced when fear is present, but the stressor is unknown to the person. Consequently, no direct outlet exists for the built-up tension; the anxiety becomes a stressor itself.

Sigmund Freud was the first theorist to emphasize the importance of anxiety in the development of human behavior. He first demonstrated the use of ego defense mechanisms as an adaptation to anxiety and believed that the necessity for their use indicated a greater or lesser degree of psychopathology. In contrast, contemporary theorists believe that psychopathology exists when the individual uses defense mechanisms as the predominant mode of dealing with anxiety, thereby obscuring reality, or when the individual uses only one or two such mechanisms to the exclusion of all others. In other words, it is acknowledged that a sparing use of a variety of mental mechanisms is within the range of healthy behavior. However, as the society becomes more complex and therefore more stressful, anxiety and its adaptations become more frequent causes and effects of mental disorders. Mental disorders specific to anxiety and to its adaptations are discussed more fully in Chapter 17. The box on p. 202 lists some medical and nursing diagnoses related to anxiety.

Table 13-1 provides an overview of anxiety throughout history.

DEFINITION AND CHARACTERISTICS OF ANXIETY

Anxiety is defined as a vague sense of impending doom, an apprehension or sense of dread, that seemingly has no basis in reality. Laypersons refer to anxiety as "being nervous."

As observed earlier, anxiety is the only emotion that is always perceived as negative. In contrast to anxiety, emotions that are usually con-

DIAGNOSES RELATED TO ANXIETY

Medical diagnoses	Nursing diagnoses* NANDA
Agoraphobia	
Simple phobia	Anxiety
Social phobia	Sleep pattern distur-
Posttraumatic stress dis-	bance
order	Posttrauma response
Sleep disorders	Ineffective individual
Depersonalization	coping
Obsessive-compulsive	Ineffective denial
disorder	

From Rawlins RP and others: *Mental health–psychiatric nursing,* ed 3, 1993, St Louis, Mosby–Year Book.
NANDA, North American Nursing Diagnosis Association.

sidered painful sometimes bring pleasure. For example, most people do not enjoy being angry. On occasion, however, it is satisfying to experience anger when one believes it is justified and shares it with others. Another characteristic of anxiety is its extreme communicability. Almost acting as a living organism, anxiety is transferred with amazing rapidity from one individual to another, often below a level of awareness.

When individuals experience anxiety, they cannot distinguish it from fear, a feeling state that occurs in response to a specific identifiable environmental threat. Because anxiety cannot be distinguished from fear, the physiological response is the same in that the autonomic nervous system is activated and the body becomes ready for "fight or flight." Since an identifiable environmental threat is not present, individuals cannot discharge the tension of anxiety by fighting or fleeing and consequently may experience such symptoms as a pounding heart and a dry mouth, the perception of which serves to increase anxiety. Furthermore, when persons become aware of being anxious, they often frantically search for a reason to explain this feeling in the hope of abolishing it. They are rarely successful, and their explanation often describes the result of the anxiety, not its cause. For example,

a young woman who believes she is anxious because of the responsibilities she must assume in the care of her young infant may really be experiencing a conflict between a desire to be dependent and the need to be independent. This in turn creates anxiety, making her decreasingly able to care for the infant. Therefore her explanation of her anxiety is not its cause but rather its manifestation.

Anxiety occurs in degrees. Although it is never seen as desired, mild anxiety serves the function of motivating and making the person more physically and mentally alert. When the level of anxiety is extremely high, the individual may be incapable of action or may react with unusual behavior or what appears to be irrational behavior. This irrational behavior is referred to as a *panic state.*

ORIGIN OF ANXIETY

Current research findings indicate that a genetic predisposition to anxiety may exist. Biochemical changes are also associated with anxiety, although it is unknown at this time whether these changes cause anxiety or result from it.

Traditionally, most authorities have taken the position that anxiety occurs as an adaptation to a threat to biological integrity, an unconscious symbolic conflict, or a threat to the self-concept.

Freud believed that anxiety is a response to the emergence of id impulses that are unacceptable to the superego. In other words, the ego detects a real or potential conflict between the id and the superego, which results in anxiety, thereby alerting the ego to the necessity for intervention. Freud believed that all persons experience anxiety initially during the birth process, when the respiratory and cardiovascular systems must undergo rapid, extensive changes to support extrauterine life. He also viewed the birth process as the prototypical separation. These two factors, the threat to life and separation, are associatively linked to each other and

Table 13-1.   Views and theories of anxiety throughout history

DATES	EVENTS
Pre-1900s	In early Greek literature, responses to anxiety were described as accepting fate, appealing to a higher being, or stoicism.
	During the Middle Ages, emphasis was placed on the identification and categorization of emotions. Anxiety was identified as a disagreeable feeling.
	The use of reason to control anxiety, which led to denial and repression, was emphasized during the Renaissance.
1900	Kierkegaard described the direct confrontation of anxiety as a way to open possibilities of freedom and self-development.
	Freud identified anxiety as central to personality development.
1950s	Peplau linked nursing actions directly to clients' security. She developed a theory of anxiety characterized by levels of anxiety that ranged from mild to panic levels.
1960s	The twentieth century is described as the "age of anxiety" because of the advent of the atomic bomb and other profound, anxiety-producing situations, such as economic insecurity, nuclear warfare, political upheaval, and changing values and standards of behaviors related to family, church, and school.
1990s	Nursing today emphasizes the relationship between anxiety and physical conditions such as cardiovascular problems, ulcers, hypertension, pregnancy, and responses to accidents and surgical procedures. Additional emphasis is placed on the effect of anxiety on clients' ability to receive information and to learn.

From Rawlins RP and others: *Mental health–psychiatric nursing,* ed 3, St Louis, 1993, Mosby–Year Book.

to the experience of anxiety. In subsequent developmental stages, Freud theorized, unconscious conflicts are perceived as life-threatening, are associated with separation, and result in anxiety.

Sullivan viewed anxiety as always occurring in an interpersonal context. That is, anxiety is generated when individuals anticipate or actually receive cues that signal disapproval from one or more significant others. This presents persons with an approach-avoidance dilemma; they want to approach or please the other person because they view this person as being significant, but to do so incurs the risk of self-disapproval, a threat to their existence as they know themselves. According to Sullivan, the human being first experiences anxiety as an infant when either the need for satisfaction, which is physiologically based, or the need for security, which is interpersonally based, is not met by the mothering one. As discussed in Chapter 12, Sullivan's theory of personality development also emphasizes the empathic linkage between the infant and the mothering one through which anxiety is readily communicated. The empathic linkage makes the infant and mothering one extremely sensitive to discomfort in each other. Because of an inability to solve problems, infants have no alternative but to believe that the mothering one's anxiety, which is communicated to them via the empathic linkage, is caused by them, even though the source of this discomfort may be external to them. This phenomenon, which all adults have experienced, by definition, during their infancy, is the basis for Sullivan's belief that anxiety is interpersonally based.

Some authorities distinguish between normal anxiety and pathological anxiety. In reality this distinction refers to the nature of the stressor that precipitates the response of anxiety rather than to the nature of the anxiety itself. **Normal anxiety** arises from a realistic apprehension of a previously unencountered situation that has symbolic meaning to the individual. For example, the anxiety a bridegroom experiences before his wedding likely arises in response to his unconscious concern about his ability to assume the role of husband and therefore his view of the wedding as a symbolic threat to his identity as an adequate male.

In contrast, **pathological anxiety** is often a response to thoughts, feelings, wishes, or desires that, if conscious, would be unacceptable to the individual or that, if known, would cause the loss of approval or love from significant others. Therefore, situations that evoke such unacceptable thoughts, feelings, wishes, or desires are associated with anxiety, against which the individual must defend to maintain a self-concept. For example, a young man who has unconscious homosexual desires that, if known to him, would be repugnant might react with great anxiety when circumstances force him to live in physical proximity with other young men.

ADAPTATIONS TO ANXIETY

Because moderate to high levels of prolonged anxiety can prove lethal to the human system, some method of relieving anxiety is essential if the system is to regain homeokinesis. The human being usually is able to relieve anxiety through a form of adaptation referred to as mental mechanisms. **Mental mechanisms** are patterns of thinking and behaving that are used to protect the individual from threatening aspects of the environment or from personal feelings of anxiety. Mental mechanisms are learned as being effective adaptations to anxiety during one of the phases of personality development. They are further developed and elaborated on as the individual grows and struggles with stressors. Thus the use of these mechanisms is a matter of re-

sorting to earlier patterns of thinking and behaving that have already proved helpful in relieving anxiety. Many of these methods of thinking and behaving are totally unconscious, whereas others are partly conscious and partly unconscious. All, however, are a means of protecting the individual from situations perceived as dangerous. In this regard these mechanisms serve a very important function by helping the person to maintain biological integrity and self-esteem.

Ego defense mechanisms are one type of frequently used mental mechanism. These are used when the individual unconsciously experiences a basic conflict between id impulses and the demands of the superego. The ego unconsciously uses some of its energy to initiate a defense mechanism that effects a compromise between the demands of the id and the superego, thereby relieving anxiety.

Another form of mental mechanism is called **security operations.** These were identified by Sullivan and are called into play when anxiety is a response to a threat to the self-concept. Security operations, as with ego defense mechanisms, operate without the awareness of the individual employing them.

Although the sparing use of mental mechanisms is considered healthy and serves the function of lowering anxiety, thereby enabling the system to regain homeokinesis, their use does take a toll. The price of this adaptation is the use of system energy, resulting in less potential energy available for growth. Furthermore, the stressor, whether a conflict or threat, is not directly addressed or resolved.

Another adaptation to anxiety is **coping mechanisms.** A coping mechanism, unlike an ego defense mechanism or a security operation, is based on a conscious acknowledgment that a problem exists. As a result, the individual engages in reality-oriented problem-solving activities designed to reduce tension. Therefore, coping mechanisms are considered more healthy adaptations than ego defense mechanism or se-

---

**GUIDELINES FOR PRIMARY
PREVENTION OF ANXIETY**

Primary prevention

Teach client to:
  Be kind to self and to appreciate self
  Be less critical of self
  Maintain high self-esteem
  Restore self-esteem when lowered
  Identify physiological symptoms of anxiety
  Share feelings when upset or anxious with a sup-
    portive person
  Manage stress with diet, exercise, rest/sleep, and
    relaxation
  Realize some anxiety is part of living
  Problem solve
Teach family to:
  Lessen demands on client when upset or anxious
  Employ listening skills
  Develop ways to be supportive

From Rawlins RP and others: *Mental health–psychiatric nursing,* ed 3, St Louis, 1993, Mosby–Year Book.

---

curity operations. For example, when a student unexpectedly fails an examination, he would be using the ego defense mechanisms of projection if he believed that he failed because the teacher was inadequate. Although this would reduce his anxiety, it would not be helpful in enabling him to pass the course. On the other hand, if this student were able to acknowledge his failure to himself, he would then be able to use the coping mechanism of going to the instructor for help. If he understands his errors, not only is his anxiety reduced, but also he is able to learn what is necessary to pass the course.

The box above lists guidelines for preventing anxiety.

Ego defense mechanisms

This section discusses frequently used ego defense mechanisms as identified by Freud. The student should remember from Chapter 12 that these defenses emanate from the unconscious and use psychic energy derived from the ego as

they protect it from anxiety. Furthermore, an ego defense mechanism may originate in more than one stage of personality development, or it may originate in one stage and be reinforced in others. Ego defense mechanisms are not clear-cut and almost never appear as isolated phenomena.

Compensation

Compensation is a pattern of adaptive behavior by which anxiety resulting from feelings of inadequacy or weakness is relieved as the individual emphasizes some personal or social attribute that overshadows the perceived inadequacy or weakness and gains social approval.

The origins of this adaptation can be seen in the young infant who substitutes the thumb or a toy for the nipple or bottle to relieve tension and compensate for some pleasurable sensations of sucking that may be lacking in quantity.

Compensation is much more complicated in adults than in infants and is usually prompted by feelings of guilt or inferiority. It may explain much of the behavior observed in adults who work zealously to promote philanthropic enterprises. Also, compensation may be operating in the behavior of a man who is very small in physical stature but who is extremely successful in the business world through his aggressive practices. It may also be one of the mechanisms operating when a young person who is paralyzed as a result of a car accident is able to achieve many honors for outstanding scholarship in college.

Displacement

Displacement is a defense mechanism used when individuals unconsciously believe they would be in great danger if their feelings about another person were known to that person. The adaptation to the resultant anxiety is the discharge of feelings onto a person or object entirely different from the one to which they actually belong. Displacement may be used by a teacher who is angry with an immediate super-

---

OF SPECIAL INTEREST

Have you ever known someone to overcome his or her anxiety about a particular situation without using a mental mechanism? People who are mentally healthy and confronted with a moderately anxiety-producing situation often do so by voluntarily repeating the anxiety-producing experience, in reality or symbolically, over and over again. What is most astounding is that they seem to enjoy this activity. Reducing anxiety by achieving mastery of a situation through repetition explains why many adults enjoy suspense movies, roller coaster rides, and similar activities while simultaneously declaring how scared they are. It also explains the pleasure children experience when they repetitively play the same game in exactly the same way or hear the same story told in exactly the same words. Sometimes the meaning of the games or stories is symbolic. In other instances, it relates directly to the anxiety-producing situation. In one family, for example, three sisters, 4, 5, and 8 years old, were aware of their parents' constant fighting even though their parents went to great lengths to be cordial with each other "in front of the girls." In view of this, their mother was shocked one day to overhear one of her daughters say to the other two, "Let's get out our doll house and play divorce again."

Can you think of an instance in which you successfully conquered your anxiety through enjoyable repetition?

---

visor and does not show these feelings in his or her presence but reacts with unreasonable anger when a pupil accidentally breaks a windowpane on that same day. The teacher may be displacing angry feelings by expressing them toward the student rather than toward the supervisor. Actually the teacher has unconsciously substituted the student for the supervisor and has displaced the feelings accordingly.

Denial

Denial is the adaptation often employed to defend the system against the stress of the sudden onset of great anxiety. It is a process whereby the individual truly does not recognize the existence of an event or feeling. Although denial is a frequently used defense in severe emotional illnesses such as schizophrenia, it is often seen as a reaction of the healthy individual when unexpectedly confronted by a disastrous situation. For example, the wife of a policeman who has just been killed in the line of duty may calmly respond to the informant, "You must have made a mistake! I had breakfast with him no more than 2 hours ago. I'm getting ready to shop now, so you'll have to excuse me."

It is important to understand that the mechanism of denial operates on a totally unconscious basis in response to the sudden onset of massive anxiety. Denial should not be confused with lying, which is a conscious effort to avoid responsibility in a situation.

Fixation

Fixation refers to the point in the individual's development at which certain aspects of the emotional development cease to advance. For reasons that are usually obscure, further development seems to be blocked. This blocking appears to arise from the individual's inability to solve problems that occurred during the specific phase of development at which progress ceased. Thus the individual is unable to achieve the developmental tasks of that phase, and since it is not possible to bypass a stage entirely, the person is always handicapped in proceeding to the stages that follow. For example, individuals who have not experienced the love and security required for the satisfactory resolution of the first stage of development may spend the remainder of their lives attempting to achieve gratification through the oral cavity. Some individuals fixated at this stage of personality development may drink huge quantities of alcohol or compulsively overeat because food and liquid intake are so closely allied to love and security in the unconscious emotional life.

Sublimation

In the mechanism of **sublimation** the energy involved in anxiety-producing primitive impulses and cravings is unconsciously redirected into constructive and socially acceptable channels. This is one of the chief mechanisms operating when a child learns to redirect the pleasurable sensations involved in expelling excrement at will into the more socially acceptable patterns of toilet training.

Sublimation is one of the more positive adaptations to anxiety and is at least partially responsible for much of the artistic and cultural achievement of civilized people. It is operating when an angry, hostile young man channels his feelings into a successful career as a boxer. Sublimation also is probably operating when a young woman who has lost her lover turns to writing poetry about love.

Reaction formation

Reaction formation can occur when individuals experience anxiety resulting from unconscious feelings or wishes that are unacceptable to them and relieve the anxiety by expressing an attitude or acting in a way that is directly opposite to how they really feel. Thus these persons are denying, in a sense of the word, their true feelings or desires. People who are extremely friendly, overly polite, and very socially correct frequently have unconscious feelings of anger and hatred toward many people. These true feelings may be evident in slips of the tongue or in biting humor.

Reaction formation sometimes develops out of rigid toilet-training experiences. Evidence of reaction formation may be observed in adults who are untidy about their homes and their personal hygiene but whose mothers required meticulous conformity to rules of cleanliness and tidiness.

Identification

Identification is a much used and extremely useful mechanism because it plays a large part in the development of a child's personality and in the process of acculturation. Through the process of identification, individuals defend against anxiety resulting from feelings of inadequacy by unconsciously taking on desired attributes found in people for whom they have admiration and affection. These individuals integrate these attributes into their own personality. Thus the little boy takes on masculine attributes that he admires in his father. Students integrate into their personality makeup the attributes they admire in their professors. Another form of identification is observed when an individual develops an unreasoning sympathy for a criminal because of an unconscious sense of guilt.

Introjection

The mechanism of **introjection** is closely related to identification. However, whereas the mechanism of identification adds to the individual's personality, introjection tends to replace all or part of the personality. This defense is based on the psychoanalytical concept of oral receptivity and refers to the unconscious, symbolic swallowing of an aspect of a significant person in response to anxiety precipitated by the real or perceived loss of this person. Introjection is operating when the child develops the superego by incorporating the parents' ideals and standards. When introjection is operating in adults, it suggests that the entire personality of a second person has been incorporated and has replaced the original personality. A psychotic client who claimed to be Moses wore a beard, let his hair grow long, talked in biblical phrases, and acted as Moses might have acted. This client incorporated what he believed to be the personality of Moses and had given up his own personality. Introjection may operate in a less constructive way than identification, especially when observed in adults. For instance, a depressed client may have unconsciously incorporated another person and attempt to commit suicide to kill the introjected person whom the client unconsciously hates.

Undoing

In the mechanism of **undoing**, the individual engages in certain behaviors as a means of symbolically canceling out unconscious thoughts or feelings that are unacceptable and therefore associated with anxiety. Although individuals are aware of their behavior, they are not aware of its purpose, and the behavior often seems irrational, even to them. Undoing is seen as the basis of compulsive behavior. Undoing behavior is frequently highly repetitive because it does not achieve its aim of actually canceling out the anxiety-producing thought or feeling. A famous example of this defense mechanism is found in Shakespeare's play *Macbeth*. Lady Macbeth, the wife of the main character, compulsively washes her hands, exclaiming, "Out, out damned spot!" after having goaded her husband into murdering the king.

Isolation

Isolation is a phenomenon in which the feeling is detached from the event in the individual's memory, enabling the person to recall the event without its attendant anxiety. This mechanism is evident in situations when an individual recounts a harrowing experience without any evidence of emotion.

Rationalization

Rationalization is a mental mechanism that is almost universally employed. It is an attempt to make one's behavior appear to be the result of logical thinking rather than the result of unconscious desires or cravings that are anxiety producing. Rationalization is used when individuals have a sense of guilt about something they do or believe or when they are uncertain about their behavior. It is a face-saving device that may or may not deal with the actual truth. Rationalization should not be confused with falsehoods or alibis, since the latter are conscious avoidance maneuvers. Rationalization is almost totally unconscious, and although it is used to put the individual in the best possible light, it does not have the deliberate aspect of other conscious avoidance maneuvers.

The person who does not want to keep an appointment because to do so would create anxiety and says that the appointment slipped his or her mind is not telling a falsehood but rather is using rationalization as a defense mechanism. Although rationalization relieves anxiety temporarily, it is not an effective mechanism of adjustment because it assists the individual to avoid facing the reality of the situation.

Repression

Repression is a widely used, completely unconscious mechanism. Painful experiences, unacceptable thoughts and impulses, and disagreeable memories are forcibly dismissed from consciousness to relieve the anxiety associated with them. The psychic energy with which they were invested becomes an active, free-floating source of anxiety in the unconscious mind. Many painful experiences are repressed during early childhood and become unconscious sources of emotional conflict in later life. Selfish, hostile feelings and sexual impulses are frequently repressed. Such repression always causes internal conflict. This repressed material may find escape through conversion into physical symptoms or into obsessions or pathological anxieties that arise without apparent reason.

Regression

Regression occurs when individuals are faced with anxiety stemming from a conflict or problem that cannot be solved by using the adaptive mechanisms with which they customarily solve problems. In such a situation, these persons may unconsciously resort to behavior that was successful at an earlier stage in their development but that they had presumably outgrown. Thus, regression is a return to patterns of behavior appropriate to an earlier developmental stage. Any retreat into a state of dependency on others to avoid facing acute problems can be called a regressive trait. "Crying on someone's shoulder" is symbolic of the infant seeking comfort on the maternal bosom. Although seeking a dependency relationship may be a benign form of regression, this mechanism also may be symptomatic of a serious mental illness.

Projection

Projection is a frequently used, unconscious mechanism that relieves anxiety by transferring the responsibility for unacceptable ideas, impulses, wishes, or thoughts to another person. The mechanism is used when the individual's own hostile, aggressive thoughts are unacceptable to him or her and thus cause anxiety. Although all people use this mechanism to some extent, it is not a healthy method of adaptation and is more frequently used by persons with a mental illness than by healthy individuals. For example, a paranoid male client may project his own inner hate of others by saying that a group of people is plotting to kill him. Less pathological use of projection is evident when a worker blames the boss for difficulties on the job or when a student blames the teacher for failure on an examination. Paranoid persons frequently project their feelings of sexual inadequacy on others. Thus a common delusion concerns the unfaithful spouse, when the actual lack of fidelity is in the mind of the accuser.

Symbolization and condensation

A symbol is an idea or object used by the conscious mind instead of the actual idea or object, which, if consciously perceived, would be anxiety producing. Instinctual desires may appear through symbols, the meanings of which are not clear to the conscious mind. For example, a man who unconsciously harbors feelings of inadequacy about his masculinity may defend against this anxiety by owning only large automobiles despite not being able to afford to purchase or operate them. The phallic symbolism of large automobiles serves to reassure this individual about his adequacy as a male.

Symbols are the language of the unconscious. Such symbols appear in dreams or fantasies and may emerge through various rituals or obsessive behavior. Symbols may become further merged by condensation to represent a wide range of anxiety-producing ideas that become lumped together so as to lose their painful significance. When they rise to the conscious level, these ideas take the form of an apparently incoherent jumble of words, the real meaning of which is hidden in the unconscious. Such condensations of thinking are frequently noted in the apparently irrational language of an individual with schizophrenia. However, these condensations have meaning and significance for the person.

Conversion

Conversion refers to the expression of emotional conflicts through a physical symptom with no demonstrable organic basis. The use of this mechanism is preceded by the use of repression, whereby the anxiety resulting from the emotional conflict was previously adapted to by repressing the conflict into the unconscious. When the conflict reappears as a physical symptom, the individual is unaware of any connection between the two phenomena. Thus a girl who is highly anxious because of chronic friction between her parents, both of whom she loves, may find herself suddenly blind. This symptom literally relieves her of the necessity of seeing such incompatibility. Similarly, a young soldier who simultaneously loves his country but abhors killing may suddenly develop a paralysis of his right hand, rendering him unable to pull the trigger of a gun.

Although the physical symptom is symbolically related to the nature of the conflict, conversion is not always expressed in a direct, easily recognized manner. Frequently it is difficult to determine which repressed conflicts in the unconscious produce a certain physical symptom. The symptom always serves to distract attention from the individual's real problems. This mechanism is entirely unconscious and is not used by mature, well-adjusted individuals.

Table 13-2 summarizes the ego defenses.

Security operations

This section discusses the security operations identified by Sullivan as protective measures against anxiety. As discussed in Chapter 12, Sullivan stressed that anxiety emanates from an interpersonal context and is highly communicable.

Apathy

The security operation of **apathy** is similar to the ego defense of isolation, in which individuals defend against anxiety by not allowing themselves to feel the emotion associated with an anxiety-producing event. Thus the individual using apathy manifests an extreme indifference to an event that would usually elicit a high degree of emotion. This security operation protected a young wife against extreme anxiety when her husband was convicted of involvement in organized crime and sentenced to 15 years in prison. Although she had no previous knowledge of his business, she was able to recount to her parents the events that transpired after his arrest without any emotion, leading them to conclude that she did not care.

Somnolent detachment

The security operation of **somnolent detachment** manifests itself by the individual falling asleep when confronted by a highly threatening, anxiety-producing experience. It has its origin in the developmental stage of infancy when the baby can be observed to fall asleep after crying fails to bring the mothering one to feed the infant. Although somnolent detachment is a primitive defense, it can be observed in adults under great stress. For example, a young woman sitting for the licensure examination in nursing falls asleep less than a half hour after the examination begins, and she fails.

Selective inattention

Selective inattention is the mechanism whereby anxiety-producing aspects of a situation are not allowed into awareness, thereby enabling the individual to maintain an adequate level of system homeokinesis. For example, the security of a woman whose husband is having an affair is threatened so she is selectively inattentive to the many clues to his behavior and is consciously surprised when he asks for a divorce to marry his lover.

Preoccupation

The security operation of **preoccupation** is manifested by a consuming interest in a person, thought, or event to the exclusion of the anxiety-producing reality. Preoccupation was used as a protective measure by a devout Christian woman who routinely made home visits in her community to invite others to worship at her church. One day she was severely bitten on her left leg by a large dog in the yard of the home she was approaching. The dog's attack caused her to fall on her right knee, and she became preoccupied with the bruise on this knee to the exclusion of concern about her mangled left leg. The anxiety she was experiencing was caused not only by the suddenness of the dog's attack, but more fundamentally by a threat to her security that was based in part on the belief that God would always protect her when she was doing His work.

Coping mechanisms

The variety and number of coping mechanisms are as great as the creativity and resources of human beings. They cannot all be listed and defined, but they can be categorized into short-term and long-term adaptations. This categorization is based not only on a time factor but also on the object and effect of the adaptation. The

Table 13-2. Ego defense mechanisms

DEFENSE MECHANISM	DEFINITION	EXAMPLE
Compensation	Exaggerating one trait to make up for feelings of inadequacy or inferiority in another dimension	A physically small man verbally bullies his employees.
Displacement	Attributing feelings to a person or object that are really directed at another person or object	A young woman kicks her cat after a telephone argument with her boss.
Denial	Failing to perceive some threatening object or event in the external world	A woman sets a place for dinner for her husband, who has just been killed.
Fixation	Remaining "stuck" in a developmental stage	A husband depends totally on his wife for most of his activities of daily living.
Sublimation	Redirecting socially unacceptable urges into socially acceptable behavior	An angry, hostile young man becomes a boxer.
Reaction formation	Substituting directly opposite wishes for one's true wishes	An adult who grew up in a very messy home is compulsively neat in his home.
Identification	Integrating desired attributes of an admired person to compensate for perceived inadequacy	A shy adolescent girl styles her hair identical to that of a popular rock star.
Introjection	Incorporating another person to avoid the threat posed by the person or by one's own urges	A psychotically depressed woman attempts suicide to kill her mother, who she states is in her stomach.
Undoing	Engaging in certain thoughts and actions so as to cancel out or atone for threatening thoughts or actions that have previously occurred	A business executive studies to become a nursery school teacher after having an abortion.
Isolation	Severing the connection between the thoughts and feelings associated with an event so the event can remain conscious without undue anxiety	A single parent talks unemotionally about her only child's recent diagnosis of a malignant brain tumor.
Rationalization	Substituting a fictitious, socially acceptable reason for the genuine, unacceptable reason for one's wishes or actions	"I would have helped you if I could, but I had to take my dog to the vet."
Repression	Forcibly dismissing anxiety-producing thoughts, feelings, or events from consciousness	A woman is unable to remember being raped by her brother when she was 10 years old.
Regression	Returning to patterns of behavior characteristic of a less anxiety-producing stage of development	A 6-year-old child begins to wet the bed at night after her mother's remarriage.
Projection	Attributing to others an objectionable trait or feeling that really emanates from oneself	"My husband is cheating on me."
Symbolization and condensation	Using a neutral idea or object to represent an unacceptable idea or object	A 40-year-old man has unconscious feelings of inadequacy as a male and spends all his money on guns and all his time polishing and cleaning them.
Conversion	Expressing unconscious emotional conflicts through a physical symptom with no demonstrable organic basis	A young woman wakes up paralyzed from the waist down on the morning of her wedding day.

student should remember that all coping mechanisms are conscious, learned adaptations to anxiety based on problem solving and result in altered behavior.

Short term

Short-term coping mechanisms are conscious maneuvers focused on the anxiety itself rather than on its source and are designed to effect a relatively immediate relief from anxiety. Consequently, short-term coping mechanisms represent avoidance or escape behaviors. A frequently used short-term coping mechanism is **suppression.** Although historically considered an ego defense machanism, suppression does not emanate from the unconscious. Rather, suppression is the conscious, intentional dismissal to the preconscious mind of impulses, feelings, and thoughts that are unpleasant or unacceptable to the individual. Suppressed material is easily recalled and is thus available to the conscious mind. A famous example of suppression is used by Scarlett O'Hara in *Gone with the Wind.* When Scarlett's sense of security is repeatedly threatened, she exclaims, "I'll think about that tomorrow." Other examples of short-term coping mechanisms are the decisions to drink or eat when anxious or to avoid conflictive situations by pleading illness. Although these maneuvers are successful in relieving anxiety, they do not help the individual to adapt effectively to similar anxiety-producing situations in the future. Furthermore, the result of a frequently used short-term coping mechanism can become a stressor itself. For example, consistent overeating can lead to obesity.

Long term

Long-term coping mechanisms are characterized by efforts to address the source of anxiety. Therefore the anxiety is not relieved immediately but rather continues while its source is being sought. Long-term mechanisms tend to represent confrontational behaviors in that the source of the anxiety is dealt with rather than avoided. An

Table 13-3. Helpful steps in working with the anxious client

STEP	RATIONALE
Observe for behaviors characteristic of anxiety.	To identify anxiety
Ask, "What are you feeling?"	To help client name the feeling
Connect the feeling with behavior.	To help client understand that he or she behaves characteristically when feeling anxious.
Explore with client what happened before he or she felt anxious.	To discover cause
Discuss alternatives for dealing with the situation (cause).	To improve patterns of handling anxiety

From Rawlins RP and others: *Mental health–psychiatric nursing,* ed 3, St Louis, 1993, Mosby–Year Book.

example of a long-term coping mechanism is the housewife's decision to attend college to prepare herself to become financially independent, thereby coping with the anxiety caused by being financially dependent on her husband.

Long-term coping mechanisms are more functional than short-term mechanisms, since they provide the individual with patterns of behavior that increase self-esteem and can be built on in future anxiety-producing situations. However, they can be used only in instances in which the individual is able to experience anxiety without too much system disequilibrium.

Table 13-3 lists steps the nurse can take when working with the anxious client.

KEY POINTS

1. Anxiety is defined as a vague sense of impending doom, an apprehension, or a sense of dread, that seemingly has no basis in reality.

2. Anxiety is always perceived as a negative feeling. It is extremely communicable, cannot be distinguished from fear by the person experiencing it, and occurs in degrees.

3. Freud believed than anxiety results from the emergence of id impulses that are unacceptable to the superego.

4. Sullivan viewed anxiety as occurring when the individual anticipates or actually receives cues that signal disapproval from one or more significant others.

5. Mental mechanisms are patterns of thinking and behaving that are used to protect the individual from threatening aspects of the environment or from feelings of anxiety. Therefore, mental mechanisms are adaptations to anxiety.

6. Ego defense mechanisms are believed to effect a compromise between the demands of the id and the superego, thereby relieving anxiety.

7. Security operations relieve anxiety by interfering with the person's ability to perceive an anxiety-producing situation, emotion, or relationship. Security operations are believed to be used when anxiety poses a threat to the self-concept.

8. Coping mechanisms are conscious problem-solving activities the individual uses to relieve anxiety.

SUGGESTED SOURCES OF ADDITIONAL INFORMATION

Beeber L and others: Peplau's theory in practice, *Nurs Sci Q* 3:6, Spring 1990.

Freud A: *The ego and mechanisms of defense,* New York, 1967, International Universities Press.

Knowles R: Dealing with feelings: managing anxiety, *Am J Nurs* 81:110, January 1981.

Musil CM, Abraham IL: Coping, thinking, and mental health nursing: cognitions and their application to psychosocial intervention, *Issues Ment Health Nurs* 8:191, 1986.

Peplau HE: The power of the dissociative state, *J Psychosoc Nurs Ment Health Serv* 23(8):31, 1985.

Sadow D, Ryder M: Anxiety reduction: lessons that benefit students and patients, *J Psychosoc Nurs Ment Health Serv* 28(9):29, 1990.

Tache J, Selye J: On stress and coping mechanisms, *Issues Ment Health Nurs* 7:3, 1985.

Trimpey ML: Self-esteem and anxiety: key issues in an abused women's support group, *Issues Ment Health Nurs* 10:297, 1989.

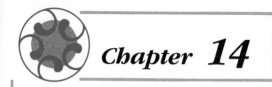

Chapter 14

Cultural Factors Influencing Mental Health and Mental Illness

Joyce N. Giger
Ruth E. Davidhizar
Sharon Evers
Charlotte Ingram

CHAPTER OUTLINE

Historical perspective
Cultural nursing assessment
Giger and Davidhizar's transcultural assessment
  model
  Communication
  Space
  Social organization
  Time
  Environmental control
  Biological variations
  Implications for nursing care

LEARNING OBJECTIVES

After studying this chapter, the student will be able to:

* Describe the communication problems encountered when caring for clients and families from multicultural backgrounds.

* Explain how orientation to time and space may affect nursing care needs of clients and families.

* Describe how cultural behavior is acquired in a social setting and the relevance of this to psychosocial development.

* Identify types of health care practices, including folk beliefs, that may have significant impact on wellness, illness, and health-seeking behaviors of persons from various cultural groups.

* Describe biological differences among individuals and families that may affect psychosociological adaptation.

* Discuss the difference between cultural sensitivity and cultural stereotyping.

* Describe the relationships between cultural factors and the symptoms of mental illness.

* Discuss why it is essential for the nurse who works in a psychiatric setting to be culturally sensitive.

KEY TERMS

Culture
Cultural values
Culturally diverse nursing care
Ethnicity
Race
Minority
Communication
Space
Social organization
Time
Environmental control
Biological variations

To understand the term *transcultural nursing,* the nurse must understand essential components such as culture, cultural values, and culturally diverse nursing care. This information can assist the psychiatric nurse in understanding how individuals are unique and thus can facilitate culturally appropriate nursing care.

Culture is a patterned behavioral response that develops over time as a result of imprinting the mind through social and religious structure and intellectual and artistic manifestations. Culture is also the result of acquired mechanisms that may have innate influences but is primarily affected by internal and external environmental stimuli. Culture is shaped by values, beliefs, norms, and practices that are shared by members of the same cultural group. Culture guides our thinking, doing, and being and becomes patterned expressions of who we are. Patterned expressions of culture are passed down from one generation to the next (Giger and Davidhizar, 1994). Other definitions of culture have been offered by Leininger (1985a), Spector (1991), and Boyle and Andrews (1989).

Culture implies a dynamic, ever-changing, active or passive process. **Cultural values** are unique, individual expressions of a particular culture that have been accepted as appropriate over time. They guide actions and decision making that facilitate self-worth and self-esteem (Giger and Davidhizar, 1994). According to Leininger (1985a), cultural values develop as a result of an individual's preferred way of acting. **Culturally diverse nursing care** implies that health care delivery is based on varying nursing approaches to provide culturally appropriate care.

Other important terms are ethnicity, race, minority, ethnic minority, and people of color. Often, ethnicity is used to imply "race." However, ethnicity includes more than the biological identification. In its broadest sense, **ethnicity** refers to groups whose members share a common social and cultural heritage passed on to each successive generation (Giger and Davidhizar, 1991).

Members of an ethnic group share a sense of identity with one another. Regardless of race, all people have a cultural heritage that makes them ethnic.

The term **race** is related to biology (Giger and Davidhizar, 1991). When members of a particular group share distinguishing physical features such as color, bone structure, or blood group, they are said to belong to a particular race. It is important to remember that ethnic and racial groups often overlap because biological and cultural similarities frequently reinforce one another (Bullough and Bullough, 1982).

One of the most frequently misused words is minority, particularly in reference to persons of color. By definition, a **minority** can consist of a particular racial, religious, or occupational group that constitutes less than a numerical majority of the population (Giger and Davidhizar, 1991).

In any society, cultural groups can be arranged into a hierarchical power structure. Dominant groups are considered to be powerful, whereas those groups considered inferior and lacking in power are referred to as minorities. Therefore the term "minority" is not always synonymous with numbers. For example, the ruling class in South Africa, which composes 2% of the population, is white (Gary, 1991). In the United States, people of color (African Americans, Latin Americans, Asian Americans) are considered minorities. However, when the world's population is considered, people of color are the majority.

Gender is another example of how "minority" is used erroneously. Females in the United States compose a larger numerical percentage (51%) than do males (49%) but are considered to be the minority (U.S. Department of Commerce, Bureau of Census, 1991).

One should understand the significance of the term *minority.* The central defining characteristic of any minority group, according to Gary (1991), is its relative powerlessness and inability to chart its own course to a better way of life.

The term *ethnic minority* is often used because it is less offensive to people of color than other terms. Supposedly, it takes into account ethnicity, race, and the relative status of the groups of persons included in the category. If not for the use of the word minority, perhaps this terminology would be less culturally offensive to some groups of people (i.e., ethnic people of color). According to Gary (1991), use of the term *people of color* might be the preferable option, particularly in situations where sensitivity to racial preferences needs to be heightened.

HISTORICAL PERSPECTIVE

Only recently has culture been considered a significant factor in the assessment, diagnosis, and treatment of individuals with a mental disorder. Several unrelated but significant events have interacted to promote a heightened awareness of sociocultural factors among mental health professionals. As a result of the vast numbers of psychiatric casualties from World War II, the U.S. population became aware of the need for greater knowledge and understanding of psychiatric illnesses. During this period, many thought that one way of developing knowledge about psychiatric illnesses was to define those behaviors that constitute mental health.

In fields such as biology or physics, the trend was to study an object as it interacted in its natural environment. A variety of scientists began to draw parallels between the environment and the subject that subsequently led to the development of various theories, including systems and stress and adaptation theories.

During the 1960s the community mental health movement was born, which promoted mental health through the provision of comprehensive mental health care in community settings. As a result, attention was focused on the parallel between the person and the environment. Variables were examined that appeared to affect mental health, such as poverty, unemployment, environmental conditions, crime, and social support systems. The 1960s also gave rise to

the civil rights movement. For the first time, U.S. population was forced to address seriously the concerns of "people of color," religiously oppressed groups, and women. The civil rights movement did more than any other movement in the United States to force people to recognize the relationship between mental health and sociocultural factors.

In recent years, psychiatric nursing has evolved with the development of the subspecialty of community mental health nursing. In community mental health nursing, the community is viewed as the focus of nursing interventions.

CULTURAL NURSING ASSESSMENT

Nurses are likely to encounter clients from diverse settings because we live in a multicultural society. Factors that influence individual health and illness behaviors must be taken into account and fully understood if culturally appropriate nursing care is to be rendered (Tripp-Reimer, Brink, and Sanders, 1984). This is especially true when the nurse is providing care to the client in a psychiatric setting. Clients in need of therapeutic interventions in primary, acute, or long-term psychiatric settings are experiencing stress and anxiety. These individuals may have difficulty discerning the value of continuing traditional beliefs and practices while developing new and more beneficial health care practices. The nurse needs to remember that cultural assessment can and does provide meaning to behaviors that might otherwise be judged in a negative way (Affonso, 1979). The nurse must understand the significance of behavior and its appropriate relationship with an individual's cultural beliefs and practices. The nurse must avoid labeling unfamiliar behavior as "pathological" or "deviant" to prevent delivering culturally inappropriate nursing care.

Transcultural nursing theories are proliferating and have begun to appear in the nursing literature in recent years (Affonso, 1979; Leininger, 1985a, 1985b). However, adequate nursing

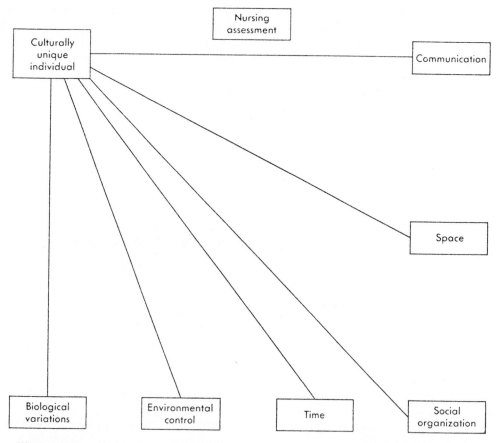

Figure 14-1

Application of cultural phenomena to nursing care and nursing practice.

From Giger JN, Davidhizar RE: *Transcultural nursing: assessment and intervention,* St Louis, 1991, Mosby–Year Book.

assessment tools have not always accompanied these theories. In response to the need for a practical assessment tool for evaluating cultural variables and their effects on health and illness behavior, Giger and Davidhizar developed a model for assessing clients using six cultural phenomena (Figure 14-1).

GIGER AND DAVIDHIZAR'S TRANSCULTURAL ASSESSMENT MODEL

Six cultural phenomena are evidenced among all cultural groups: (1) **communication,** (2) **space,** (3) **social organization,** (4) **time,** (5) **environmental control,** and (6) **biological variations.** These phenomena vary across cultures by application and use. The six cultural phenomena are presented individually along with specific data to be collected in each area (Figure 14-2). The nurse must keep in mind that a comprehensive nursing assessment is necessary for both the clinician and the researcher to provide culturally appropriate nursing care in psychiatric settings. The box on pp. 220 and 221 outlines a transcultural assessment model.

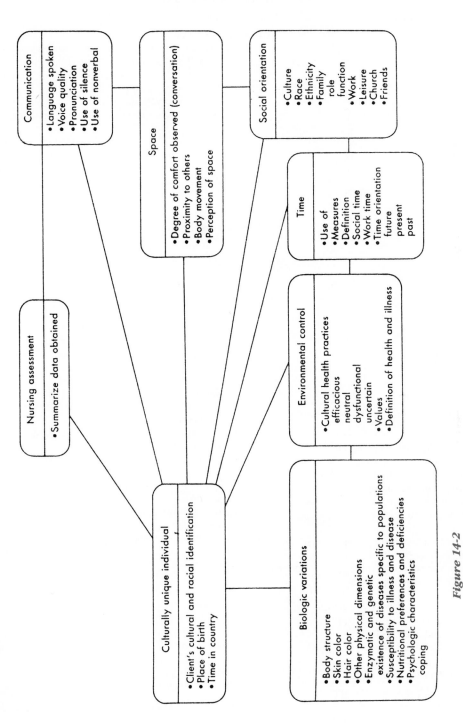

Figure 14-2

Transcultural assessment model.

From Bobak IM, Jensen MD: *Maternity and gynecologic care*, ed 5, St Louis, 1993, Mosby–Year Book.

A TRANSCULTURAL ASSESSMENT MODEL

Culturally unique individual

1. Place of birth
2. Cultural definition
   What is . . .
3. Race
   What is . . .
4. Length of time in country

Communication

1. Voice quality
   a. Strong, resonant
   b. Soft
   c. Average
   d. Shrill
2. Pronunciation and enunciation
   a. Clear
   b. Slurred
   c. Dialect
3. Use of silence
   a. Infrequent
   b. Often
   c. Length
      (1) Brief
      (2) Moderate
      (3) Long
      (4) Not observed
4. Use of nonverbal communication
   a. Hand movement
   b. Eye movement
   c. Moves entire body
   d. Kinesics (gestures, expressions, stances)
5. Touch
   a. Startles or withdraws when touched
   b. Accepts touch without difficulty
   c. Touches others without difficulty
6. Ask these and similar questions:
   a. How do you get your point across to others?
   b. Do you like communicating with friends, family, and acquaintances?
   c. When asked a question, do you usually respond (in words or body movement, or both)?
   d. If you have something important to discuss with your family, how would you approach them?

Space

1. Degree of comfort
   a. Moves when space invaded
   b. Does not move when invaded
2. Distance in conversations
   a. 0 to 18 inches
   b. 18 inches to 3 feet
   c. 3 feet or more
3. Definition of space
   a. Describe degree of comfort with closeness when talking with or standing near others
   b. How do objects (e.g., furniture) in the environment affect your sense of space?
4. Ask these and similar questions:
   a. When you talk with family members, how close do you stand?
   b. When you communicate with co-workers and other acquaintances, how close do you stand?
   c. If a stranger touches you, how do you react or feel?
   d. If a loved one touches you, how do you react or feel?
   e. Are you comfortable with the distance between us now?

Social organization

1. Normal state of health
   a. Poor
   b. Fair
   c. Good
   d. Excellent
2. Ask these and similar questions:
   a. How do you define social activities?
   b. What are some activities that you enjoy?
   c. What are your hobbies, or what do you do when you have free time?
   d. Do you believe in a Supreme Being?
   e. How do you worship that Supreme Being?
   f. What is your function (what do you do) in your family unit/system?
   g. What is your role in your family unit/system (father, mother, child, advisor)?
   h. When you were a child, what or who influenced you most?
   i. What is/was your relationship with your siblings and parents?
   j. What does work mean to you?
   k. Describe your past, present, and future jobs.
   l. What are your political views?
   m. How have your political views influenced your attitude toward health and illness?

Time

1. Orientation to time
   a. Past oriented
   b. Present oriented
   c. Future oriented
2. View of time
   a. Social time
   b. Clock oriented

A TRANSCULTURAL ASSESSMENT MODEL—cont'd

3. Physiochemical reaction to time
   a. Sleeps at least 8 hours a night
   b. Goes to sleep and wakes on a consistent schedule
   c. Understands the importance of taking medication and other treatments on schedule
4. Ask these and similar questions:
   a. What type of timepiece do you wear daily?
   b. If you have an appointment at 2 PM, what time is acceptable to arrive?
   c. If a nurse tells you that you will receive a medication in "about a half hour," realistically, how much time will you allow before calling the nurse's station?

Environmental control

1. Locus of control
   a. Internal locus of control (believes that the power to effect change lies within)
   b. External locus of control (believes that fate, luck, and chance greatly affect how things turn out)
2. Value orientation
   a. Believes in supernatural forces
   b. Relies on magic, witchcraft, and prayer to effect change
   c. Does not believe in supernatural forces
   d. Does not rely on magic, witchcraft, or prayer to effect change
3. Ask these and similar questions:
   a. How often do you have visitors at your home?
   b. Is it acceptable to you for visitors to drop in unexpectedly?
   c. Name some ways your parents or other persons treated your illnesses when you were a child.
   d. Have you or someone else in your immediate surroundings ever used a home remedy that made you sick?
   e. What home remedies have you used that worked? Will you use them in the future?
   f. What is your definition of "good health"?
   g. What is your definition of illness or "poor health"?

Biological variations

1. Conduct a complete physical assessment, noting:
   a. Body structure
   b. Skin color
   c. Unusual skin discolorations
   d. Hair color and distribution
   e. Other visible physical characteristics (e.g., keloids, chloasma)
2. Ask these and similar questions:
   a. What diseases or illnesses are common in your family?
   b. Describe your family's typical behavior when a family member is ill.

c. How do you respond when you are angry?
d. Who (or what) usually helps you to cope during a difficult time?
e. What foods do you and your family like to eat?
f. Have you ever had any unusual cravings for:
   (1) White or red clay dirt?
   (2) Laundry starch?
g. When you were a child, what types of foods did you eat?
h. What foods are family favorites or are considered traditional?

Nursing assessment

1. Note whether the client has become culturally assimilated or observes own cultural practices.
2. Incorporate data into plan of nursing care:
   a. Encourage the client to discuss cultural differences; people from diverse cultures who hold different world views can enlighten nurses.
   b. Make efforts to accept and understand methods of communication.
   c. Respect the individual's personal need for space.
   d. Respect the rights of clients to honor and worship the Supreme Being of their choice.
   e. Identify a clerical or spiritual person to contact.
   f. Determine whether spiritual practices have implications for health, life, and well-being (e.g., Jehovah's Witnesses may refuse blood and blood derivatives; an Orthodox Jew may eat only kosher food high in sodium and may not drink milk when meat is served).
   g. Identify hobbies, especially when devising interventions for a short or extended convalescence or for rehabilitation.
   h. Honor time and value orientations and differences in these areas. Allay anxiety and apprehension if adherence to time is necessary.
   i. Provide privacy according to client's personal need and health status (NOTE: the perception and reaction to pain may be culturally related).
   j. Note cultural health practices.
      (1) Identify and encourage efficacious practices.
      (2) Identify and discourage dysfunctional practices.
      (3) Identify and determine whether neutral practices will have a long-term negative effect.
   k. Note food preferences.
      (1) Make as many adjustments in diet as health status and long-term benefits will allow and as dietary department can provide.
      (2) Note dietary practices that may have serious implications for the client.

Developed by Geneva Turner. From Giger JN, Davidhizar RE: *Transcultural nursing: assessment and intervention*, St Louis, 1991, Mosby–Year Book.

Communication

Communication often appears to be the most insurmountable problem when working with clients from diverse multicultural backgrounds in psychiatric settings. According to Foster (1989), communication patterns are formed indelibly by culture. People learn to think, feel, believe, and strive for what their culture considers proper (Porter and Samovar, 1985). Culture not only determines appropriateness of the message but influences all the components of communication. A cultural assessment of communication requires an evaluation of:

1. Dialect
2. Style (language, social situation)
3. Volume (silence)
4. Touch
5. Context of speech (emotional tone)
6. Kinesics (gestures, stances, eye behavior)

Dialect

Dialect differs between and among cultural and ethnic groups. Although dialect is directly impacted by culture and ethnicity, it is also influenced by geographical location. For example, in the South it customary to say "cut the lights off," whereas in the North one would say "turn the lights off."

Language styles

Language styles may vary significantly among people of different cultures. Words may have different meanings. For example, when the nurse is interacting with an African American client, the phrase "that's bad" when used by the client may actually mean "that's good." Language style becomes a more complicated phenomenon in a psychiatric setting regardless of cultural heritage. For example, a schizophrenic client might interpret the phrase "people who live in glass houses should not throw stones" as "if you live in a glass house, and you throw stones, you may break it" (Haber, 1992). An individual not familiar with the U.S. language style may also interpret the phase literally. In another example, a foreign nurse greets a client with, "How are you feeling?" and the client responds, "I feel like a million dollars." The nurse notes in the assessment that the "client is having delusions of grandeur." Since many psychiatrists practicing in the United States are not American born or educated, lack of familiarization with the language style creates the opportunity for a misdiagnosis. It is also important for the nurse to learn that language styles vary not only between and among various cultures but also within cultures.

Negative interrogatives are perceived as a cultural phenomenon of communication for some ethnic and cultural groups. For example, the avoidance of the word "no" may be a cultural phenomenon for some Afghans, Chinese Americans, and Vietnamese Americans. Afghans will not use the word "no" when conversing because they believe it conveys disrespect. In addition, they do not like others to use this word when conversing with them (Lipson and Omidian, 1992). Some Chinese Americans may use positive responses in answer to negative interrogatives when replying to a question. With these clients, "yes" may not necessarily imply "understanding" or "compliance." For example, the nurse says, "Will you not hit other clients when you are in the day room?" and the client responds "yes." When interacting with these clients, it is essential to clarify the meaning of the word "yes" (Chung, 1977).

A common misconception is that persons of the same culture can understand each other because of cultural similarity. An example is the belief that all African Americans understand black English. However, if an African American from Bronx, New York, were to spend 1 hour with an African American from South Central Los Angeles, there would be many differences in the use of black English.

Volume of speech

Volume of speech is also a variable that has cultural significance. A nurse must learn to evaluate and interpret factors such as loudness, softness, shouting, and silence in a cultural context. Interestingly, there are high-volume and low-volume cultural groups. High-volume cultural groups include Irish Americans, who are frequently perceived as using high volume to communicate not because of anger but rather as part of their cultural background (Greely, 1981). Some Jewish Americans tend to be expressive when communicating and frequently use low volume for emphasis (Novak and Waldoks, 1981). Other low-volume cultures include Chinese Americans, Navajo Indians, and Japanese Americans. It is essential that the nurse avoids mislabeling cultural behavior as signs of pathology, such as "withdrawn," "depressed," "aggressive," or "passive."

The use of silence has more significance in some cultures than in others. Not all silence has a negative connotation, indicating a lack of understanding, disinterest, or inattentiveness. On the other hand, silence does not always imply comprehension, empathy, or involvement. Culture can and does influence, for example, whether a client will question health care providers about health and illness conditions or remain silent. Silence may be used by some cultural groups to promote communication, to pass time, as a method of controlling others, or as a defense mechanism. For example, an Asian American responding to auditory hallucinations may remain silent and hyperalert instead of verbalizing concerns. In a psychiatric setting, the nurse must distinguish between cultural factors and pathological behaviors. The cultural significance of silence may also be related to gender and the roles assigned because of gender in certain cultures. For example, a female Chinese American client often will rely on her husband to communicate her needs even when capable of communicating fluently.

Touch

Touch is often used to facilitate communication. Spanish, Italian, French, Jewish, and South American cultures are considered more tactile, whereas English, German, and Navajo Indian cultures are generally considered less tactile (Montagu, 1971). Some cultural groups may interpret touch as intrusive or having sexual connotation. Different rules and meanings apply to touch depending on the sex of the person involved. Whether it is permissible to touch or be touched may vary in cultures in relation to health situations. In the United States, some female nurses perceive their male clients as being less responsive and receptive to touch or any form of closeness than female clients. A double standard may exist because male clients could be more receptive to touch, but female nurses are more comfortable with the closeness and touch of female clients (Lane, 1989).

Because touch is considered mystical or magical in some cultures, casual touching is considered taboo. For example, touch may be viewed by Mexican Americans and Native American Indians as "undoing" of an evil spell, as a means of prevention of harm, or as a method of healing.

Context of speech

The use of emotion in communication is often referred to as the context of speech and varies across cultural groups. Small talk, a derivation of verbal communication, is an important cultural consideration when working with persons from diverse backgrounds. Small talk is important to establish a therapeutic relationship. For example, Mexican Americans may engage in small talk before approaching the business of an interview. Laughter is a valuable mode of communication, and its importance varies across cultural groups. For example, in the Navajo culture, when the newborn laughs for the first time, members of the tribe gather and give small gifts and prepare a small feast to mark the occasion (Hanley, 1991). Smiling may also have cultural significance. In India, smiles are exchanged between social equals only in the most informal situations, whereas in the United States, social smiles are frequently exchanged even among strangers (Ramakrishna and Weiss, 1992).

Kinesics

The use of gestures, stances, and eye behavior is a form of communication referred to as kinesics. Kinesics behavior is extremely important in the development of a successful therapeutic relationship. A nurse may be able to bridge an interaction by certain gestures or postures. In the United States, if one wishes to convey an attentive posture, one leans toward the individual. Since the meaning of gestures differs from culture to culture, gestures used in conversation should be deliberately studied to avoid offending the client from a different cultural background. For example, in the United States, when an individual extends the hands with the palms up, this gesture is considered acquiescence. With certain cultural groups, however, this gesture may have sexual implications (Mehrabian, 1981).

Posture can give clues about an individual's self-esteem, whereas an individual's walk may give indications about self-concept (Haber, 1992). For example, if the client has a robotlike, cogwheel gait, the client may have a side effect from a phenothiazine. A client who has rigid boundary movements could be a schizophrenic with a fragmented, fragile self-concept (Sideleau, 1992). Although it is essential to understand the psychodynamic implications related to posture, an individual's gait may be related to a cultural phenomenon. For example, some cultural groups such as the Vietnamese will cross their arms over the chest, lower their heads, and bend their upper torso slightly forward when greeting someone entering the room. This behavior continues throughout life as a form of respect. A Vietnamese American client might maintain this posture in a clinical psychiatric setting, particularly when conversing with a nurse or a psychiatrist who may be viewed on a higher social, economic, and educational level than the client.

An accepted behavior in the United States is to look directly into the individual's eyes when speaking. However, this practice may seem strange to some cultures. It is thought that African Americans engage in a direct eye contact more often than whites (Murray and Huelskoetter, 1987; Tripp-Reimer and Lively, 1992). However, some African Americans have been socialized through a long history of hostile, punitive interactions with whites to avoid direct eye contact. Even today, some African Americans engage in direct eye contact only with personal acquaintances. In India, direct eye contact is avoided with people in higher or lower socioeconomic groups. Although some Chinese Americans avoid overt expressions of anger, they may narrow their eyes to communicate anger. It is common practice for some Chinese Americans to avoid direct eye contact during interactions because excessive eye contact may indicate rudeness. In India, eye contact may carry sexual connotations and may be restricted with persons of the opposite sex (Sue, 1981).

Blinking as a mode of communication probably receives very little serious attention. However, blinking may have significant cultural meaning. For some Alaskan Eskimos, blinking may indicate agreement (Davidhizar, 1988). In a psychiatric setting, blinking may also indicate anxiety or evasiveness. It is important for the nurse to make a distinction between pathological factors and cultural practices of blinking when assessing clients.

Implications for nursing care

Psychiatric nurses should remember that communication is a product of culture and thus must be considered in a cultural context. Nonetheless, it is essential to balance what is happening in a psychiatric setting with the cultural significance of behavior. Although basic communication can be especially problematic, it becomes even more complicated when pathological and cultural variables are added. An individual's personal beliefs, values, and mores can affect communication and may influence health. Personal communication must be modified to meet cultural needs. If a client and/or the family does not speak English, the nurse needs to use special approaches that will allow the family's health care needs to be addressed and culturally appropriate nursing care to be rendered. Such approaches might include using interpreters to convey not only the client's and family's needs, but also culturally specific health care instructions. Communication through a third party can also compound the problem of sending a message clearly. Sometimes translation can be so literal that the actual intent of what is being said is lost in the translation. A translator should serve two vital functions: as a translator and as a client advocate translating and interpreting the implications of the communication.

Space

The area that surrounds the person's body is referred to as *personal space* and includes both distance between persons and distance from objects present in the environment. An individual's comfort level usually is related to personal space, and discomfort is experienced when it is violated. Personal space is an additional requirement and varies in situations. In addition, dimensions of personal space comfort zones are culturally determined and are influenced by the need for territoriality.

Territoriality

Territoriality involves feelings or attitudes about a spatial area. An individual must be in control of some space and be able to establish rules for this space. The concept of territoriality meets the needs for security, privacy, autonomy, and self-identity (Orland, 1978). The nurse must consider three important aspects of territoriality when planning care: a physical space of one's own, a personal space, and a territory of expertise or role (Hayter, 1981). When territoriality comfort boundaries are encroached on, the nurse may be presented with almost insurmountable obstacles to rendering culturally appropriate care. The need for territoriality cannot be fully addressed unless individuals are allowed opportunities to defend their space against misuse by others (Roberts, 1978). When an individual feels in control of personal space, a sense of security, self-worth, and privacy is developed that enhances the individual's ability to become autonomous in seeking self-identity.

Interpersonal zones

The classic 1966 work of Hall delineates four interpersonal zones: (1) intimate zone, (2) personal zone, (3) social-consultative zone, and (4) public zone. The *intimate zone* involves interactions closer than 18 inches and is reserved for close personal relationships involving activities such as comforting, protecting, and lovemaking. The *personal zone* encompasses distances of 18 inches to 4 feet and is usually space that is reserved for family and friends. Touch is generally permitted and tolerated in the intimate and personal zones. The *social-consultative zone* encompasses distances from 4 to 12 feet and for all practical purposes is maintained in business situations by people who are working together or in casual gatherings. In this zone, sensory involvement and communication with other people are less intense. The *public zone* ranges from 12 feet and beyond and is outside the sphere of personal involvement. It is essential to remember that culture may be a determinant in the wide variations that exist across the dimensions of interpersonal zones.

Perception of space

To develop an understanding about the perception of space, one must first understand that the phenomenon of space can be understood only as it relates to sight, sound, touch, and smell. For example, Japanese Americans are more perceptive to visual stimuli and as such are able to screen out various information into relevant or irrelevant categories. Additionally, Japanese Americans are quite comfortable with simple paper walls as an acoustic screen. Most white Americans would not be able to tolerate a room with simple paper screen walls because the sound would be almost unbearable. It may also be a cultural phenomenon that certain individuals and/or racial groups are more aware of subtle changes in skin temperature. For example, if insufficient space exists to dissipate the heat in a room, the feelings or sensations of crowding will be evident for some cultural groups more rapidly than for others.

Space and culture

Dimensions of the personal space comfort zone vary from culture to culture. For example, French Americans are uncomfortable with a distance of 2 to 3 feet because it is viewed as too formal. On the other hand, some African Americans may feel uncomfortable when personal space is invaded (Evans and Howard, 1973; Watson, 1980). Clients in some psychiatric settings may feel "crowded" or have a sense that their personal space is collapsing inward. Placing an individual in an isolation room could also serve to collapse a client's space inward. The time required for certain clients to report a sense of "overcrowding" after being placed in an isolation room varies. Clients from some cultural groups may be accustomed to extremely small spaces and may not find the space of an isolation room objectionable. For example, the small space may not bother clients from very heavily populated countries such as China, Japan, or Jamaica.

Implications for nursing care

Nurses need to respect, preserve, and protect the client's need for distance. When the client is able to control and maintain personal space, a sense of autonomy is supported, thereby increasing the sense of security. The use of space varies with the individual; however, cultural heritage often has some bearing on certain aspects of a person's use of space. In the United States, most individuals have the Western need to be territorial; however, this has traditionally not been a value of other groups, such as American Eskimos. Culture also has a profound impact on the client's reaction to close contact with others. For example, Chinese Americans have traditionally been a noncontact group. Some Chinese Amer-

icans associate closeness, increased eye contact, and touch as being offensive or impolite.

Social organization

The term social organization refers to the manner in which a cultural group organizes itself around the family unit. How an individual acts in certain situations (cultural behavior) is a socially acquired phenomenon. Family structure and organization, religious values and beliefs, and role and role assignment may all relate to ethnicity and culture. Socially acquired behavior may vary in a cultural setting and consequently can affect nursing care. Knowledge of the family structure and organization, religious values and beliefs, and role and role assignments can all provide valuable information in assisting the family in achieving goals.

Culture as a totality

Most anthropologists believe that to develop an understanding about the totality of culture, it is necessary to view cultural in a total social context. Holism is an integral concept that requires that human behavior not be isolated from the context in which it occurs. If the nurse is to develop an operational definition of the term culture, it is important to remember that culture must be viewed in its totality, as a functional, integrated whole whose parts are interrelated but significantly independent (Giger and Davidhizar, 1991). Terms germane to developing a keen understanding of the totality of culture include culture bound, ethnocentrism, homogeneity, bicultural, biracial, and stereotyping.

Culture bound. From the moment we are born, we begin to learn a specific culture. In a sense, children from their very beginning of existence on earth are imprisoned without knowing it. Anthropologists call this particular phenomenon culture bound. Culture bound describes an individual living with a certain reality that is considered *the* reality. In most cases, as individuals, we have learned ways to interpret the world based on acculturation. As a result, people who share the same frame of reference are often able to make unique interpretations about things in their world. In many ways, nurses are culture bound by their profession. Nurses are likely to bring to the health care environment a unique scientific approach, the nursing process, to determine and resolve health care problems. Nurses presuppose that the nursing process is unique in its orientation and perhaps the best and only way to meet clients' needs. However, it is important to remember that the nursing process may not necessarily take into account alternative health services, such as folk remedies, holistic health care, therapeutic touch, and spiritual interventions.

Ethnocentrism.   Ethnocentrism is a perception that one's way or world view is best. Individuals view the world from their own unique cultural perspective. Nurses can and do become ethnocentric. Often, nurses are convinced that their approach to the world is scientifically based, whereas that of the client is not. It is essential to remember that nurses' ways are not necessarily the best and that other people's ideas are not "ignorant" or "inferior." Ideas held by some lay people may be valid for them and, more important, will influence their health care behavior and consequently their health status.

Homogeneity.   A homogeneous society does not exist in the United States. If such a society did exist, all individuals would share the same attitudes, interests, and goals. When homogeneity does occur, the phenomenon is referred to as *ethnic collectivity.* Individuals who are reared in ethnic collectivity share a bond that includes common origins, a sense of identity, and a shared standard of behavior. It is thought that these values are often acquired from experiences that are perceived to be cultural norms and that determine the thoughts and behaviors of individual members (Giger and Davidhizar, 1991; Harwood, 1981).

Bicultural.   When a person crosses two cultures, lifestyles, and sets of values, it can be said that this individual is bicultural. These in-

dividuals may be caught in the conflict that is created by attempting to adapt to the value system inherent to both cultures. Nonetheless, as ethnic, racial, and cultural groups intermingle and intermarry, a bicultural society may be formed.

Biracial.   When an individual crosses two racial and cultural groups, the individual is considered biracial. To be both biracial and bicultural creates an almost insurmountable mental dilemma for an individual. For the individual who is biracial, physical attributes such as color, shape of eyes, or hair may have a profound impact on acceptance by others. The problem associated with biracialism is the individual's inability to identify or find acceptance in any one of the biologically related racial groups. It is the total exclusion and the sense of not belonging to any one particular racial group that create the dilemma. For example, an African American who is an octoroon, a person with one-eighth black blood, would encounter difficulty living as a white or black person. If this person embraced the African American race and culture, this individual might be ostracized because of the lightness of the skin by other African Americans. On the other hand, if this individual embraced the white race and culture, some white Americans might ostracize the individual because legally this individual is termed black.

Stereotyping.   Stereotyping is the assumption that all people in a similar cultural, racial, or ethnic group are alike and share the exact same values and beliefs. An excellent example of stereotyping is when an African American nurse is assigned to care for an African American client simply because of ethnicity and race. It is stereotypical when the assumption is held that all African Americans are alike and therefore the African American nurse is more likely to be more sensitive to the needs of the African American client. Race and ethnicity do not, in and of themselves, make us "resident experts" on the belief and value systems of other individuals. Likewise, when the assumption is made that all Jewish clients tend to be stoic in response to pain, the assumption is a stereotype. Whether we engage in stereotyping because of scientifically proved research-based data or because of past associations and experiences, stereotyping can ultimately lead to faulty data gathering and faulty interpretation.

Family systems and cultural significance

It is a culturally significant phenomenon for some cultural groups to view the family constellation as the most important social organization. Some cultural groups tend to extend the family boundaries beyond the traditional nuclear family. For example, many Chinese, Mexican, Vietnamese, Italian, and Puerto Rican Americans hold the family unit supreme to other social organizations. In such cases, family causes take on more significance than personal, cultural, or national causes (Giger and Davidhizar, 1990). The concept of family as a "super organic unit" is a view of the family held by some cultural groups, such as the Vietnamese. The Vietnamese view of family as super organic unit is profoundly different from the individualization of the nuclear family concept common in the United States (Stauffer, 1991).

Role of gender and cultural significance

There is a growing awareness of the need to consider gender as a cultural factor that has a significant relationship to health, health-seeking, and illness behaviors. Mental health problems would be no exception. For example, in traditional Chinese society, the idea that women must have a subordinate role to men dates back to the first millennium BC (Mo, 1992). Traditional Chinese believe that the universe developed from two complementary opposites, "yin" (ingam), the female, and "yang" (yeuhung), the male. For some traditional Chinese Americans, the yin represents the dark, cold, wet, passive, weak feminine aspect of humankind. In stark contrast, the yang represents the bright, hot, dry, active, strong masculine aspect of humankind (Mo, 1992). In traditional societies, "written" and "unwritten" roles dictate the behavior of girls and women.

In the United States, although we are a highly evolved technological country, we still hold traditional beliefs about the role of women in society. For example, even today, women in military service engaging in active combat during wartime is an oddity.

It is important to remember, however, that although women appear to be an oppressed group, gender norms also have psychological consequences for male members of the society. Additionally, a rapid change in gender roles has occurred in the United States over the last several decades.

Gender is a factor that may influence the type of mental health problems that individuals experience. Women are more inclined to have major depressive illnesses, phobias, and eating disorders than their male counterparts. Men, on the other hand, tend to engage more often in alcohol abuse and violent behaviors. Although several explanations may exist for these phenomena, most experts agree that cultural norms channel the expression of feelings and conflicts differently for women than men.

Impact of immigration and acculturation on the family system

Interestingly, immigration to the United States and acculturation by many families into the mainstream of American life has resulted in varying degrees of modification of cultural behavior. In many cases, if assimilation or accommodation is to occur, patterns of cultural behavior must be modified to fit into the dominant culture. Some individuals, by virtue of cultural heritage, believe that mental illness or deprivation in emotional health is a normal condition that requires no medical intervention. On the other hand, some people with a differing cultural perspective believe that mental health is extremely important.

Therefore, when a deprivation of mental health occurs, these people are more likely to seek medical asssistance.

Religion and religious views and cultural significance

Religion is a social phenomenon of major importance to most individuals, regardless of race, ethnicity, or cultural heritage. As human beings, we have a profound need to believe in a Supreme Being with infinite, extraordinary powers. Many religions today, regardless of cultural heritage, are based on the organization of religion into basic church types. Religious church groups generally fall into two categories: (1) the church type and (2) the withdrawal group type.

The *church-type structure* is broadly based and represents the normative spiritual values of the society that most people adhere to by virtue of their membership in the society, such as Hinduism in India, Catholicism in Spain, or the Church of England. The church-type structure is a comprehensive system that allows for individual variations. The uniqueness of the church-type structure is that it generally does not make rigid demands on members. The church-type structures include individual churches that may be identified with an ethnic group rather than with a social class, such as the black church or the Amish church, particularly when these represent the black or Amish life experiences.

The second type of religious structure is the *withdrawal group,* which believes personal commitment and experience are more important than the family and the community functions of religion. In withdrawal groups, individuals make a choice and place that choice above the family or community functions of religion. Groups such as Jehovah's Witnesses or Mormons have a more intense or unbending commitment than that held by the average person. In a psychiatric care setting, these individuals may be assessed as having "delusions of religiosity." The challenge to the nurse is to balance pathological behavior with appropriate cultural expressions of religion.

Family roles and cultural significance

Family member roles are often expressed as patterns of wants, goals, feelings, attitudes, and actions that family members have for themselves and others in the family. Roles usually are related to social class and cultural norms. In some cultures, specific roles for men and boys and specific roles for women and girls may be stressed. For example, an East Indian Hindu woman ranks far below men in social status. A socialized role expectation of East Indian Hindu women would be typified as one of faithfulness and servility to her husband. In fact, East Indian Hindu women are deprived of inheritance if a male descendant is not produced. Likewise, children are similarly socialized at a very early age as to roles in the family. If a very young child is made to feel guilty or ashamed of his or her role, it is likely that the child will develop a poor self-concept.

Role reversals occur in U.S. society because of the country's pluralistic nature. When families, out of dictated needs, are forced to reverse roles, much stress and anxiety probably accompany the reversals. For example, after arriving in the United States, many Vietnamese Americans are forced to reverse traditional roles. Those who were traditionally the "providers" became the "recipients." For example, Vietnamese American women initially on arriving in the United States are more likely to gain employment. Jobs traditionally identified as "women's jobs," such as maids, sewing machine operators, and food service workers, are more plentiful than male-oriented unskilled jobs. Thus the Vietnamese American male is forced to reverse roles with the wife, becoming the recipient instead of the provider. Likewise, Vietnamese American children often assume the role of translator for non-English-speaking parents. Because Vietnamese American children have assimilated very rapidly into the U.S. society, they are more likely than their parents to find gainful employment. Such role reversals have caused intergenerational conflicts for Vietnamese American families (Gold, 1992).

Implications for nursing care

When one family member is receiving care, the family represents the environment in which care is given. The family also has needs that should be addressed. Although one family member may be the identified client, the family should be regarded and treated as a whole. Whether the family is viewed as the environment or as the client, it is essential to incorporate cultural considerations when using the nursing process in developing a plan of care. When the extended family is considered important by a cultural group, the nurse must be considerate of this value. Variables in gender role behaviors according to culture are another important consideration. In a matriarchal culture, the wife or mother is responsible for many family decisions, including when to seek health care. Therefore, if the nurse does not consult the matriarch of the family for advice on the client's care, the entire family probably will resist and become noncompliant. For example, although in 1992 48% of African Americans were reported to be married-couple families, the view held by some African Americans is that the family still is matrifocal (U.S. Department of Commerce, Bureau of Census, 1991).

Time
Concept

Since the beginning of time on Earth, time has been the greatest mystery of all. For most individuals the concept of time is familiar regardless of cultural heritage. Wessman and Gorman (1977) conclude that through an awareness of the conception of time, the products of the human mind, that is, time itself, seem to possess an existence apart from the passage of time, which is perceived as personal and inexorable. Nevertheless, the one certainty of life on Earth is that days and nights come and go and that with each passing day, aging occurs. In this sense, time is perceived as real, as something concrete and as having direct effects. However, time can also be perceived as being "not real," since it is also an abstract concept (i.e., cannot be touched, seen, smelled, or heard).

Scientific definition

For decades, many scientific disciplines have attempted to define the concept of time. Some sciences, such as the mathematical and physical sciences, have defined time as a dimension with only a location or reference function. In contrast, scientists in the biological sciences have defined time as an essential ingredient in many of life processes, such as gestation, healing, and metamorphosis.

Time has two distinct, although related, meanings. One way that time may be viewed is duration. In this sense, duration is an interval of time. On the other hand, the concept of time may be seen as that of specified instances and points in time. These two meanings are related because a point in time is identified as being the end of a time interval that starts at an arbitrary or fixed reference point, such as the birth of Christ or the founding of Rome.

Differentiation between past-, present-, and future-oriented cultures

Persons in cultural groups may be either past, present, or future oriented in regard to time perspective. Individuals who focus on the past strive to maintain tradition and have little motivation for formulating future goals. Although some people in the Appalachians are viewed as present oriented, many hold to traditions and values that have been passed from generation to generation (Tripp-Reimer, 1982). Old Order Amish may be viewed as past-oriented individuals (Wenger, 1989). Some Navajo Indians may be viewed as present-oriented individuals, but many hold a past time orientation and tend to cling to traditional values and beliefs (Hanley, 1991).

Present-oriented cultures include African Americans, Puerto Rican Americans, Chinese Americans, and Mexican Americans. Present-oriented individuals do not necessarily adhere to strict time-structured schedules and may adopt an attitude that an acceptable lateness can include up to 30 minutes after the scheduled time for an event. This perception of time can be traced back to West Africa, where time encompassed events that had already taken place (Mbiti, 1970).

People who have a future time orientation use the present to achieve future goals. A person oriented to the future may appear cold because future tasks may appear more important than people.

Time orientation and significance on compliance with treatment regimens

Persons with a present time orientation are often noncompliant with medical regimens. For example, since Arabic time orientation is primarily on the present and dictated by need, Arab Americans are often late and tend to miss scheduled appointments (Meleis and Sorrell, 1981). This is also true for Chinese American women (Kim, 1988; Yeun, 1987). Present time orientation may also result in nonadherence to feeding schedules, visiting hours, and follow-up appointments.

Implications for nursing care

It is essential to remember that time has important implications for nursing care. The nurse who is able to gain an understanding about the importance of time as a cultural variable with significant impact on clients and ultimately on the client's care is more likely to be able to provide quality care. According to Sideleau (1992), psychiatric clients have impairment in regard to (1) the passage of time (time passes too quickly or too slowly), (2) recognition of distinct divisions in time (the ability to distinguish night and day), and (3) adherence or attention to time schedules. In addition, a distortion in time perception may be found among drug abusers and persons undergoing stressful events. For exam-

ple, individuals who use hallucinogenic and excitatory drugs may experience temporal contraction and spatial expansion. This distortion of time perception often causes these clients to arrive early for appointments. On the other hand, individuals influenced by the effects of tranquilizers experience time expansion and space contraction. These clients are more likely to arrive late for appointments.

Although all these phenomena can be experienced by a client in a psychiatric setting, it is essential that the nurse determine if the faulty time perception is caused by the disorder or by a cultural phenomenon. In Barrow, Alaska's northernmost city, the sun sets on Dec. 21 and does not rise again until May 10. On June 21 the sun rises and does not set again until Aug. 2. People would be confused as to whether it was day or night without the aid of a mechanized timepiece. It is thought that in Alaska the extended periods of daylight and darkness give rise to seasonal, geographically related behaviors. For example, in extended periods of daylight in summer, one may see small children playing in the streets at 2 AM. Because of the extended periods of darkness in the winter, people may sleep late and engage in behaviors more appropriately related to nighttime activities (Lefever and Davidhizar, 1991). Similarly, by virtue of their cultural heritage, some people would have extreme difficulty adhering to a fixed time schedule.

Environmental control
Concept

Environmental control refers to the ability of an individual or group representing a particular culture to plan activities that control nature. At the same time, environmental control refers to the individual's perception of the ability to direct factors in the environment (Giger and Davidhizar, 1991).

The definition of environmental control implies that the concept of environment is broader than just the place where an individual resides or merely where treatment occurs (Giger and Davidhizar, 1991). Environment encompasses relevant systems and processes that affect all individuals (Haber and others, 1987). Systems may be viewed as organized structures that impact and influence the individual. Individuals and the environment enjoy a reciprocal relationship in the sense that a continuous exchange of matter and energy occurs between the two. This exchange may be purposeful and goal directed or the exchange may be viewed as dysfunctional when the exchange has no purpose and lacks goal direction. When this occurs, a dyssynchronous relationship develops (Giuffra, 1987).

Health status reflects a balance between the individual and the environment. For example, in the United States, people are becoming more health conscious. They are eating nutritiously, exercising, reducing stress, and subscribing to preventive health care services available in the community.

Distinction between illness and disease

Scientists, physicians, and anthropologists have begun to make a distinction between the concepts of illness and disease. Individual experiences relating to illness do not necessarily correlate with the biomedical interpretation of disease. For the most part, illness can and does occur in the absence of disease. Approximately 50% of visits made by individuals to physicians are for complaints without a definite medical basis. Illness is culturally shaped in the sense that culture influences expectations and perceptions of illness and disease (Kleinman, Eisenberg, and Good, 1978). For example, some people in the Appalachians attribute mental illness to "bad nerves," "getting old," or being "odd-turned" (Lewis, Messner, and McDowell, 1985).

The term *health care behavior* is inclusive. Health is defined as an individual's social and biological activities related to maintaining acceptable health status or manipulating and/or altering unacceptable conditions (Bauwens and Anderson, 1988).

Cultural health practices versus medical health practices

In the broadest sense, cultural health practices may be categorized as efficacious, neutral, dysfunctional, or uncertain (Pillsbury, 1982). By Western medical standards, efficacious cultural health practices are viewed as beneficial to health status. This is so even when these practices differ greatly from modern Western scientific practices (Giger and Davidhizar, 1991). For example, some Chinese Americans subscribe to the theory of yin and yang, whereas some Mexican Americans hold beliefs that are very similar about "hot and cold" illnesses and conditions. One example is avoiding hot foods because of a stomach condition such as an ulcer. This practice is consistent with Western medical treatment (i.e., bland diet for ulcer treatment). In contrast to efficacious practices, neutral cultural health practices have no effect on the individual's health status. Neutral health care practices may have no direct physiological effect on the individual, but they should not be dismissed as irrelevant. Pillsbury (1982) noted that such practices may be extremely important because they are often linked to beliefs integrated into individual behavior. Examples of neutral health practices include African Americans placing a knife under the bed to cut pain or Navajo Indians sprinkling salt around the sick bed. Such practices may not have a physiological impact on the condition, but the psychological impact may be of great benefit to the client.

Health care practices that are termed dysfunctional are viewed as harmful to the individual. In a psychiatric setting, an example of a dysfunctional health care practice is consuming white dirt in an effort to ward off illness or prevent evil spirits from entering the body.

Williams and Jelliffee (1972) developed a cultural assessment system that included a category of cultural health practices with unknown effects. For the most part, these practices are considered uncertain as to their effect on the individual. In other words, such practices may or may not have harmful implications for the individual. For example, some Navajo Indians and some Mexican Americans believe that an infant should not be provided the opportunity to self-view the image in the mirror until age 1 year. Some African Americans believe that it unwise to cut the hair of a boy until he is about 15½ months old. It is uncertain as to whether such practices might create maladaptation at some future time in life.

Nevertheless, the nurse must combine cultural healing practices with traditional healing practices when possible. For example, it would be appropriate to invite a shaman (a tribal medicine man) to the hospital to perform rituals such as "bless the medication" for a client.

Values and their relationship to health care practices

Values may be defined and viewed as individualized sets of rules by which individuals live and are governed. At best, values serve as the cornerstone for beliefs, attitudes, and behaviors. Cultural values are often acquired unconsciously as a direct result of efforts exerted as an individual assimilates into the dominant culture. In the classical work of Kluckhohn and Strodbeck (1961), value orientations were defined as "complex but definitely patterned principles . . . which give order and direction to the ever-flowing stream of human acts and thoughts as they relate to the solution of common human problems." It is possible for an individual to hold a different value orientation from the mainstream of the cultural group. However, despite differences in value orientation within a cultural group, dominant value orientations can be identified for most persons of a particular cultural group.

Locus of control construct as a health care value

The locus of control construct originated in the social learning theory and is defined as follows (Rotter, 1966):

When a reinforcement is perceived as following some action but not being entirely contingent upon (personal) action, then in our culture it is typically perceived as a result of luck, chance, and fate, as under the control of powerful others, or unpredictable because of the great complexity of the forces surrounding [the individual]. When the event is interpreted in this way by an individual, we have labeled this belief in external control. If a person perceives that the event is contingent upon his own behavior or his permanent characteristics, we have termed this a belief in internal control.

This definition presupposes that individuals who believe that a contingent relationship exists between actions and outcomes subscribe to a belief based on internal feelings of control. For example, persons who subscribe to beliefs based on *internal* locus of control and who believe that a correlation exists between excessive drinking and alcoholism may elect not to drink even casually. Individuals who hold beliefs related to internal locus of control are likely to act to influence future behaviors and situations. In the United States, many middle-class white Americans are viewed as having an internal locus of control.

Individuals who believe that outcomes are controlled by fate, chance, or luck rather than by individual actions subscribe to feelings of *external* locus of control. These individuals are likely to believe that their actions are subjugated to and dictated by nature and the environment. Individuals who believe that efforts and rewards are uncorrelated and who have an external locus of control are less likely to take action to change the future. Some Navajo Indians, Appalachian Americans, African Americans, Chinese Americans, and Mexican Americans have an external locus of control (Kluckhohn and Strodbeck, 1961; Tripp-Reimer, 1984).

Folk beliefs and significance of cultural beliefs

Some cultural groups subscribe to a system of folk beliefs. In Western medical practices, folk medicine may be referred to as "third-world beliefs." Some health care professionals unfamiliar with these beliefs and practices view them as "strange" or even "weird."

Distinction between natural and unnatural illnesses. Some cultural groups view illness and disease as natural or unnatural events. Natural events keep balance between nature and humankind and as such are thought to be designed by God. Natural laws are thought to give life predictability (Snow, 1981).

Unnatural events are thought to upset the balance of nature and at their worst represent forces of evil and the Devil. Unnatural events lack predictability because they exist beyond the parameters of nature and are beyond the control of "mere mortals." This view is in stark contrast to traditional Western medical beliefs. For example, a client in a pyschiatric care setting who has complaints of reptiles crawling or wriggling in the stomach may be diagnosed as having visceral or somatic hallucinations. Therefore the nurse must remember that some individuals believe that illness is a result of witchcraft. People who supposedly possess supernatural power are thought to be able to alter the health status of others. Cultural groups that may subscribe to this belief include Mexicans and Mexican Americans, African Americans, Haitians, Trinidadians, and some southern whites (Snow, 1981).

Implications for nursing care

Variations in health care beliefs and practices cross not only ethnic and cultural boundaries but social boundaries as well. Culture influences an individual's expectations and perceptions regarding health, illness, disease, and symptoms related to disease. Cultural beliefs and cultural values can also influence how one copes with illness, disease, or stress (Bauwens and Anderson, 1992). In addition, individuals from all aspects of society may use folk medicine either alone or in conjunction with a scientifically based medical system. The importance of folk medicine and the level of practice vary among the different ethnic and cultural groups depending on education and socioeconomic status (Bullough and Bullough, 1982).

In contrast to the scientifically based health care system in the United States, folk medicine is characterized by a belief in either supernatural powers or external forces of some form. Snow (1983) says that it does not matter whether an individual comes from a rural background when it comes to selecting health care providers. Folk medicine is still used widely in the African American community because of humiliation in the mainstream health care system, lack of money, and lack of trust in health care workers (White, 1977). Even today some African Americans go to physicians simply because of the control of medicines and not because they believe the physician is superior in knowledge or training (Murray and Huelskoetter, 1987).

According to McKenzie and Christman (1977), witchcraft, voodoo, and magic have always been an integral aspect of folk medicine systems. The nurse should not hastily dismiss folk medicinal practices and beliefs. At times, folk medicine has been used with satisfactory results. In one case a young child whose back was badly burned had not responded to traditional medical interventions. The grandmother enlisted the assistance of a "firetalker" whose rituals of exorcism "mystically" effected a cure (Ingram, 1993).

Biological variations

Biological differences exist between individuals in different cultural groups. In general, biological variations are less understood than other cultural variations. Today, knowledge is developing rapidly in this area. The body of scientific knowledge that exists about biological racial differences is part of the emerging field known as *biocultural ecology*. Biocultural ecology explores the biological differences between individuals of various racial and cultural groups and the biologically adaptive efforts necessary for homeostasis (Bennett, Osborne, and Miller, 1974). Although biocultural ecology concepts have existed in disciplines such as sociology and medical anthropology, it is only recently that the nursing literature has begun the documentation of this field. The emergence of transcultural nursing is a phenomenon of the last two decades, but nursing research into the impact of biological variations on culturally sensitive nursing care remains an area yet to be explored.

Dimensions of biological variations

Undoubtedly a direct relationship exists between race and body structure, skin color, other visible physical characteristics, enzymatic and genetic variations, physiological jaundice, electrocardiographic patterns, susceptibility to disease, and nutritional deficiency. However, the relationship, if any, between race and mental health is ambiguous. The data available tend to suggest that socioeconomic factors, environmental conditions, educational level, migration, separation, and divorce all contribute to symptoms of mental illness more than race, ethnicity, or culture. Gaitz and Scott (1974) noted that although cultural factors may influence mental health scores in research studies, scores are not indicative of whether one cultural or racial group has more or fewer incidences of mental illness than another.

Psychological characteristics

For cultural groups with a low socioeconomic status, the lack of money does affect mental health. For example, low socioeconomic status affects housing, education, physical health, political influence, communication, and social exclusion of groups such as Mexican Americans. The concept of social exclusion is related to poor assimilation of a cultural group into a larger society. The individual who has broad exposure to other lifestyles, cultures, environments, and ideas is more likely to be able to solve problems and fit into a larger society.

Feelings of insecurity can also be related to cultural background. For example, the psychological adjustment of American Indians who grew up on a reservation and now go away to college may be difficult. Poor adjustment may be attributed to this person living in an isolated environment and now being assimilated into the mainstream of society.

A consistent, systematic attack on problems of mental illness has not occurred around the world. Although no cultural group seems immune to mental illness, feelings of racism have prevented a thorough study in all societies. Some authorities contend that psychiatry has not seriously discussed the possibility that racism may be a manifestation of an individual psychological disorder (Pouissant, 1975).

Mental illnesses and treatment vary with cultural groups. For example, psychiatric institutions in Japan are small, whereas in the United States they are much larger. Various societies have placed differing demands on those persons seen as different or having a mental illness. For example, in Russia an individual with political views that differ from the mainstream may be diagnosed with "sluggish schizophrenia." Thus, it is important to remember that the concept of *deviance* varies among cultures. The concept of deviance is useful in understanding the interactions that occur among a person, the cultural environment, and mental health. Social scientists continue to differ on a precise definition of deviance. The term generally is used to describe behavior that violates the dominant cultural norms of a given society.

Racial and ethnic differences cause deviations in the clinical presentation of certain psychiatric disorders. Significant racial differences have been noted among proposed biological markers for various psychiatric disorders, such as serum creatinine phosphokinase, platelet serotonin, and HLA-A2 determinations.

Racial and ethnic differences have been noted in response to psychotropic drugs. For example, certain drugs cause higher blood levels in Asians and thus require modified dosages. Lawson (1986) reports that third-world patients are routinely given smaller doses of neuroleptics because some racial groups metabolize drugs more slowly and therefore experience a greater drug effect. Habits such as drinking and smoking are known to speed drug metabolism, and thus whites and blacks drinking significantly more alcohol than Asians is an important consideration. Lefley (1990) claim that black patients are significantly misdiagnosed as psychotic. Since they are viewed as more violent, they receive more medication and spend more time in seclusion than whites, Hispanics, or Asians. The higher dose of medication prescribed for blacks may result more from staff perception than a decision based on serum levels and careful observation (Keltner and Folks, 1992).

In the United States the incidence of mental illness has been found to vary among racial groups in such conditions as posttraumatic stress disorder (PTSD). Black veterans of the Vietnam War were found to have PTSD at a higher rate than white veterans. Diagnosis, as well as treatment, of PTSD among blacks is complicated by a tendency to misdiagnose black patients. This is caused by the varied manifestations of PTSD and the client's frequent use of alcohol and drugs (Allen, 1986).

We now know that alcohol is metabolized differently in persons in different groups. Also, alcohol is metabolized differently depending on race. For example, in whites, alcohol is metabolized by the liver enzyme dehydrogenase. In Asians, it is metabolized by aldehyde dehydrogenase, which works faster, often causing circulatory and unpleasant effects such as facial flushing and palpitations (Kudzma, 1992). With alcohol use, facial flushing occurs in 45% to 85% of Asians versus 3% to 29% of whites (Chan, 1986). In addition, caffeine, a component of many drugs as well as coffee, tea, and colas, appears to be metabolized and excreted faster by whites than by Asians (Grant, 1983).

In the United States, schizophrenia has been consistently overdiagnosed and affective disorders have been underdiagnosed, particularly among blacks and lower socioeconomic groups

(Gurland, 1976; Taylor and Abrams, 1978; World Health Organization, 1976). Causes of such misdiagnoses of schizophrenia include overreliance on the classic thought disorder symptoms. For affective disorders, a lack of clearly defined boundaries between normal and abnormal mood and failure to realize that these clients can manifest cognitive thought processes are the causes. Also, Jones and Gray (1986) reported that blacks were misdiagnosed as a result of cultural differences in language and mannerisms; the white staff had difficulty understanding black clients. Research is needed on how cultural and racial differences may affect diagnosis as well as establishing baseline behaviors and symptomatology for racial groups.

Use of mental health services is another area that needs study. Services must be based on the levels of need for the different groups. Equitable care between ethnic and racial groups is an important sociological problem (Lopez, 1981).

Implications for nursing care

A better understanding of the differences among various cultures in the area of mental health and treatment could facilitate more culturally appropriate mental health care. Griffith and Griffith (1986) identified that mental health professionals should give more consideration to cultural issues such as racism as they affect individuals psychologically. Although rice and tea may not be the most potent tools of modern psychiatry, they may play an important role in making psychiatric care more acceptable to the acutely disturbed Asian or Pacific American individual. It is important that the nurse appreciate that caring for patients from different cultural groups may require different care methods, but the nurse must avoid stereotypes in the assessment of the patient.

KEY POINTS

1. Culture has a profound impact on how and to whom we communicate our health care needs.

2. Culture can and does dictate spatial needs and requirements for an individual.

3. Culture can give clues as to the meaning of wellness, health-seeking, or illness behaviors.

4. Developing an understanding of folk beliefs and practices and their relevance to cultural behavior is essential to the delivery of culturally appropriate nursing care.

5. Persons may have either a past-, present-, or future-oriented reference to time that can profoundly impact their adherence to and compliance with treatment regimens.

6. Although a clear relationship between race and mental health has not been established, biological variations do exist in relation to the manner in which the body metabolizes medication or responds to treatment.

SUGGESTED SOURCES OF ADDITIONAL INFORMATION

Affonso D: Framework for cultural assessment. In Clark AL, editor: *Childbearing: a nursing prospective,* ed 2, Philadelphia, 1979, FA Davis.

Allen I: Posttraumatic stress disorder among black veterans, *Hosp Community Psychiatry* 37(1):55, 1986.

Bauwens E, Anderson S: Social and cultural influences on health care. In Stanhope M, Lancaster J, editors: *Community health nursing: process and practice for promoting health,* ed 3, St Louis, 1992, Mosby–Year Book.

Bennett KA, Osborne RH, Miller RJ: Biocultural ecology. In *Annual Review of Anthropology,* Palo Alto, 1974.

Boyle JS, Andrews MM: *Transcultural concepts on nursing care,* Glenview, Ill, 1989, Scott, Foresman.

Bullough V, Bullough B: *Health care for the other Americans,* New York, 1982, Appleton-Century-Crofts.

Chan AW: Racial differences in alcohol sensitivity, *Alcohol Alcohol* 21(1):93, 1986.

Chung HJ: Understanding the Oriental maternity patient, *Nurs Clin North Am* 12:67, March 1977.

Davidhizar R: Personal communication, 1988.

Evans G, Howard R: Personal space, *Psychol Bull* 80:335, 1973.

Foster R: *Family-centered nursing care of children,* Philadelphia, 1989, Saunders.

Gaitz C, Scott J: Mental health of Mexican Americans: do ethnic factors make a difference? *Geriatrics* 1(11):110, 1974.

Gary F: Sociocultural diversity and mental health nursing. In Gary F, Kavanagh C: *Psychiatric nursing,* Philadelphia, 1991, Lippincott.

Giger J, Davidhizar R: Transcultural nursing assessment: a method of advancing nursing practice, *Int Nurs Rev* 37(1), 1990.

Giger J, Davidhizar R: *Transcultural nursing: assessment and intervention,* St Louis, 1991, Mosby–Year Book.

Giger J, Davidhizar R: *Transcultural nursing: assessment and intervention,* ed 2, St Louis, 1994, Mosby–Year Book.

Giuffra M: Sociocultural issues. In Haber J and others, editors: *Comprehensive psychiatric nursing,* ed 3, New York, 1987, McGraw-Hill.

Gold S: Mental health and illness in Vietnamese refugees, *West J Med* 157(3):290, 1992.

Grant DM: Variability in caffeine metabolism, *Clin Pharamacol Ther* 33:591, 1983.

Greeley A: *The Irish Americans,* New York, 1981, Harper & Row.

Griffith E, Griffith A: Racism, psychological injury, and compensatory damage, *Hosp Community Psychiatry* 37(1):71, 1986.

Gurland B: Aims, organizations, and initial studies of the cross-national project, *Int J Aging Hum Dev* 7:283, 1976.

Haber J: Therapeutic communication. In Haber J and others: *Comprehensive psychiatric nursing,* ed 4, St Louis, 1992, Mosby–Year Book.

Haber J, Guiffra M: Sociocultural factors related to mental health/mental illness. In Haber J and others: *Comprehensive psychiatric nursing,* ed 4, St Louis, 1992, Mosby–Year Book.

Haber J and others: *Comprehensive psychiatric nursing,* New York, 1987, McGraw-Hill.

Hall E: *Hidden dimension,* New York, 1966, Doubleday.

Hanley C: Navajo Indians. In Giger J, Davidhizar R: *Transcultural nursing: assessment and intervention,* St Louis, 1991, Mosby–Year Book.

Harwood A, editor: *Ethnicity and medical care,* Cambridge, Mass, 1981, Harvard University.

Hayter J: Territoriality as universal need, *J Adv Nurs* 6:79, 1981.

Ingram C: Personal communication to Joyce Newman Giger, February 1993.

Jones B, Gray B: Problems in diagnosing schizophrenia and affective disorders among blacks, *Hosp Community Psychiatry* 37(1):61, 1986.

Keltner N, Folks G: Psychopharmacology update: culture as a variable in drug therapy, *Perspect Psychiatr Nurs* 28(1):33, 1992.

Kim YY: Intercultural personhood: an integration of Eastern and Western perspectives. In Samovar LA, Porter RE, editors: *Intercultural communication: a reader,* ed 5, Belmont, Calif, 1988, Wadsworth.

Kleinman A, Eisenberg L, Good B: Culture, illness, and care, *Ann Intern Med* 88:251, 1978.

Kluckhohn F, Strodbeck F: *Variations in value orientation,* Elmsford, NY, 1961, Row, Peterson.

Kudzma E: Drug responses: all bodies are not created equal, *Am J Nurs* 92:48, December 1992.

Lane P: Nurse-client perceptions: the double standard of touch, *Issues Ment Health Nurs* 10:1, 1989.

Lawson W: Racial and ethnic factors in psychiatric research, *Hosp Community Psychiatry* 37:50, 1986.

Lefever D, Davidhizar R: American Eskimos. In Giger, J, Davidhizar R, editors: *Transcultural nursing: assessment and intervention,* 1991, St Louis, Mosby–Year Book.

Lefley H: Culture and chronic mental illness, *Hosp Community Psychiatry* 41:277, 1990.

Leininger M: *Qualitative research methods in nursing,* New York, 1985a, Grune & Stratton.

Leininger M: Transcultural care diversity and universality: a theory of nursing, *Nurs Health Care* 6(4), 1985b.

Lewis S, Messner R, McDowell R: An unchanging culture, *J Gerontol Nurs* 11(8):20, 1985.

Lipson J, Omidian P: Health issues of Afghan refugees, *West J Nurs* 157(3):271, 1992.

Lopez S: Mexican-Americans' usage of mental health facilities: underutilization reconsidered. In Baron A, editor: *Exploration in Chicano psychological injury and compensatory damage,* New York, 1981, Praeger.

Mbiti SS: *African religions and philosophies,* New York, 1970, Anchor.

McKenzie J, Christman N: Healing herbs, gods, and magic, *Nurs Outlook* 25(5):325, 1977.

Mehrabian A: *Silent messages: implicit communication of emotion and attitude,* Belmont, Calif, 1981, Wadsworth.

Meleis A, Sorrell: The Arab American in the health care system, *Am J Nurs* 81(6):1180, 1981.

Mo B: Modesty, sexuality, and breast health in Chinese-American women, *West J Med* 157(3):260, 1992.

Montagu A: *Touching: the significance of the human skin,* New York, 1971, Columbia University.

Murray R, Huelskoetter: *Psychiatric/mental health nursing,* East Norwalk, Conn, 1987, Appleton & Lange.

Novak W, Waldoks M: *The big book of Jewish humor,* Philadelphia, 1981, Harper & Row.

Orland L: The need for territoriality. In Yura H, Walsh MB, editors: *Human needs and the nursing process,* New York, 1978, Appleton-Century-Crofts.

Pillsbury B: Doing the month: confinement and convalescence of Chinese women after childbirth. In Kay M, editor: *Anthropology of human birth,* Philadelphia, 1982, FA Davis.

Porter RE, Samovar LA: Approaching intercultural communication. In Samovar LA, Porter RE, editors: *Intercultural communication: a reader,* ed 4, Belmont, Calif, 1985, Wadsworth.

Pouissant AF: Interracial relations. In Freeman AM, Kaplan HI, Sandock BJ, editors: *Comprehensive textbook of psychiatry,* ed 2, vol 2, Baltimore, 1975, Williams & Wilkins.

Ramakrishna J, Weiss M: Health, illness and immigration: East Indians in the United States, *West J Med* 157(3):265, 1992.

Roberts SL: *Behavioral concepts and nursing throughout the life span,* Englewood Cliffs, NJ, Prentice Hall.

Rotter JB: Generalized expectancies for internal versus external control of reinforcement, *Psychol Monogr* 80(1):1, 1966.

Sideleau B: Space and time. In Haber J and others: *Comprehensive psychiatric nursing,* ed 4, St Louis, 1992, Mosby–Year Book.

Snow L: Folk medical beliefs and their implications for the care of patients: a review based on studies among black Americans. In Henderson G, Primeaux M, editors: *Transcultural health care,* Reading, Mass, 1981, Addison-Wesley.

Snow L: Traditional health beliefs and practices among lower class black Americans, *West J Med* 139(6):820, 1983.

Spector R: *Culture diversity in health and illness,* ed 3, Norwalk, Conn, Appleton & Lange.

Stauffer R: Vietnamese Americans. In Giger J, Davidhizar R, editors: *Transcultural nursing: assessment and intervention,* St Louis, 1991, Mosby–Year Book.

Sue D: *Counseling the culturally different: theory and practice,* New York, 1981, John Wiley & Sons.

Taylor MA, Abrams B: The prevalence of schizophrenia: a reassessment using modern diagnostic criteria, *Am J Psychiatry* 135:945, 1978.

Tripp-Reimer T: Barriers to health care: variations in interpretation of Appalachian client behavior by Appalachian and non-Appalachian health professionals, *West J Nurs Res* 4(2):179, 1982.

Tripp-Reimer T: Research in cultural diversity, *West J Nurs Res* 6(3):353, 1984.

Tripp-Reimer T, Lively S: Cultural considerations in mental health nursing–psychiatric nursing. In Rawlins R, Williams S, Beck C: *Mental health–psychiatric nursing: a holistic approach,* ed 3, St Louis, 1992, Mosby–Year Book.

Tripp-Reimer T, Brink P, Saunders J: Cultural assessment: content and process, *Nurs Outlook* 32(2), 1984.

US Department of Commerce, Bureau of Census: *The black population,* March 1991.

Watson M: *Proxemic behavior: a cross-cultural study,* The Hague, Netherlands, 1982, Moutons.

Wenger F: President's address, *Transcultural Nurs Soc Newslett* 9(1):3, 1989.

Wessman A, Gorman B: The emergence of human experience and concepts of time. In Gorman BS, Wessman AE, editors: *Personal experience of time,* New York, 1977, Plenum.

White EH: Giving health care to minority patients, *Nurs Clin North Am* 12:27, 1977.

Williams C, Jelliffee D: *Mother and child health: delivering the service,* London, 1972, Oxford.

World Health Organization: *Schizophrenia: a multinational study,* Geneva, 1976, WHO.

Yeun J: Asian Americans, *Birth Defects* 23(6):164, 1987.

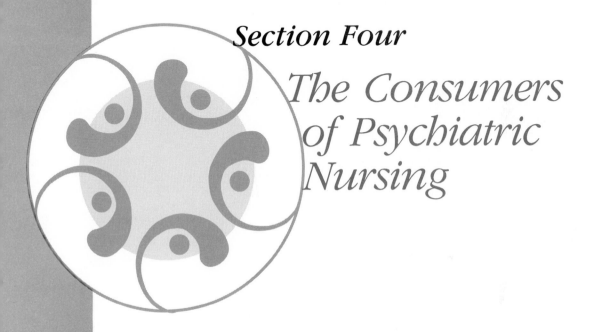

Section Four

The Consumers of Psychiatric Nursing

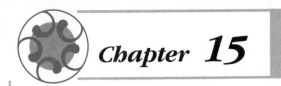

Chapter 15

Individuals with Thought Disorders

LEARNING OBJECTIVES
After studying this chapter, the student will be able to:

* Describe the symptoms exhibited by a person with the medical diagnosis of schizophrenia.

* Discuss the causative factors associated with thought disorders.

* State the major medical treatment for persons with schizophrenia.

* Describe the behaviors the nurse is most likely to observe in an individual who has a thought disorder.

* State examples of nursing diagnoses likely to be applicable to an individual with a thought disorder.

* State and explain nursing interventions likely to be effective with an individual who has a thought disorder.

* Develop a hypothetical plan of nursing care for an individual with a thought disorder.

KEY TERMS
Schizophrenia
Positive symptoms
Negative symptoms
Delusions
Loosening of associations
Hallucinations
Affect
Disturbance in volition
Ambivalence
Withdrawal
Genetics
Neurophysiology
Biochemistry
Dopamine hypothesis
Stress
Antipsychotic medications
Psychomotor retardation
Psychomotor overactivity
Dual diagnosis
Malnutrition
Self-care
Thought processes
Self-perception
Self-concept
Social ineptitude
Coping
Client and family teaching
Discharge planning
Nurse-client relationship
Social support

To cope effectively with the demands of living in a highly complex society, a person must be able to filter, process, and adapt to countless internal and external stimuli. After engaging in these processes, the person then must test reality by consensually validating perceptions with others whose opinions are trusted. When, because of physiological dysfunction or a consistently high level of anxiety, the person is not able to perform these functions, a pattern of reality distortion becomes established. When an individual's distorted perceptions of reality result from and contribute to disturbed thought processes, that individual may have **schizophrenia.**

Although not all authorities agree that the cluster of symptoms currently labeled as schizophrenia represents the same syndrome, all agree that this is one of the most serious forms of mental illness. For the vast majority of persons affected, schizophrenia results in a chronic disability that lasts a lifetime. The personal, social, and economic tragedy of this illness can be appreciated best when one understands that the onset of schizophrenia characteristically is during late adolescence or young adulthood. Furthermore, schizophrenia is a relatively common mental illness. It is estimated that 2 million Americans have schizophrenia and that 1% of the population of the Western world will be diagnosed as having schizophrenia by the time they reach age 55.

HISTORICAL PERSPECTIVE

The thought disorder known today as schizophrenia undoubtedly has existed throughout human history. However, the deviant behavior associated with this disorder was not always viewed negatively. Some primitive societies elevated those who saw visions and heard voices to a position of prominence, believing they had supernatural powers.

Not until the end of the nineteenth century was formal research into the cause and nature of nervous and mental disease conducted. The pioneer of that effort was Jean Charcot (1825-1893), the great French neurologist whose clinics attracted students from every country in the world.

In 1883 Emil Kraepelin (1856-1926), a German professor of psychiatry, published the first edition of *Psychiatrie,* the English translation of which changed the whole view of classifications of mental disorders in America. Kraepelin classified human behavior on the basis of symptomatology and labeled what is now called schizophrenia *dementia praecox.* This label reflected Kraepelin's belief that the deterioration associated with the illness was inevitable, progressive, and irreversible. Eugene Bleueler (1857-1939), a Swiss psychiatrist, elaborated the concept of dementia praecox by recognizing underlying disturbances in the thought processes and therefore renamed the syndrome schizophrenia in 1911. His description of schizophrenia was refined and enlarged over the years but remained essentially the same until 1980, when the American Psychiatric Association published the third edition of the *Diagnostic and Statistical Manual of Mental Disorders* (DSM-III). This manual describes the illness in behavioral terms, and the manual's multiaxial approach allowed, for the first time, a holistic assessment of the individual.

Although a necessary first step, descriptions of a disorder do not necessarily provide direction for treatment. Over the centuries many modalities have been adopted to treat persons with thought disorders, with varying degrees of success. For example, in 1933 Dr. Manfred Sakel developed insulin shock therapy, a procedure in which a series of hypoglycemic shocks are induced by injections of insulin. This treatment, as well as other somatic therapies such as hydrotherapy, has been almost completely replaced by the use of antipsychotic medications and behaviorally oriented interventions. These treatment modalities, although not curing thought disorders, have proved sufficiently safe and effective in controlling symptoms that it was hoped many individuals with thought disorders could be maintained in the community with only infrequent, limited hospitalization.

This hope is far from being fully realized. The average length of hospitalization of individuals with thought disorders has been drastically reduced, but the number and frequency of readmissions remain high. Furthermore, the quality of life of the individual and family is often very poor when the person is not hospitalized. Currently, much research is being conducted to determine not only those factors that contribute to the development of thought disorders, but also those factors necessary to enable individuals with thought disorders to live in a satisfying, satisfactory way in the mainstream of community life.

SCHIZOPHRENIA

No laboratory tests are available to determine conclusively whether a person has schizophrenia. The diagnosis is made solely from the person's symptoms and clinical history. This medical diagnosis is not always easy to determine because a wide cluster of symptoms is associated with schizophrenia and many of these symptoms can result from other disorders. Therefore the psychiatrist's first task is to exclude the presence of any other illness that would explain the client's symptoms.

The onset of schizophrenia may be acute or insidious, and precipitating factors may or may not be present. The symptoms of schizophrenia are often classified as either positive or negative. **Positive symptoms** *reflect the presence of unusual behavior,* specifically distortions in both the content and form of thought and in perception. **Negative symptoms** *reflect the absence of behavior normally expected,* specifically in the dimensions of affect, definition of self, volition, interpersonal relations, and in some clients psychomotor behavior. Some persons with schizophrenia exhibit only positive symptoms; others display only negative symptoms; and many exhibit some of both types. As a result, it is believed that future research is likely to demonstrate that

the syndrome called schizophrenia is several different, although related, illnesses.

The most common symptom associated with distortions of content of thought is **delusions.** Delusions are false beliefs out of keeping with the individual's level of knowledge and cultural group; the belief is maintained against logical argument and despite objective evidence to the contrary. Delusions characteristic of schizophrenia include delusions about one's thoughts, feelings, and activities being controlled by some external force (delusion of being controlled) and delusions about one's thoughts being broadcast into the external world (thought broadcasting), inserted from the external world into one's mind (thought insertion), or removed from one's head by some external source (thought withdrawal). Persecutory, religious, and somatic delusions may occur.

Distortions in the form of thought are manifested by **loosening of associations** (derailment), whereby the individual's idea or trend of thought skips off one track onto another that is completely unrelated. As a result, the person's speech may be unintelligible to the listener even though individual words are understood.

One of the most dramatic symptoms of schizophrenia is related to distortions in perception and is called **hallucinations.** Hallucinations are false sensory perceptions in the absence of an actual external stimulus. Although any of the five senses may be involved in a hallucinatory experience, auditory hallucinations, often of a persecutory nature, are most characteristic of schizophrenia.

One of the most prominent negative symptoms of schizophrenia is a disturbance in affect. The term **affect** refers to the feeling tone of the individual. The person with schizophrenia characteristically exhibits a blunt or flat affect, in contrast to healthy individuals, whose affect conveys a feeling indicative of their emotional state and congruent with the content of what they are saying. One observes that the feeling tone conveyed by individuals with schizophrenic disorders does not enhance what they are saying. It is not unusual to spend much time talking with persons with schizophrenia without learning what they are feeling, despite much of the conversation having been their attempt to describe their feelings. It is also not unusual for individuals to convey a feeling tone inappropriate to the content of what they are saying; for example, a person who has schizophrenia may laugh while stating how upset and sad he or she feels.

Individuals with schizophrenia also have a very poorly defined sense of self and experience extreme confusion about such issues as who they are in relation to both their environment and other people, and what their purpose and role are in the larger scheme of things. When acutely ill, the person literally may not be able to differentiate between where the self begins and ends and where others and the environment begin and end. This very frightening feeling is referred to as a *loss of ego boundaries.*

Disturbance in volition refers to the individual's inability to engage in self-initiated, goal-directed activity. This symptom impacts greatly on the ability to engage in self-care, recreational, and work activities. It is often accompanied by **ambivalence,** in which the person exhibits approach-avoidance behavior resulting from simultaneously experiencing two mutually exclusive emotions such as love and hate.

Impaired interpersonal functioning is one of the most obvious and distressing symptoms of schizophrenia. Individuals with schizophrenia tend to withdraw into their own subjective world. **Withdrawal** is manifested behaviorally by an increasing aversion to interpersonal interactions and often is the symptom that causes the most distress to the client's family. In the extreme, this symptom develops into *autism.* Autism is a form of thinking that does not take reality factors into account and therefore makes it impossible for the person to relate to others in the environment. The individual's autistic world is unique to the person and consequently difficult for others to understand. One can appreciate the nature of autistic thinking to some degree by recalling adolescents' frequent daydreaming. The process is similar in that both autistic thinking and daydreaming are designed to meet unfulfilled needs. A major difference is that the daydreamer can easily call the self back to the world of reality, whereas the individual engaged in autistic thinking cannot.

Finally, the individual with schizophrenia typically displays abnormal psychomotor behavior, which is manifested as either physical and mental overactivity or inactivity.

See Table 15-1 for a summary of the positive and negative symptoms of schizophrenia.

Once the medical diagnosis of schizophrenia is made, the individual's behavior is further categorized into types of schizophrenia. Psychiatrists have subclassified schizophrenia into five major types, depending on the predominant patterns of behavior displayed. These subclassifications are the disorganized, the catatonic, the paranoid, the undifferentiated, and the residual types. The *disorganized type* is characterized by severe personality disintegration, including hallucinations, inappropriate behavior (e.g., silly laughter), and regression. The *catatonic type* is characterized by an acute stupor associated with a sudden loss of animation and a tendency to remain motionless in a stereotyped position; this behavior may alternate with periods of excitement and explosive overactivity. The *paranoid type* is characterized by suspiciousness and ideas of persecution of grandeur called *paranoid delusions.* The *undifferentiated type* is characterized by the prominence of psychotic symptoms that fall into more than one subtype or that do not meet the criteria for any one subtype. The *residual type* is the diagnosis used for individuals who no longer exhibit overtly psychotic symptoms but do exhibit inappropriate behavior characteristic of schizophrenia.

Whether it is possible to help an individual with schizophrenia to achieve a satisfactory and satisfying life depends on several factors:

1. *Character of prepsychotic personality.* The prepsychotic personality includes the effectiveness of the individual's adaptation

Table 15-1.   Positive and negative symptoms of schizophrenia

Symptom	Description
Positive	
Delusion	False belief out of keeping with individual's level of knowledge and cultural group that is maintained against logical argument and despite objective evidence to the contrary
Loosening of association	Idea or trend of thought skipping off one track onto another that is completely unrelated
Hallucination	False sensory perception in absence of actual external stimulus
Increased psychomotor activity	Increase in physical and mental activity
Negative	
Disturbance in affect	Blunt or flat feeling tone
Disturbance in sense of self	Poorly defined conception of who one is and what is meaning of one's life; loss of ego boundaries
Disturbance in volition	Inability to engage in self-initiated, goal-directed activities
Disturbance in interpersonal functioning	Withdrawal from others; autism in extreme situations
Decreased psychomotor activity	Decrease in physical and mental activity

before becoming mentally ill, the type of interests that were maintained, and the coping mechanisms that were used.

2. *Nature of the onset of illness.* Did the illness develop insidiously over a long period as the result of progressively more unsatisfactory methods of coping with life's problems, or was the onset rapid and precipitated by a situation external to the individual's life?

3. *Timing and nature of treatment.* Was treatment sought early in the illness, and was treatment individualized and personalized?

An individual who has adapted reasonably well to the stressors of life before becoming ill will have a better chance of recovery, at least of returning to the prepsychotic level of effectiveness, than will someone who has never adapted effectively and therefore has limited system energy. Someone whose illness has developed slowly and insidiously has a less optimistic future than does someone whose illness was precipi-

tated only after experiencing great stress emanating from the environment.

Persons who receive help very soon after the development of the illness and are given individalized, skilled, and highly personalized care have a good chance of making a social recovery. This is much less true of persons who receive treatment after the illness has been full-blown for a year or more.

Authorities suggest that expectations for recovery should be in terms of social recovery and not necessarily in terms of cure. During remission, these individuals may maintain a marginal adjustment, still retaining an essentially shallow affective response and shyness. They can be thought of as interpersonally fragile and may require professional help from time to time. Many require a daily maintenance dose of one of the antipsychotic medications.

Schizophrenia increasingly is viewed as a chronic, long-term illness with periods of remission and periods of exacerbation. This view is seen as realistic and therapeutic rather than pessimistic and stigmatizing because it encourages the client, family, and all health care professionals to develop attainable goals. This view implies a focus on rehabilitation strategies that emphasize the acquisition of skills that aid functioning rather than focusing on aspects of living with which the client is unable to cope.

CAUSATIVE FACTORS

Although much progress has been made in describing the biological and behavioral characteristics of people with schizophrenia, the precise cause of this tragic illness remains elusive. Nevertheless, it is currently believed that schizophrenia is an outcome of complex interactions of multiple biological and psychosocial factors. Awareness of the etiological complexity of schizophrenia is a relatively new phenomenon.

Until recently, the cause of schizophrenia was believed to be primarily psychosocial and psychodynamic in nature. For example, Freud believed the etiology was related to a particularly unsatisfactory oral stage of psychosexual development that severely hampered the individual's ego development. Sullivan also theorized that the seeds of schizophrenia were sown during infancy when the baby was subjected to inconsistent and inadequate nurturing, resulting in massive levels of anxiety that interfered with the development of a sense of self. In the 1950s much research was devoted to describing the familial relationships of those with schizophrenia. The concept of the "schizophrenogenic" family arose from these studies. This type of family was described as engaging in dysfunctional relationships characterized as overprotective, cold, critical, and withholding of affirmation. These dysfunctional patterns of relating were thought to be major factors in causing schizophrenia. An unfortunate outcome of these theories was blaming parents, particularly mothers, for the illness of their children.

Theories that claim that faulty interpersonal relationships are primary factors in the development of schizophrenia are no longer seen as valid. A causal relationship between dysfunctional interpersonal relationships and schizophrenia has not been demonstrated. Furthermore, many believe that some dysfunctional relationships observed in certain families of persons with schizophrenia result from the unremitting stress experienced by these families as they try to cope with the illness.

Biological factors

Biological factors associated with schizophrenia include those in the realms of **genetics, neurophysiology,** and **biochemistry.**

Genetic factors

Psychiatric genetics is a specialty that focuses specifically on the role of human heredity in the transmission of mental illness. Several methodologies are typically used in the field of psychiatric genetics. These include family studies, twin studies, adoption studies, and genetic linkage analysis.

Family studies. Family studies are based on the concept that, if a disorder is genetically determined, blood relatives of individuals with a mental illness are more likely to have inherited the predisposing gene or genes for the same mental illness than are family members related by marriage or adoption. Thus the goals of family studies are to determine the frequency of mental illness among family members and the patterns of genetic transmission.

The risk of people in the general population developing schizophrenia is 0.5% to 1%. Family studies have demonstrated a much higher incidence of schizophrenia in individuals who have a family history of schizophrenia. The risk is greatest for those persons who are genetically close to the family member with schizophrenia. For example, when a sibling has schizophrenia, the risk of another sibling developing this illness is 8%; when one parent has schizophrenia, the risk of an individual developing this disorder increases to 12%; when both parents have this illness, the risk rises to 40%. These findings have led some authorities to conclude that genetic factors play a major role in the development of schizophrenia. Other authorities, however, argue that such conclusions cannot be drawn, since it is not possible to separate the effects of the familial and cultural environments from the effects of heredity.

Other studies that suggest a genetic basis for schizophrenia include those related to persons' ability to follow smoothly a moving object with their eyes. Persons with schizophrenia characteristically demonstrate abnormalities in performing this neurological test. This same defect is found in unusually high proportions in the healthy relatives of a person with schizophrenia, but not in the healthy relatives of persons with other illnesses, such as Parkinson's disease and multiple sclerosis, that cause the same defect.

Therefore, it is believed that a common genetic defect may exist in individuals with schizophrenia and their families that manifests itself in different ways in different family members.

Twin studies. Twin studies have been used to compare the rates of mental illness between identical and fraternal twins. If a mental disorder is genetically transmitted, it is more likely that identical twins will share the same mental disorder than will fraternal twins or siblings, since identical twins are genetically alike. Several studies have shown that if one identical twin has schizophrenia, a 50% likelihood exists that the other twin will also have the disease. With fraternal twins, when one has schizophrenia, the risk of the other twin developing this illness decreases to 17%.

Despite the convincing evidence of twin studies, it should be noted that if genetic transmission were the sole causative factor of schizophrenia, the identical twin of an individual with schizophrenia would always develop schizophrenia as well, since identical twins have the same genes. Furthermore, twin studies, as with studies of the rate of schizophrenia among close family members, do not account for the role of environment in the development of schizophrenia.

Adoption studies. To separate the influences of heredity and environment, some researchers have used adoption studies to examine the relationship between the incidence of schizophrenia among persons separated at birth from their parent with schizophrenia. These studies have found that the offspring of an individual with schizophrenia are more likely to develop this disorder than other adopted individuals whose biological parents did not have this illness. In addition, some studies have shown that a child without a familial history of schizophrenia who is adopted and reared by an individual with schizophrenia is not at any greater risk for developing the disorder than anyone else in the general population.

Many authorities maintain that the results of adoption studies offer the most compelling evidence that schizophrenia is genetically transmitted. However, other experts caution that the number of individuals studied is too small to allow definitive conclusions to be made.

Genetic linkage studies. Genetic linkage studies have received increased attention in the last decade. Recent technological advances have allowed experts to locate genes on a human chromosome map. More than 900 genes have been mapped thus far. With this information scientists use various linkage markers to locate the genes associated with certain diseases on specific chromosomes. For example, linkage analysis has established that the gene for Huntington's chorea is located on chromosome number four. Advances in gene mapping allow for more accurate genetic counseling as well as improvement in the overall quality of genetic analysis.

Some psychiatric genetic experts have argued that the genetic influences on schizophrenia are complex and do not conform to the classic Mendelian pattern of transmission as do some physical illnesses in which genetic transmission occurs in predictable patterns. In addition, these experts argue that schizophrenia is actually a group of related but separate illnesses. Recently, one group of scientists engaged in a genetic linkage study of many individuals diagnosed as having schizophrenia. They reported that a link appears to exist between schizophrenia and an abnormally functioning gene or genes on chromosome number five. However, another group of scientists found no association between schizophrenia and chromosome number five, although they did not believe that their findings necessarily contradicted the findings of the first study. Rather, they proposed that the individuals in the first study may have been affected by a form of the illness related to chromosome number five, whereas those in the second study may have had a different form of schizophrenia.

Neurophysiological factors

The recent availability of sophisticated brain-imaging equipment and techniques has enabled researchers to study the brains of people with schizophrenia at various points during the illness and with and without medication. These studies have yielded much information. For example, studies using the computed tomography (CT) scan have shown abnormalities of brain structure in 20% to 50% of persons with schizophrenia. These abnormalities include larger cerebral ventricles and greater atrophy of cortical and cerebellar tissue than in healthy subjects. However, these findings are not limited to individuals with schizophrenia and therefore cannot be the specific cause of the illness.

Magnetic resonance imaging (MRI) studies suggest that the frontal lobes of those with schizophrenia are smaller than average. Atrophy in the temporal lobes of the brain of persons with schizophrenia is also suggested by these studies.

Positron emission tomography (PET) allows the brain to be studied as it works. Some of these studies have demonstrated that those with schizophrenia have low metabolic activity in the frontal lobes of the brain, especially in the prefrontal area of the cerebral cortex. This is the area of the brain that governs planning and abstract thinking and controls social judgment and expression of feeling.

It is not certain how these brain abnormalities are related to the symptoms, much less the cause,

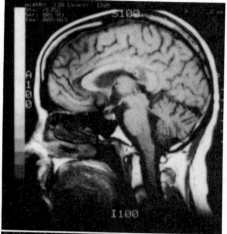
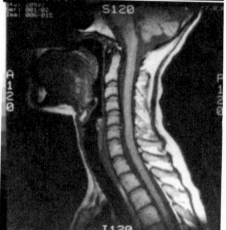

Figure 15-1

A, Magnetic resonance imaging (MRI) helps identify biological factors in psychiatric disorders such as schizophrenia. **B,** MRI can be used to help with the diagnosis of schizophrenia.

From Chipps EM et al: *Neurologic disorders,* St Louis, 1992, Mosby–Year Book.

of schizophrenia. Nevertheless, some researchers believe that the negative symptoms of schizophrenia are related to enlarged ventricles and frontal lobe deficiencies.

Biochemical factors

After the chance discovery of various psychotropic drugs in the 1950s, experts attempted to *transmitters,* natural chemicals necessary for the transmission of nerve impulses in the brain.

Scientists have identified the presence of many neurotransmitters in the brain. The central nervous system neurotransmitters can be classified into three major categories: the amino acids, the biogenic amines, and the neuropeptides. Each of these three major categories has several subcategories. For example, the biogenic amines include the catecholamines termed dopamine, norepinephrine, and epinephrine. The biogenic amines also include acetylcholine, histamine, and serotonin.

One of the most widely known hypotheses relating neurotransmitters to mental illness is the **dopamine hypothesis.** This hypothesis proposes that the symptoms of schizophrenia result from overactivity of the neurotransmitter dopamine in the central nervous system. In 1963 Carlsson and Lindqvist were the first to suggest that antipsychotic drugs diminished dopaminergic activity through a blockage of dopamine in the mesolimbic and mesocortical tracts of the brain. The mesolimbic and mesocortical tracts are associated with intellectual and emotional functioning, and it is thought that some symptoms of schizophrenia, such as hallucinations and delusions, involve these two systems.

Recently, scientists have suggested that it is unlikely that schizophrenia results only from a single neurochemical problem. The neurotransmitter systems of the brain are interactive systems that continuously influence one another. Therefore, experts have begun to examine the role of neurotransmitters other than dopamine in determining schizophrenic symptoms, such as the biogenic amines norepinephrine and serotonin and the neuropeptides termed endorphins.

Other biochemical factors demonstrated to be related to schizophrenia are low-platelet monoamine oxidase (MAO), viral and immunological deficits, and elevated serum creatine phosphokinase (CPK). The significance of these findings is not clear, but they do point to the need for continued research.

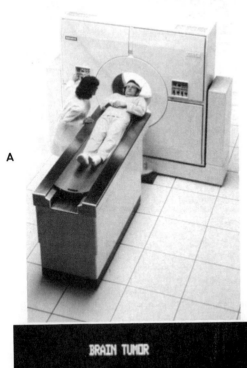

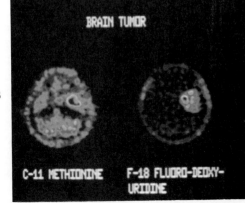

Figure 15-2

A, Clinical setting for positron emission tomography (PET). **B,** PET scans provide information about abnormalities in brain function that can be related to schizophrenia.

From Chipps EM et al: *Neurologic disorders,* St Louis, 1992, Mosby–Year Book.

identify how these medications acted to relieve symptoms of mental illness. One of the earliest areas of investigation focused on discovering the action of psychotropic medications on *neuro-*

Psychosocial factors

Any interpersonal or social factor that impedes optimum personality development can potentially interact with a biological predisposition to schizophrenia and precipitate the onset of the illness, exacerbate its symptoms, or impede its resolution. Despite the growing evidence linking biological factors with the development of schizophrenia, many authorities believe that psychosocial factors are also powerful contributors to the development of schizophrenia.

Psychosocial **stress** has been extensively studied as a factor contributing to the development of schizophrenia. Little evidence indicates that stress causes schizophrenia, but increasing data demonstrate that stress is associated with relapse. Specifically, a high level of expressed emotion (EE) in one or more family members of individuals with schizophrenia has been associated with an increase in symptoms.

Other psychosocial factors associated with schizophrenia are a low socioeconomic level, minority status, and environmental crowding. Whether these factors combine with a biological predisposition to the illness to cause schizophrenia or whether they are the result of the illness is the subject of much debate.

MEDICAL TREATMENT

The major medical treatment for persons with schizophrenia is the use of **antipsychotic medications.** This category of medication is discussed in detail in Chapter 10.

Although natural and synthetic chemical substances had been used for centuries in an effort to normalize behavior, it was not until 1953 that relatively safe and effective psychotropic medications were developed. In 1956 the most useful of the new medications, chlorpromazine, was introduced. It was marketed under the name of Thorazine and today is only one of several medications that are effective in diminishing the psychotic symptoms associated with schizophrenia; thus these medications are referred to as antipsychotic drugs. Over the years, clinical experience with the use of these medications has shown that they are particularly effective in reducing the positive symptoms of schizophrenia, that is, delusions, loosening of associations, and hallucinations. They are less effective and sometimes ineffective in ameliorating the negative symptoms.

Although it is known that not every individual is helped by these medications, it is not possible to determine at diagnosis which clients will be helped and which will not. Therefore an antipsychotic medication is initially prescribed for the vast majority of individuals experiencing an acute exacerbation of symptoms. Standard practice is to maintain clients on moderate doses of antipsychotic drugs for as long as possible, since relapse rates increase dramatically once medication is stopped. The nurse should be very aware, however, that the incidence of side effects increases as dosage and duration of use increase.

Drug manufacturers often make claims that a drug is specifically useful in alleviating a particular symptom, implying that major differences exist between drugs within a given chemical group. Clinicians, on the other hand, more often report that the drug's effect seems to be idiosyncratic to the individual and that if a drug in one chemical group is not successful in alleviating the symptomatology without adverse effects, success can often be achieved by the administration of an antipsychotic drug from another chemical group.

Despite the general success of the antipsychotic medications in ameliorating the symptoms of schizophrenia, 10% to 20% of persons with this illness are not helped by the most frequently prescribed drugs. Many of these "treatment-resistant" individuals are clients who are severely ill and who exhibit the negative symptoms of schizophrenia. A relatively new medication, clozapine, is now in use in the United States and has promise for helping these clients.

Clozapine is considered an "atypical" antipsychotic medication in that it does not produce the same extrapyramidal side effects typical of the other antipsychotic agents. However, clozapine has caused the potentially lethal adverse reaction of agranulocytosis. Since the risk of developing agranulocytosis is not related to age, sex, or dose, it is not possible to predict who will exhibit this symptom. However, it is known that agranulocytosis most often occurs between the sixth and eighteenth week of treatment.

Because of its potential to cause agranulocytosis, clozapine currently is available only to selected individuals for whom the potential benefits are judged to outweigh the risks. White blood cell (WBC) counts are required weekly for as long as clozapine treatment continues. Therefore, clients must be willing and able to have blood drawn weekly. If the WBC count shows a significant decrease from the previous count or if the count drops to less than 3500, the physician must institute a protocol established by the manufacturer of the medication. This may include immediate discontinuation of the drug. The nurse must be alert to any signs of fever, sore throat, lethargy, or weakness in a client receiving clozapine treatment, since these symptoms may signal a depressed WBC count.

It is too soon to determine whether clozapine will prove to be a sufficiently effective treatment to warrant the health risk and the cost of both medication and laboratory tests for large numbers of persons with schizophrenia.

NURSING CARE OF INDIVIDUALS WITH THOUGHT DISORDERS

Nursing assessment

When assessing an individual with a thought disorder, it is important for the nurse to remember that the medical classification of schizophrenia into five types has little practical significance for designing a plan for nursing care. The nurse must attempt to understand the needs of the person rather than to focus on diagnostic entities.

For purposes of clarity, typical behaviors of persons with thought disorders are discussed by categories. Although behaviors in each category are presented as separate entities, they are highly interrelated and are adaptations to similar stressors. Further, behavior designed as an adaptation to one stressor often becomes a stressor itself in another dimension. Therefore, nursing care directed at altering one behavior will inevitably have an effect on others.

Health perception–health management

Behaviors related to unmet physical needs may or may not be related to the client's emotional problems. It cannot be overemphasized that emotional illness provides no immunity to physical illness. Therefore, in the initial assessment it is imperative that the nurse determine the degree of the client's general physical health. Complaints of physical discomfort must be thoroughly investigated to determine whether they are related to physical illness or to the individual's emotional state.

CLINICAL EXAMPLE

Barry is a 52-year-old white male who is well known to the mental health system. He is readmitting himself to the hospital because of overwhelming feelings of anxiety and a reemergence of auditory hallucinations. He tells the nurse that he stopped taking his medication about a month ago because he was feeling so much better and the price of cigarettes had gone up so he used the money he normally spent on his medication to buy cigarettes. As the nurse listens, she observes that Barry is short of breath and coughing. His vital signs are within normal range. Even though the nurse knows that dyspnea is a common symptom of anxiety, she encourages the physician on duty to order a chest radiograph. The radiograph reveals a tumor in the lower lobe of Barry's left lung.

The individual may not spontaneously report a long-standing physical condition such as diabetes or hypothyroidism caused by a thyroidectomy, either of which may require daily medication. The nurse should be alert to indications of these and other physical conditions by observing for such evidence as scars or injection marks.

Because of the nature of thought disorders, the nurse may find various physical problems that are a consequence of the thought disorder. For example, because of **psychomotor retardation** or **psychomotor overactivity,** the person may have circulatory problems evidenced by peripheral edema or may be verging on a state of exhaustion.

When making the initial assessment, the nurse must determine whether the person has taken any psychotropic medications and, if so, the type, dosage, and frequency. The purpose of these medications is to alter emotional states biochemically, which brings about altered behavior. In addition, the medications themselves may have side effects that are reflected behaviorally. It is important to differentiate between behavior induced by medications and behavior reflecting the emotional state, since the subsequent intervention differs.

In addition to the use of psychotropic medications, an increasing number of persons with thought disorders use street drugs, often in an effort to decrease their symptoms. Therefore a comprehensive assessment includes ascertaining whether the individual takes nonprescribed mind-altering drugs. Persons with a thought disorder who also are addicted to mind-altering drugs are referred to as mentally ill chemical abusers (MICAs) or clients with a **dual diagnosis.** Although the treatment of persons with a thought disorder and the treatment of individuals

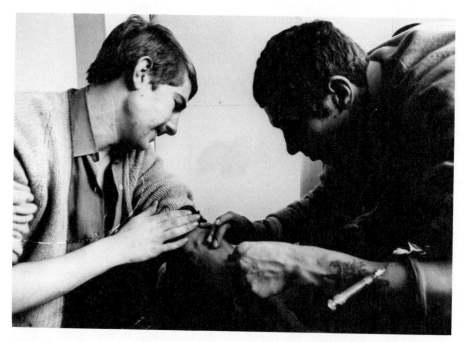

Figure 15-3
An increasing number of persons with thought disorders use street drugs.
From Ray O, Ksir C: *Drugs, society, and human behavior,* ed 6, St Louis, 1993, Mosby–Year Book.

with substance abuse (see Chapter 19) are well known and relatively effective, determining effective treatment of persons with both these disorders simultaneously represents one of the greatest challenges to contemporary mental health care.

Nutritional-metabolic

Malnutrition caused by psychomotor retardation, suspiciousness, or generalized neglect of activities of daily living is often seen in persons with thought disorders. Even though clients might not be able to tell the nurse their usual weight, the nurse can observe whether clothing fits properly. If an individual has been taking psychotropic medications for a time, especially the phenothiazines, the person may be overweight because these medications stimulate the appetite. Obesity should not be seen as evidence of a sound nutritional state; many obese people are malnourished because food high in caloric value frequently has limited nutritional value.

CLINICAL EXAMPLE

Peggy asked the nurse to help her undress for the physical examination. The nurse was surprised to discover that Peggy needed help because her husband had fastened her dress with safety pins so it would not fall off her shoulders.

NURSE: This dress seems very large for you.

PEGGY: I know it doesn't fit, but I like the color.

NURSE: I like the color, too. Did it ever fit?

PEGGY: A while ago.

NURSE: Have you lost a lot of weight recently?

PEGGY: Uhhh . . .

NURSE: What food do you usually eat?

PEGGY: I don't eat anything but hard-boiled eggs. They can't poison them.

Elimination

Elimination is not necessarily a problem for most individuals with a thought disorder. However, the nurse must ascertain the client's pattern of elimination as part of a comprehensive health assessment. Clients who are severely ill may be incontinent of urine and/or feces, not because of loss of sphincter control but because of an inability to decide to go to the bathroom.

Activity-exercise

It is unusual for an individual with a thought disorder to exhibit normal psychomotor behavior, that is, both mental and physical activity congruent with the requirements of the situation. Rather, the person frequently exhibits retardation or overactivity in the psychomotor realm. An extreme example of psychomotor retardation is seen in persons who are in a catatonic stupor. These persons move very slowly and can take hours to walk the distance of a city block or to eat a meal. Concomitantly, they speak very slowly, which reflects an extreme slowing down of mental processes. The term *retardation* as used in this context does not mean the client has an intellectual deficit. Individuals with a thought disorder do not necessarily have an intellectual impairment, although this may appear to be the case because of their temporarily diminished ability to comprehend and respond to mental stimuli.

CLINICAL EXAMPLE

Pam was not able to go to the dining room for meals because it took her more than an hour to walk the 50 yards from the ward to the dining room. She would slowly place her left foot forward and, while it was suspended, would recite, "Go, go, flow, flow," before she set her foot down. She would then raise her right foot and say, "Back, back it's a hack," before placing her right foot down. After two series of these rituals, Pam would rapidly move back two steps. Therefore, for every four steps forward, she would take two steps backward.

Psychomotor overactivity is manifested by loud, rapid talking (pressure of speech) and frequent, rapid, gross motor movements that seem aimless. Despite the quantity of activity, fine motor movements are usually impaired. This person literally finds it impossible to sit still and frequently paces, swinging the arms and talking continuously.

When questioned about recreational activities, many clients with a thought disorder will report that their only recreation is listening to the radio or watching television. These passive activities are solitary and do not require much concentration. Other clients enjoy reading but not material that evokes emotional responses such as romance novels. Once again, reading is a solitary activity and nonverbally discourages social approaches from others.

Neglect of all areas of **self-care** is often the first sign of an impending psychosis. It is not unusual for the individual with a thought disorder to neglect personal hygiene and become poorly groomed and inappropriately dressed. Such clients often have many unmet physical needs because they have not attended to their basic needs for food, water, or shelter and have not sought health care.

CLINICAL EXAMPLE

Mrs. Smith brought Wendy, her 26-year-old daughter, to the hospital emergency room, stating that Wendy needed help. Wendy sat quietly next to her mother. She appeared disinterested in what was going on around her and stared blankly at the wall. Wendy's general appearance was inappropriate for her age. She looked soiled and disheveled and wore a printed housedress of the style usually worn by women three times her age. Her red hair was dirty and was held off her face by a headband. Mrs. Smith said she was exhausted by arguing with Wendy about the need for her to take a bath and change her clothes. Mrs. Smith said she hoped someone else could do something with Wendy. Wendy made no comment to her mother's statement.

As is true with self-care, the individual with a thought disorder is unlikely to be able to engage in the activities required to maintain a home,

such as cleaning, shopping, and transacting normal business activities such as paying rent.

Sleep-rest

Almost all persons with a thought disorder experience a disturbance in their normal sleep pattern. For some, an inability to sleep is a prodromal symptom of an impending psychosis. During the assessment, it is important for the nurse to determine the usual sleep pattern of the client and whether this has changed in the recent past.

CLINICAL EXAMPLE

When asked how much sleep he normally needed, Ben told the nurse he had not slept more than 2 hours a day for the last week. He said that the voices were much louder when he woke up so he tried to prevent their return by not going to sleep.

Cognitive-perceptual

Decision making and judgment are both typically impaired in individuals with thought disorders. These persons may be observed vacillating over seemingly simple decisions such as whether to go outdoors or what to wear if they do.

As its name indicates, the major impairment experienced by people with thought disorders is in relation to their **thought processes.** Their inability to think abstractly is dramatically manifested through psychological tests that require the client to explain proverbs. For example, when asked the meaning of "a rolling stone gathers no moss," the client is likely to say, "When a stone rolls down a hill it will not catch on the grass because it is moving." If asked what brought the client to the hospital, the client is likely to reply, "A bus."

Delusions, regardless of their nature, are another indication of altered thought processes. Many clients, especially if they have been ill for some time, have learned not to divulge their delusional thinking to an individual whom they are meeting for the first time. Therefore the nurse who is making the initial assessment may be unaware of these delusions.

Auditory and visual hallucinations may be symptoms affecting persons with a thought disorder. The individual experiencing hallucinations rarely offers this information spontaneously. Rather, the person will be observed cocking the head to one side as if listening, staring into space as if watching something, and talking as if to someone, although no one is present.

The client and family may be totally ignorant about the illness and its treatment. Even worse, they may have numerous incorrect beliefs about the illness that they learned as a result of society's misinformation about mental illness. It is important for the nurse to learn what the client and family understand about the illness and its treatment as the first step in designing a plan for teaching.

CLINICAL EXAMPLE

Margarita, an 18-year-old Hispanic female, was brought to the hospital by the police because she had been walking nude down the street. Her mother arrived a few minutes later and sat in the waiting room while Margarita was examined by the physician. Ms. Jones, one of the admitting nurses, observed that the mother was in great distress and continuously fingered rosary beads. Since another nurse was with Margarita and the physician, Ms. Jones sat with Margarita's mother.

NURSE: This situation seems to be very upsetting to you.

MOTHER: My poor baby, my poor baby!

NURSE: I know Margarita's behavior is frightening, but it's likely that she will act more normally in a few days.

MOTHER: She will burn in hell!

NURSE: Burn in hell?

MOTHER: To be naked is to sin. She will have to repent.

NURSE: I think Margarita was naked because she is sick, not because she is a sinner.

MOTHER: She's not sick—she's a whore. (Sobbing) I love her.

Ms. Jones reported this interaction to the nurse who was admitting Margarita so a plan for teaching about mental illness could be developed.

Self-perception/self-concept

Individuals with a thought disorder characteristically have a distorted **self-perception** and a poor **self-concept.** These clients may believe they are simultaneously omnipotent (all powerful) and powerless. This belief is normal during the first stage of psychosexual development but in usual circumstances is outgrown as the child develops. Unfortunately, persons with thought disorders often see themselves as responsible for events over which they had no control but for which they wished. In addition, they often have a distorted image of their appearance and are often preoccupied with a body part, such as the nose or breasts.

The self-concept is a relatively enduring view of self as worthy, worthless, or nonexistent. In the acute phase of a psychosis, many persons with a thought disorder see themselves as nonexistent.

CLINICAL EXAMPLE

As Ms. Heinrich interviewed Sonny as part of the admission process of the mental health unit, he got up from the chair and walked at a normal pace into the wall. After bumping himself against the wall, he returned to his seat, but then repeated this behavior several times. When Ms. Heinrich asked Sonny why he continued to hurt himself by walking into the wall, he replied, "It doesn't hurt. I don't know why I can't get through."

Role-relationship

It is not unusual to hear someone describe a conversation with a client who has a thought disorder with phrases such as, "I feel there is an intangible wall between us" or "I just can't seem to get through to him." This reaction is often the result of the client's blunt or flat affect, whereby the feeling tone associated with the client's words does nothing to enhance their meaning.

Because the client's grasp on reality is tenuous and because he or she may be stimulated by intrapsychic phenomena such as voices or visions, the client may strike out at things or persons in the environment. Even though the nurse has learned in social situations to associate aggressive, physical behavior with the feeling of anger, this seemingly hostile behavior on the client's part is more likely to be an adaptation to feelings of anxiety or fear.

Social ineptitude is a prominent feature of the behavior of individuals with thought disorders. They often have not been able to learn many rudimentary social skills that healthy adults take for granted. Such common occurrences as meeting people for the first time can precipitate overwhelming anxiety and may lead to highly inappropriate behavior. These persons may go to great lengths to avoid social situations and activities such as dating and team sports. Instead, they prefer to engage in solitary activities, which enables them to keep their anxiety at a manageable level but also increases their social ineptitude. They often report that they have few if any friends; the nurse may observe that few if any people visit or inquire about the client's welfare.

The social ineptitude of these clients partly stems from and is compounded by their communication problems, which in turn result from their thought disorder. As previously stated, these individuals think in a very concrete, personalized manner and consequently have difficulty understanding and appropriately responding to the superficial chatter characteristic of most social situations.

CLINICAL EXAMPLE

The nurse at the mental health clinic was interviewing Sam, a 20-year-old African American who recently had been discharged from the hospital and was registering at the clinic for continuing care. Even though Sam was very cooperative in answering questions, he had an expressionless look, spoke with a flat affect, and did not volunteer information.

NURSE: Do you have any friends?

SAM: I've got lots of friends.

NURSE: Tell me about them.

SAM: (Slowly) Well, there's John, and then there's Mike.

NURSE: Who are John and Mike?

SAM: John's the mailman. I see him every day. He's got a neat uniform and cart he uses to push the mail around.

NURSE: And Mike?

SAM: He's my landlord. He comes up to my place on the first of the month, real prompt, to get my rent.

NURSE: Do you spend time talking with John or Mike?

SAM: No. But I spend my money with Mike.

Many people believe that persons with thought disorders are not at risk for suicide. Nothing could be further from the truth! In fact, the rate of suicide is increasing in young adults with chronic schizophrenia. Some authorities believe that the decision to commit suicide is related to clients' realization that they are likely to suffer from the disabilities associated with the disorder for the remainder of their lives. Therefore the nurse should be alert to any indication that the client has lost hope. (See Chapter 16 for an in-depth discussion of behaviors associated with thoughts of suicide.)

Sexuality-reproductive

The nurse can expect to find altered sexual behavior in individuals with a thought disorder. This usually results from their impaired social relationships. In some instances the client reports having been a victim of rape or child abuse. If this is the case, the effect of these experiences on the client needs to be thoroughly explored during treatment.

Coping–stress tolerance

Not surprisingly, most persons with a thought disorder give many indications of ineffective **coping** skills. Neuroscientific studies indicate that although stress is not likely to cause schizophrenia, persons with this disorder are particularly vulnerable to many forms of stress. Some persons with a thought disorder may report that they became ill because they were unable to cope with a recent loss or change. This event may be as minor as a change in office or as catastrophic as the unexpected loss of a home because of a fire.

In addition to having limited internal resources for coping with stress, persons with a thought disorder often have few external resources to depend on during times of stress. This is not surprising when one remembers that these persons elicit little social support and are stigmatized by society.

CLINICAL EXAMPLE

Henry was a conscientious 26-year-old accountant who did nothing but go to work and clean his efficiency apartment. He had been employed by the same firm for the past 3 years. Although he had no friends in the company, his boss valued him because his work was accurate and on time and he was always willing to work overtime during tax season. Two months ago the owner of the firm announced they would be moving to another, less expensive office building. Henry was assigned a new office without a window (which he had in his previous office) because it was assumed he would not mind. After 1 week of working in his new office, Henry became psychotic and was admitted to the local hospital.

Value–belief

Because of their thought disorder, clients are often perplexed about their existence, its meaning, and its goal. It is not unusual for a client to state being simultaneously "at one with the universe but all alone in this world."

Nursing diagnosis

As with all nursing diagnoses, the nursing diagnoses for the individual with a thought disorder are based on the themes identified during the assessment phase of the nursing process.

Accepted NANDA* nursing diagnoses that may be specifically applicable to the individual with a thought disorder include:
Altered health maintenance
Ineffective management of therapeutic regimen
Noncompliance with medication regimen
High risk for infection
High risk for injury
Altered nutrition: high risk for more than body requirements
Altered nutrition: less than body requirements
Activity intolerance
Self-care deficit, bathing/hygiene; dressing/ grooming; feeding; toileting
Diversional activity deficit
Impaired home maintenance management
Sleep pattern disturbance
Pain
Chronic pain
Sensory/perceptual alteration (specify) (visual, auditory, kinesthetic, gustatory, tactile, olfactory)
Knowledge deficit (specify)
Altered thought processes
Decisional conflict (specify)
Fear
Anxiety
Hopelessness
Powerlessness
Body image disturbance
Personal identity disturbance
Self-esteem disturbance; situational low self-esteem; chronic low self-esteem
Altered role performance
Social isolation
Impaired social interaction

---

*North American Nursing Diagnosis Association.

Altered family processes

Impaired verbal communication

High risk for violence: self-directed or directed at others

Sexual dysfunction

Ineffective individual coping

Spiritual distress

To develop a nursing diagnosis that fulfills its function of providing direction for planning nursing care, the nurse is encouraged to postulate and state etiological or antecedent factors and connect the two phrases by using the term "related to." For example:

Social isolation related to suspicion of others

Planning and implementing nursing care

The plan for nursing care is derived from the nursing diagnoses and includes the objectives of the care, the nursing interventions, and outcome criteria. To be effective, the plan needs to be highly individualized. The suggestions that follow should be seen as general guidelines to be used if they are appropriate to the client's needs. All too often clients are required to conform to the dictates of a standardized nursing care plan rather than receiving care specifically designed for them.

In general, the objectives of all nursing care for the individual with a thought disorder should relate to helping the person to increase functional adaptations to reality, particularly in regard to activities of daily living; decrease dysfunctional adaptations, particularly in regard to the tendency to withdraw; and learn to identify and avoid those stressors that are particularly noxious to the individual.

Since the client's nursing diagnoses are often interrelated, stemming as they do from similar etiologies or antecedents, the student should see that appropriate nursing interventions are also interrelated. In other words, by intervening in one dimension, the nurse will also affect other dimensions.

Health perception–health management

The nurse has a major responsibility to monitor the intended effects, side effects, and adverse reactions of all medications prescribed for the client. In addition, clients with a thought disorder and their families have a right and a responsibility to know about and understand the illness and its treatment. This is particularly true in regard to medication. It is important for the nurse to provide **client and family teaching** regarding the name, dosage, intended effects, side effects, and adverse reactions to the medication. Most antipsychotic agents have troublesome side effects that may lead the client to stop taking them when the most distressing symptoms of the illness abate. Research has shown that along with lack of social support, discontinuing medication is a frequent reason for relapse and rehospitalization.

Side effects are not the only reason clients stop taking their medication. Lack of money and lack of understanding of the medication are other factors. For example, one client was not taught the name of his medication. Rather, he was taught to recognize it by color and shape. When he renewed his prescription a month later, he received a generic brand of the prescribed medication. Since the client did not recognize the pill, he did not take it, thereby following the instructions he had been given. Fortunately, this client kept his next clinic appointment, and the nurse was able to explain the reason for the difference in the pills. In addition, she wrote out the generic and brand names of the prescribed medication and encouraged the client to keep this paper in his wallet.

Persons who are withdrawn often are unaware of or do not report symptoms of physical illness; they may offer no complaints even when the condition is a painful one. The nurse must be constantly alert to clients' physical condition so that interventions can be appropriate and timely. In addition, the nurse should teach clients where they may receive appropriate health care in emergencies.

Nutritional-metabolic

Because of their thought disorder, many clients may be unable to plan and cook a meal, resulting in inadequate nutrition. It is perfectly appropriate for the nurse to initiate such plans by helping the client to prepare lists or by arranging to have food preparation and intake supervised by others. For an overactive individual, foods that are high in caloric and protein value, that require little preparation, and that can be eaten easily are to be encouraged. Milk shakes are an example of a food that meets these criteria. The nurse's interest in the client's food intake often enhances their relationship because of the symbolic link between food and security.

Activity-exercise

It is often necessary for the nurse to take the initiative in stimulating the client's interest in recreational activities. It is important to know something of the client's background so the nurse can initiate conversations in which the client can participate. When the client begins to trust the nurse, participation in some recreational activity can be encouraged. This may be accomplished by extending an invitation such as, "I need a partner for a game of table tennis; come and join me in a game." Initially, it may be best for the nurse to limit the activity to only the client invited. As the client develops more confidence, however, other participants should be added.

Some clients with a thought disorder may have difficulty in accomplishing even the most basic elements of self-care. Although it is important for the nurse to help the client take responsibility for personal hygiene and grooming, the nurse temporarily may have to assist the client with toileting, bathing, and dressing. The therapeutic value of a client being clean, well groomed, and appropriately and attractively dressed should not be underestimated, since this appearance is likely to elicit the deeply needed, positive reflected appraisals of others. Assisting the client with these basic activities also has the potential for initiating a positive relationship with the client and therefore should not be viewed as just one more task to be accomplished as quickly as possible.

Since most clients spend only a short time in the hospital, adequate and appropriate **discharge planning** becomes very important. Although the physician often makes the decision about when the client is ready for discharge and the social worker assumes primary responsibility for establishing referrals to community agencies, the nurse is an essential part of the treatment team in planning, implementing, and evaluating the discharge process. For example, the nurse should collaborate with the physician by sharing observations of the client's behavior over a 24-hour period as they determine the client's ability to function in the community. The nurse should collaborate with the social worker in learning where the client will be living and what skills the client needs to master in order to function effectively in this setting. With this knowledge, the nurse then can assist the client in learning these skills before they are needed. It is also important for the nurse to share with the treatment team an assessment of the client's self-care abilities. Finally, it is vital that the nurse, along with all other members of the treatment team, encourage and facilitate the active participation of the client and family in planning for discharge.

Sleep-rest

As more is learned about schizophrenia as a brain disease, accumulating research indicates that in the acute phase of the illness, the client benefits from sleep, rest, and a nonstimulating environment. However, as the acute symptoms of the illness are stabilized by antipsychotic agents, the same client may have to be encouraged to become involved with activities and other people and spend less time sleeping and resting. The goal is for the client to receive an optimum amount of sleep, which is often achieved by establishing a flexible schedule that takes into account the client's premorbid sleeping routine.

Cognitive-perceptual

Clients with a thought disorder always manifest impaired thought processes. When communicating verbally with the client, the nurse should avoid the use of long, involved sentences. Many persons with a thought disorder are easily confused and have a limited attention span. Short phrases are more effective and specific words more helpful than generalizations. For instance, *ice cream* is more meaningful than *dessert,* and *ham* is more specific and concrete than *meat.*

Many clients with a thought disorder experience hallucinations. Since these experiences are often frightening, the client may ask the nurse to confirm their existence. In such a situation, it is therapeutic to answer truthfully by saying, for example, "No, Mr. Jones, I do not see the face of Christ on the wall, although I understand that you do because of your illness." Such a reply simultaneously presents reality, avoids an argument, and reassures the client that the experience is a symptom of the illness.

Many clients also have delusions. When the client talks about delusions, it is not therapeutic for the nurse to try to explain them away or to argue about them. Such an approach will result in the client becoming increasingly adamant about these false beliefs and perhaps hostile and suspicious. If the nurse can appreciate the necessity of the delusion to preserving the client's fragile personality organization, the nurse will understand the futility of trying to change such ideas through logic. Generally, it is wise to listen to the client without commenting on the content of the delusions.

The nurse must avoid the temptation to exploit the negativism displayed by some clients. For example, the nurse may think it helpful to request the client to walk backward when the nurse wants the opposite action. Similarly, making use of delusional and hallucinatory content to direct the client's behavior should be avoided. If, for instance, the client believes that he hears the voice of his mother, the nurse may be tempted to say that his mother just told him to eat his lunch. These "techniques" are never therapeutic, since they diminish whatever trust the client may have in the nurse. Their use is also likely to increase the client's confusion and encourage withdrawal.

As already implied, clients and their families almost always have a knowledge deficit in regard to the illness and its treatment. More than any other member of the treatment team, the nurse has the responsibility to develop, implement, and evaluate a plan to address these knowledge deficits if the client can be expected to make an effective adjustment in the community.

Self-perception/self-concept

The development of a positive self-concept depends on positive reflected appraisals of significant others combined with the person's ability to test reality accurately. Because of their illness and subsequent behavior, persons with thought disorders are likely to have received negative reflected appraisals from significant others and be unable to test reality accurately. Therefore, they often have a poor self-concept and low self-esteem. Consequently, one of the most therapeutic interventions a nurse can implement is to develop a **nurse-client relationship** in which the nurse becomes a significant other. This is not always possible in the inpatient setting because of the short time the client is likely to be hospitalized. However, even in the hospital, the nurse can interact with the client in a consistent, accepting manner. In community-based treatment settings, the nurse often does have the opportunity to develop a nurse-client relationship and should take advantage of the opportunity to do so.

Although the nurse-client relationship is a vehicle through which many other interventions can be implemented successfully, it has value in and of itself, since it can provide a corrective emotional experience in which the client experiences, over time, the unconditional positive regard of another human being who communicates in a healthy functional way.

Meticulous honesty and fairness on the nurse's part are of primary importance when establishing and maintaining a relationship with a client who has a thought disorder. Once a promise is made, the nurse is obligated to carry it out. A response should be given to all the client's requests and questions. If the client makes a request that the nurse cannot comply with, a suitable answer is, "I am sorry, but I am not allowed to carry out such a procedure." If no answer is possible, the client should be informed that the question will be referred to an appropriate person who can give an answer or that the answer is truly not known.

Role-relationship

The client's inability to initiate and sustain satisfactory human contact is often characteristic of a thought disorder. Therefore, interpersonal experiences must be planned for and provided. However, the client's consistent affective indifference or emotional impoverishment may make it difficult for the nurse to express warmth and demonstrate spontaneous interest in the client. It is often possible to achieve this warmth and interest if the nurse understands that the client feels lonely, isolated, and hungry for human contact but is often incapable of inviting a friendly approach from another person. Only when the nurse approaches the individual with an accepting attitude and with friendliness can the nurse be a source of therapeutic help.

The nurse is often in a position to help clients develop social skills by assisting them to participate in small group activities with others. This is a particularly effective intervention when the focus of the group is a topic or a task in which the client has some interest and ability. Not only can small group activities help clients develop social relationships, but they also can be a vehicle to learn needed knowledge and skills and receive positive feedback about their achievements. The many objectives that can be achieved simultaneously through small group activities are the reason this intervention is employed so often in both hospital and community treatment settings.

Just as clients need help in developing **social support,** families of clients also need such assistance. The nurse can and should be instrumental in developing a relationship with the client's family, teaching them about the client's illness, and referring them to lay support groups such as the local chapter of the Alliance for the Mentally Ill.

The physical and emotional safety of clients should always be of paramount concern. During the acute phase of the illness the client may lash out at others, either physically or verbally. This behavior almost always stems from distortions of reality caused by the illness that result in the client becoming very frightened. It is important for the nurse to learn to recognize behaviors that indicate the client is losing control and to intervene at that point to try to prevent assaultive behavior. For example, the client who repetitively approaches the nurses' station to ask what time it is may be behaviorally asking for the nurse to pay attention. The nurse who responds to this behavior in a caring, concerned way and takes the time to explore with the client why he or she is worried about the time may be able to avert an assaultive act.

Because not all instances of assaultive behavior can be prevented, the nurse needs to know the policies of the institution and the state laws governing interventions such as seclusion and restraint. In addition, the nurse and other staff need to be adept at placing clients in restraints or seclusion should these actions be necessary. When staff members are not skilled at these procedures, their anxiety is communicated to the client and contributes to the client's fear, thereby worsening the situation. In addition, staff members who are not skilled at physically restraining clients are more likely to inadvertently injure the client and themselves during the procedure.

Clients who have recovered from the acute phase of their illness sometimes have developed enough insight into their disorder to realize that it is a chronic illness. This realization, in turn, might depress them and lead to thoughts of suicide. The nurse needs to be very vigilant in observing for changes in behavior that may indicate suicidal thoughts. One young man who had been ill for many years killed himself by jumping off the roof of his apartment house. At the psychological autopsy, his parents reported that their son had never been as cheerful or functional as he had been in the 2 weeks before his suicide. Although it is understandable that lay persons would not be concerned about positive changes in behavior, the nurse and other mental health professionals must understand that abrupt, dramatic changes in behavior, even positive changes, are often signals of suicidal ideas and should be investigated.

Sexuality-reproductive

A common side effect of the phenothiazine antipsychotic medications is a decrease in libido that may result in impotence in men. For some clients, especially young males, this side effect can be very distressing and serve as an assault on an already fragile self-concept. The client needs to be taught that this symptom is related to the medication and not to his masculinity. Further, the nurse should work with the physician in decreasing the dosage of the medication to the lowest effective level so that this and other side effects can be minimized.

It is important for all people to understand the necessity for monogamous sexual relationships and the use of condoms when having sex to minimize the risk of contracting blood-borne pathogens such as human immunodeficiency virus (HIV) and hepatitis B. It is imperative for the nurse to teach individuals with thought disorders about how to protect themselves from these

pathogens, since they are sometimes not capable of using the best judgment in selecting sexual partners. At worst, they can be sexually victimized by others who take advantage of their poor judgment.

Coping–stress tolerance

Although stress is not believed to cause schizophrenia, it has been demonstrated that an inability to cope with stress leads to relapse. Therefore the nurse has an important role in helping the client to identify situations that cause stress and to learn how to cope with or avoid

---

KEY INTERVENTIONS FOR CLIENTS WITH THOUGHT DISORDERS

Teach clients and their families about the illness and its treatment.
Encourage and facilitate compliance with the treatment regimen.
Observe client carefully for symptoms related to medication and to unreported physical illness.
Assist client to secure adequate nutritional intake.
Stimulate client's interest in recreational activities.
Assist with and teach self-care.
Actively participate in discharge planning with other treatment team members, including the client and family.
Help client develop a flexible schedule to achieve optimum sleep.
Communicate effectively by using short phrases and specific, concrete words.
Assure clients who are hallucinating that this experience is a symptom of their illness.
Do not argue with clients who talk about their delusions.
When possible, develop a nurse-client relationship.
Assist clients to participate in relevant small group activities.
Ensure the safety of clients.
Teach clients how to decrease their risk of contracting blood-borne pathogens during sexual activity.
Help clients identify situations that cause stress and assist them to learn how to cope with or avoid them.
Encourage and facilitate involvement with religious groups when beneficial to the client; help the client to avoid exploitation.

them. A common example is large family gatherings such as during the holiday season. Often the lack of structure and unpredictability of the situation, the noise of many people talking, and the well-meaning attempts of some to include the client in conversation combine to provide more interpersonal stimulation than the client can handle. If this type of situation causes stress, the nurse can help the client practice appropriate social responses to questions and comments and means by which to excuse oneself appropriately from the activities.

Value-belief

Many persons with thought disorders derive great comfort from becoming involved with religious groups whose beliefs provide hope for the future. In addition to finding the group's beliefs helpful, clients undoubtedly benefit from a sense of belonging to a group where they feel accepted. The nurse should encourage and facilitate such involvement. Unfortunately, however, clients with thought disorders can also be exploited by others who capitalize on their need to explain their existence. The nurse can be helpful in assisting clients to "reality test" the benefits they are receiving against what they are giving. At the very least, clients in such a situation should be encouraged to seek legal advice if they are requested by any group to contribute their paycheck or otherwise sign away any belongings.

NURSING CARE PLAN: *An Individual with a Severe Thought Disorder*

CASE FORMULATION

Frances B. was 19 years of age when she was admitted to a psychiatric hospital. The only child of missionary parents, she was born in a mission station in Africa. Her father was a quiet-spoken man who was rigidly consistent in the practice of his religion. Her mother was more practical and tolerant but was frightened by her husband's anger whenever she deviated from the practices he deemed right. They were very busy with the work of the mission and had little time to spend with their daughter.

During the first 5 years of her life, Frances's only playmates were native children. She reportedly had always displayed an attitude of superiority toward them. On entering a church-supported boarding school in the United States at age 5, she had difficulty with her classmates. She was inclined to be too critical of them and insisted

on lecturing them about personal matters. When she was 12 years old, she had a long siege of pneumonia, after which she lost weight and was chronically anemic and undernourished. She spent many hours in prayer and wrote endless letters to her parents, most of them consisting of long quotations from the Bible. She insisted on wearing old, worn clothing to school and bitterly criticized her classmates for not doing likewise.

Although her parents returned to the United States on furlough every year, they could spend only a few days with Frances because they had many church meetings to attend.

Frances's social behavior improved somewhat during high school in that she no longer offended her classmates. However, she made few friends. She adopted a stray dog

Continued.

NURSING CARE PLAN: *An Individual with a Severe Thought Disorder—cont'd*

to which she was greatly attached and spent most of her free time taking long walks with it. She showed a preference for mathematics and biblical history.

Frances began the freshman year of college about 11 months before her admission to the hospital. Although her grades in college were good, she had a reputation for being a strange girl who avoided others, smiled a great deal to herself, and showed no interest in the opposite sex. Her parents, while on furlough from Africa, visited her during the Christmas holidays, and her mother expressed fear that she was not emotionally well. Frances displayed little interest in her parents' visit, despite not having seen them for more than a year.

During the commencement activities that spring, Frances disappeared from the campus for several days; later it was learned that she had spent that time at an evangelical camp meeting. She remained on the campus during the summer months to take some advanced courses in mathematics. During this time she roomed with two other young women. Her roommates were in the habit of discussing their love interests in Frances's presence, and she suddenly displayed an unusual interest in their conversations. Among other things, she inquired about various matters of sex and how to approach boys. A few nights later she told one of the girls that she saw the face of her future husband in the light fixture. She scrutinized the fixture for several hours, during which she sat in a trancelike state with a smile on her face. Early the next morning she spoke to a 13-year-old newsboy and informed him that she

would marry him. When he made light of her statement, she became upset, struck him in the face, and chased him down the street. Returning to her room, she tore out the light fixture, removed her clothing, and became unmanageable.

On being admitted to the psychiatric hospital, she refused to answer questions. She smiled to herself and identified the admitting physcican as "Herbert." She insisted on having the window opened because "they are playing the wedding march." Her speech was incoherent; she was hallucinating and stated that she was hearing voices that questioned her moral standards.

For the first few days after hospitalization, Frances talked at length about a fantasized courtship in which she was the central character. She carried on a dialogue, at one time representing the lover, at another time the maiden. After this she entered a long period of silence, during which she was mute and resistive and refused food. Occasionally she said, "If thy eye offend thee, cut it out." One evening she almost succeeded in enucleating her right eye with the thumb and forefinger of her right hand. She continued to talk incoherently, laughed a great deal, and made little attempt to keep herself clean.

Nursing Assessment

The history of Frances's life experiences reveals little information about her as a child. We do know that her father was perceived as an authoritarian individual who placed the welfare of the mission above all else. It is quite possible that even as an infant, Frances's care was relegated to employed

NURSING CARE PLAN: *An Individual with a Severe Thought Disorder—cont'd*

native women who may not have remained in the household consistently. In the development of a sense of personal security, the first 5 years of a child's life are crucial. The type of mothering person by whom the child is nurtured is of the greatest importance, especially in developing a sense of trust.

At age 5 Frances was sent to a boarding school. Although this was probably the best plan her parents could develop, it was apparently not helpful to Frances. Authorities believe that this period in a child's life is of great significance in the scheme of psychosexual development. During this period the child is beginning to identify with the parent of the same sex, has discovered that the sexual organ is a source of pleasurable sensations, and has recognized the structural difference between the genitalia of boys and girls. When a child in this age period is removed from the parents, he or she is apt to feel banished as a punishement for some transgression. Since sexual longings and fantasies have occupied some of the child's thoughts and since the child realizes that these are frowned on by the parents, it is natural for the child to feel that the banishment is related to "bad" thoughts.

Frances undoubtedly felt banished by being sent to boarding school. It is possible that Frances believed that she was being punished. Even when parents are not a source of comfort and security for a child, the child mourns their loss when separated from them because they are the only significant reality known. Thus it is reasonable to believe that Frances passed through a period of loneliness and bereavement at being de-

prived from the only mothering person she knew.

Initially, children protest this separation by crying or by other aggressive acting-out behavior. After several days of hopelessness and withdrawal from activity, the child usually becomes detached and seems unwilling to resume a close relationship with any adult, even if the lost person returns. This detached attitude could be altered if the parent returned and remained with the child consistently. However, Frances undoubtedly developed a detached attitude toward other people and attempted to isolate herself personally to avoid anxiety resulting from fear of being cast aside and abandoned a second time. Her subsequent attachment to a dog suggested that she could not trust another person with her love and therefore gave it to an animal who made no demands and gave her unconditional devotion.

After Frances had a serious illness at age 12, she began to spend long hours in prayer, wrote letters to her parents filled with quotes from the Bible, and wore her shoddiest clothing to school. This behavior suggests that she was seeking to gain the favor and forgiveness of her parents. Perhaps she felt unworthy of anything better when she chose to wear old, shoddy clothing to school and again was seeking to atone for fantasized sin.

Her interest in the sexual affairs of other girls of her age and the inappropriate proposal of marriage may have indicated the inability of Frances's ego to develop an effective adaptation to the stressors of adolescence. She obviously had a limited capacity to evaluate clearly the realities of the situa-

Continued.

NURSING CARE PLAN: *An Individual with a Severe Thought Disorder—cont'd*

tion in which she found herself. In addition, she was not able to repress hostile aggressive drives effectively and expressed these feelings freely by tearing out the light fixture.

When Frances saw the face of her future husband in the light fixture, she was exhibiting a severe mental symptom called visual hallucinations. Hallucinations are one example of the symptoms experienced by individuals with an active psychosis.

They are an example of being out of touch with reality. The person experiencing hallucinations is reacting to an internal stimulus that is unrelated to the real situation. This person's behavior becomes extremely confusing when the person reacts part of the time to external stimuli and part of the time to internal stimuli.

Nursing Diagnosis

The assessment data, including present behavior, past life experiences, and an understanding of the underlying dynamics, led to the development of the following nursing diagnoses for Frances:

Impaired social interaction related to fear of abandonment

Sensory/perceptual alteration (visual) related to hallucinations.

Self-care deficit, dressing/grooming, related to feelings of worthlessness

Self-care deficit, feeding, related to feelings of worthlessness

Planning and Implementing Nursing Care

The boxed material on pp. 268 and 269 is a sample nursing care plan designed for Frances. Because this client was so acutely ill on admission, all the objectives are short term.

The logical starting point in carrying out the plan was the establishment of a positive relationship with Frances. It was hoped that this relationship would lead to the development of some communication with her.

Because the nurse knew that persons with thought disturbances are highly fearful of rejection, the approach to Frances was unhurried, warm, friendly, and accepting. The nurse found it necessary to make repeated verbal overtures and to modify her own nonverbal messages to Frances before Frances was able to respond.

It was decided that the entire responsibility for the nursing care of Frances during the first weeks of her hospital experience would be assigned to a few carefully chosen nurses. This decision was made because the staff recognized that Frances needed to develop a feeling of security and to learn to trust other people. Security can be enhanced by limiting the number of individuals with whom such ill persons come in contact and by keeping their daily routines much the same for several months. In the beginning, few demands were made on Frances.

It is recognized that the attitude of the people with whom persons with a mental illness come in contact during the early part of their illness has a significant effect on their recovery. Persons such as Frances require consistent acceptance, sincere interest, and constant encouragement from nurses and the other members of the professional staff.

Although communication with Frances was difficult because she used language in a highly personal way, it was important for the

NURSING CARE PLAN: *An Individual with a Severe Thought Disorder—cont'd*

nurse to spend time sitting with her and talking to her even though she rarely responded verbally. The nurse used simple, uncomplicated, direct statements when talking to her.

These nursing interventions were related to the plan for development of a satisfactory relationship with a significant other, which would in turn decrease Frances's fears of abandonment. In addition, much of her behavior was symptomatic of an individual who felt unworthy and guilty, and Frances's self-esteem obviously was badly shattered. Thus the nurse's efforts were focused on trying to assist Frances to develop a more positive attitude toward herself. This was partially achieved by the attention provided for her and the sincere, interested way in which it was given. Self-esteem was also enhanced through the mechanism of assisting her to improve her grooming.

Early in Frances's hospital experience, a nurse needed to assume much responsibility for bathing and dressing her, but in time Frances was encouraged to assume more and more responsibility for this activity herself. The nurses gently suggested that she would enjoy visiting the beauty parlor. At first they accompanied her on these trips and remained with her while she was there.

The dietary intake for persons who refuse food is always of great concern. Because Frances regressed when she was first admitted, the nurses tried to help her in feeding herself by making suggestions such as, "Pick up your fork" and "Put the food in your mouth." This plan was used because it was thought that she was unable to make the necessary decisions herself. However, it was eventually necessary to spoon-feed her. The nurses used an unhurried, relaxed manner and fed her from a tray in her own room.

During the spoon-feeding periods the nurses gave Frances many opportunities to take the spoon in her own hand and assume some of the responsibility for feeding herself during a part of the meal. After a few weeks she was encouraged to return to the dining room and take her meals with others.

The problem of self-destruction was especially distressing. Criticism and reprimands for this behavior were withheld because the nurses realized that it would confirm Frances's opinion that she was indeed a bad person. The close personal attention Frances received when she was first admitted solved the problem of self-destruction during the early part of her hospitalization. However, she was helped to reestablish her own inner controls, and the nurse served as an external authority until Frances was able to accept responsibility for her own safety.

Evaluation

Evaluation of the plan of nursing care and its implementation was based on outcome criteria established at the time the plan was formulated. Since the nurse knew that Frances's illness had developed slowly and insidiously, the outcome criteria the nurse established reflected the expectation of small but significant gains. The nurse continuously reassessed the client as she provided care. As anticipated, after 2 weeks Frances was able to accept most of the responsibility for her own grooming and ate in the dining room with the other clients. In addition, days elapsed without any evidence

Continued.

NURSING CARE PLAN: *An Individual with a Severe Thought Disorder—cont'd*

of hallucinations, and her self-destructive behavior had stopped.

After 1 month Frances showed little evidence of accepting her assigned nurse as a significant other. Although she did call the nurse by name and seemed to recognize her at most times, she rarely appeared for their meetings at the agreed time. Frances's nurse was discouraged about this and arranged to have the nursing care plan reviewed at a team meeting. In view of this client's history with significant others and her progress in other areas, the team believed that the nurse's outcome criteria for this diagnosis were unrealistic in terms of time. As a result, the nurse revised this aspect of the care plan

to indicate a 6-week time frame.

After 6 weeks, Frances's behavior did indicate a beginning level of trust in her assigned nurse. At that time the nurse reassessed the client's condition, developed revised nursing diagnoses, and designed a new plan of care that indicated long-term goals. She was careful to develop outcome criteria that were realistic in light of Frances's lifetime of dysfunctional adaptation. It was anticipated that Frances could be expected to recover sufficiently to be discharged to a sheltered living situation, but she probably would require a maintenance dose of the prescribed antipsychotic medication.

NURSING CARE PLAN FOR FRANCES B.

Nursing diagnosis	Objective (rationale)	Nursing interventions	Outcome criteria
Impaired social interaction related to fear of abandonment	Client will trust another human being. (Development of trust in at least one other human being is a prerequisite to experiencing a sense of security and overcoming a fear of abandonment, leading to increased social interaction.)	Assigned nurse establishes relationship with client. Approach client in a calm, friendly manner. Orient client to purpose and structure of relationship. Determine times and places for meeting three times a day for 20 minutes. Convey consistent acceptance of client as an individual who has value and worth. Use simple, direct statements when talking with client.	Within 1 month, client: Calls nurse by name. Shows evidence of beginning trust in assigned nurse by appearing for meetings on time.

NURSING CARE PLAN FOR FRANCES B.—cont'd

Nursing diagnosis	Objective (rationale)	Nursing interventions	Outcome criteria
Sensory/perceptual alteration (visual) related to hallucinations	Frequency of hallucinations will diminish. (Decreased frequency of hallucinations indicates increased contact with reality.)	Sit silently with client if she is hallucinating. Administer antipsychotic medication as prescribed. Observe for side effects and adverse reactions to medications. Reassure client about side effects. Record medications given. Observe for and record changes in behavior indicative of hallucinations.	Within 2 weeks, client manifests behavior indicative of hallucinations only when exposed to numerous external stimuli, such as two persons talking to her at same time.
	Client will not engage in self-destructive acts. (Self-destructive acts are not only physically injurious but also indicate dysfunctional adaptations.)	Restrain client as necessary. Do *not* reprimand client if she attempts to injure self.	Within 2 weeks, client does not attempt to injure self.
Self-care deficit, dressing/grooming, related to feelings of worthlessness	Client will assume responsibility for bathing and dressing appropriately. (An ability to engage in self-care activities is essential to feeling competent to function in the community.)	Establish and implement routine for bathing and dressing. Bathe client as necessary. Dress client as necessary. Encourage client to assist with bathing and dressing.	Within 2 weeks, client shows interest in activities of bathing and dressing, as manifested by such statements as "I'll wash my own face."
Self-care deficit, feeding, related to feelings of worthlessness	Client will be adequately nourished. (Adequate nutrition is essential to physiological homeokinesis.)	Ascertain and serve, if possible, client's favorite foods. Present food in small amounts. Help client eat by providing simple directions. Spoon-feed if necessary. Allow client to eat at her own pace. Record amount eaten. Encourage client to go to dining room, and accompany if she indicates desire to go.	Within 2 weeks client eats 1800 calories among three well-balanced meals in the dining room.

KEY POINTS

1. Schizophrenia is one of the most serious forms of mental illness.

2. The symptoms of schizophrenia are often classified as either positive or negative. Positive symptoms reflect the presence of unusual behavior; negative symptoms reflect the absence of behavior normally expected.

3. Common symptoms of schizophrenia include delusions, loosening of associations, hallucinations, a blunt or flat affect, a poorly defined sense of self, disturbance in volition, ambivalence, withdrawal, and abnormal psychomotor activity. Because of the variety of symptoms associated with schizophrenia as well as other factors, many authorities believe research will demonstrate that schizophrenia is actually several different, although related, illnesses.

4. The precise cause of schizophrenia is not known. It is currently believed that this illness is an outcome of complex interactions of multiple biological and psychosocial factors. Awareness of the etiological complexity of schizophrenia is a relatively new phenomenon.

5. The major medical treatment for persons with schizophrenia is the use of antipsychotic medications.

6. Nursing interventions need to be individualized and based on the client's nursing diagnoses. Interventions frequently indicated include:

    Teaching the client and family about the illness and its treatment

    Closely monitoring the client's reaction to the prescribed medication

    Assisting with and teaching self-care

    Actively participating in discharge planning

    Developing a nurse-client relationship

    Encouraging and assisting clients to participate in relevant small group activities

    Ensuring the client's safety

    Helping clients to identify and cope with or avoid stressful situations

SUGGESTED SOURCES OF ADDITIONAL INFORMATION

Arieti S: *Understanding and helping the schizophrenic,* New York, 1980, Basic Books.

Baker AF: Living with a chronically ill schizophrenic can place great stress on individual family members and the family unit: how families cope, *J Psychosoc Nurs* 27(1):31, 1989.

Bellack A, Mueser K: A comprehensive treatment program for schizophrenia and chronic mental illness, *Community Ment Health J* 22:175, Fall 1986.

Breier A and others: National Institute of Mental Health longitudinal study of chronic schizophrenia, *Arch Gen Psychiatry* 48:239, March 1991.

Breslin NA: Treatment of schizophrenia: current practice and future promise, *Hosp Community Psychiatry* 43:877, September 1992.

Brooker C: The health education needs of families caring for a schizophrenic relative and the potential role for community psychiatric nurses, *J Adv Nurs* 13:1092, 1990.

Davidhizar R, McBride A: Teaching the client with schizophrenia about medication, *Patient Educ Counseling* 7:137, 1985.

Davis KL and others: Dopamine in schizophrenia: a review and reconceptualization, *Am J Psychiatry* 148:1474, November 1991.

Fenton WS, McGlashan TH: Natural history of schizophrenia subtypes, *Arch Gen Psychiatry* 48:978, November 1991.

Garza-Trevino ES and others: Neurobiology of schizophrenic syndromes, *Hosp Community Psychiatry* 41:971, September 1990.

Gerace L: Schizophrenia and the family: nursing implications, *Arch Psychiatr Nurs* 2:141, June 1988.

Hamera E and others: Patient self-regulation and functioning in schizophrenia, *Hosp Community Psychiatry* 42:630, June 1991.

Hamera E and others: Symptom monitoring in schizophrenia: potential for enhancing self-care, *Arch Psychiatr Nurs* 6:324, December 1992.

Kahn ME, White EM: Adapting milieu approaches to acute inpatient care for schizophrenic patients, *Hosp Community Psychiatry* 40:609, June 1989.

Lebrun LJ and others: Schizophrenic outpatient education, *Can Nurse* 87(5):25, 1991.

Lefley HP: Expressed emotion: conceptual, clinical, and social policy issues, *Hosp Community Psychiatry* 43:591, June 1992.

Lucas M: Understanding schizophrenia, *RN* 52, October 1990.

McEnany GW: Psychobiology and psychiatric nursing: a philosophical matrix, *Arch Psychiatr Nurs* 5:255, October 1991.

Middlemiss MA, Beeber LS: Update on psychopharmacology: issues in the use of depot antipsychotics, *J Psychosoc Nurs* 27:36, June 1989.

Mulaik JS: Noncompliance with medication regimens in severely and persistently mentally ill schizophrenic patients, *Issues Ment Health Nurs* 13:219, 1992.

O'Connor FW: Symptom monitoring for relapse prevention in schizophrenia, *Arch Psychiatr Nurs* 5:193, August 1991.

Olfson M and others: Inpatient treatment of schizophrenia in general hospitals, *Hosp Community Psychiatry* 44:40, January 1993.

Plante TG: Social skills training: a program to help schizophrenic clients cope, *J Psychosoc Nurs* 27:6, March 1989.

Rosenthal TT, McGuinness TM: Dealing with delusional patients: discovering the distorted truth, *Issues Ment Health Nurs* 8:143, 1986.

Seymour R, Dawson N: The schizophrenic at home, *J Psychosoc Nurs* 26:28, January 1986.

Simpson RBC: Expressed emotion and nursing the schizophrenic patient, *J Adv Nurs* 14:459, 1989.

Sulliger N: Relapse, *J Psychosoc Nurs* 26:20, June 1988.

Sullivan HS: *Conceptions of modern psychiatry,* New York, 1953, Norton.

Thompson LW: The dopamine hypothesis of schizophrenia, *Perspect Psychiatr Care* 26(3):18, 1990.

Torrey EF: Management of chronic schizophrenic outpatients, *Psychiatr Clin* 9(1):143, 1986.

Williams CA: Patient education for people with schizophrenia, *Perspect Psychiatr Care* 25(2):14, 1989.

Williams CA: Perspectives on the hallucinatory process, *Issues Ment Health Nurs* 10:99, 1989.

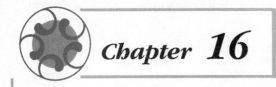

Chapter 16

Individuals with Mood Disorders

LEARNING OBJECTIVES

After studying this chapter, the student will be able to:

- Describe the symptoms exhibited by a person with the medical diagnosis of a mood disorder.
- Differentiate between the emotion of grief and the mood of depression.
- Discuss the causative factors associated with mood disorders.
- State the desired effects, side effects, and adverse effects of antidepressant medications, lithium carbonate, and electroconvulsive therapy.

- Describe behaviors the nurse is most likely to observe in an individual who is depressed.
- State examples of nursing diagnoses likely to be applicable to an individual who is depressed.
- State and explain nursing interventions likely to be effective with an individual who is depressed.
- Develop a hypothetical plan of nursing care for an individual who is depressed.
- Describe behaviors the nurse is most likely to observe in an individual who is elated and overactive.
- State examples of nursing diagnoses likely to be applicable to an individual who is elated and overactive.
- State and explain nursing interventions likely to be effective with an individual who is elated and overactive.
- Develop a hypothetical plan of nursing care for an individual who is elated and overactive.

KEY TERMS

Mood disorders
Electroconvulsive therapy
Depressive disorders
Bipolar disorders
Grief
Depression
Catecholamine hypothesis
Neuroendocrinology
Hypertensive crisis
Parnate-cheese reaction

All human beings are familiar with the emotions of joy and sadness. Healthy adults experience these emotions in a predictable way, usually in response to an external stimulus. For example, graduating from college or achieving a promotion may cause great joy, whereas the death of a parent may precipitate sadness. These emotions are experienced by healthy adults to an extent and for a length of time appropriate to the situation. In contrast, individuals with **mood disorders** experience a great depth of joy or sadness, seemingly unrelated to external stimuli, and for a long period. Furthermore, these emotions pervade the person's entire being and may fluctuate widely from one to another.

There is great concern in the United States about the increasing number of adults who experience mood disorders. Of particular concern is the incidence of depression, which has been accelerating rapidly since the 1970s and shows no sign of abating. A recent study by the National Institute of Mental Health indicates that 6% of the U.S. population experiences depression during any 6-month period. Middle-aged females and elderly persons of both sexes are particularly vulnerable to severe depression.

Mood disorders seriously interfere with the quality of life enjoyed by the affected person and the family. In addition, depression increases the risk of death by suicide. Nurses in all settings have a responsibility to recognize and appropriately intervene in situations where the individual is experiencing a mood disorder.

HISTORICAL PERSPECTIVE

Mood disorders, especially depression, have been documented since ancient times. An Egyptian papyrus of 1500 BC contains a discourse on old age and says of it that "the heart grows heavy and remembers not yesterday." The Old Testament records the erratic behavior of King Saul as his moods fluctuated between elation and depression. If he were alive today, this influential person would undoubtedly bear the medical diagnosis of bipolar disorder.

In 1896 Emil Kraepelin identified the illness known today as bipolar disorder and called it manic-depressive psychosis. He was among the first to recognize the cyclical nature of this disorder.

Hippocrates (460-375? BC), the greatest of the old Greek physicians, knew the symptoms of depression well and believed it resulted from a surplus of black bile, which is termed *melancholē* in the Greek language. The English word *melancholy* is derived from this Greek word.

Treatment of mood disorders was not effective until the development of the convulsion-producing drug pentylenetetrazol (Metrazol) by Meduna, followed by the introduction of **electroconvulsive therapy** by Cerletti and Bini in 1938. Electroconvulsive therapy was first developed as a treatment for persons with thought disorders; however, it has been found to be most effective for persons with depression. Although still in use today, electroconvulsive therapy (electrotherapy) has been supplanted as the primary treatment for mood disorders by the psychotropic agents, specifically the antidepressant medications and lithium carbonate.

MOOD DISORDERS

Mood disorders are subdivided into the medical diagnoses of **depressive disorders** and **bipolar disorders.**

Individuals medically diagnosed as having a depressive disorder experience an all-pervasive depressed mood or loss of interest or pleasure in all, or almost all, activities for at least 2 weeks. Associated symptoms include appetite disturbance, resultant change in weight, sleep disturbance, psychomotor agitation or retardation, decreased energy, feelings of worthlessness and guilt, difficulty thinking or concentrating, and recurrent thoughts of death.

To be medically diagnosed as having a bipolar disorder, the individual must have a history of one or more manic episodes, usually with a history of episodes of major depression. During manic episodes, the elated mood may be so pronounced and sustained that the individual expresses the belief that every good thing is possible or will soon be consummated and every wish will be fulfilled. Ideas emerge in an easy, fluid manner; thinking seems to be effortless; memory is quickened; and the individual shows a quick but superficial wit. The person has an apparent sense of self-security, and fears are pushed to the background. The individual may be aggressive, opinionated, and ready to talk with conviction on anything and everything. Ideas pour out so rapidly and with such ease that the tongue cannot give them full expression. Thus the individual may utter only segments of ideas and may jump from one to another in a rapid barrage. The person is hyperalert and has a tendency to argue. The person is apt to be domineering and becomes irritable, denunciatory, and hypercritical of everything that interferes with the desire for free action. The individual is likely to become overactive and to have a decreased need for sleep. When limits must be set for behavior, the person sometimes becomes noisy, belligerent, and violent. Insight is always poor. This person's interest is in the outside world rather than in the self. Ideation is concerned with the environment. In fact, the individual can almost be said to be at the mercy of the environment.

Surprising as it may seem, at another time such an aggressive, overactive individual may exhibit quite different behavior. Within a few months the person may be sad, may have difficulty in thinking and expressing thoughts, and may be very slow in physical responses, or the individual may exhibit agitation. Such a person may have difficulty in formulating answers, may lose the ability to concentrate, and may be unable to choose a direct line of action. The individual may be tormented by a sense of insecurity or by ideas of remorse and self-abasement or may be overcome by a sense of guilt. The person may complain of a total lack of affection and of a loss of interest in the things for which he or she formerly had much concern. The individual may feel that he or she is lost or being punished. Such a person may have an overpowering sense of futility, a "feeling of emptiness," and a desire to retreat from everything, to seek oblivion, and to end life. The danger of suicide is the outstanding feature of this condition, and this alone justifies the greatest caution and consideration in care and treatment.

The probability of recovery from a single episode of overactivity or depression is great. Recurrences are to be expected, although second and third attacks need not necessarily occur. An attack of overactivity in early adult life generally means more attacks later. Depressions are most likely to occur in the later years of life.

It is never safe to predict the probable duration of any given attack. Great variations exist, and even the same individual may have both short and long periods of elation and depression. The average length for all untreated attacks of elation is about 6 months; for untreated depressive episodes it is generally longer. When depressive periods show a strong element of fear, anxiety, and hypochondriasis, the condition may endure for many years. Likewise, elation may become chronic, particularly in older individuals, if it is associated with organic changes in the brain such as arteriosclerosis. Current treatments, including maintenance levels of lithium carbonate as a preventive measure, have shortened the length of attacks in both elation and depression.

An outstanding feature of mood disorders is that even after repeated attacks, intellectual capacities are rarely impaired. During remissions of this disorder, individuals are usually able to carry on their regular occupation and live an entirely normal life.

Although a bipolar disorder is a common type of mood disorder, some individuals have severe mood disturbances that do not meet the criteria for this diagnosis. However, the principles stated in the following discussion are applicable to all individuals with mood disturbances, regardless of their medical diagnosis.

DIFFERENTIATION BETWEEN THOUGHT DISORDERS AND MOOD DISORDERS

It is sometimes difficult for students of nursing to differentiate between the overactivity demonstrated by one individual with thought disorders and the overactivity that the manic individual exhibits. Both these individuals may be physically overactive, and at times both may talk excessively. The individual who exhibits catatonic behavior may fluctuate from being almost stuporous to exhibiting explosive overactivity. In such a situation the individual is probably responding to inner thoughts and feelings that are not related to reality but that are threatening, upsetting, and disturbing. This type of overactivity is especially difficult to understand because disharmony often exists between the mood and the ideas expressed. The person may smile inappropriately or laugh while speaking of the disturbing thoughts that are uppermost in the mind. The person may experience terrifying visual or auditory hallucinations.

In contrast, the overactivity of an individual displaying manic behavior is characterized by glib, argumentative speech that may be humorous but may change quickly to sarcasm and verbal abuse. Such a person may appear to have boundless energy. The individual is usually irrepressible, demanding, and irritable. The person frequently expresses ideas of grandeur and delusions of having great power and wealth. There is a dominant tone of euphoria even though the person may demonstrate an underlying mood of sorrow. Some authorities believe that the overactivity of the manic individual is actually a defense against depression. The professional person usually finds that manic overactivity can be understood because the client main-

tains some contact with reality except in the most extreme examples of this illness.

Withdrawal and depression may be difficult for the beginning student of nursing to differentiate because individuals affected by these states are usually physically inactive. However, the individual with a thought disturbance who is withdrawn demonstrates a disharmony of thought, feeling, and behavior. Although there may be a persistent mood, it has little apparent relationship to the situation in which persons find themselves or to their past experiences. In contrast, everything about the depressed individual conveys this feeling to the observer. The way the person sits, the facial expression, the voice quality, and the ideas expressed all suggest hopelessness and a sense of impending doom. Depressed individuals remain well aware of reality, and their feelings seem understandable to individuals working with them.

Some authorities believe that the attempt to differentiate these behavioral reactions is actually an artificial and unwarranted exercise. These authorities suggest that such reactions may be aspects of one broad disease entity.

DIFFERENTIATION BETWEEN GRIEF AND DEPRESSION

Although **grief** is a human condition characterized by a disturbance in mood, it is a normal, common, necessary reaction to the loss of a highly valued individual or object. The nurse may help grieving persons to cope with the sense of loss and guilt by encouraging them to talk about their feelings. The goal is to assist these individuals to integrate this emotional reaction with similar experiences in their past and to learn from it.

Depression is a profound disturbance in mood that shares some characteristics with grief; however, it differs in many ways. Depression is not as common an expression as grief, but it occurs frequently. All nurses should be able to differentiate between the normal reaction called grieving and the pathological elaboration of grief, which is called depression. The nurse needs to recognize that normal grieving should be encouraged and that it usually terminates within months or a year without professional help. In contrast, depression is not self-limiting, usually does not improve without professional help, and is dangerous for the individual because of the potential for suicide.

Table 16-1 contrasts grief and depression in terms of cause, symptoms, and outcome.

CAUSATIVE FACTORS

Deviations in mood extreme enough to be categorized as either mania or depression have no specific causative factors that can be identified with scientific certainty. However, the cause of mood disorders has been the subject of much

research over the last decade. It is currently believed that multiple, complex biological and psychosocial factors interact in such a way as to result in these disorders.

Biological factors
Genetic factors

Family studies indicate a higher than expected incidence of depression and bipolar disorder among close relatives of individuals who have these disorders. Twin studies have shown that when one identical twin has a mood disorder, the other twin is also affected in 67% of the cases; the rate decreases to 20% in fraternal twins. Adoption studies have shown that a greater incidence of clinical depression is found among the biological parents of adopted adults with bipolar disorder than in their adoptive parents. Although all these studies point to a genetic pre-

Table 16-1. Difference between grief and depression

GRIEF (BEREAVEMENT)	DEPRESSION
1. Grief is a disturbance in mood that is normal, universal, and necessary in an individual's life experience.	1. Depression is a disturbance in mood that is a pathological elaboration of grief. It is related to grief but is not the same.
2. Grief is a reaction to the *real* loss of a highly valued object that may be tangible or intangible.	2. Depression is a reaction to the actual, threatened, or imagined loss of a valued object, tangible or intangible. It is an overwhelming response to what the individual considers a catastrophic loss.
3. Grief is self-limiting and gradually diminishes over a period of about a year, except in elderly persons, who may need 2 years. Except in the early, acute stage, grief is not incapacitating.	3. Depression is not self-limiting and goes beyond grief in duration and intensity. Depression is prolonged, severe, and increasingly incapacitating in all areas of the individual's life.
4. The three phases of normal grieving are: a. Shock and disbelief b. Developing awareness of the pain of the loss, which eventually results in crying c. Restitution, which involves the mourning experience and eventual elevation of the memory of the lost object to a degree of perfection. New objects replace the lost one at the end of this phase.	4. Depression does not enter the phase of restitution within weeks or months. Professional help is often required.

disposition of mood disorders, the findings are not sufficiently definitive to warrant the conclusion that mood disorders are caused by a specific gene or genes.

Biochemical factors

Psychopharmacological discoveries led experts to examine the role of neurotransmitters in depression. The two major classes of antidepressant medications, the tricyclics and the monoamine oxidase (MAO) inhibitors, were both discovered in the 1950s. Some experts proposed that these drugs acted to relieve symptoms of depression through their effects on the group of neurotransmitters termed the catecholamines, including dopamine, norepinephrine, and epinephrine. Norepinephrine was identified as particularly linked to symptoms of depression.

The **catecholamine hypothesis** of depression proposes that some forms of depression are associated with catecholamine deficiency, particularly norepinephrine, in the brain. In contrast, manic states, in which the individual is highly overactive rather than depressed, may be related to an excess of catecholamines in the brain. Recent studies on the relationships among neurotransmitter systems, depression, and bipolar disorder indicate that several neurotransmitter systems may be involved. For example, the biogenic amines acetylcholine and serotinin may be involved in depression. Experts also agree that several neurotransmitter systems may interact in a complex fashion to produce the symptoms of depression and of bipolar disorder.

The term **neuroendocrinology** refers to the study of the relationships between the nervous and endocrine systems. Psychiatric neuroendocrine studies have explored the relationship of mental illness to a variety of hormones whose secretions are regulated by neurotransmitter systems. For example, some studies have indicated that depressed individuals may show cortisol hypersecretion. Adrenocorticotropic hormone (ACTH) is responsible for the regulation of cortisol secretion.

Psychosocial factors

Psychodynamic factors

Psychoanalytically oriented theorists believe that extreme mood disturbances are closely related to the infant's early feeding experiences. During this period the mother who provides food and attention is both an object of love and a source of frustration for the infant. Ambivalent feelings of both love and hate for the mothering person may exist in this early period and may remain throughout life. In adult life, ambivalent feelings are directed toward the environment and the significant persons in the environment. Individuals who develop extreme mood disturbances such as elation and depression are thought to be reacting to the unconscious loss of a real or fantasied love object that was incorporated at an early phase of personality development. The individual first responds as if mourning for the lost love object and eventually begins to express hostility because of feeling abandoned. The aggressive overactivity of mania is thought to be a defense against the real problem of depression.

In depression, individuals are thought to turn their hostility toward themselves. They believe that they are at fault, that they are responsible for the loss of the love object, and that they are unworthy; thus they hate themselves. They are said to be at the mercy of a punishing, sadistic superego. Such individuals have many narcissistic love needs. Their adult relationships are likely to be immature and dependent. The lifelong problems with which these individuals struggle are hostility and the feelings of guilt that the hostility precipitates when their security is threatened.

Cognitive factors

In the 1970s psychologist Aaron Beck introduced a cognitive model of depression. This model proposes that depressed individuals have learned during their early life to view themselves in a negative way and to interpret life events as related to themselves. This learned pattern of thinking lies dormant until it is activated by environmental stressors and results in a distorted view of these stressors as confirming the person's worthlessness and responsibility for their existence. This type of thinking manifests itself as depression.

A related theory is the *learned helplessness theory,* first proposed by Overmeir and Seligman. This theory states that depression-prone persons have learned to view life as negative and unlikely to change and to view themselves as the cause of the negative events. Because they view change as impossible, these persons feel and act helpless, thereby precipitating depression.

MEDICAL TREATMENT

Mood disorders are very amenable to treatment. The primary treatment is the use of antidepressant medications in the client with depression and lithium carbonate in the client with bipolar disorder (Figure 16-1). Statistics show that about 70% of the persons who receive these medications greatly improve.

Antidepressant medications

The antidepressants fall into two main chemical structures: the tricyclic antidepressants and the MAO inhibitors. Unfortunately, it takes several weeks for antidepressant medications to have a therapeutic effect. Therefore, individuals who are suicidal are best hospitalized during this period, not only for their protection but also to allow the professional staff to assess the onset of the drug's effect, which clients often do not report because of their depression.

Side effects

Dryness of the mouth is experienced by all who take any of the antidepressants. Other common side effects include difficulties in visual accommodation, perspiration about the head and neck, and postural hypotension that often leads to injuries. A mild degree of urinary retention or constipation may also occur. These drugs aggra-

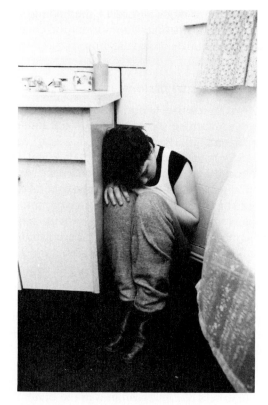

Figure 16-1
Depression is a serious, debilitating disorder that often responds to antidepressant medication.
From Ray O, Ksir C: *Drugs, society, and human behavior,* ed 6, St Louis, 1993, Mosby–Year Book.

vate glaucoma. In addition, MAO inhibitors may also produce a variety of central nervous system symptoms that may include tremor of the upper extremities, convulsions, twitching, and ataxia. If such symptoms appear, they can be easily controlled by decreasing the dosage.

Adverse effects

Adverse effects of the tricyclic antidepressants include exacerbation of the psychosis and cardiac dysrhythmias. The most serious and potentially lethal adverse effect of the MAO inhibitors is a **hypertensive crisis.** Monoamine oxidase is essential in the metabolism of tyramine, a substance contained in many frequently eaten foods that exerts a pressor effect. When a client is taking an MAO inhibitor, particularly tranylcypromine (Parnate), and eats a food containing tyramine, the tyramine cannot be metabolized, and this can cause a hypertensive crisis. This syndrome is often referred to as the **Parnate-cheese reaction.** Foods containing tyramine that must be avoided include aged cheese, whiskey, beer, cream, chocolate, canned figs, coffee, licorice, Chianti and sherry wines, live yeast or yeast extracts such as yogurt, fava beans, soy sauce, pickled herring, pickles, chicken liver, sauerkraut, smoked salmon, snails, and raisins. These dietary restrictions should be maintained for at least 2 weeks after the medication is discontinued to allow for its complete resynthesis.

MAO inhibitors potentiate epinephrine, so clients who are taking these drugs must be warned to avoid other drugs containing ephedrine because this combination may cause extreme hypertension. Examples of typically used over-the-counter medications that must not be taken include many cold remedies and antihistamines.

Finally, MAO inhibitors should not be administered with the tricyclic antidepressants. If a client's medication is changed from one category of antidepressant to another, a lag period of at least 2 weeks should elapse to avoid an adverse synergistic effect.

Lithium

Another widely used psychotropic drug is lithium. This drug is now recognized as effective in the treatment of mania and in preventing the recurrence of bipolar disorder when given on a maintenance basis. About three fourths of the individuals who have a definite diagnosis of bipolar disorder improve remarkably when treatment with lithium is properly carried out. The optimum dose of lithium is based on both the clinical response and the serum lithium level. The usual dose for a patient in an acute manic

state is 600 mg three times a day. The desired serum lithium level is 1.0 to 1.5 mEq/L. Maintenance doses are usually 900 to 1200 mg daily. The desired maintenance serum lithium level is 0.6 to 1.2 mEq/L.

Lithium does not impair intellectual activity, consciousness, or range or quality of emotional life. However, the toxic levels of lithium are close to the therapeutic levels. Adverse effects of lithium, or lithium toxicity, can be monitored by measuring serum lithium levels. Thus, facilities for prompt, accurate serum lithium level determinations should be readily available to the client. Clinical symptoms of an adverse reaction to lithium include nausea, abdominal cramps, vomiting, diarrhea, thirst, and polyuria. These symptoms can occur at lithium levels less than 2 mEq/L. If the drug dosage is not reduced at the first sign of toxicity, serious central nervous system and cardiovascular system damage may ensue. Recent studies have shown that prolonged use of lithium even without symptoms of adverse reactions may lead to renal tubule damage, cardiac toxicity, and thyroid imbalance. Therefore, long-term treatment with lithium requires blood tests at least every 3 months to determine not only the lithium level but also renal and thyroid functions. Despite its effectiveness, lithium is prescribed cautiously and is unlikely to fulfill its initial promise of completely preventing the recurrence of bipolar disorder.

Electroconvulsive therapy

Electroconvulsive therapy (ECT) is sometimes prescribed for severely depressed individuals who have not improved after an adequate trial of antidepressant medications and whose depression manifests itself in agitated behavior. ECT is also used for individuals who are actively suicidal and for whom no other intervention has been effective. Very little is known about how ECT achieves its results.

ECT is a fairly simple procedure to administer. It consists of applying controlled electrical current to the individual's frontal lobes through electrodes placed on the temples to produce a generalized seizure. The treatment is given in the early morning after 8 to 12 hours of fasting. Atropine or another anticholinergic agent is given before the treatment. An intravenous line is placed in a peripheral vein, and access to this vein is maintained until the client is fully recovered. The anesthetic methohexital is given first, followed by succinylcholine for muscle relaxation. Ventilatory assistance is provided with a positive-pressure bag using 100% oxygen. The electrocardiogram, blood pressure, and pulse rate should be monitored throughout the procedure. Stimulus electrodes are placed either bifrontotemporally (bilateral) or with one electrode placed frontotemporally and the second electrode placed on the ipsilateral side (unilateral). Bilateral ECT may be more effective in certain clients or conditions. It has been established, however, that unilateral ECT, particularly on the nondominant side, is associated with a shorter confusional period and fewer memory deficits. Also, a brief pulse stimulus is associated with fewer cognitive defects than the traditional sine wave stimulus. Seizure threshold varies greatly among clients and may be difficult to determine; nevertheless, the lowest amount of electrical energy to induce an adequate seizure should be used. Seizure monitoring is necessary and may be accomplished by an electroencephalogram or by the "cuff" technique. In this technique a blood pressure cuff is placed on an arm or leg and is inflated above systolic pressure before the injection of a muscle relaxant. In unilateral ECT the cuff should be on the same side as the electrodes to ensure that a bilateral seizure occurred.

The number of treatments in a course of therapy varies. Six to 12 treatments are usually effective. The standard practice is to administer the treatment three times weekly.

The major side effects of ECT are spotty but persistent memory loss and transient posttreatment confusion. The severity of the confusion is greatest after bilateral sine wave treatment and least when nondominant, unilateral pulsed ECT

is administered. Likewise, greater memory loss occurs from bilateral sine wave treatment than from unilateral pulsed ECT. Although most clients report that their memory returns several weeks after the last treatment, a significant number experience long-term memory deficits, either for events before the onset of treatments or for events occurring for the months after treatment. Clients vary widely in their reaction to this memory disturbance. Some are not concerned about it, whereas others are very distressed.

In general, the nurse's role when ECT is prescribed is the same as for preoperative and postoperative care. This includes facilitating informed consent, which is just as important as for the surgical patient. In addition, the nurse can be instrumental in reassuring both the client and the family that the acute confusion and memory loss will lessen after the course of treatment is concluded.

NURSING CARE OF INDIVIDUALS WHO ARE DEPRESSED

Nursing assessment

For purposes of clarity, typical behaviors of persons with depression are discussed by categories. Although behaviors in each category are presented as separate entities, they are highly interrelated and are adaptations to similar stressors. Further, behavior designed as an adaptation to one stressor often becomes a stressor itself in another dimension. Therefore, nursing care directed at altering one behavior will inevitably have an effect on others.

Health perception–health management

Individuals who are depressed usually have numerous somatic complaints. It is believed that many people who seek medical help for diffuse, vague complaints such as headaches, gastrointestinal problems such as "fullness," and chest pains have an underlying depression. Nevertheless, all somatic complaints should be thoroughly investigated. Depressed individuals who are inactive are prone to develop physical disorders because of their inactivity. The most common of these are fecal impaction, peripheral edema, and pneumonia. Infections are frequent, but the depressed person tends to ignore the symptoms of these illnesses.

Nutritional-metabolic

A marked change in weight over a relatively short time is often associated with the client's physical complaints. Some less severely depressed persons turn to food and alcoholic beverages as a coping mechanism and thus gain large amounts of weight. Although eating and drinking may provide temporary solace, the resultant overweight becomes an additional stressor, further convincing persons of their worthlessness. Severely depressed individuals are more likely to lack appetite, as well as lacking the energy to buy and prepare food. Thus it is not unusual for them to lose a large amount of weight rapidly. They may not be aware of the amount of weight loss, but the observant nurse will make note of poorly fitting clothes.

Elimination

Constipation often occurs in persons who are depressed and may result in fecal impaction. This problem is most likely to occur in individuals whose depression manifests itself in psychomotor retardation.

Activity-exercise

The depressed individual may exhibit psychomotor retardation, with every word and action requiring monumental effort. On the other hand, this individual may display agitation, often pacing the floor and wringing the hands. When agitation is present, it usually indicates the presence of anxiety as well as depression.

The appearance of persons who are depressed is almost always unkempt, and they often have not bathed recently, since they lack the energy required for bathing and grooming. Furthermore, their unattractive appearance is congruent with their mood.

CLINICAL EXAMPLE

Priscilla is a 35-year-old manager of an exclusive clothing boutique. She was always immaculately groomed and fashionably dressed, as befitted her position. She was also very hard working and rarely took a vacation. Much to the surprise of her co-workers, Priscilla announced one Friday afternoon that she was going to take a 2-week vacation beginning the next Monday. This news resulted in much gossip among the sales personnel because they had long suspected Priscilla was having an affair. When Priscilla did not return to work as planned, Belinda, the assistant manager, became concerned and tried unsuccessfully to reach her by telephone. When she still had not come to work or called in the next 2 days, Belinda went to Priscilla's apartment. After she repeatedly rang the doorbell, the door slowly opened. Belinda was shocked at Priscilla's appearance. It looked as if she had not washed her hair or changed her clothes in at least a week. Belinda convinced Priscilla to let her be taken to the hospital. The psychiatric clinical nurse specialist who interviewed Priscilla discovered that Priscilla's married lover had told her a month before that he was not able to leave his wife and marry Priscilla as he had promised.

Just as the depressed individual's self-care deteriorates, so does the ability to care for the environment. Even the most basic activities associated with cleaning, washing dishes and clothes, and caring for pets and plants go unattended. The result of this lack of attention is often a dirty, cluttered environment, which in turn acts as a further stressor. One community mental health nurse reported making a home visit to a depressed client because he had failed to keep several clinic appointments. The nurse found the client sitting in his living room among several houseplants that were dead from lack of water. The client's environment reflected his depressed mood to such an extent that the nurse had difficulty in not feeling sad herself.

Sleep-rest

Regardless of the severity of the depression, the individual will almost always report changes in sleep patterns. Less severely depressed persons find they sleep for longer intervals and more frequently than usual. More severely depressed persons report they have little difficulty falling asleep but awaken in the early hours of the morning, usually between 3 and 4 AM. At that time their feelings of loneliness, overwhelming anxiety, and worthlessness are most pronounced. Time seems to move very slowly, and they believe daylight will never come. Repeated episodes of early morning wakefulness may make them fearful of going to sleep in the evening. No matter how much sleep depressed individuals have had, they complain of constant fatigue. The simplest task often seems insurmountable, requiring more mental and physical energy than the person possesses.

Cognitive-perceptual

Most individuals who are depressed maintain contact with reality but view themselves and the world around them in the most pessimistic light. This symptom is more reflective of a disturbance in emotional processes than in cognition processes. However, severely depressed individuals experience difficulty in concentration and sometimes have self-accusatory delusions. For example, clients may believe they are responsible for a natural disaster such as an earthquake, since they view the earthquake as evidence that God is trying to swallow them up. Such clients are experiencing a disturbance in cognition processes.

CLINICAL EXAMPLE

Mrs. Bishop lives in a geographical area plagued by tornadoes. When the last tornado struck, Mrs. Bishop believed the loss of her house resulted from her sinful nature, as evidenced by her not having gone to church for the past five Sundays. When well-meaning neighbors pointed out that all their homes were destroyed, and therefore Mrs. Bishop could have not been at fault, Mrs. Bishop was not reassured but rather responded with increased guilt for the destruction of the entire community.

Self-perception/self-concept

Low self-esteem is a predominant characteristic of individuals who are depressed. These feelings of worthlessness are likely to be long-standing but become more severe and prominent when the individual becomes ill. As a result, the depressed individual attends to situations and reactions of others that reinforce this belief and ignores or rationalizes those that indicate the person has value.

CLINICAL EXAMPLE

Ronald Webster, a 52-year-old handyman, came home one evening with the news that he was offered the job of superintendent of the apartment building in which he had faithfully and effectively worked for the last 20 years. Mrs. Webster was ecstatic because of the increase in pay this job would mean. Ronald told her to calm down because he might not take the job. When she asked why not, he replied, "They really don't want me. They just couldn't get anyone else."

The depressed individual almost always feels helpless, hopeless, and powerless to change the situation. Expressions of these feelings include statements such as, "I feel worthless, rotten, no good," "Life is a struggle," or "I don't deserve to be taken care of, I'm just a burden to everyone."

Role-relationship

The individual with depression expresses despair, gloom, a sense of foreboding, and feelings of guilt, sadness, and shame. These feelings are so overwhelming that the nurse can sense them even before the person describes them.

Needless to say, depressed persons report that they find no pleasure in any activity, even those they had previously enjoyed.

Although lay people often associate crying with depression, this expression of anguish may not be present in severely depressed individuals. Sometimes these persons may sob, but tearlessly. At other times, they may not cry, but their faces wear tortured expressions.

Although not every depressed individual harbors suicidal thoughts, almost every person who attempts suicide is depressed. Consequently, every depressed client should be considered as potentially suicidal unless reason exists to believe otherwise.

Some authorities believe that all individuals who contemplate suicide give clues of their intention. Common clues include a dramatic change in behavior, giving away treasured possessions, or actually talking about their intentions. The common belief that a person who talks about suicide never attempts suicide is a fallacy. People usually talk about the thoughts uppermost in their minds. Individuals allude to suicide because they are thinking about it. Persons who make statements about life not being worth living, who suggest that they may not be around much longer, or who have actually injured themselves should be considered at risk for suicide.

A person who is depressed is at the greatest risk for suicide after the depression has begun to lift. Suicide attempts at this time are common because the individual has sufficient mental and physical energy to plan and implement a self-destructive act while still being sufficiently depressed to desire death.

Another common fallacy about suicide is that questioning depressed individuals about the presence of suicidal thoughts will give them the idea that this might be a solution to their problems. Nothing could be further from the truth. If the individual were so responsive to suggestion, it would be a relatively easy matter to suggest that life is worth living. The nurse should never hesitate to ask depressed persons if they are contemplating suicide, especially if their behavior raises that suspicion in the nurse's mind.

Sexuality-reproductive

Understandably, the individual who is depressed often has sexual dysfunction. Many of these persons have never had satisfactory, satisfying sexual activity because of their pervasive feelings of worthlessness. Even those who previously had a satisfactory sexual life frequently report current lack of interest in and lack of energy to engage in sexual activity. Many depressed women who continue to have sex merely submit to the act as passive partners, perhaps creating increased interpersonal dysfunction. Another consequence of this behavior may be an unplanned pregnancy, which compounds the stressors the woman is already experiencing. Some severely depressed individuals report bemusement about why their sexual partner would even be interested in having sexual relations with them.

Coping–stress tolerance

Persons who are depressed have ineffective coping skills. Not only are they unable to deal with the stressors of daily living, but they tend to incorporate even the most generalized stressors as evidence of their incompetency and worthlessness, thereby increasing their depression.

Value-belief

Individuals with depression may think they are being punished by God for real or imagined sins. Other persons may feel a deep sense of alienation from any source of spiritual support. Individuals who had an active spiritual life before becoming ill are particularly likely to be spiritually distressed because of the incongruency between their beliefs and how they feel.

Nursing diagnosis

As with all nursing diagnoses, the nursing diagnoses for the individual who is depressed are based on the themes identified during the assessment phase of the nursing process.

Accepted NANDA nursing diagnoses that may be specifically applicable to the individual with depression include:

Altered health maintenance

High risk for infection

Altered nutrition: high risk for more than body requirements

Altered nutrition: less than body requirements

Constipation

Activity intolerance

Fatigue

Self-care deficit, bathing/hygiene, dressing/ grooming

Impaired home maintenance management

Sleep pattern disturbance

Knowledge deficit (specify)

Hopelessness

Powerlessness

Self-esteem disturbance; situational low self- esteem; chronic low self-esteem

Dysfunctional grieving

High risk for violence: self-directed

Ineffective individual coping

Spiritual distress

To develop a nursing diagnosis that fulfills its function of providing direction for planning nursing care, the nurse is encouraged to postulate and state etiological or antecedent factors and connect the two phrases by using the term "related to." For example:

Impaired home maintenance management related to lack of energy

Planning and implementing nursing care

The plan for nursing care is derived from the nursing diagnoses and includes the objectives of the care, the nursing interventions, and outcome criteria. The plan needs to be highly individualized. The suggestions that follow should be seen as general guidelines to be used if they are appropriate to the client's needs.

In general, the objectives of all nursing care for the individual who is depressed should relate to helping the person to increase self-esteem.

Since the client's nursing diagnoses are often interrelated, stemming as they do from similar etiologies or antecedents, the student should see that appropriate nursing interventions are also interrelated. In other words, by intervening in one dimension, the nurse will also affect other dimensions.

Health perception—health management

Because depressed individuals tend to be very inactive, they frequently become chilled without appearing to realize it. Therefore, they need to be supplied with extra clothing and encouraged to wear it.

The inactivity of depressed individuals also makes them susceptible to infection and gastro-intestinal and circulatory problems. The nurse can help prevent these problems by ensuring that the client maintains adequate food and fluid intake and engages in as much physical activity as possible. This is easier said than done. The nurse most likely to be successful offers fluids routinely and small amounts of food frequently rather than insisting the client eat three full meals at regularly scheduled times. With severely depressed persons, even the simple act of walking down the hall will not take place unless the client is encouraged to do so and accompanied by a member of the nursing staff. The nurse who works with a depressed client needs to have much patience and be willing to take the time required to provide individualized care.

Nutritional-metabolic

Many depressed individuals present a difficult feeding problem. It is helpful if the nurse can discover why food is being refused. These individuals may refuse to eat because they believe they are unworthy of receiving food. Some may say that they do not deserve food because they have not paid for it. Still others seek to destroy themselves through starvation. Many of these individuals have simply lost a desire for food, along with all the other interests they formerly had in life. Inactivity also contributes to a lack of interest in food.

Finding a way to combat the depressed individual's failure to eat depends on the reason for which the food is being refused. If failure to eat is caused by a feeling of unworthiness or the thought that the food has not been paid for, the person may be reassured by being told that the food is prepared for the group and all are expected to eat regardless of whether they pay or not. It might be helpful to provide an opportunity for such an individual to wash dishes or to do some other simple tasks to give a feeling of "paying" for the food.

Activity-exercise

Patience is the keynote in working with depressed individuals who are so greatly retarded in the spheres of thinking, feeling, and acting that every movement or word requires great effort and much time. The same question often needs to be asked more than once, and the nurse must wait patiently for the answer. A large part of the therapeutic value of the hospital situation is that decisions can be made for the individual. Thus the nurse should avoid asking questions as, "Do you want to take your bath now?" A more positive approach would be, "Your bath is ready now. I will help you with it."

Encouraging depressed individuals to take pride in their personal appearance is part of their care. This is difficult to achieve because it is in opposition to their tendency toward self-depreciation. Careful supervision of personal hygiene with attention to supplying clean clothing and helping them dress neatly is important in increasing self-esteem. Women need to be encouraged to accept appointments at the beauty parlor and men to go to the barbershop regularly. If a depressed individual is hospitalized because of being actively suicidal, it may be safer to ask the barber or beauty operator to come to the unit where the person is hospitalized rather than to send him or her to the operator.

Sleep-rest

If the client is unable to sleep at night, warm tub baths, warm milk, and hypnotic drugs may be of benefit. However, treatment with antidepressant medications is usually most effective in alleviating the symptom of sleep disturbance.

Cognitive-perceptual

Because depression can be effectively treated, most clients will be taking antidepressant medication. The nurse is responsible for teaching the client and family about the intended effects, side effects, and adverse effects of the prescribed medication. Of particular importance is helping the client to understand that it may take weeks before the medication begins to have an effect. The client also must understand the dietary and over-the-counter medication restrictions that must be observed when taking certain types of antidepressants.

Self-perception/self-concept

The need that many inexperienced nurses feel to "cheer up" the person who is depressed is not helpful and often actually causes the client to feel more guilty and unworthy than ever. When caring for a depressed individual, such statements as, "Buck up," "Let's see you smile," or "There is a silver lining in every cloud" are not helpful. Gaiety and laughter have a tendency to make such a person feel more guilty and thus more morose. The nurse can be most helpful by being friendly in a kind, understanding, businesslike way. Attempts at changing the client's mood through logical suggestions are fruitless and should be avoided. Sometimes just sitting beside the client without trying to carry on a conversation is helpful. At other times it is effective to talk, even though the client may not answer.

One of the methods by which a nurse may contribute to the care of some depressed individuals is to provide them with tasks that will help relieve feelings of guilt. Depressed individuals have been known to ask for such menial tasks as scrubbing the floor or the walls. Such tasks may provide a release for the depressed individual's guilt and a means of atonement for real or imaginary sins. They most certainly contribute to increased physical activity, which often results in increased feelings of well-being. Although providing such experiences is controversial and contrary to the usual recommended treatment plan, it has proved to be of great value to selected individuals. Such work assignments for depressed persons should not be carried out unless they have been approved by the treatment team.

Role-relationship

The potential for depressed persons to injure or destroy themselves is one of the most serious problems with which the nurse must cope. The most effective methods for dealing with this problem vary, depending on the situation and the individual. However, every nurse should be fully acquainted with some basic principles concerning the care of the self-destructive individual.

Self-destructive tendencies are probably treated most effectively by developing an environment to help the individual bear the emotional pain. Instead of removing all the potentially dangerous items from the environment, an attempt can be made to meet the client's emotional needs. This may be done by assigning a staff member, preferably a skillful psychiatric nurse, to remain constantly with the individual. The nurse helps the client participate in occupational, social, and recreational activities. Subtly and appropriately, ways are identified to reassure the individual that he or she is a worthwhile, useful human being. Acutely depressed individuals should be constantly supervised, but the focus of the supervision should be to help clients deal with their feelings. The emphasis should be on supplying safe opportunities for participation in the daily routine.

Sometimes an attempt is made to ensure clients' safety by removing from the environment all the equipment with which they might injure themselves. This is extremely difficult because every piece of clothing, all eating utensils, cigarettes, furniture, bathroom equipment—literally everything an individual needs in the process of daily living—could be used if individuals wished to injure or destroy themselves. One client strangled herself by using a toothbrush to fashion a tourniquet from her long, braided hair; another client dived headlong into the toilet and suffered a serious head wound; a third client destroyed herself by using the armholes of her knitted underwear as a noose; and a fourth client injured herself seriously by setting fire to her dress with a cigarette. If the philosophy of making the environment safe were carried to its logical conclusion, the client would be placed in an absolutely barren room with a pallet on which to lie. At best this procedure of environmental control is only a preventive measure.

Depriving clients of freedom to move about may increase their self-destructive tendencies, convincing them that their worst fears are true and that they are worthless and unworthy or that they have committed an unforgivable crime and are being justly punished. An illustration of such an occurrence is an incident in which a nurse was playing cards with a young man who was actively suicidal and confined to an empty seclusion room, dressed only in trousers. As both sat cross-legged on the floor, over a period of hours the client dealt the cards a few inches to the right and the nurse unconsciously shifted her position to accommodate to the cards. This client eventually succeeded in shifting the nurse's position so that he had free access to the door, which he fled through and proceeded to fling himself through a window. This incident illustrates that even with all precautions, prevention of suicide is not always possible, and its occurrence may be increased by establishing an environment that serves as a constant reminder to clients of their destructive wishes. Although there is no question that the actively suicidal client should be closely supervised, the hospital staff should emphasize the client's participation in safe activities with others rather than the environmental modifications so often unsuccessfully employed.

If individuals are able to believe that people are truly interested in them, if their needs for recognition and emotional support are being met, and if they are accompanied by staff who help them talk about their concerns, the incidence of attempts at self-destruction is greatly lessened.

KEY INTERVENTIONS FOR CLIENTS WHO ARE DEPRESSED

Treat the client as an individual who has worth and dignity.

Ensure adequate nutrition and activity to maintain physiological stability.

Assist with self-care activities as a means of increasing self-esteem.

Avoid attempts to "cheer up" the client.

Be alert to indications of suicidal ideations, which most often occur when the depression begins to lift.

Teach the client and family about the illness and its treatment.

NURSING CARE PLAN: *A Depressed Individual*

CASE FORMULATION

Carol B., 29 years of age, has been married 3 years and has one child 14 months of age. Family history reveals nothing significant.

Five years before marriage, Carol had a period of nervousness and depression that lasted about 3 months. This was precipitated by an unfortunate love affair. At that time she was attending summer school at a local university, where she met a young man. He had encouraged her to believe he was greatly interested in her, but at the school outing that ended the summer session, he ignored her and danced with another girl. Carol came home, said little or nothing to her parents, and the following morning was found in bed in a stupor. She had taken 12 1-grain phenobarbital tablets. She was rushed to a hospital, given emergency treatment, and then transferred to a mental health treatment center, where she remained 2 weeks.

The present attack began about 6 weeks before admission. Again the onset was rather abrupt. Her husband returned home from work one evening and found Carol sobbing. After much urging on his part, she confessed that she was crying because she was a bad mother and a poor housekeeper. The husband naturally assured her that she was quite the contrary, but this only brought more sobbing and self-deprecation. She worried excessively about a small scar on her baby's temple that was caused by chicken pox. She accused herself of "marking" the child. The family suspected that she was merely tired from her spring housecleaning and hired a helper to come in and care for the baby. Her sister-in-law was called in to act as a companion. For 3 weeks Carol remained at home. She complained of inability to concentrate and prayed much of the time. The

Continued.

NURSING CARE PLAN: *A Depressed Individual—cont'd*

well-meaning sister-in-law attempted to encourage her by suggesting that she "snap out of it," but this comment merely served to agitate Carol. She was finally taken to her parents' home in the country. On two occasions she was found walking along the country road, and when questioned as to her destination, she merely stated that she wanted to "run away from everything." Her husband came to visit her one Sunday afternoon and took her for a car ride back into the city. She requested him to stop at their home, since she wanted some extra clothes for the baby. She went to the kitchen and, before the husband could realize what she was about to do, cut both her wrists with a carving knife. She was admitted to a short-term treatment unit in a community mental health center after receiving emergency treatment for her wounds.

On the day of admission she was able to give a clear account of her actions but responded in a dull manner. She frequently interjected the remark that she should be dead but that she was too big a coward to take her own life. She accused herself of being a rank failure and asserted that she should never have been born. She frequently announced that there was no sense in bothering about her, since she would die the next day. She cried but did not shed many tears. She complained of a "numb" feeling in her head, inability to sleep, and loss of appetite. The physical examination was entirely negative.

Nursing Assessment

The history provides little information about the present episode of depression. However, it does provide information about the first attack, which came as a result of the failure of an interpersonal relationship of great importance to Carol and the loss of a beloved object, a cherished lover. At that time she attempted suicide by taking an overdose of sleeping pills.

Psychoanalytically oriented theorists believe that individuals who resort to self-destruction are frequently fixated at the oral stage of psychosexual development. During the late oral period of the child's development, the loved object (the mother or the mother's breast) is unconsciously introjected. Later in life, a loved object may unconsciously represent the original object that was introjected. When Carol first attempted suicide, she may have been seeking relief from suffering or punishment for herself, or she may have been attempting to kill the introjected person.

This young woman's child was in the toilet-training period. At this period in development the child becomes more self-assertive and begins to defy the mother. This mother may have viewed the change in her child from a dependent, passive organism requiring constant tender guidance to a self-assertive individual as a loss. In a sense, Carol had lost a dependent organism and gained a demanding child. She may have been overwhelmed with the new responsibilities brought about by the child's development. Thus she blamed herself for being a bad mother and a poor housekeeper and having caused a small scar on the baby's temple.

Carol's physical symptoms were those usually found in depressed individuals: in-

NURSING CARE PLAN: *A Depressed Individual—cont'd*

ability to sleep, loss of appetite, complaints of a numb feeling in the head, and crying without tears. Her emotional responses were also those frequently found among depressed individuals: inability to concentrate, self-accusatory ideas, suicidal ideas, and feelings of unworthiness. Characteristically, she was able to give a clear account of all the experiences relating to her illness.

Nursing Diagnosis

The assessment data, including present behavior, past life experiences, and an understanding of the underlying dynamics, led to the development of the following nursing diagnoses for Carol:

High risk for violence: self-directed related to feelings of guilt and worthlessness

Sleep pattern disturbance related to depression

Self-care deficit, feeding, related to lack of appetite

Planning and Implementing Nursing Care

The boxed material on pp. 290 and 291 is an example of a plan of nursing care that could be designed for Carol B. Because she was actively suicidal, individual nursing care was provided for her. Nurses or other staff members with proved ability to work successfully with depressed individuals were chosen to be with her at all times until she recovered from the acute phase of the depression. They recognized the importance of showing Carol that they cared about her and set about to achieve this. Their goals for her care were to protect her from her self-

destructive tendencies and to encourage her to discuss her feelings about the problems that concerned her.

These staff members adopted a kind, courteous, firm, hopeful attitude toward Carol. In this way they tried to convey the impression that she was not a hopeless case as she insisted. They listened carefully to everything she said and answered her questions carefully without disputing or agreeing with her expressions of worthlessness. They accepted her silences when she did not wish to talk. They avoided using meaningless statements such as, "Cheer up," or "You know your family loves you!"

The staff members who worked closely with Carol were aware of her physical needs for food, fluid intake, and rest. They found that she ate better if served food on a tray in her room rather than going to the dining room with the other clients. If at night she wanted to sit up and talk or walk up and down the corridors, the staff member who was assigned to stay with her accompanied her in these activities.

When Carol accused herself of being a rank failure, the nurse tried to help her recognize that she was improving and had demonstrated abilities and skills since coming to the treatment center. This was an attempt to improve her self-esteem.

The staff made decisions for Carol until she was able to make them for herself. They tried to develop a congenial, pleasant living atmosphere for her. They encouraged her to become interested in some activities available in the occupational therapy department and accompanied her there whenever she felt well enough to go.

Continued.

NURSING CARE PLAN: *A Depressed Individual—cont'd*

Evaluation

Evaluation of the plan of nursing care and its implementation was based on outcome criteria established when the plan was formulated. Since the nurse knew that the most significant factor in alleviating the symptoms of acute depression is the prescribed antidepressant medication and that this medication requires 2 to 4 weeks to have an effect, she did not expect to see changes in Carol's behavior until then.

For several days after admission, Carol remained sad and indifferent. She ate only when coaxed. She never inquired about the welfare of her child and was indifferent toward her husband during visiting hours. Al-

though she was not particularly untidy, she was rather slipshod in appearance and made no attempt to comb her hair or keep herself presentable. She took little or no interest in unit activities or in the other clients.

In the second week of Carol's hospital stay, she began to show improvement. After being in the hospital for 1 month, she began clamoring for discharge, insisting that she must go home to take care of her family. She was cheerful and industrious, teaching flower arranging to a small group of women in occupational therapy.

Carol's nurse joined other members of the treatment team in recommending discharge to the aftercare clinic.

NURSING CARE PLAN FOR CAROL B.

Nursing diagnosis	Objective (rationale)	Nursing interventions	Outcome criteria
High risk for violence: self-directed related to feelings of guilt and worthlessness	Client will be protected from self-destructive tendencies. (Until antidepressant medication works, the client needs to be protected from herself.)	Assigned nurse(s) remain with client at all times. Administer prescribed antidepressant medication. Observe and listen carefully for clues of suicidal intention; record same. Encourage constructive activity, such as occupational therapy (OT) and recreational therapy (RT). Comment positively on accomplishments.	Within 4 weeks, client: No longer expresses desire to kill self. Acknowledges positive comments by nurse about client's accomplishments, for example, by saying, "Thank you." Spontaneously attends OT and RT activities.
	Client discusses her feelings and problems. (An ability to discuss feelings and problems makes them amenable to reality testing and problem solving.)	Reflect client's statements to encourage conversation. Sit with client in silence if she does not wish to talk.	With 2 weeks, client: Spontaneously approaches nurse to express feelings. Shows evidence of attempting to problem solve.

NURSING CARE PLAN FOR CAROL B.—cont'd

Nursing diagnosis	Objective (rationale)	Nursing interventions	Outcome criteria
		Convey interest in what client says.	
		Do not argue with expressions of worthlessness.	
		Avoid platitudes, such as, "tomorrow will be a better day."	
		Encourage problem-solving technique.	
Sleep pattern disturbance related to depression	Client's periods of sleep at night will increase. (Uninterrupted sleep enhances physiological stability and indicates a decrease in depression.)	Discourage naps during the day.	Within 4 weeks, client sleeps from 10 PM to 6 AM without awakening.
		Remove client from environmental stimuli (e.g., TV) 1 hour before bedtime.	
		Do not discuss charged issues at bedtime.	
		If client awakes at night, do not scold; be reassuring and remain with her.	
Self-care deficit, feeding, related to lack of appetite	Client's food and fluid intake will increase. (Optimum food and fluid intake enhances physiological stability and indicates a decrease in depression.)	Offer small amounts of easily chewed, nutritional food at mealtimes.	Within 4 weeks, client eats three meals a day without needing to be encouraged to do so.
		Offer 6 ounces of water or juice in plastic cup every 2 hours.	
		Record amount of food and fluid taken.	

NURSING CARE OF INDIVIDUALS WHO ARE ELATED AND OVERACTIVE

Nursing assessment

Health perception–health management

The individual who is overactive and elated may have numerous physical health problems that may or may not be related to the mental illness. Because of overactivity and distractibility, it is unlikely that the client would seek health care for preexisting, unrelated health problems. Therefore, it is important that the nurse assess whether such conditions exist.

Because of overactivity and irritability when thwarted, the individual is likely to become involved in altercations with others or accidents that may result in physical trauma. Injuries can range from superficial bruises to broken bones. However, the individual who is elated is unlikely to complain of discomfort.

Nutritional-metabolic

As with many other individuals who have a mental illness, the elated, overactive individual may be malnourished. Overactivity consumes much energy, and the person cannot concentrate long enough on one task to purchase, prepare, or eat food. For the same reason the individual rarely consumes sufficient fluid. Consequently, an overactive individual often loses much weight and may become severely dehydrated.

Elimination

Constipation, fecal impaction, and bladder distention are common problems related to inadequate food and fluid intake and not taking time to use the bathroom.

Activity-exercise

The elated, overactive individual moves constantly and finds it almost impossible to sit or stand in one spot for more than a few seconds. As a result, the person's hygiene needs are often unmet. In addition, the person's appearance is often dramatically bizarre. Frequently the individual dresses in clothing that is not only inappropriate to the setting or the season but is also very brightly colored. Females, in particular, adorn themselves with flowers in their hair, large pieces of ornate jewelry, and an abundance of sloppily applied makeup. One client appeared for admission to a northeastern psychiatric hospital in February dressed in a long, bright-yellow ball gown and a wide-brimmed straw hat. Around her shoulders she wore a foxtail stole. Her only concession to the 20-degree weather was a pair of checkered mittens. By the time she arrived at the hospital, this individual was almost suffering from hypothermia but had no sense of discomfort.

As with any individual who has alterations in self-care, the elated, overactive individual has great difficulty in home maintenance. The person is able to give little attention to maintaining the environment in a clean, safe condition.

Sleep-rest

Exhaustion and death have been known to occur in overactive, elated individuals who do not receive treatment. Many of these individuals are so alert to all environmental stimuli that they sleep only 1 to 2 hours out of every 24.

Cognitive-perceptual

The elated, overactive individual is hyperalert to the environment and seemingly cannot block out stimuli. Consequently, the person is unable to maintain sustained attention to anything, sometimes for any longer than a few seconds. In addition, this individual characteristically shows very poor judgment. Because of feelings of grandiosity and their impulsivity, such persons may bankrupt themselves and their family by charging thousands of dollars for such items as clothing, cars, jewelry, and furniture despite not needing or being able to afford these items. This characteristic often leads the family to seek treatment for the person. One such individual sold the family clothes dryer to a visitor who admired it. His lack of judgment was displayed not only by selling the dryer, but also by delivering it filled with a load of partially dried clothes.

Self-perception/self-concept

Although the elated, overactive individual gives the impression of feeling all-powerful, in reality the person feels powerless and out of control. The content of speech and nature of behavior are likely to be antisocial and in conflict with the values the individual espouses when well. Family and friends may emphasize how uncharacteristic such behavior is for this person.

Role-relationship

The mood expressed by the elated, overactive individual is euphoria, although many authorities believe that this mood state is a defense against an underlying depression. The jovial, good-natured euphoria the client expresses can quickly turn into irritability and anger when desires or activities are thwarted.

The constant movement of elated, overactive individuals is accompanied by excessive talking. The content of their verbalizations may not be immediately understood by the listener, since their thoughts occur faster than they can speak and tend to fly from one topic to another. However, with concentration the listener can usually accurately guess the missing words and make sense of what the person is saying, unlike when conversing with an individual with a thought disorder.

When the elated individual is left alone, the content of speech is likely to be jovial and humorous, often with many sexual references and puns. When the stream of talk is interrupted even by as simple an event as being asked a question, the good-natured banter may suddenly turn to biting sarcasm, pointed profanity, and vulgarity.

Elated individuals are very adept in discovering a physical or personality defect in the person with whom they are speaking, particularly one about which the person is sensitive. They seem to take delight in repeatedly calling attention to this defect.

Sexuality-reproductive

The individual who is overactive and elated often becomes sexually preoccupied and may engage in frequent sexual activity with several partners. These partners may be persons whom the individual knows, or they may be prostitutes. In either situation, this promiscuous sexual activity puts the person at great risk for becoming infected with a blood-borne pathogen.

Coping–stress tolerance

Because of their illness, these individuals' usual coping mechanisms do not work, and therefore they are subject to decreased stress tolerance. In addition, their behavior is almost always a major stressor to their social system, particularly the family.

CLINICAL EXAMPLE

Mr. Matthews was a successful car salesman. He, his wife, and their four children lived in a two-story brick colonial-style home in the best section of town. Mr. Matthews had been acting strangely for the last 2 weeks. For example, although he came home for dinner every evening as usual, he would talk incessantly during the

meal and then leave to go back to work despite not being needed there. This afternoon his wife came home to find Mr. Matthews showing the house to a young couple. After they left, Mrs. Matthews asked who they were. Mr. Matthews replied that he had sold the house to them and that she was to pack because they were leaving for Saudi Arabia in the morning so he could begin work at an oil refinery, where he expected to earn at least "a million dollars a year."

Value-belief

Clients who are overactive and elated often report a "special closeness" with God. They may believe that God has called them to a special task or that they have been supernaturally endowed with special powers. Rather than indicating an increased spirituality, these grandiose beliefs are symptoms of the illness.

Nursing diagnosis

Accepted NANDA nursing diagnoses that may be specifically applicable to the individual with overactivity and elation include:
Altered health maintenance
High risk for injury
Altered nutrition: less than body requirements
Constipation
Self-care deficit, bathing/hygiene; dressing/ grooming; feeding
Impaired home maintenance management
Sleep pattern disturbance
Knowledge deficit (specify)
Altered thought processes
Self-esteem disturbance; situational low self-esteem; chronic low self-esteem
Impaired social interaction
Altered family processes
Impaired verbal communication
High risk for violence: directed at others
Ineffective individual coping
To develop a nursing diagnosis that fulfills its function of providing direction for planning nursing care, the nurse is encouraged to postulate and state etiological or antecedent factors

and connect the two phrases by using the term "related to." For example:

Self-care deficit, dressing/grooming, related to overactivity and inability to sustain attention to a task

Planning and implementing nursing care

The plan for nursing care is derived from the nursing diagnoses and includes the objectives of the care, the nursing interventions, and outcome criteria. To be effective, the plan needs to be highly individualized. The suggestions that follow should be seen as general guidelines to be used if they are appropriate to the client's needs.

Individuals who are elated and overactive require skillful, tactful nursing care. In general, the objectives of all nursing care for the individual who is elated and overactive should relate to protecting the client and others from the overactive behavior until the prescribed medications take effect.

Since the client's nursing diagnoses are often interrelated, stemming as they do from similar etiologies or antecedents, the student should see that the appropriate nursing interventions are also interrelated. In other words, by intervening in one dimension, the nurse will also affect other dimensions.

Health perception—health management

The nurse needs to be vigilantly aware of the physical needs of a client who is elated and overactive. In addition to ensuring adequate food and fluid intake, the nurse must monitor elimination and intervene appropriately if indicated.

Because overactive individuals are unlikely to report an illness or injury, it is especially important for a complete physical examination to be completed as soon as possible after admission to the mental health care delivery system. Thereafter the nurse must be alert for signs and symptoms of physical illness that may or may not be related to the client's overactivity.

Nutritional-metabolic

Elated, overactive individuals may not take time to sit down to eat. For such clients the nurse should serve food that can be carried about in the hands. Sandwiches, fruit, and cupcakes are dietary items that may be "eaten on the run." Elated, overactive individuals require a high caloric intake and should have between-meal nourishment. Nurses should not disregard the need for fluids even though water fountains are usually available; the overactive individual often does not take time to drink and should have water offered each hour.

If the individual is served food on a tray and will take time for self-feeding, the equipment on the tray should be simple and unbreakable. As in every other aspect of the care of these overactive, elated persons, the nursing procedures must be individualized to meet specific needs. At times the elated individual may get along well in the dining room setting. However, these clients usually are so stimulated by the dining room situation that it is more helpful if they are served on a tray in their room.

Activity-exercise

It is useless to attempt to hurry the elated individual because such an approach will result in anger and hostility. Thus the attitude of having all the time in the world to accomplish a task will be much more effective. Quiet persuasion is one of the chief aids in getting the elated individual to cooperate.

Because all elated, overactive individuals are stimulated by environmental factors, one of the nurse's first responsibilities is to simplify their surroundings and, insofar as possible, provide a sedate environment for them. The client's room should be as far away from other daily activities as possible and yet easily accessible to the nurse, who needs to be constantly aware of the individual and his or her behavior. Pictures and colorful drapes probably should be removed because they may be too stimulating and may be destroyed in a burst of excitement. The same is true of unnecessary furniture such as a small table or a light chair, either of which may be used as a weapon if the client becomes extremely irritated.

Although these individuals should be encouraged to carry out their own personal hygiene, they need to be supervised closely. Some overactive, elated individuals are too ill to assume any responsibility for their physical care and may need to have much of it done by the nurse. Other, less excited individuals can take much responsibility for their own cleanliness and grooming if someone skillful directs their activities. Such individuals may become playful and mischievous in the bathroom. Because of poor judgment, these individuals have been found washing their hair in the toilet bowl, throwing water about with gay abandon, or in various other ways reducing the bathroom to a shambles. For this reason such individuals should not be left alone in the bathroom.

Keeping overactive persons warmly dressed during cold weather is sometimes difficult because clothing may be an irritating factor. Excited individuals may tear off clothing that impedes the movement of arms and legs. They often appear totally unaware of body temperature and must be safeguarded against becoming chilled.

Overactive individuals may react with a tremendous burst of energy for which they must find some outlet. Usually such individuals are admitted to a hospital because the outlets they have chosen for their energy have been dangerous to them or to the family. The nurse is confronted with the task of controlling or redirecting this excessive energy into more acceptable channels.

An excellent outlet for the excessive energy of individuals who are only mildly elated is writing. Most of these people are eager to write their life stories or to disclose the deficiencies of the political system to the world and thus will readily put paper and pencil to use. Many mildly elated individuals will be content to spend hours over their manuscripts.

Physical activities provided for these individuals should require large sweeping movements, since they will become annoyed and lose interest in anything requiring fine, discriminative skills. Games such as table tennis, croquet, badminton, and medicine ball are often helpful as outlets for energy, provided no element of competition is present. In competitive games the elated client becomes overly stimulated and excited.

Cognitive-perceptual

As with any client who has a mental illness and for whom a psychotropic medication is prescribed, the client who is overactive and elated must be taught about the nature of the illness and the prescribed medication. Education is not possible during the acute phase of the illness. However, as the overactivity lessens, the client is often very amenable to learning since basic thought processes are not impaired. Furthermore, learning that the illness has a biological basis over which the person has little control is likely to alleviate any fear and diminish any guilt the client may be experiencing. Many clients with bipolar disorder are able to learn to identify early signs and symptoms of a relapse so as to seek treatment before their behavior becomes destructive.

It is particularly important to teach the client about the prescribed medication. If the client is taking lithium, the nurse must emphasize the necessity to have blood levels determined as instructed and must ensure that the client and family understand the symptoms of lithium toxicity.

Role-relationship

The euphoria of overactive clients can easily turn to irritability and anger, which in turn may result in destructive, threatening behavior. When clients begin to threaten destructive behavior, they should be assisted to a room that is away from the center of activity and should remain there until their emotions are under control. The nurse needs to be aware of and carefully follow the legal procedures and institutional policies regarding the use of restraint and seclusion as a therapeutic intervention. Fortunately, with the availability of effective psychotropic medications, the necessity to restrain mechanically or seclude overactive individuals occurs less frequently than in the past.

More important than managing destructive, threatening behavior is learning how it can be prevented. The first step in learning to prevent problem behavior is to identify situations that are upsetting to such individuals and to discover how to keep these from occurring. The nurse needs to learn to recognize the signs of an approaching emotional outburst and to employ measures that will help individuals to handle negative feelings without acting out against the environment. Destructive behavior is rare when an attempt is made to recognize and meet emotional needs and when personnel recognize the importance of developing positive interpersonal relationships with persons who have a mental illness.

Whether the nurse can help elated, overactive clients depends greatly on the manner with which the nurse approaches them. The nurse's tone of voice is of primary importance. A firm, kind, low-pitched voice that carries a coaxing quality probably is most effective. The nurse who uses a loud, demanding tone not only is likely to be ineffective but also is likely to provoke hostile, aggressive behavior from the client.

Consistent fairness and honesty in dealing with elated, overactive clients are essential if rapport with them is to be maintained over time. Although they deserve and must have simple, honest explanations, long discussions and explanations should be avoided.

In dealing with overactive, elated individuals, the nurse must recognize that the behavior is a result of an illness and will be replaced by socially acceptable behavior when the person is well again. The inexperienced nurse may be embarrassed by the loud talking, the vulgarity and profanity, the destructive activity, and the overt sexual behavior. However, part of the skillful care of such a person includes understanding why he or she behaves in such a way. With understanding comes acceptance of behavior.

The nurse who is accepting of the elated individual's behavior will not scold or shame the client for the uninhibited actions or become angered by the pointed, biting remarks because the nurse will understand that they are a part of the illness.

KEY INTERVENTIONS FOR CLIENTS WHO ARE ELATED AND OVERACTIVE

Be alert to signs and symptoms of physical illness and injury that the client is not likely to report.

Ensure adequate nutrition by providing high-calorie foods that can be "eaten on the run."

Decrease environmental stimuli.

Redirect excessive energy into acceptable outlets such as writing and noncompetitive games that require large sweeping movements.

Teach the client and family about the illness and its treatment.

Protect the client and others from the client's destructive behavior, whether physical, social, or economic.

NURSING CARE PLAN: *An Overactive Individual*

CASE FORMULATION

Maurice H., 48 years of age, was an unmarried real estate salesman who was an only child. His mother had a mental illness at 46 years of age, which was probably depression of midlife. He had been educated in private schools and earned a college degree in business administration. During his junior year in college, he failed to win a scholarship and became morose, sleepless, and nervous for 2 months. A few years after finishing college, he entered an auto sales contest and won first prize, a trip to Hawaii. While on this trip, he became overactive and insisted on eating every meal at the captain's table, where he told obscene stories and embarrassed the women passengers. He participated in frequent brawls with the stewards and complained to the purser on the slightest provocation. On disembarking, he refused to return to his home city. He demanded the most pretentious accommodations at the hotel, and when these were unavailable, he entered into a noisy altercation with the manager that resulted in his being hospitalized because of his behavior. He remained there for 3 months and then returned to his parents' home.

The present attack began about 6 weeks before Maurice sought help. At that time he was engaged in selling real estate in a new subdivision. He became extremely active, arose early, and approached prospective clients at bus terminals, waiting rooms, and hotel corridors. He talked in such a convincing manner that he made a good sales record in the first week. He continued to send in many deposits, bragged about his sales ability, argued noisily with his fellow salesmen, and finally was arrested because he failed to pay his fare on a city bus. He then entered a damage suit against the company for $100,000. The attorney who was approached realized the absurdities of his claims and convinced him to seek help.

Immediately after going to the mental health center, Maurice demanded to see the head physician and requested permission to use the telephone. He was fairly coherent but was circumstantial in his conversation. When asked a simple question, his reply was a long, rambling, digressive account. After being continually reminded to answer the question, he did so, only to return to another long digression.

Although Maurice believed he was being abused, he harbored no other delusional ideas and at no time was confused or hallucinatory. His intellect was keen and his memory, particularly for trivial things, remarkable, but he had no insight into his abnormal exultation and irritability and his judgment was poor. He made unreasonable demands of the personnel at the clinic and, if refused, became abusive, sarcastic, and irritable. At this time it was discovered that when a client had refused to make a down payment on a lot, Maurice had drawn the sum out of his own bank account and had forged a signature on the sales contract. This explained his amazing sales success.

Maurice spent much of his time while in the short-term treatment unit of the mental health clinic writing letters to the mayor, various attorneys, and influential citizens. He wrote on odd pieces of paper with pencil in a broad, sweeping hand, underlining many words and capitalizing others. Every day he

Continued.

NURSING CARE PLAN: *An Overactive Individual—cont'd*

met the physicians at the door of the unit and began to revile them. He particularly enjoyed arguing with the physicians, demanding evidence to prove that he was insane and consistently denying all charges of misbehavior. In a loud voice he promised to have the director of the center removed and the physicians exposed as quacks. He was suggestively lewd in his conversation with all female staff except one young woman to whom he proposed marriage.

Throughout the 4 weeks he spent in the short-term treatment unit, Maurice was the constant focus of commotion, a chronic critic of everything and everybody about him, collecting and hoarding papers, combs, magazines, and all sorts of trash and getting into quarrels with others. Occasionally he was very agreeable and jolly, particularly if he was allowed to do all the talking. On these occasions he was fond of reciting parodies of famous poems in a quick, witty fashion. Some of these he had not quoted since his high-school days.

Nursing Assessment

This client's mother suffered from a midlife depression. Too little is known about this situation to do more than suggest that the mother was unable to give her son the sense of security he required as an infant to develop into a well-adjusted adult. The mother's depression also raises the possibility of this individual having an inherited predisposition to mood disorder.

Maurice H. first experienced a depression at about the age of 21 when he failed to win a scholarship in college. To him this failure to achieve a prized goal represented a failure in life, and he became depressed in an unconscious effort to punish himself. For 2 months he had typical symptoms of a mild depression. He was morose, sleepless, and nervous.

A few years later, Maurice won a coveted prize in an auto sales contest. This award was a trip to Hawaii that eventually resulted in Maurice's hospitalization for 3 months because of his overactivity. In this instance he probably developed anxiety over his company's high expectations. He may have reasoned that they would undoubtedly expect more and bigger sales records from him now that he had been able to achieve the award of a trip. The anxiety about being able to fulfill the future expectations of his company changed into guilt feelings that in turn caused him to feel that somehow he should be punished. To guard against the depressed feelings that arose from a sense of failure and a need to be punished, he developed overactivity and elation, the defense against depression.

Several years later, Maurice once more became involved in a competitive selling activity. His need to succeed started the chain reaction again. Anxiety about succeeding caused him to be concerned about the possibility of failing, and this in turn led to the depressed feelings that accompany a loss. The loss was the anticipated failure in selling, which in his own mind had already occurred. Thus the unconscious defense against depressed feelings was again used. He became expansive, overactive, argumentative, sarcastic, and irritable; made unrea-

NURSING CARE PLAN: *An Overactive Individual—cont'd*

sonable demands; and became a constant center of commotion. In a sense, he did not give himself time to become depressed because he was too busy striking out against his environment.

Typically, Maurice was not delusional and did not experience hallucinations. Thus he was constantly in touch with reality. His intellect was as keen as ever, and his memory was intact.

Some inexperienced people might conclude that this man did not have a mental illness. However, he was unreasonable and sometimes abusive when he did not get his own way. He also wrote letters to outside authorities because he believed he should not be undergoing treatment, and he constantly sought to expose the clinic personnel for their inefficient handling of the situation. He had no insight into his condition, and his judgment was impaired.

Nursing Diagnosis

The assessment data, including present behavior, past experiences, and an understanding of the underlying dynamics, led to the development of the following nursing diagnoses for Maurice H:

High risk for violence: directed at others related to elation and overactivity

Self-care deficit, feeding, related to overactivity

Planning and Implementing Nursing Care

The plan of nursing care developed for Maurice H. is summarized on pp. 301 and 302.

The members of the staff assigned to care for Maurice were chosen carefully because his verbally hostile, physically aggressive behavior was difficult to accept. Not all staff members were able to control their feelings about his vulgar comments or to understand objectively why it was impossible for him to control his behavior. In addition, he related more positively to some individuals than to others. Finally, some staff members enjoyed working with him and others did not. All these factors were considered in the choice of staff to work with him.

The staff decided that it would be best for Maurice to be cared for in a unit of the treatment center where a single room was available. In such a room it was possible to eliminate all but the essential furnishings. The single room was helpful in avoiding the overstimulation that might have resulted from sleeping accommodations where he would have been involved with other clients.

Maurice's recreational activities needed to be controlled because it was obvious that he became loud and disruptive when involved in competitive games. He became angry when he scored lower than other players in a game and accused them of cheating. These accusations usually brought on loud arguments and sometimes fights.

When it was necessary for the staff to intervene in such an altercation, they took advantage of his distractibility. They subtly redirected his attention away from the argument to an activity that could be carried on in his room with one other person who was able to tolerate his rapid conversation and accept his pointed criticism.

Continued.

NURSING CARE PLAN: *An Overactive Individual—cont'd*

The staff members were careful to avoid scolding or threatening Maurice when he initiated fights with other individuals. They avoided comparing his behavior with that of other, better controlled individuals or even with his own behavior on a day when he was less noisy. The staff realized that his problem behavior was part of his illness.

Maurice responded negatively to any staff member who attempted to speak to him somewhat sharply or who commanded him to do anything. They learned that he could not be hurried and that their approach was much more effective if they were quiet, friendly, patient, and courteous to him and used a pleasant, businesslike tone of voice. On one occasion when a staff member did order him to comply with a hospital rule, he refused and did not let the individual forget the incident.

The staff discovered that it was unwise to encourage Maurice when he was reciting or singing parodies or telling jokes. When some staff members did laugh at his jokes, he became much louder and more ribald. It was necessary for them to intervene by accompanying him to his room before he became so excited that he lost control.

In talking to this man, the staff avoided getting into long, complicated discussions or giving elaborate explanations. Instead, short sentences with specific, straightforward responses to his questions seemed to satisfy him and avoid arguments.

The staff members were careful when praising Maurice. They found that he sometimes turned the words of praise around and used them in a different context to refute a point they had been trying to make with him some time previously.

They were aware of his physical needs and realized that he frequently did not eat enough. This problem arose because his attention was distracted from the food or he left the dining room early before finishing the meal. Likewise, he sometimes had dry, cracked lips because he failed to maintain his fluid intake. Maurice was weighed every week, and when his weight had dropped below a desired point for 2 consecutive weeks, his food was served in his room on a tray. A staff member remained with him during the meal and encouraged him to eat. Removing him from the dining room eliminated the many distracting features present in a group. At the same time, Maurice was placed on a schedule so that fluids were offered to him every hour.

Crayons, paper, and pencils were made available to him in his room, and he was encouraged to write and sketch there in the hope that these more sedentary activities would lessen his hyperactivity. The staff members were careful to explain to him in an honest, straightforward manner why he was not encouraged to join the rest of the clients in the dining room. Likewise, all other restrictions on his behavior were explained so that he could understand the reason for them and realize that he was not being rejected as a person.

Evaluation

After receiving the prescribed amount of the medication lithium carbonate for 2 weeks, Maurice gained some control of his

NURSING CARE PLAN: *An Overactive Individual—cont'd*

behavior and became quieter and more amenable to suggestion. The professional staff did not believe that he was well enough to leave the hospital permanently. However, at the request of his mother, he was allowed to go home at the end of 4 weeks with the understanding that he would continue taking lithium carbonate for 1 year and have the

blood levels of this medication checked weekly by a physician.

Although the nurse who had primary responsibility for this client's nursing care continuously reassessed his behavior, she did not engage in a complete evaluation because Maurice was discharged after 4 weeks.

NURSING CARE PLAN FOR MAURICE H.

Nursing diagnosis	Objective (rationale)	Nursing interventions	Outcome criteria
High risk for violence: directed toward others related to elation and overactivity	Client will not injure himself or staff. Client will control his hostile language and physical aggressiveness. (Protection of client and others from client's destructive activity is necessary to ensure safety and prevent social alienation.)	Administer prescribed medication; observe carefully for signs of lithium toxicity. Arrange for daily blood work and check results against norms. Carefully select three staff members to work with client per shift. Reduce all environmental stimuli by: Assigning client to single room Avoiding competitive games Providing activities for client in his room Do not interrupt when client is singing or reciting. Ignore client's jokes. Speak in calm, direct manner using simple short sentences. Do not argue.	Within 4 weeks, client: Talks with one other person for 15 minutes without sarcasm or hostility. Does not attempt to hit other clients or staff unless provoked.

Continued.

NURSING CARE PLAN FOR MAURICE H.—cont'd

Nursing diagnosis	Objective (rationale)	Nursing interventions	Outcome criteria
Self-care deficit, feeding, related to overactivity	Client will be adequately nourished and hydrated. (Adequate food and fluids are essential to promote physiological stability.)	In addition to meals, provide high-calorie nutritional snacks that can be eaten standing or walking, such as milk shake and hamburgers. Offer 6 ounces water or juice every hour. Weigh weekly. Observe for signs of dehydration. Feed in room if client is unable to stay in dining room long enough to finish meal.	Within 1 week, client: Shows signs of adequate hydration. Consumes sufficient calories to avoid weight loss.

KEY POINTS

1. Depressive disorders and bipolar disorder are two types of mood disorders.

2. The cause of mood disorders is believed to be an interaction of multiple, complex biological and psychosocial factors.

3. Antidepressant medications have replaced electroconvulsive therapy as the primary medical treatment for individuals who are depressed.

4. Electroconvulsive therapy is still used for selected individuals who have not improved after an adequate trial of antidepressant medications or who are actively suicidal.

5. Assessment of the individual who is depressed reveals psychomotor retardation, pessimism, lack of self-care, despair, suicidal thoughts, low self-esteem, physical complaints, and feelings of helplessness and hopelessness.

6. Increasing the individual's self-esteem is the central objective of all nursing care for the client who is depressed.

7. Self-destructive tendencies in the client who is depressed are probably treated most effectively by developing a safe, supportive environment.

8. Assessment of individuals who are elated and overactive reveals constant movement, poor judgment, euphoria, excessive talking, irritability, hyperalertness, malnourishment, and the feeling of being all powerful.

9. Protecting the individual and others from the client's overactive behavior is the goal of all nursing care for the person who is elated and overactive.

10. When the euphoria of overactive clients turns to irritability and anger, it is most important for the nurse to know how to prevent destructive, threatening behavior.

SUGGESTED SOURCES OF ADDITIONAL INFORMATION

Abraham IL and others: Depression: nursing implications of a clinical and social problem, *Nurs Clin North Am* 26:527, September 1991.

Akiskal H, Tashjian R: Affective disorders. II. Recent advances in laboratory and pathogenic approaches, *Hosp Community Psychiatr* 34(9):822, 1983.

Akiskal H, Webb W: Affective disorders. I. Recent advances in clinical conceptualization, *Hosp Community Psychiatry* 34(8):695, 1983.

Assey J: The suicide prevention contract, *Perspect Psychiatr Care* 23(3):99, 1985.

Blythe M, Pearlmutter D: The suicide watch: a re-examination of maximum observation, *Perspect Psychiatr Care* 21:90, July/September 1983.

Brenners DK, Harris B, Wetson PS: Managing manic behavior, *Am J Nurs* 87:620, May 1987.

Buckwalter KC, Babich KS: Psychologic and physiologic aspects of depression, *Nurs Clin North Am* 25:945, December 1990.

Busteed E, Johnstone C: The development of suicide precautions for an inpatient psychiatric unit, *J Psychosoc Nurs Ment Health Serv* 21:15, May 1983.

Bydlon-Brown B, Billman R: At risk for suicide, *Am J Nurs* 88:1358, October 1988.

Calarco MM, Krone KP: An integrated nursing model of depressive behavior in adults: theory and implications for practice, *Nurs Clin North Am* 26:573, September 1991.

Campbell L: CE depression: acute care in the hospital, *Am J Nurs* 86:288, March 1986.

Capodanno A, Targum S: Assessment of suicide risk: some limitations in the prediction of infrequent events, *J Psychosoc Nurs Ment Heath Serv* 21:11, May 1983.

Crockett MS: CE depression: a case of anger and alienation, *Am J Nurs* 86:294, March 1986.

Field W: Physical causes of depression, *J Psychosoc Nurs Ment Health Serv* 23:6, October 1985.

Harris E: CE lithium: in a class by itself, *Am J Nurs* 89:190, February 1989.

Hauenstein EJ: Young women and depression: origin, outcome, and nursing care, *Nurs Clin North Am* 26:601, September 1991.

Keltner NL, Folks DG: Psychopharmacology update: alternatives to lithium in the treatment of bipolar disorder, *Perspect Psychiatr Care* 27(2):36, 1991.

Lahaie U: Seasonal affective disorder, *Can J Psychiatr Nurs* 9, January-March 1990.

Maurer F: Acute depression treatment and nursing strategies for this affective disorder, *Nurs Clin North Am* 21:413, September 1986.

McEnany GW: Managing mood disorders, *RN* 28, September 1990.

McEnany GW: Psychobiological indices of bipolar mood disorder: future trends in nursing care, *Arch Psychiatr Nurs* 4:29, February 1990.

Minot SR: CE depression: what does it mean? *Am J Nurs* 86:284, March 1986.

Schlesser M, Altshuler K: The genetics of affective disorder: data, theory, and clinical application, *Hosp Community Psychiatry* 34(5):415, 1983.

Simmons-Alling S: New approaches to managing affective disorders, *Arch Psychiatr Nurs* 1:219, August 1987.

Thomas MD, Sanger E, Whitney JD: Nursing diagnosis of depression, *J Psychosoc Nurs Ment Health Serv* 24:6, August 1986.

Vogel P: Lithium and the thyroid, *J Psychosoc Nurs Ment Health Serv* 24:8, February 1986.

Wright J, Beck A: Cognitive therapy of depression: theory and practice, *Hosp Community Psychiatry* 34(12):1119, 1983.

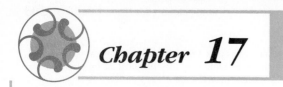

Chapter *17*

Individuals with Anxiety Disorders

LEARNING OBJECTIVES

After studying this chapter, the student will be able to:

* Describe the symptoms exhibited by a person with the medical diagnosis of anxiety disorder, somatoform disorder, or dissociative disorder.

* Discuss the causative factors associated with anxiety disorders.

* State the desired effects, side effects, and adverse effects of anxiolytic medications.

* Discuss the treatment technique of psychotherapy.

* Describe behaviors the nurse is most likely to observe in an individual experiencing an anxiety disorder.

* State examples of nursing diagnoses likely to be applicable to an individual who is experiencing an anxiety disorder.

* State and explain nursing interventions likely to be effective with an individual who is experiencing an anxiety disorder.

* Develop a hypothetical plan of nursing care for an individual who is experiencing an anxiety disorder.

KEY TERMS

Anxiety disorders
Panic disorders
Phobia
Agoraphobia
Social phobia
Simple phobia
Obsession
Compulsion
Obsessive-compulsive disorder
Posttraumatic stress disorder (PTSD)
Generalized anxiety disorder
Somatoform disorders
Dissociative disorders
Anxiolytic
Supportive psychotherapy
Uncovering or insight psychotherapy
Mental ventilation
Desensitization
Transference
Countertransference

Most people live normal, relatively anxiety-free lives by successfully adapting to stress and its resultant anxiety through the use of various strategies and compromises, both conscious and unconscious. Nevertheless, there is a large group of individuals for whom these defenses are not effective. In fact, data recently released by the National Institute of Mental Health indicate that during any 6-month period, 8.3% of the U.S. population has an anxiety disorder. These persons must continually focus on activities and behaviors designed to control intolerable anxiety in an unsuccessful effort to achieve a state of physical and emotional homeokinesis. In the past this group of individuals has been labeled "neurotic" by both the health care delivery system and the lay public. This term has been replaced by the more descriptive phrase **anxiety disorders.**

Because individuals with anxiety disorders are in touch with reality and often recognize the inappropriateness of their behavior, many nurses have difficulty accepting them as persons in need of health care. To achieve a more understanding attitude toward these individuals, it is important to develop some knowledge about the emotional conflicts with which they struggle and the ways in which they use symptoms to cope with the anxiety that stems from these conflicts (Figure 17-1).

HISTORICAL PERSPECTIVE

Although the emotion of anxiety has been recognized since ancient Greek times, the disorders stemming directly from an inability to adapt to stress and the subsequent anxiety were not brought into focus until the early twentieth century. At that time Sigmund Freud (1856-1939) identified the role anxiety plays in the unconscious life of the individual and demonstrated how it affects the person's perception of reality and subsequent behavior.

During the Victorian era in which Freud practiced, many women had a condition called *hysteria*. This malady manifested itself by unexplain-

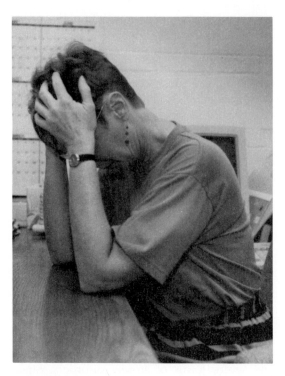

Figure 17-1
Persons suffering from anxiety sometimes need help to overcome their emotional conflicts.

able fatigue and weakness, "swooning," and other forms of dramatic behavior. Today these persons would be diagnosed as having a dysfunction stemming from overwhelming anxiety. Freud developed the technique of psychoanalysis, through which he helped these patients to explore their unconscious minds for the emotional conflicts that were expressed in these symptoms. He discovered that the nature of these conflicts frequently centered on real or fantasized aggressive sexual acts. Given the culture of the day in which women were expected to assume a passive, dependent role, they understandably had little opportunity to resolve these conflicts, which were expressed by symptoms indicative of passivity and dependency.

The manifestations of anxiety disorders have changed over the years. It is rare today to encounter an individual who exhibits the classic symptoms of hysteria, although phobic disorders are common. This change in symptomatology has led authorities to believe that the specific behaviors unconsciously chosen by the individual to express emotional conflict are determined in part by societal sanctions. For example, fainting at the sight of blood would not be culturally acceptable today, but an inordinate and irrational fear of heights evokes sympathy in this age of skyscrapers and jet travel.

The incidence of dysfunctions related to overwhelming anxiety has also greatly increased over the last three decades. Unquestionably this increase is related to the increased stress associated with the highly complex, postindustrial society in which we live. In fact, the last half of the twentieth century is often called "the age of anxiety."

Only persons with the severest form of anxiety disorders have ever been hospitalized. Therefore, until recently, nurses have not had much experience in providing care for individuals with less severe forms of anxiety disorders. Since mental health care has moved into the community, however, nurses now have the opportunity and the challenge of intervening therapeutically with these individuals on an outpatient basis.

ANXIETY DISORDERS

Anxiety disorders are characterized by symptoms of extreme anxiety and avoidance behavior. The DSM-III-R categorizes these disorders into seven main groups: panic disorders, with or without agoraphobia; agoraphobia; social phobia; simple phobia; obsessive-compulsive disorder; posttraumatic stress disorder (PTSD); and generalized anxiety disorder. The proposed revisions in the DSM-IV (see Appendix B) differentiate between panic disorder and panic attack, change the term "simple phobia" to "specific phobia," and add three diagnoses: acute stress disorder, anxiety disorder due to a general medical condition, and substance-induced anxiety disorder. These changes and additions are de-

signed to reflect more accurately the clinical symptoms exhibited by persons with anxiety disorders.

Panic disorders are characterized by recurrent attacks of intense fear or discomfort that may or may not be obviously associated with a situation consciously perceived as anxiety provoking by the individual. Symptoms experienced during an attack are shortness of breath or smothering sensations; dizziness, unsteady feelings, or faintness; choking; palpitations or accelerated heart rate; trembling or shaking; sweating; nausea or abdominal distress; hot flashes or chills; chest pain or discomfort; fear of dying; and fear of going crazy or of doing something uncontrolled during the attack.

A **phobia** is a specific pathological fear reaction out of proportion to the stimulus. The painful feeling has been automatically and unconsciously displaced from its original internal source and has become attached to a specific external object or situation. The phobia may be focused on anything that in some manner suggests death, disease, or disaster.

Agoraphobia is a fear of open spaces. The incidence of its occurrence is increasing. The individual manifests agoraphobia by expressing dread at being left alone or going out of the home. The person avoids crowds and public places because he or she anticipates some dreadful form of collapse. Agoraphobia is particularly incapacitating because it greatly interferes with the individual's ability to live a normal life.

Social phobia is a persistent fear of any group situation in which persons believe they are the focus of attention and in which they fear they will act in a way that will be humiliating or embarrassing. The most common social phobia is the fear of public speaking. Individuals who have this fear often are terrified that they will collapse in front of the audience or will become mute.

Simple (or specific) **phobia** is characterized by a persistent fear of a specific object or situation. The person may fear open places, narrow corridors, small rooms, running water, staircases, high places, various animals, or any other specific object or situation. When exposed to the feared object or situation, the individual immediately responds with symptoms of overwhelming anxiety, which disappear just as quickly when the person is removed from the object or situation. Therefore this person goes to great lengths to avoid such exposure.

An **obsession** is an undesired but persistent thought or idea that is forced into conscious awareness. The thought is charged with great but unconscious emotional significance. Such a thought may include repetitive doubts, wishes, fears, impulses, admonitions, and commands. A **compulsion** is an unwanted urge to perform an act or a ritual that is contrary to the individual's ordinary conscious wishes or standards. All these intrusive ideas and compelling urges and fears appear in consciousness as though independently self-created.

The individual with an **obsessive-compulsive disorder** is driven to think about or to do something that the person recognizes as being inappropriate or foolish. Persons have an excessive preoccupation with a single idea or a compulsion to carry out and to repeat over and over again certain acts against their better judgment. Underlying these compulsive or obsessive states is a personality that is usually conscience driven, sensitive, shy, meticulous, and precise about bodily functions, dress, religious duty, and daily routine. Obsessive-compulsive disorder is a serious emotional illness because the imperative ideas so control individuals that they become slaves to their morbid preoccupation and can scarcely carry on their normal work and social activity.

Posttraumatic stress disorder (PTSD) is characterized by the reexperiencing of the terror associated with a psychologically distressing event experienced at an earlier time in the person's life. The nature of this event is always one outside the range of common human experiences, such as war, natural disaster, rape, or other unusual situations that threaten the survival of the person or loved ones. The flashbacks of the experience and the accompanying terror are often precipitated by a stimulus linked to the original event. For example, the backfiring of an automobile can reawaken the anxiety originally experienced when the individual served in the military. This disorder was highly publicized in the late 1970s and early 1980s, since many Vietnam veterans were afflicted with it.

Generalized anxiety disorder is characterized by unrealistic or excessive anxiety and worry about two or more life circumstances that are usually developmentally determined. For example, a middle-aged parent may be consumed with fear that he will become bankrupt and that he will not live to see his child graduate from college. In contrast, adolescents may be unrealistically anxious about their performance in sports, extracurricular activities, or academics.

Although they are not anxiety disorders, a brief description of somatoform disorders and dissociative disorders is included here because they occur as dysfunctional adaptations to anxiety.

SOMATOFORM DISORDERS

Most **somatoform disorders** are characterized by the presence of long-standing, generalized physical symptoms in the absence of demonstrable organic pathology. These include *body dysmorphic disorder,* in which a person who is normal in appearance has a preoccupation with some imagined defect in appearance, such as the shape or size of the nose; *hypochondriasis,* in which the individual is preoccupied with the fear of having, or the belief that he or she has, a serious disease, as a result of numerous vague physical symptoms; *somatization disorder,* in which the person seeks constant medical attention for treatment of recurrent and multiple somatic complaints not caused by any physical disorder; and conversion disorder.

Conversion disorder is an example of a somatoform disorder. This is a purposeful although unconscious psychological mode of reaction in which the individual uses a physical symptom as a disguise in an attempt to solve some acute problem or fulfill some desire, the open or conscious gratification of which is unacceptable to the individual. Conversion represents a primitive instinctual mechanism to which a person resorts when he or she is incapable of adjusting through the usual methods of rational volitional activity.

The person who uses a conversion disorder unconsciously selects a set of symptoms that symbolizes the problems. These symptoms are dictated by suggestion or by some previous acquaintance with persons who had the actual problem. Paralysis, blindness, and epilepsy are afflictions frequently affecting the person using conversion. The symptoms are physical, but no underlying pathophysiology can be demonstrated.

No matter what form the symptoms take, a characteristic feature of conversion is the individual's attitude of indifference toward the handicaps. An air of contentment seems to surround individuals with conversion disorder. They seem to be more relieved than distressed, an attitude that at once suggests that they are more comfortable with the physical problem than with the mental torment.

DISSOCIATIVE DISORDERS

Dissociative disorders are characterized by a disturbance or alteration in the functions of identity, memory, or consciousness, all of which are normally integrated in the healthy individual. The most dramatic dissociative disorder is multiple personality disorder.

Multiple personality disorder is characterized by the existence within the person of two or more distinct personalities, each of which recurrently takes control of the person's behavior. Each personality is distinct unto itself, often representing opposite attitudes and behaviors. This disorder is believed to be caused by violent trauma in early childhood, probably sexual in nature, which resulted in massive anxiety that threatened to destroy the individual. As a defense, the individual "split off" parts of the personality.

Not surprisingly, multiple personality disorder occurs predominantly, although not exclusively, in women and is now thought to be more common than previously believed. It is unusual for the person to have only two personalities; the typical female has 13 to 15, and the typical male has five to eight personalities.

Each personality may or may not be aware of some or all of the other personalities. Consequently, each is likely to be unable to account for periods of time during which the other personalities were in control.

Multiple personality disorder has been brought to the attention of the public through various case histories published as books. The best known of these are *The Three Faces of Eve* and *Sibyl*. Unfortunately, this disorder is often incorrectly associated with schizophrenia by the lay person.

CAUSATIVE FACTORS

No specific causative factor of anxiety disorders has been identified. Nevertheless, an increasing amount of research indicates the probability that a physiological or neurochemical predisposition is associated with the development of anxiety disorders. Some authorities hypothesize that a genetic hyperactivity occurs in the central noradrenergic system. This view is supported by a significant incidence of anxiety disorders occurring in close relatives of those with such a disorder.

Because individuals with an anxiety disorder characteristically believe their symptoms are indicative of an impending catastrophe, some theorists believe that a cognitive dysfunction exists.

Specifically, it is theorized that the individual has learned to interpret normal increases in autonomic function as abnormal. For example, an increase in heart rate is perceived by the person with an anxiety disorder as evidence of an impending heart attack.

Behaviorists believe that the person associates increased anxiety with the situation or site in which the anxiety first occurred. The person then subsequently generalizes this experience to other situations or sites that are the same or similar, either symbolically or in reality.

Psychodynamically oriented authorities postulate that the anxiety disorder represents a conflict between two divergent drives or desires that have been repressed into the unconscious mind. This conflict is believed to represent primitive impulses unacceptable to the person and the simultaneous need for acceptance by significant others. This conflict does not necessarily cause difficulty as long as the individual has sufficient psychic energy to keep it repressed. However, when energy is diverted by the necessity to cope with other stressors, the ego can no longer effect a compromise between these clashing desires, and anxiety threatens to become conscious. At this point, symptoms develop as an adaptation to the emergent anxiety. This theory helps to explain why symptomatology often first appears during adolescence, when the individual must adapt to potent developmental stressors. In addition, the emergent, tumultuous sexuality of adolescence activates repressed, unresolved sexual conflicts.

It is believed the symptoms of anxiety disorders are designed simultaneously to alleviate the anxiety and to obscure the nature of the conflict. Thus the symptoms are socially acceptable symbols of the original conflict. For example, the compulsive handwasher is conscious of his irrational fear of germs but is totally unaware of his unconscious sexual longing for his mother. By compulsively washing his hands 10 times after toileting, he experiences relief from the anxiety

caused by his conflict. Unfortunately, this relief is only temporary because his action did not directly address the source of the anxiety. Thus the ritual must be repeated at frequent intervals.

The wide range of theories that attempt to explain the development of anxiety disorders illustrates the inseparability of the human system and the fallacy of seeking a singular cause for these disorders.

MEDICAL TREATMENT
Anxiolytic medications

The word **anxiolytic** refers to the ability to relieve anxiety or simple emotional tension. Unfortunately, anxiolytic medications are often referred to as *minor tranquilizers*. This term is misleading in that these medications do not have a tranquilizing effect but are potent chemical agents that have a major effect on the body chemistry. The false belief that anxiolytic medications are minor tranquilizers undoubtedly has led to their being inappropriately prescribed for individuals who do not have a mental illness but who are experiencing the anxiety associated with crisis states. These medications often are abused by individuals who seek relief from anxiety. This practice is dangerous because these medications not only create a physiological disequilibrium but may also create a false sense of well-being, decreasing the person's motivation to address and solve those problems from which the anxiety stems.

Anxiolytic medications are most appropriately used to (1) treat individuals with delirium tremens, (2) relieve anxiety in individuals experiencing moderate situational stress (e.g., preoperatively), (3) potentiate anticonvulsant medications, (4) relieve muscle spasm, and (5) reduce high to moderate levels of endogenous anxiety to a moderate or mild level, rendering the client able to benefit from psychotherapy.

All anxiolytic medications have the potential for creating physical and emotional dependence.

Withdrawal symptoms similar to those experienced following withdrawal from barbiturates and alcohol have occurred following abrupt discontinuation of these medications, especially diazepam. Therefore the dosage of the drug should be gradually tapered before its discontinuation, especially with clients who have taken large doses of anxiolytic medications over an extended time.

Anxiolytic medications have a limited number of side effects. Sedation occurs when large doses are given, and the client needs to be warned not to engage in activities that require complete mental alertness. Ataxia is occasionally observed. Adverse effects occur infrequently; the most serious are those in which a paradoxical reaction in the form of acute excitement, anxiety, hallucinations, increased muscle spasticity, insomnia, or rage occurs. The medication should be discontinued if these symptoms appear.

Psychotherapy

Unquestionably, anxiolytic medications have been helpful in reducing tension and providing the client with a degree of emotional comfort. Behavior modification and desensitization also are recognized as efficient and effective intervention techniques. In addition to these interventions, many persons can be helped to understand the source of their symptoms through the treatment technique of psychotherapy. Psychotherapy can be conducted by any prepared mental health professional. As nurses gain additional knowledge and skill in this treatment modality, they sometimes assume responsibility for its implementation.

Any procedure that promotes the development of courage, inner security, and self-confidence can be called psychotherapy. However, the traditional use of this term is limited to sustained interpersonal interactions between the psychotherapist and client in which the goal is to help the client to develop behaviors that are more functional. Psychotherapy is not a fixed technique; it is more an art than a science, and its

methods must be adapted and modified to fit the individual situation. In plain language, it is a form of mental exploration. It is universally acknowledged that one cannot standardize psychotherapy, that it must be individualized, and that it will vary from client to client.

Psychotherapy falls into two general types: supportive psychotherapy and "uncovering" or "insight" psychotherapy. **Supportive psychotherapy** helps the individual cope with problems and includes such techniques as diagnosis, advice, education, guidance, counseling, and assurance. **Uncovering or insight psychotherapy** involves exploring and bringing to consciousness the source of repressed and suppressed conflicts and experiences that operate at unconscious levels to cause anxiety. Uncovering psychotherapy gives meaning to abnormal or irrational feelings and dysfunctional behaviors.

The type of psychotherapy used depends on the therapist's assessment of the interrelationship of several variables. Chief among these variables are the extent and severity of the client's dysfunction, the client's goals, intellectual ability, and personal and interpersonal resources. Generally, clients with little ego strength, few resources, and limited intellectual capability are candidates for supportive psychotherapy. Supportive psychotherapy requires the psychotherapist to assume a direct role by offering direction and guidance. Clients may not develop an understanding of the dynamics underlying their behavior, but they can learn behaviors that are more functional.

Clients who give evidence of available ego strength, a viable support system, and at least average intelligence can often benefit from uncovering or insight psychotherapy. During this type of psychotherapy, clients are encouraged to talk about their life experiences. They are encouraged to talk freely about anything that comes to mind, as long as they relate their own ideas and concerns. This random talk allows the client to follow freely the associations that come to mind and is accurately described as **mental ven-**

tilation. The therapist will note that the client dismisses quickly or avoids mentioning certain occasions and events except in a superficial way. These sensitive areas are then explored more fully. The client is encouraged to talk about them freely until they no longer cause excess emotion, a process known as **desensitization.**

The client is guided to an understanding of how repressed feelings are related to his or her behavior. This is done in a simple, clear style, thereby helping the client to gain insight into the exact nature of the problem. Thus the process of reeducation begins.

It should be noted that a client who initially requires supportive psychotherapy may be able to increase self-esteem to the point where uncovering or insight psychotherapy is indicated. A skilled psychotherapist has the ability to make this assessment and to respond accordingly.

Regardless of the type of psychotherapy employed, clients are encouraged to face their distressing problems; they are urged to think of them instead of running away from them, to become familiar with them rather than to "forget" them, and to approach their solution in a candid, open manner. Clients are encouraged to take an active part in their own therapy. If all goes well, clients should take more and more constructive steps in the management of their own treatment. They can then answer some of their questions and make their own decisions. Therapists measure therapeutic success by the degree to which they make themselves less and less necessary.

The most important element in any psychotherapeutic process is the relationship between the therapist and the client. The client must have confidence in the therapist and some respect for the therapist's knowledge and experience. A word of assurance alone may be the deciding factor in relieving many anxious clients of their fears. Such a relationship depends on a positive rapport between the therapist and the client.

A very important aspect of the therapist-client relationship is the unconscious attitude of the client toward the therapist. The therapist is cast into a variety of roles, including that of a parent. The client's attitude may be competitive or even erotic. This shifting toward the therapist of desires, feelings, and relations originally experienced by the client with his or her own parents, siblings, and other persons is known as **transference.** Therefore, every nuance of feeling, ranging from trustful dependence to open hostility, may be directed toward the therapist. When the client's attitude toward the therapist appears to be favorable, the transference is regarded as being positive. Resistant or antagonistic attitudes of the client toward the therapist imply a negative transference. The client's transference reaction to the therapist may elicit an unconscious counterresponse by the therapist. This attitude of the therapist toward the client is called **countertransference.**

The development of a transference reaction between the client and the psychotherapist is often viewed as a positive sign, since it indicates that the therapist has become significant to the client, thereby establishing the potential for the client to benefit from a corrective emotional experience. For example, if clients respond to the psychotherapist in the clinging, dependent manner that they learned in early life was necessary to maintain their mother's love, the psychotherapist can subtly but consistently encourage clients to make their own decisions while still conveying approval. Through this process clients can learn that they can take steps toward independence without jeopardizing the highly valued relationship with the psychotherapist. Clients may or may not be helped to become aware of their transference reaction and the process engaged in by the therapist to use the transference therapeutically.

A countertransference reaction is rarely, if ever, seen as having therapeutic potential except as it provides the therapist with an understanding of the psychodynamics underlying the client's behavior. In other words, by becoming aware of personal reactions to the client, the therapist can better understand the unconscious purpose of the client's behavioral patterns. An example of a nontherapeutic countertransference is when the client behaves toward the psychotherapist as if the therapist were the parent (transference), and the psychotherapist unconsciously responds by treating the client as if he or she were a child for whom all decisions need to be made (countertransference). Since both transference and countertransference occur on an unconscious level, and since countertransference is not desired, many teachers of psychotherapy require their students to undergo psychotherapy themselves as a means of discovering their own emotional vulnerabilities and increasing their own overall level of self-awareness. Whether or not a psychotherapist has undergone personal psychotherapy, supervision of psychotherapy by a skilled colleague is necessary to identify and prevent countertransference. The occurrence of the transference and countertransference phenomena is a testimony to the fundamentally human nature of the psychotherapeutic process.

In summary, the success of the psychotherapeutic process depends to a large extent on the quality of the interpersonal experience between the client and the therapist. The therapy can be a success only if the therapist succeeds in motivating clients toward promoting their own well-being on their own behalf rather than to please another person.

NURSING CARE OF INDIVIDUALS WITH AN ANXIETY DISORDER

Nursing assessment

Although each anxiety disorder has its unique features, it is possible to cite some commonalities about the behavior of all persons with typical anxiety disorders. For purposes of clarity, behaviors of persons with anxiety disorders are discussed by categories. Although behaviors in each category are presented as separate entities, they are highly interrelated and are adaptations to similar stressors. Further, behavior designed as an adaptation to one stressor often becomes a stressor itself in another dimension.

Health perception—health management

The individual with an anxiety disorder almost always has many physical complaints that are generally focused on the vital organs of the body. Tightness of the stomach, fast-beating heart, a feeling that the heart may suddenly stop, no appetite, loose bowels, and a heavy feeling in the abdomen are frequent complaints of the individual seeking assistance. Palpitation, a feeling of shortness of breath, compression sensations in the head, tight sensations in the throat, numbness in the extremities, and a constant feeling of exhaustion are other typical experiences reported by individuals with anxiety disorders. These symptoms usually frighten such persons; they cannot concentrate on work, feel depressed, and harbor fears of sudden death or insanity. Frequently, many of these symptoms appear at one time and cause the individual to respond with a panic reaction or acute fear. Consequently, anxiety about the anxiety compounds the stress.

CLINICAL EXAMPLE

Cynthia is a 35-year-old assistant professor of history who is finishing her doctoral dissertation. She has worked on the doctoral degree for the past 6½ years and is near completion of the dissertation. Yesterday she received a form letter from the dean of the graduate school informing her that she had only one semester left to complete the requirements for the degree. Knowing she was almost finished with her dissertation, Cynthia gave little thought to the letter. This morning she awoke with massive anxiety, a pounding heart, difficulty in breathing, and chest pains. She was sure she was having a heart attack and called her physician, who instructed her to go immediately to the local emergency room. By the time Cynthia arrived at the hospital, her symptoms had subsided. She told the triage nurse she had had these symptoms before when she looked down from a high place and now copes with her terror of heights by staying away from such places.

Activity-exercise

The motor behavior of the individual with an anxiety disorder may or may not be altered. However, individuals who are highly anxious often exhibit motor restlessness in the forms of pacing and wringing of their hands. Persons with obsessive-compulsive disorder often display ritualistic behaviors in which an activity is repeated in exactly the same manner for a specified number of times. For example, to be at work on time, one business executive arose 3 hours earlier than necessary because she was compelled to return to her house from her car 10 times to check that every window was closed and locked.

The individual with an anxiety disorder often does not voluntarily engage in recreational activities because of emotional and physical fatigue and an inability to control the environment in which the activity takes place. One avid baseball player who developed a phobia about dogs had to stop playing ball completely because of his fear that a dog would wander onto the field and send him into a panic.

Self-care may or may not be affected, but it is always altered when the focus of the anxiety relates to a self-care activity. For example, an individual who is phobic about running water must go to great lengths to bathe from a basin rather than taking a shower.

Home maintenance is often altered. Since the individual with an anxiety disorder is chronically fatigued, altered home maintenance may be reflected by a disorderly, dirty environment. In other cases the person is driven to maintain an immaculately clean and tidy environment in an effort to ward off anxiety resulting from a phobia about dirt or germs.

Sleep-rest

Regardless of the severity of the anxiety experienced, the person will almost always report changes in sleep patterns. Usually the anxious individual has great difficulty falling asleep but, once asleep, has difficulty arising in the morning. Regardless of the amount of sleep, the individual reports constant fatigue.

Cognitive-perceptual

The individual with an anxiety disorder maintains contact with reality. In fact, this characteristic serves as a stressor, since persons are often well aware that their fears and behavior are not based on reality and that they may appear foolish to others.

Individuals experiencing obsessive-compulsive disorder will report the existence of one or more obsessive thoughts that torment them and over which they believe they have no control.

The individual with an anxiety disorder often exhibits a hyperalertness to environmental stimuli. The person is easily startled by an unexpected movement and experiences increased anxiety when unable to control the events in the environment.

Self-perception/self-concept

The outstanding feature of anxiety disorders is the individual's awareness of anxiety, either continuously or in response to a specific object or situation. The person will report overwhelming feelings of impending doom. These feelings are so distressing that the individual will go to any length to avoid or diminish them. In extreme situations, individuals have been known to attempt suicide, not for the purpose of ending their lives, but rather with the goal of relieving their anxiety.

CLINICAL EXAMPLE

April is a 27-year-old manager in a nationally known company. She had joined this company immediately after her graduation from college and had worked many long hours to achieve her present position. April developed an anxiety disorder 2 years ago. She routinely takes prescribed anxiolytic medication and is engaged in psychotherapy with a psychiatrist. Last week April's boss asked her to take a 2-week trip across the United States to learn how another branch office was handling a particular production problem. April had never flown before, but she did not share this information with anyone at work because she feared they would think she was too immature and inexperienced to keep her job. On the scheduled day, April took a 3-hour flight and arrived safely at her hotel. However, she was tired and somewhat disoriented because of the time change. Even though the local time was only 4 PM, April ate dinner and went to bed. She awoke at midnight in an acute anxiety attack with a compulsion to jump from the window of her tenth-floor room.

Helplessness, hopelessness, and powerlessness over the symptoms associated with the anxiety disorder are often reported by the client. When the symptoms are severe, individuals may attempt to relieve their anxiety by engaging in behaviors normally outside their value system. For example, many anxious individuals attempt to self-medicate by drinking alcohol, which may provide some temporary relief from anxiety. If the person's value system dictates abstinence from alcohol, resorting to this measure further compounds the anxiety.

The self-esteem of persons with an anxiety disorder is often low because they believe they should be able to control their behavioral and emotional responses to anxiety-producing stimuli, although they are simultaneously aware that they are incapable of doing so. Consequently, they are likely to be self-critical and report that they are "weak" and have little self-control or self-discipline.

Role-relationship

The interpersonal relationships of persons with anxiety disorders are frequently strained. Family and friends have had much experience in attempting to reassure the client, all to no avail. Furthermore, they may have had increasing difficulty tolerating the person's idiosyncratic ways. For example, one middle-aged secretary with a fear of germs was forced to share an office with several others in a typing pool. She offended her co-workers by covering her coffee mug with plastic wrap between sips to protect its contents from germs in the air. She also scrupulously cleaned her typewriter keys with a strong disinfectant

every morning in case someone had touched them in her absence. When this woman's rituals became so time-consuming that she was unable to complete her assigned work, her job was threatened and she sought help from the local mental health clinic.

Nursing diagnosis

As with all nursing diagnoses, the nursing diagnoses for the individual with an anxiety disorder are based on the themes identified during the assessment phase of the nursing process.

Accepted NANDA nursing diagnoses that may be specifically applicable to the individual with an anxiety disorder include:

Fatigue
Diversional activity deficit
Impaired home maintenance management
Sleep pattern disturbance
Knowledge deficit (specify)
Altered thought processes
Decisional conflict (specify)
Fear
Anxiety
Hopelessness
Powerlessness
Self-esteem disturbance; situational low self-esteem; chronic low self-esteem
Altered role performance
Impaired social interaction
Ineffective individual coping
Defensive coping

To develop a nursing diagnosis that fulfills its function of providing direction for planning nursing care, the nurse is encouraged to postulate and state etiological or antecedent factors and connect the two phrases by using the term "related to." For example:

Diversional activity deficit related to fear of going outdoors

Planning and implementing nursing care

The plan for nursing care is derived from the nursing diagnoses and includes the objectives of the care, the nursing interventions, and outcome criteria. To be effective, the plan needs to be highly individualized. The suggestions that follow should be seen as general guidelines to be used if they are appropriate to the client's needs.

In general, the objectives of all nursing care for the individual with an anxiety disorder should relate to helping the client lower anxiety and/or to develop functional adaptations to the anxiety.

Since the client's nursing diagnoses are often interrelated, stemming as they do from similar etiologies or antecedents, the student should see that the appropriate nursing interventions are also interrelated. In other words, by intervening in one dimension, the nurse will also affect other dimensions.

Many health professionals who work skillfully and empathically with psychotic individuals find that they are not nearly so effective when giving care to those who express anxiety through physical symptoms or ritualistic behavior. Much of the difficulty in dealing with anxious persons originates in an unconscious attitude toward persons with these problems and in a failure to understand the true nature of the illness. Because such individuals are aware of their surroundings, are not carrying on a conversation with unseen people, and complain of physical symptoms that have no organic basis, some professionals may feel unsympathetic toward them and may believe that they are "attention seekers" and that they could "snap out of it" if they really tried.

It is important to realize that all symptoms stemming from anxiety disorders develop because of an overwhelming *unconscious* conflict and that the symptoms have great unconscious significance. The word unconscious has been stressed, since it is necessary to realize that the individual does not clearly understand why the symptom has developed or what is gained by using the symptom repeatedly. The client does realize that the symptom helps relieve unbearable anxiety and tension.

To make an intelligent, therapeutic plan of care, the nurse needs to understand the nature of the person's conflict and the meaning of the symptoms. The plan of care and treatment should be developed collaboratively by the staff who will be involved with the individual. The type of treatment required and the goals to be established should be developed in conjunction with the individual. Whatever the treatment goals may be, the individual requires a consistent approach from all staff involved.

Health perception–health management

It is usually wise to listen completely and with an accepting attitude when the anxious person describes physical symptoms. Comments should be directed toward eliciting more information about the complaints. The nurse must remember that these clients can and do become physically ill and deserve medical attention if any reasonable doubt exists concerning the cause of the complaint. However, hospitalization on a medical unit may be unfortunate for some persons who have already focused most of their attention on physical symptoms that have no organic basis. Such individuals may become more tense, anxious, and fearful in a setting that emphasizes physical problems.

The nurse must realize that the discomfort and pain the individual complains of are actually present even though no organic basis can explain the existence of the symptoms. Experts are beginning to recognize that fear plays a significant role in causing pain. Since fear is prominent in the symptomatology of many anxiety-ridden people, it is not difficult to realize that they actually feel the pain of which they complain. The nurse must understand that emotionally conditioned pain is as distressing as pain that results from true physical disease.

Activity-exercise

One of the most helpful approaches to the care of anxious clients is to assist them to develop interests outside themselves. Thus, recreational and occupational therapies are significant in their treatment. Many anxiety-ridden individuals have never been able to enter into games or group activities. It is important to help them learn to play games and to participate in group activities. This provides opportunities to release tensions as well as to develop new interests. Recreational and occupational activities are usually more successful if they are focused on interests that the individual has had in the past.

In suggesting that an anxious person participate in some social activity, it is unwise to ask, "Would you like to go swimming with the group?" Such a question will often bring the flat answer "no" or a long recital about why the individual cannot possibly go. A more effective approach would be, "The group is going swimming. I hope that you will go with us." If the objective is to have the individual participate in a game of table tennis, more positive results will be obtained if the tennis paddle is placed in the client's hand by the nurse, who might say, "We need one more person to play this game. Come and play." This approach is more apt to elicit participation if the client wants to play.

The individual with morbid fears and compulsions usually presents a challenging nursing problem. Some nurses who have no understanding of the forces that play a part in developing such symptoms may assume the attitude that the client's many maneuvers are ridiculous. Nurses have been known to force phobic persons to touch a doorknob even though it was well known that they were morbidly afraid of the dirt and germs they believed they would contact by touching the object. Other nurses have made it impossible for clients to go into the bathroom to carry out the handwashing rituals that were so important to them in releasing tensions and fears.

When phobic and compulsive individuals are not allowed to carry out the procedures they feel are necessary, they have no way of releasing tension. A high level of unreleased tension may culminate in a panic state. Nurses should make it possible for individuals to carry out the anxiety-releasing rituals they have developed. The rituals carried on by these individuals are essential for them if they are to develop a feeling of security in the situation. Because such rituals are time-consuming, time must be allowed for the individual to perform such ritualistic maneuvers.

Cognitive-perceptual

Many uninformed health care professionals, as well as the individual's relative and friends, attempt to discuss the symptoms experienced by the person with an anxiety disorder in a reasonable way in the hope of altering the behavior. This form of pressure does nothing to help the individual and may actually create more anxiety and lowered self-esteem. The nurse can intervene effectively in such a situation by teaching the client, friends, and family about the nature of the disorder. Many pamphlets are available that describe anxiety disorders in terminology that can be understood by lay persons. In addition, an increasing number of communities have self-help groups for clients and their families to which the nurse can refer interested individuals.

Self-perception/self-concept

Even with a cognitive understanding of the disorder, the individual with an anxiety disorder often has low self-esteem because of an inability to control the symptoms. Techniques such as imagery, diaphragmatic breathing, biofeedback and relaxation, and assertiveness training are often useful in preventing the onset of symptoms or alleviating them. Teaching these techniques is within the scope of nursing practice. If the client is able to master them and they are successful in preventing or reducing anxiety, the client will feel in more control of the situation and is likely to experience increased self-esteem.

In general, it is helpful if anxious individuals are provided with an opportunity to succeed in the activities in which they participate, thereby building self-esteem and self-confidence. Giving deserved praise and recognition for activities performed well is one way of reassuring and encouraging persons with anxiety disorders.

Role-relationship

Short-term hospitalization is usually helpful for persons who exhibit severely dysfunctional behavior because the environment is neutral, they are removed from the significant members of the family who may be associated with much emotional tension, and they are able to feel more secure when the routine is simple, makes few demands, and can be fairly accurately anticipated.

Such individuals need a warm, friendly, empathic nurse who accepts them as people in need of help and who helps them feel that they are worthwhile human beings. Scolding or sarcastic remarks serve only to reinforce their need to protect themselves by the use of their symptoms.

Some nurses ignore symptoms that stem from anxiety, and often this becomes synonymous with ignoring the individual. Since anxious persons are using symptoms to ask for help, ignoring them increases their need to use the symptoms more frequently.

Encouraging the anxious individual to talk about concerns and feelings is an important aspect of care. However, the nurse should avoid asking, "How are you today?" For anxious persons, this question is often an invitation for another outpouring of physical complaints. A much more helpful way to begin a conversation might be to comment on some neutral topic that is of mutual interest.

KEY INTERVENTIONS FOR CLIENTS WITH ANXIETY DISORDERS

Investigate the basis for all physical complaints but do not overemphasize them.

Assist clients to develop interests outside themselves.

Allow clients sufficient time to carry out compulsive behaviors.

Provide education about the disorder and its treatment to the client, family, and friends.

Teach techniques designed to prevent or alleviate anxiety.

Relate to client in a supportive, reassuring, and understanding manner.

NURSING CARE PLAN: *A Ritualistic Individual*

CASE FORMULATION

Herbert B., 47 years of age, and his wife, Jane, 46 years old, came to the community mental health center to ask for help. Mr. B. was well oriented and intelligent, had good insight, and otherwise appeared to be mentally normal. He gave the following history.

An only child, Mr. B. reported that he remembers his childhood as being uneventful. However, he also stated that his mother was a meticulous housekeeper who was known in her community as fanatical about main-

taining correct standards of behavior and observing religious customs.

During his college days, Mr. B. had become emotionally upset and had worried excessively. His pastor was consulted, and after several conferences, he was able to resume his schoolwork and graduated at age 21 as an accountant. He stated that he had always been very conscientious, worried a great deal about body cleanliness, and was known for his concern about keeping his room and clothing in perfect order. He was

Continued.

NURSING CARE PLAN: *A Ritualistic Individual—cont'd*

always prompt in appearing at his office and never left his desk before 5 PM. His fellow workers regarded him as very fussy, and his employer always remarked about the neatness of his desk and files, a comment that greatly pleased him. At home any irregularity in household routine upset him. His wife was fully aware of his rigid regard for rules and his scrupulousness. She spoke freely about their marital relations being unsatisfactory and disturbing. She had given up any hope of improving the situation by discussing it with him because he became extremely anxious when she introduced the topic. She also stated that she was "thankful" they never had any children, since she was sure that the "mess" that children normally make in the house would be intolerable for her husband.

Four months before he came to the center, Mr. B. had been assigned the responsibility of making out the income tax report for his firm, which dealt in stocks and bonds. This assignment was made on March 1, and he realized that he had but 6 weeks before the returns were to be filed. He worked under great pressure, and almost every day he remained in the office until late at night. With a day to spare, he entered the final figures on a roll of paper from an adding machine. Badly in need of sleep and rest, he seized this roll, thrust it into his overcoat pocket, and dashed for the midnight bus. He intended to show the slip of paper to his wife as evidence that his job was completed. On reaching his home, he could not find the roll. In a frenzy he searched his clothing and ran out on the street searching the sidewalk

but failed to find it. He went to bed in an anxious, fearful state and sought his physician's help the next day. He remained under medical care for several weeks.

On returning to work, Mr. B. found that he had developed an overwhelming compulsion. He could no longer pass a piece of crumpled paper on the floor or sidewalk without picking it up and inspecting it. During rush hour he was greatly humiliated and embarrassed by the necessity of bending over and picking up odd bits of paper. On several occasions he was knocked down by a hurrying passerby while carrying out this compulsion. A wastebasket full of discarded paper literally threw him into a panic. His only relief was obtained by waiting until after office hours when he could go over each item piece by piece. His physician recommended treatment in the community mental health center.

Nursing Assessment

It is significant that Herbert B.'s mother was a fastidious housekeeper and fanatical about observing religious customs and maintaining correct standards of behavior. Undoubtedly, such a mother would insist that a child achieve perfection in toilet training at a very early age. In addition, she would rear him to behave in a rigidly correct manner and would covertly encourage him to repress instinctual thoughts and desires.

A young man who at the age of 21 is known to be overly concerned about orderliness, is overly conscientious, and is worried about bodily cleanliness is already well on the road

NURSING CARE PLAN: *A Ritualistic Individual—cont'd*

to developing compulsive symptoms to control unconscious anxiety by employing persistently repetitive acts. This behavior, as with all human behavior, has purpose and meaning for the individual who employs it, even though the forces producing it are unconscious.

Despite Herbert's early tendencies to be upset by household irregularities, he married. He and his wife managed to work out a relationship that could be tolerated. However, according to his wife, their sexual relationship was unsatisfactory and such an upsetting topic to her husband that she avoided discussing it. His basic problem focused, in part at least, on his unresolved conflict about his role as a marital partner. This conflict was relieved to some extent by his fastidious attitude toward his body. Such problems probably originated in the attitudes that were learned during the habit-training period.

Not until he was 47 did Herbert's symptoms become so severe that he required treatment. This was precipitated by the loss of a scrap of paper on which was recorded a final total of a complicated accounting problem he had been assigned to complete. Interestingly, he was attempting to elicit his wife's approval for a successful task accomplished. Since he did not have her approval as a sexual partner, her approval about some other aspect of life was very necessary. The loss of the paper probably represented much more than simply the loss of a list of figures. Symbolically it must have represented the loss of love and approval. This would account for his extreme fear and anxiety. The tax report had been completed before he left the office. Thus a duplicate of the figures probably could have been found. The loss must have been symbolic of the loss of something more important and irreplaceable.

In compulsive individuals the repetitive act has a symbolic significance reminiscent of a magic ritual designed to eradicate the possible effect of unacceptable instinctual impulses. It also represents a type of self-punishment, since the individual recognizes compulsive acts as being unreasonable and ridiculous. Despite the individual's partial insight, the tension and anxiety mount until the urge to repeat the act to control the tension becomes irresistible.

As with most severely anxious individuals, Mr. B. was well oriented, intelligent, and intellectually normal except for his compulsive behavior. This is an example of an individual whose personality is intact except in the one area that is involved with the compulsive behavior. However, despite the normal aspects of his personality, he was almost totally incapacitated by the need to examine every scrap of paper.

Nursing Diagnosis

The assessment data, including present behavior, past life experiences, and an understanding of the underlying dynamics, led to the development of the following two nursing diagnoses for Herbert B.

Ineffective individual coping related to anxiety stemming from unconscious conflicts

Altered role performance related to

Continued.

NURSING CARE PLAN: *A Ritualistic Individual—cont'd*

client's inability to discuss the couple's sexual relationship.

Planning and Implementing Nursing Care

The boxed material on p. 321 illustrates a nursing care plan for Herbert B. After assessing his needs and formulating nursing diagnoses, the nurse participated in a meeting of the mental health team that discussed Mr. B. As a result of this discussion, a collaborative decision was made not to hospitalize him. Rather, the psychiatrist prescribed diazepam, and the nurse made an appointment for Mr. B. to see a staff psychologist for psychotherapy three times a week. In addition, she made an appointment with him for 1 hour twice a month after one of his therapy sessions. Although the nurse's goal was not to engage in psychotherapy with this client, she did have the goal of monitoring his reaction to his medication and to the family system. She was aware that as Herbert B. was able to change his behavior, his relationship with his wife would also be altered.

The nurse maintained close communication with the psychologist who was engaged in psychotherapy with the client to be able to reinforce the direction he was taking and not inadvertently interfere with their relationship.

Evaluation

After 4 weeks of biweekly appointments with Herbert B., the nurse was assured that he was taking his medication regularly and was not experiencing adverse reactions. Although he reported that he still felt a mild degree of anxiety almost continuously, he was able to overcome the urge to examine every scrap of paper he saw.

As Herbert B.'s behavior changed as a result of increased insight, family disequilibrium ensued. By the end of 4 months of psychotherapy, Herbert B. had developed a beginning awareness of the relationship between his compulsion and his early childhood experiences, especially those with his mother. Although he still maintained his fastidious behavior, he grew to understand that his fear of sexual relations with his wife was related to his unconscious association of her with his mother. He became able to consider initiating a conversation with his wife about their sexual relationship. However, the first time he introduced the subject, his wife rejected his attempt by saying she did not have time to talk that evening. The nurse understood this behavior as a signal of family disequilibrium and communicated this to the mental health team. At this time the decision was made to offer this couple family therapy in addition to continuing individual psychotherapy for Herbert B. It was also decided that there was no longer any reason for him to continue meeting with the nurse.

As a result of these decisions, the nurse made an appointment for Mr. and Mrs. B. with the staff social worker and made plans to discontinue her routine appointments with Mr. B. in four more visits. Even though she was not engaged in psychotherapy with this client, the nurse understood that their relationship was meaningful to him and must not be terminated abruptly or thoughtlessly.

NURSING CARE PLAN FOR HERBERT B.

Nursing diagnosis	Objective (rationale)	Nursing interventions	Outcome criteria
Ineffective individual coping related to anxiety stemming from unconscious conflicts	Client will experience a decrease in anxiety. (Overwhelming anxiety prevents problem solving and the development of new, more functional adaptations to stressors.)	Teach client about actions and side effects of prescribed antianxiety medication. Meet twice a month with client to monitor his response to medication. Keep wastebaskets out of room in which nurse and client meet. Listen attentively to client's complaints.	Within 1 month client gives evidence of taking medication regularly and does not experience incapacitating side effects. Within 4 months client gives evidence of decreased anxiety by: Reporting a decrease in anxiety Being able to resist urge to examine scraps of paper Not developing a new compulsion
	Client will develop insight into his underlying unconscious conflicts. (Awareness of underlying unconscious conflicts can lead to their resolution.)	Refer to staff psychologist for psychotherapy. Meet twice a month with client's psychotherapist.	Client meets regularly with psychotherapist. Psychotherapist keeps nurse apprised of process of relationship with client.
Altered role performance related to client's inability to discuss the couple's sexual relationship	Client will increase meaningful communication with his wife. (Meaningful communication between spouses is necessary to establish and maintain a satisfactory and satisfying marital relationship.)	View family as a system. Understand that as client alters his behavior, system will enter disequilibrium. Monitor degree of family equilibrium and report to mental health team. Rehearse with client ways he might initiate conversations with his wife using techniques such as role playing.	Within 4 months client reports attempts to communicate meaningfully with his wife.

KEY POINTS

1. Anxiety disorders are characterized by symptoms of extreme anxiety and avoidance behavior.

2. Somatoform disorders are characterized by longstanding, generalized physical symptoms in the absence of demonstrable physical disease.

3. Dissociative disorders are characterized by a disturbance in the normal integration of identity, memory, or consciousness.

4. No specific causative factor of anxiety disorders has been identified. It is believed that they probably result from an interaction of biological, cognitive, and psychodynamic factors.

5. Medical treatment of anxiety disorders includes the use of anxiolytic medications and psychotherapy.

6. Psychotherapy is a sustained interpersonal interaction between the therapist and client in which the goal is to help the client develop more functional behaviors.

7. Assessment of the person who is anxious often reveals numerous physical complaints, motor restlessness, disinterest in recreational activities, changes in sleep patterns, a disorderly or overly neat home environment, overwhelming feelings of impending doom, strained interpersonal relationships, low self-esteem, and a sense of helplessness, hopelessness, and powerlessness.

8. The goal of all nursing care for the individual with an anxiety disorder is to help the client lower anxiety and develop functional adaptations to the anxiety.

SUGGESTED SOURCES OF ADDITIONAL INFORMATION

Calarco MM: Managing Myra's madness, *Am J Nurs* 89:346, March 1989.

Carroll P, Maher VF: Legal issues in the care of patients with anxiety, *Adv Clin Care* 6:16, September/October 1991.

Curtis GC, Glitz DA: Neuroendocrine findings in anxiety disorders, *Endocrinol Metabol Clin North Am* 17:131, March 1988.

DiMotto JW: Relaxation, *Am J Nurs* 84:754, 1984.

Gagan J: Imagery: an overview with suggested application for nursing, *Perspect Psychiatr Care* 22:20, January-March 1984.

Federici CM, Tommasini NR: The assessment and management of panic disorder, *Nurse Pract* 17:20, March 1992.

Gournay KJM: The failure of exposure treatment in agoraphobia: implications for the practice of nurse therapists and community psychiatric nurses, *J Adv Nurs* 16:1099, 1991.

Greenberg W: The multiple personality, *Perspect Psychiatr Care* 20:100, July-September 1982.

Hagerty BK: Obsessive-compulsive behavior: an overview of four psychological frameworks, *J Psychosoc Nurs Ment Health Serv* 19:37, January 1981.

Jorn N: Repression in a case of multiple personality disorder, *Perspect Psychiatr Care* 20:105, July-September 1982.

Karl GT: Survival skills for psychic trauma, *J Psychosoc Nurs Ment Health Serv* 27:15, April 1989.

Kent F: *Coping with phobias,* New York, 1980, Harper & Row.

Kneisl CR: Combatting anxiety, *RN* 50, August 1990.

Knowles R: Dealing with feelings: managing anxiety, *Am J Nurs* 81:110, 1981.

Moores A: Frightened of fear, *Nurs Times* 83(13):34, 1987.

Peplau HE: The power of the dissociative state, *J Psychosoc Nurs Ment Health Serv* 23:31, August 1985.

Tilley S, Weighill VE: How nurse therapists assess and contribute to the management of alcohol and sedative drug use among anxious patients, *J Adv Nurs* 11:499, September 1986.

Waddell KL, Demi AS: Effectiveness of an intensive partial hospitalization program for treatment of anxiety disorders, *Arch Psychiatr Nurs* 7:2, February 1993.

Whitley GG: Ritualistic behavior: breaking the cycle, *J Psychosoc Nurs* 29(10):31, 1991.

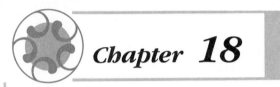

Chapter 18

Individuals with Physiological Stress Responses

• Develop a hypothetical plan of nursing care for an individual experiencing a physiological stress response.

LEARNING OBJECTIVES
After studying this chapter, the student will be able to:

• Describe the characteristics of physiological stress responses.

• Discuss the causative factors associated with physiological stress responses.

• Describe behaviors the nurse is most likely to observe in an individual experiencing a physiological stress response.

• State examples of nursing diagnoses likely to be applicable to an individual experiencing a physiological stress response.

• State and explain nursing interventions likely to be effective with an individual who has a physiological stress response.

It is well known that the functions and reactions of the mind and body are inextricably related. For example, when the individual experiences the emotion of fear, the body reacts in preparation for fight or flight. However, a physiological reaction does not depend on the person's awareness of the emotion. A physiological response still occurs even when the person is unaware of the emotion. In fact, the existence of this response often serves to further obscure the emotion. This process is termed **somatization.** For example, the woman whose self-image depends on her behaving as a loving mother but who experiences rage about the dependency of her children would find her self-image threatened if she became aware of this emotion. Therefore her rage is kept out of awareness in an effort to protect the integrity of her self-concept. However, this woman may develop stomach pains as a physiological response to her rage. By experiencing and focusing on this physical symptom, this mother would divert her attention from her emotions.

When the somatization process is sustained and organic changes occur, the individual is said to have a **physiological stress response.** Although it is important for the nurse to be aware of the emotional concomitants of all physical illnesses, the nurse also must have some understanding of the etiological dynamics of physical illnesses believed to be associated with stress. Only with this understanding will the nurse be able to provide care likely to meet the individual's needs.

HISTORICAL PERSPECTIVE

Medical historians have found evidence that from the earliest times human beings have known that a relationship exists between the mind and the body. However, beliefs about the nature of this relationship have changed over time. For example, some primitive people believed that deviant behavior and physical illnesses were caused by the invasion of the individual by evil spirits. This belief led to the prac-

tice of trephination, in which holes were bored into the skull of the afflicted person to facilitate departure of the evil spirit. Accompanying this surgical procedure were elaborate rituals performed by a revered member of the community known as a priest, witch doctor, or shaman. This procedure was sufficiently successful to justify its continued use over many centuries. Modern authorities believe that the socially sanctioned, unconditional trust in the healer was the primary factor in reversing the disease process. The importance of this factor in the healing process is still seen as basic to effective intervention, whether physical or psychological.

Other beliefs that have supported the mind-body relationship were that deviant behavior and some forms of physical illness were caused by the individual's sinning and that a physical imbalance of body fluids or humors caused emotional problems.

Early beliefs about the mind-body relationship attempted to postulate a singular cause of either physical or behavioral dysfunction. None of these early theories took a holistic view of human beings as interrelated systems in which alterations in one component inevitably result in compensatory alterations throughout the entire system, affecting the entire system. Such is the case with physiological stress responses.

In the past, these stress-related illnesses were referred to as **psychosomatic illnesses.** Unfortunately, this term has been incorrectly incorporated into the language as meaning that the physical illness is not real but rather a product of the person's imagination designed to elicit attention and sympathy. No belief could be farther from the truth, and the health care team must never assume that persons with these illnesses are not really sick or are merely looking for attention through their physical symptoms.

PHYSIOLOGICAL STRESS RESPONSES

Physiological stress responses are believed to have an emotional cause, to affect one body system, and to involve innervation of the autonomic nervous system. Affected individuals have a physical illness with evidence of organic alteration. They are often acutely ill and may have life-threatening exacerbations of the illness.

The individual often has little or no insight into the emotional conflicts underlying the illness and may resent any implication that they are present. Understandably, the person is very distressed by the physical symptoms and seeks medical treatment of them, unlike individuals with a conversion disorder. Because the symptoms interfere greatly with the ability to function and may be life-threatening, the individual is often highly motivated to diminish or eradicate them. Consequently, the person can be helped to identify the relationship between stressors and exacerbations of the illness even without gaining an awareness of the unconscious emotional conflict.

It is beyond the scope of this text to discuss each of these stress-related illnesses in depth. The student should be aware that many excellent references are available from which much may be learned about each of these disease entities. Discussion in this chapter is limited to the disorders most often encountered in general nursing practice and illustrative of different body system involvement.

Gastrointestinal system

Peptic ulcer is a very common syndrome in a highly industrialized society such as the United States. The diagnosis of peptic ulcer encompasses both *gastric ulcers* and *duodenal ulcers,* although evidence indicates that emotional factors play a greater role in the development of duodenal ulcers, which tend to occur more in men than in women and in younger age groups. Duodenal ulcers stem from sustained gastric hypermotility and marked increase in gastric secretions, which eventually erode the lining of the stomach. Clinically the individual complains of epigastric pain that occurs within 1 to 4 hours after the last meal and is relieved by eating or by taking antacids. If alterations in diet and taking nonprescription remedies do not help, the per-

son is likely to seek medical help, since the pain becomes severe enough that it cannot be ignored. Hospitalization may be necessary, either for establishing the diagnosis or for treatment. Although medical treatment is always conservative if possible, the presence of bleeding or intractable pain may indicate the need for surgical removal of the affected part of the stomach or severance of a branch of the vagus nerve. Unfortunately, when this occurs, the individual may subsequently develop another, even more severe form of physiological stress response.

The personality characteristics of persons who develop a peptic ulcer are those of individuals who see themselves and are seen by others as strong, independent, hard working, and unemotional. Despite their occupational successes, these persons are tormented by feelings of not having done well enough and constantly strive to achieve even higher goals. Authorities believe that underlying these behaviors are strong dependency needs in conflict with the individual's self-image that therefore cannot be directly expressed. If these needs are met, it is a result of fortuitous accident rather than goal-directed behavior.

The initial onset of the illness as well as subsequent exacerbations tend to be precipitated by stressful life events that bring the dependency-independency conflict closer to the surface of consciousness. One man experienced his first episode of duodenal ulcer attack at the time of his marriage when he left his parents' home to establish a home with his wife. Despite marrying an attractive, caring woman whom he loved very much, the very act of marriage abruptly changed his role from that of son to that of husband, or symbolically from child to adult. The first gastrointestinal episode was successfully treated through diet modification and medication, and the symptoms subsided. The second attack occurred after the birth of their first child, a son, 4 years later. Once again, it can be seen that the birth of a child, particularly a son whose infantile dependency the father may have identified with, put increased pressure on this man to act as a strong, responsible adult while simultaneously decreasing direct opportunities to have his dependency needs met. As in the previous attack, conservative medical treatment was successful in alleviating the ulcer symptoms, although they were more severe and took longer to disappear than in the initial episode. Interestingly, when their second child, a daughter, was born 4 years later, no exacerbation of ulcer symptoms occurred. The third and most severe episode of ulcer symptoms took place about a year after this man's father died. The father died as a result of bowel cancer, which was treated by colostomy and radiation but nevertheless metastasized. During the course of his illness, the father moved in with his son and daughter-in-law because of his increased need for physical care and supervision. Although the daughter-in-law provided most of the care, the son frequently willingly helped, especially with more personal tasks such as bathing. The father died in the home, and during the following year the son was deeply involved in settling his father's complex estate. After this task was completed, he once again experienced ulcer symptoms so severe that surgical removal of two thirds of his stomach was ultimately required. It can be conjectured that the death of this man's father was unconsciously seen by him as the ultimate proof of his adulthood, which he was not able to withstand because he maintained a large reservoir of unmet dependency needs, and his father's death symbolically cut off all hope of having those needs met.

Although peptic ulcer is a common form of gastrointestinal physiological stress response, other illnesses such as ulcerative colitis and chronic constipation also fall into this category.

Cardiovascular system

A health problem of increasing incidence, particularly among black Americans, is *essential hypertension*. Essential hypertension is a sustained elevation of systolic and diastolic arterial blood pressure in the absence of any of the demonstrable known causes of arterial hypertension. Although persons with essential hypertension may remain asymptomatic for years, if the syndrome is sustained, organic alterations, particularly renal damage, may occur. Often the acceleration of the disease with resultant complications occurs in conjunction with life crises. It is believed that tremendous amounts of repressed rage that have no acceptable outlet are the emotional dynamics underlying the development of essential hypertension. The mental mechanism used by the individual is usually denial, since the person also has a need to conform with the expectations of others, especially authority figures, as a means of meeting dependency needs. Feeling and expressing rage are therefore highly anxiety producing, and the individual often has a calm, placid exterior. The frequency of occurrence of essential hypertension in the black population has led investigators to explore genetic factors simultaneously with cultural factors as major etiological predeterminants.

Respiratory system

A major physiological stress response affecting the respiratory system is *bronchial asthma*. Bronchial asthma is caused by bronchial obstruction that does not interfere with inspiration but causes difficulty in expiration. This results in the characteristic asthmatic wheeze that sounds so similar in all persons that it is almost diagnostic. The underlying cause of the bronchial obstruction may be an infectious process, an allergic reaction, or an idiopathic bronchospasm. When an underlying disease process such as a bacterial infection is present, other symptoms such as an elevated temperature and white blood count are also present and require treatment if the asthmatic episode is to be alleviated. In some persons, however, no demonstrable physiological cause for the asthmatic episode exists, and here emotional factors are believed to play a major etiological role in the occurrence of the illness.

The personality characteristics of the individual with asthma seem to include strong dependency needs directed toward the mother or mother figure, with simultaneous anger toward this individual, which elicits unconscious fears of abandonment. Some psychoanalytically oriented authorities claim that the characteristic asthmatic wheeze is a symbolic cry for the mother. During an acute asthmatic attack, the individual is a clinging, dependent person whose behavior is justified to self and others on the basis of the life-threatening symptoms. Therefore the dependency needs of the person may be met during the acute episode, but unfortunately these temporary episodes of need fulfillment do little to alter the underlying personality dynamics, and thus future episodes are not prevented. Continued episodes of asthma result in pulmonary changes that may not be reversible and may affect the vital capacity of the person's respiratory system.

Integumentary system

The integumentary system serves a unique function in the ego psychology of an individual in that it is the only body system equally visible both to the person and to others. Because of this, the skin represents the self to others in the environment. An awareness of this fact is reflected in such sayings as, "He's too thick [or thin] skinned" or "You can't tell a book by its cover."

The skin is richly endowed with sense receptors for pain, pressure, and temperature sensations. As a result, many emotional states are reflected in skin changes; the blush of embarrassment and the paling that accompany fear are examples. These common skin changes are perceived by others as nonverbal clues to the individual's emotional state, frequently despite verbal reassurances to the contrary. In healthy interpersonal relationships, the skin acts as a friendly ally in communicating to others what is being felt and therefore enhances the probability of having the individual's needs met. When the skin is involved in a physiological stress response, however, it becomes a means of self-disclosure representing the individual's unconscious conflict between a repressed emotion and

the simultaneous need to have others acknowledge and respond to this emotion.

Numerous *dermatological conditions* can cause a person severe discomfort in the form of itching, pain, or disfigurement. Although their exact cause often is unknown, an amazing number of these maladies respond well to the treatment of a dermatologist, who may attempt various remedies before finding one that seems to help. Although not denying the positive benefits of the physical treatment received, many authorities believe that the major benefit is achieved from the sustained, concerned interest in the individual and the illness frequently shown by dermatologists that indirectly helps to meet the person's immediate needs. Exacerbations of skin rashes and severe itching are closely related to occurrences of stressful life events. These persons seem to respond to such events without undue emotional upset but rather react by somatization, on which they and others can focus their concern. Many psychiatrists believe that skin somatization is one of the most primitive ego defenses available and therefore are very cautious in pursuing aggressive physical and psychological treatment unless the individual is in great pain or unable to perform activities of daily living. The rationale underlying this conservative approach is that if the person is enabled to give up this defense without a considerable increase in ego strength, he or she might be forced to resort to an even more serious and incapacitating defense.

Musculoskeletal system

The most common and severe form of physiological stress response that affects the musculoskeletal system is *rheumatoid arthritis* (Figure 18-1). This disease results in marked organic damage and affects not only the joints but also other tissues. Its onset may occur at any age, and it affects females more frequently than males. The personality characteristics of persons affected by this disease almost universally include masochistic, self-sacrificing behavior, which is in

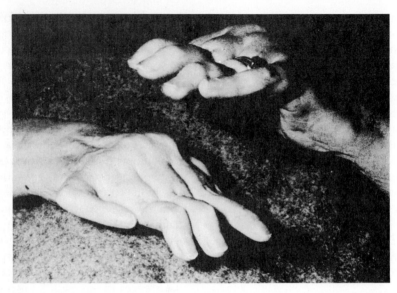

Figure 18-1

Rheumatoid arthritis.

From Hood GH, Dincher JR: *Total patient care,* ed 8, St Louis, 1992, Mosby–Year Book.

response to a rigid, punitive superego and a weak ego organization. Their family background frequently gives evidence of maternal deprivation, leaving them with many unmet dependency needs. Before becoming ill, these individuals indirectly express their emotional needs by being helpful and kind and willing to do almost anything for others, thereby receiving positive feedback from their social system. Under usual circumstances, therefore, their dependency needs are minimally met through environmental and interpersonal support, allowing them to remain healthy until such time as this support is withdrawn. Many individuals report that an event such as the death of a spouse or the loss of a job immediately preceded the initial onset of the illness.

Treatment of these persons is exceedingly complex. Many of them reflect their emotional conflict by denying the severity of their illness and either refuse treatment or are unreliable in following the treatment regimen. Conversely, some quickly become highly dependent on family, friends, and health care personnel despite their symptoms perhaps being only mildly debilitating.

CAUSATIVE FACTORS

Although a consensus seems to exist among authorities regarding the major role a person's emotions play in the development of certain physical illnesses, the exact nature of that role is not yet determined. One widely accepted theory postulates that repressed conflicts are stimulated by intrapsychic or interpersonal events and lead to an overall increase in the individual's level of anxiety. An automatic physical concomitant to an increase in anxiety is innervation of the autonomic nervous system. In other words, the person who is anxious becomes physically ready to engage in *flight or fight.* However, since the emotional conflict that is the basis for the anxiety and the subsequent physical response is unconscious, the individual has no outlet for the physical response, as would be possible if the conflict were conscious or if the danger were external. Consequently the state of physical readiness for flight or fight does nothing to resolve the underlying emotional conflict. If this phenomenon is sustained, a cyclical pattern is established. This pattern results in physiological alterations such as a peptic ulcer, which is caused by increased gastric acid secretion and gastric hypermotility as compensatory to the initial decreased gastric acid secretion and hypomotility caused by the flight-or-fight reaction. As the individual perceives physical discomfort, anxiety may further increase, thereby compounding the problem. The originator of this theory is a physician named Franz Alexander, whose works on the subject remain classics in the field.

A second theory postulates that certain personality types are particularly prone to the development of certain physical illnesses. An example of this theory is the designation of a specific personality type that is considered to place the individual in a high-risk category for myocardial infarction. These persons are seen to be highly competitive and overly ambitious, and they deny any need for dependency. This personality syndrome is manifested by hard work, aggressive behavior, and much risk taking as a means of "getting ahead." These persons frequently have many individuals dependent on them but no one on whom they feel they can depend.

A third theory places emphasis on the *symbolism* of the illness. For example, a person who unconsciously feels great rage at significant others and the environment in general but who does not see expression of this rage as acceptable may develop ulcerative colitis. Since ulcerative colitis is an illness in which persons have frequent bowel movements requiring, at the very least, alterations in their and others' activities, one might say that they are symbolically defecating on those around them, a very hostile act indeed.

A fourth theory is referred to as *organ weakness.* This theory postulates that all human beings have one body system that is relatively less healthy than the others. If a person has underlying unconscious problems that interfere with effective functioning but at the same time has sufficient ego strength so that a flight from reality is not necessary, this person may develop a physical illness as a means of coping with the unconscious problem. The type of physical illness developed will be determined by the body system that is most physiologically vulnerable.

Regardless of which theory or combination of theories proves to be correct, they all have several concepts in common, the understanding of which will prove invaluable to the nurse in caring for persons with physiological stress responses:

1. Persons who develop physiological stress responses have *unconscious* emotional conflicts that increase their anxiety and interfere with their efforts to meet their needs effectively.
2. The physical symptoms of the illness are a result of or an expression of this unconscious conflict and serve as a means of lowering the person's anxiety.
3. The illness is real in that demonstrable organic changes exist that may be life-threatening.

It is also generally accepted that the onset of the illness is associated with a real or perceived stressful life event. The physical symptoms occur as a response to this stress and mask the emotional turmoil with which the person cannot cope, thereby achieving the purpose of lowering anxiety. This benefit is termed the **primary gain.** In our society, however, the individual also may experience unexpected and unintended benefits from the illness. These benefits may be such factors as having one's dependency needs indirectly met, receiving attention and special consideration, or being relieved of responsibility. These benefits are **secondary gains,** which tend to reinforce the pattern of somatization.

NURSING CARE OF INDIVIDUALS WITH A PHYSIOLOGICAL STRESS RESPONSE

Nursing assessment

Although each physiological stress response has its unique features, it is possible to cite some commonalities about all persons with physiological stress responses. For purposes of clarity, typical behaviors of persons with physiological stress responses are discussed by categories. Although behaviors in each category are presented as separate entities, they are highly interrelated and are adaptations to similar stressors. Further, behavior designed as an adaptation to one stressor often becomes a stressor itself in another dimension.

Health perception–health management

The nature of physiological stress responses implies that an alteration always occurs in at least one physiological process. The nature and severity of the alteration are determined by the body system affected and the degree of organic change that has occurred.

Nutritional-metabolic

To the extent that the illness affects the gastrointestinal system, the individual will be at risk for altered nutrition and all resulting complications. Nutritional alterations are not inevitable, however, since many of these persons are able and willing to adhere to the numerous diet restrictions imposed by their illness.

Elimination

Bowel elimination is likely to be altered in illnesses affecting the gastrointestinal tract. In clients with inflammatory bowel disease, such as ulcerative colitis and Crohn's disease, the threat of diarrhea might interfere with normal activities.

Activity-exercise

The motor behavior of the individual with a physiological stress response may or may not be altered. However, when the musculoskeletal system is involved, as in rheumatoid arthritis, alterations in motor behavior caused by pain may be the major symptom. In illnesses affecting the respiratory system, activity intolerance may be present because of decreased vital capacity.

Recreation patterns are frequently altered as an adaptation to the actual or potential limitations caused by the illness. For example, one individual who was an avid outdoorsman stopped going on camping trips after developing ulcerative colitis. This illness required him to have a special diet and be close to toilet facilities, neither of which was easily achieved in the woods.

Self-care behaviors obviously are always altered when the person is acutely ill. They may or may not be altered at other times, depending on the nature of the disorder.

Home maintenance may or may not be altered depending on the nature of and symptomatology associated with the physiological stress response. Understandably, individuals who are acutely ill are likely to be unconcerned about their environments. At other times, many persons are able to adjust their environments to accommodate their needs in regard to safety and hygiene.

Cognitive-perceptual

Thought processes are not affected by physiological stress responses. However, this does not mean that individuals with physiological stress responses may not also have alterations in these processes related to other factors.

With all physiological stress responses, the individual and family need information about the illness and its treatment. However, it is important for the nurse to assess the level of knowledge the client and family already have, since some persons with physiological stress responses characteristically become experts about their illness and its treatment. In contrast, other individuals claim to have no knowledge of the disease despite having been affected over time.

Self-perception/self-concept

Even though physiological stress responses are believed to have an emotional cause, it is unlikely that the nurse will observe behaviors indicative of alterations in emotional processes, since the physical symptoms associated with the illness serve the purpose of symbolically expressing the person's underlying emotions. At the same time, however, the individual is likely to express great anxiety about the nature of the treatment for the illness and its outcome. These expressions of anxiety tend to focus on physical symptoms and divert attention from any underlying emotional conflict.

Unquestionably an individual who is physically ill for a time undergoes a change in self-concept. When the illness is a reaction to stress, the problem of maintaining one's self-concept is often compounded. Many persons with a physiological stress response have unmet dependency needs, which they deny because these needs do not reflect their view of themselves. They often appear to be fiercely independent persons. When their illness thrusts them into an unavoidable position of dependency, they may become quite anxious, further compounding their symptomatology. Medical dramas on television occasionally depict a successful businessman or politician who is hospitalized for a physiological stress response such as a duodenal ulcer but who attempts to continue working by dictating letters and carrying on business over the telephone.

CLINICAL EXAMPLE

Mrs. Boyer is a 40-year-old woman who has had rheumatoid arthritis for 5 years. Although all her joints have been affected at one time or another, her most lingering symptoms are in her hands. One year ago the Boyers moved into their "dream home," which Mrs. Boyer designed. Although they are very pleased with the house, the landscaping is not yet finished. This is very upsetting to Mrs. Boyer, since they are expecting guests from out of town for their daughter's wedding in 2 days. Yesterday, a load of topsoil for the garden was delivered and dumped beside the driveway. Mrs. Boyer spent the day shoveling the dirt into the garden. This morning she awoke with an acute exacerbation of her arthritis, which necessitated an increase in medication and bed rest. Mrs. Boyer is so incapacitated that it is unlikely she will be able to attend her daughter's wedding.

Role-relationship

Interpersonal processes are almost always affected in the domains of family processes, role performance, and social interaction. An individual with a physiological stress response often becomes the focus of attention within the family because of the dramatic, disabling, and long-term nature of the physical symptoms. It is not unusual for both client and family to report that he or she "is not the same person" as before the onset of the illness. For example, an individual who previously had been generous and outgoing may become demanding and intolerant of others' needs after becoming ill. If the illness is disabling, the person is unlikely to be able to fulfill a work role. This may be a major source of frustration to all concerned and an economic stressor on the family.

CLINICAL EXAMPLE

Ethel Larson is a 20-year-old college senior who has ulcerative colitis. She is an honors student and president of the senior class. At the annual class picnic, held at a nearby lake, several of Ethel's friends rented a rowboat. Ethel asked to go along, but once they were out on the lake, she frantically asked the rowers not to go too far from shore in the event she had to go to the bathroom. Two of the other girls later talked with each other about their anger at Ethel for ruining their boat ride. They questioned why Ethel had asked to go along but agreed neither felt comfortable in saying anything to her.

Coping–stress tolerance

By definition, individuals with a physiological stress response tend not to deal with stressors of daily living through reality testing and problem solving. Rather, they adapt to these stressors by somatization. In addition, the secondary gains of their illness are likely to remove them from the source of the stress, thereby further decreasing opportunities to problem solve. Therefore the nurse is likely to observe that such clients are very concerned and preoccupied with their physical symptoms to the exclusion of any psychosocial stressors they may be experiencing.

CLINICAL EXAMPLE

Jane had lived with and cared for her elderly mother for as long as she could remember. The afternoon of her mother's death, Jane had a severe asthmatic attack that required her to be hospitalized. The next day Jane's brother inquired whether Jane would be well enough to go to their mother's funeral the following day. The nurse was astounded because Jane had never mentioned that her mother had died.

Value-belief

Whether deeply held values and beliefs are affected is determined by several factors, including the extent to which the illness either relieves or creates anxiety, the degree to which the organic changes are life-threatening, the extent to which the illness is disabling in ways meaningful to the individual, and the number and type of secondary gains the individual experiences. If the illness creates more anxiety than it relieves, is life-threatening, causes disability that is stressful, and does not elicit secondary gains, the individual is likely to express feelings of helplessness, hopelessness, and powerlessness. However, because physiological stress responses are thought to shield the person from awareness of unconscious emotional conflicts, these persons more often experience a deeper sense of purpose and meaning, and perhaps spirituality, than they had before their illness.

Nursing diagnosis

As with all nursing diagnoses, the nursing diagnoses for the individual with a physiological stress response are based on the themes identified during the assessment phase of the nursing process.

Accepted NANDA nursing diagnoses that may be specifically applicable to the individual with a physiological stress response include:

Impaired skin integrity
Diarrhea
Activity intolerance
Impaired physical mobility
Fatigue
Self-care deficit, bathing/hygiene; dressing/grooming
Diversional activity deficit
Impaired home maintenance management
Ineffective breathing pattern
Chronic pain
Knowledge deficit (specify)
Fear
Anxiety
Body image disturbance
Self-esteem disturbance; situational low self-esteem; chronic low self-esteem
Altered role performance
Altered family processes
Ineffective individual coping

To develop a nursing diagnosis that fulfills its function of providing direction for planning nursing care, the nurse is encouraged to postulate and state etiological or antecedent factors and connect the two phrases by using the term "related to." For example:

Altered role performance related to inability to work as a typist because of severe pain in fingers

Planning and implementing nursing care

The plan for nursing care is derived from the nursing diagnoses and includes the objectives of the care, the nursing interventions, and outcome criteria. To be effective the plan needs to be highly individualized. The suggestions that follow should be seen as general guidelines to be used if they are appropriate to the client's needs.

In general, the objectives of all nursing care for the individual with a physiological stress response should relate to assisting the client to regain physiological homeokinesis and to develop alternative methods of coping with stress.

Since the client's nursing diagnoses are often interrelated, stemming as they do from similar etiologies or antecedents, the student should see that the appropriate nursing interventions are also interrelated; in other words, by intervening in one dimension, the nurse will also affect other dimensions.

The care of persons with physiological stress responses is usually directed by a physician whose emphasis is on the reduction of physical symptoms and the prevention of further organic damage. However, because of the nature of the illness, close collaboration with a psychiatrist is often necessary. Once the acute physical symptoms have abated, the psychiatrist may continue to treat the individual on an outpatient basis in an attempt to help the person deal with underlying emotional problems. The nurse is usually involved in providing care when the person is hospitalized for an exacerbation of the illness or in follow-up care in the home.

Health perception–health management

The methods used by the nurse in carrying out physical care are often pivotal factors in enhancing or impeding the overall treatment goals. The nurse must fully understand and accept that persons with a physiological stress response are physically ill and that their symptoms may reach life-threatening proportions. Nurses must not convey the attitude that they believe these individuals would improve if they merely exerted more control over their emotions.

During acute episodes of the illness, meeting the client's physical needs is of primary importance, even if in so doing the nurse is supporting a dysfunctional emotional adaptation. For ex-

ample, a couple whose tension-laden relationship exacerbates the wife's physical symptoms should not be encouraged to discuss their relationships during the acute episode of the wife's illness.

The secondary gains achieved by the individual as the result of being physically ill need to be minimized once the acute episode has passed. The nurse can be instrumental in working with the client to strengthen or develop coping mechanisms that do not involve somatization.

Cognitive-perceptual

As with any client, the person who has a physiological stress response can be helped to feel in control of the situation by adequate explanations of what to expect during diagnostic and treatment procedures. Some clients, however, become increasingly anxious if they are given too much information, and their dependency needs are best met by trusting in the judgment of their physician and nurse. Therefore the amount and nature of information offered to the client should be primarily determined by an assessment of the anxiety level. Certainly the client's questions should be answered, but the degree of elaboration should be gauged by the response to the answer rather than by the nurse's need to engage in health teaching.

Self-perception/self-concept

Most physical illnesses, regardless of cause, present a potential threat to clients' perception of themselves as independent adults. Persons with physiological stress responses often have underlying conflicts between dependency and independency needs, and the imposed dependence that results from the illness may stimulate great anxiety. In such instances the nurse can be helpful if she or he meets the individual's needs for dependence in an indirect way while simultaneously acknowledging the client's status as a responsible adult. An example of such an intervention is the nurse who wisely addresses the client with a peptic ulcer as Mr. Smith instead of

John. At the same time, Mr. Smith's dependency needs can be indirectly met by the nurse's administering the prescribed antacid instead of leaving it at the bedside or asking the client to ring the call light every half hour so the nurse can bring the medicine. By spontaneously making frequent contact with the client, the nurse is indirectly expressing a willingness to take care of this client without his having to assume the responsibility of asking for help. The administration of oral medication or food, especially milk, has great symbolic significance, since eating is the vehicle through which people have their dependency needs first met.

The nurse has many opportunities to engage in conversation with the hospitalized person. Nurses can be of emotional assistance to clients if they encourage these persons to talk about their feelings. It must be understood, however, that many feelings are unacceptable to clients, and therefore the nurse's acceptance of them and their feelings is of primary importance. As in communicating with any client, nurses are most helpful when they are accepting and nonjudgmental. Reflecting or restating what the client has said is an appropriate communication technique to employ, since a direct interpretation may be very threatening and raise the client's anxiety level and perhaps thereby increase the severity of physical symptoms.

Role-relationship

Working with the client's family is necessary to aid them in understanding the complexity of the illness and its treatment. The effect of the family on the client and the effect the client and the illness have on the family is a process often explored in family therapy under the guidance of a skilled therapist.

Many persons are not aware of the interpersonal resources available to them within their social system. Persons with physiological stress responses can often benefit from help in identifying existing interpersonal resources and in enlarging their social network, thereby increasing the possibility of having their emotional needs met by a greater number and larger variety of people.

KEY INTERVENTIONS FOR CLIENTS WITH PHYSIOLOGICAL STRESS RESPONSES

Convey an attitude of acceptance and understanding.
Meet all physical needs of the client during acute exacerbations of the illness, even if doing so supports dysfunctional adaptations.
Minimize secondary gains once the acute phase of the illness is resolved.
Use the client's level of anxiety as a gauge to determine the amount and specificity of health teaching.
Acknowledge the client as a responsible adult while indirectly addressing dependency needs.
Encourage clients to talk about their feelings to the extent possible.
Assist the client and family to enlarge their social network.

NURSING CARE PLAN: *An Individual with Asthma*

CASE FORMULATION

Martha B. is a 25-year-old single woman who has had asthma since age 2. Although respiratory infections have always precipi- tated an asthmatic attack, many instances of asthmatic episodes have been unaccompanied by an infectious process. Martha is the only child of an attractive 45-year-old woman

NURSING CARE PLAN: *An Individual with Asthma—cont'd*

who has never married and who is not sure who Martha's father is. Martha and her mother live together in a well-furnished two-bedroom apartment in a middle-class neighborhood of a large city.

Since age 16 Martha's mother has engaged in prostitution and become pregnant several times. For reasons that are not clear, at the time she was pregnant with Martha, she decided not to have an abortion as she had on previous occasions. After Martha was born, the mother set up housekeeping in an apartment that she furnished with the child's needs in mind.

By the time Martha was 5 years old, her mother had become so successful in her occupation that she no longer was a streetwalker but rather made appointments with her customers by telephone and therefore had advance notice as to when she would not be home. At those times she left Martha with her grandmother, a warm, kind woman who seemed unaware of her daughter's activities. Martha's grandmother lived alone, and she was always delighted to have Martha visit. When Martha and her mother were together, they seemed to enjoy each other and have a mutually satisfying relationship.

After Martha graduated from high school, she took a position as a clerk in a large plastics company located in the heart of the city. She has remained with this company but has never accepted offers of promotion. Therefore her salary is essentially at the same level as it was when she was hired because the only raises she has received were several cost-of-living increments. For this reason she feels unable to leave her mother's home and rent her own apartment.

The event preceding Martha's latest and most severe asthmatic attack was the death and burial of her grandmother. When notified of her grandmother's death, Martha responded quite stoically and made all the funeral arrangements because her mother was out of town. On the day of the funeral, Martha began to cry softly. However, by the time the family assembled at the cemetery, she was severely dyspneic and had to be rushed from the gravesite to the emergency room of the local hospital. The emergency room staff were very familiar with Martha and her family situation, although they did not know of her grandmother's death.

By the time Martha arrived at the emergency room, she was in acute physiological distress, gasping for air and wheezing so loudly that she could be heard throughout the waiting room. Her mother expressed genuine concern but also stated that "this couldn't have happened at a worse time because I have to leave town tonight." She begged the hospital personnel to admit Martha so she wouldn't have to worry while she was away.

Nursing Assessment

Martha's family situation contained all the elements sufficient for the development of idiopathic asthma. It can be conjectured that Martha's mother was a very immature person lacking in self-esteem who engaged in prostitution as one means of reinforcing her feelings of worthlessness. If this were true, it is likely that her decision not to terminate her pregnancy with Martha was an unconscious attempt to provide herself with a consistent person who would need and value her. Unfortunately, this rarely succeeds, since chil-

Continued.

NURSING CARE PLAN: *An Individual with Asthma—cont'd*

dren require more attention and love than they can give during their formative developmental periods. Martha undoubtedly believed that her mother's frequent absences were a result of some failing on Martha's part, while at the same time she experienced much anger at her mother for not providing her with the emotional support she needed. This issue could not be openly confronted, since to do so would incur the risk of abandonment, thereby dooming forever the possibility of having her needs met by her mother. On the other hand, the grandmother seemed able to meet some of Martha's needs, although her relationship with her own daughter was not growth producing, as evidenced by their lack of communication.

Although she was 25 years old, Martha's developmental maturity apparently was not congruent with her chronological maturity. Rather than struggling with age-appropriate developmental tasks, Martha's inability to establish herself in her own apartment indicates she was still struggling with dependency issues characteristic of the developmental phases of childhood. To the extent that Martha's grandmother was able to meet some of Martha's dependency needs, Martha was able to function. When the grandmother died, Martha lost the only stable, consistent person in her life and was unequipped to cope successfully with this developmental stressor. Therefore her wheezing was interpreted as a desperate cry to be cared for.

Nursing Diagnosis

Based on the nursing assessment that in-

cluded prior knowledge of the family dynamics and an understanding of the dynamics underlying physiological stress responses, the nurse formulated the following nursing diagnosis for Martha B:

> Ineffective breathing pattern related to unconscious feelings of anger at being abandoned by grandmother who died

Planning and Implementing Nursing Care

A sample nursing care plan for Martha B. is found in the boxed material on p. 337.

The immediate objective was to restore physiological homeokinesis, so Martha was given the prescribed bronchodilator by intramuscular injection. Within 10 minutes she was breathing more easily and was noticeably more comfortable. This could have been accomplished in the emergency room, but in view of the family situation, the physician had decided to hospitalize her.

After her immediate physical needs were met, it was decided that Martha could benefit from constant attention from a member of the nursing staff. Therefore a student nurse who was studying the nursing care of individuals with physiological stress responses was assigned to stay with Martha. Although one could argue that this intervention would result in secondary gains, it was believed appropriate during this crisis.

Under supervision of her instructor, the student nurse encouraged Martha to express her feelings and was careful to respond in an empathic way even though she knew that Martha's grandmother had not intentionally abandoned her. She also attempted to meet Martha's dependency needs through such in-

NURSING CARE PLAN: *An Individual with Asthma—cont'd*

terventions as offering her liquids to drink without waiting to be asked. Although Martha was allowed out of bed, the student brought her a basin of water and a towel so she could bathe in bed if she wished.

Evaluation

Martha responded so well to the interventions of medications and consistent attention that the health care team decided that she would be a good candidate for psychotherapy. This treatment option had never been

offered to Martha on any previous admission, but with the death of her grandmother it was feared that Martha would not have the resources to cope with her situation if she were not given more assistance. Martha's mother would also be invited to begin family therapy with her daughter. Although the staff were not optimistic about the mother agreeing to participate, they thought it was important that she be offered this help not only for Martha's well-being, but for the mother's as well.

NURSING CARE PLAN FOR MARTHA B.

Nursing diagnosis	Objective (rationale)	Nursing interventions	Outcome criteria
Ineffective breathing pattern related to unconscious feelings of anger at being abandoned by grandmother who died	Physiological homeokinesis will be restored. (Asthma is a life-threatening illness.)	Administer prescribed bronchodilator. Observe for respiratory distress. Plan physical care to conserve client's energy.	Within 20 minutes of receiving medication, dyspnea decreases.
	Client's dependency needs will be met in a manner appropriate to her chronological age. (Meeting the client's dependency needs while acknowledging her as an adult helps to temporarily resolve her dependency/independency conflict, leading to decreased need to somatize.)	Establish relationship with client by giving undivided attention. Anticipate client's needs; for example, offer juice at regular intervals.	Within 48 hours, client is symptom free.
	Client will express her feelings. (Expression of feelings leads to decreased need to somatize.)	Listen attentively and nonjudgmentally to client's expressions of loss.	

KEY POINTS

1. Physiological stress responses are believed to have an emotional cause, to affect one body system, and to involve the autonomic nervous system.

2. Persons who develop physiological stress responses have unconscious emotional conflicts that increase their anxiety and interfere with their efforts to meet their needs effectively.

3. The physical symptoms of the illness are a result of or an expression of an unconscious conflict and serve as a means of lowering the person's anxiety. This process is called primary gain.

4. The illness is real in that demonstrable organic changes exist that may be life-threatening.

5. Meeting the client's physical needs is of prime importance during acute episodes of the illness.

6. Meeting the client's dependency needs while also acknowledging the individual's status as a responsible adult is a major part of the nurse's role.

7. The nurse can be helpful to clients experiencing a physiological stress response by encouraging them to talk about their feelings and listening in an accepting, nonjudgmental manner.

8. The nurse is helpful when working with the client's family to help them understand the complexity of the illness and its treatment.

SUGGESTED SOURCES OF ADDITIONAL INFORMATION

Alexander F: *Psychosomatic medicine,* New York, 1954, Norton.

Byrne DG: Personal determinants of life event stress and myocardial infarction, *Psychother Psychosom* 40(1-4):106, 1985.

Castleberry K: Rules for disease: an interactional model for psychosomatic illness in families, *Issues Ment Health Nurs* 9:363, 1988.

Clochesy JM: Stress-related gastrointestinal disorders, *J Adv Med Surg Nurs* 1(4):21, 1989.

Deter HC, Allert G: Group therapy for asthma patients: a concept for the psychosomatic treatment of patients in a medical clinic, *Psychother Psychosom* 40(1-4):95, 1983.

Dunbar F: *Emotions and bodily changes,* New York, 1954, Columbia University Press.

Haggarty J, Drossman D: Use of psychotropic drugs in patients with peptic ulcer, *Psychosomatics* 26:277, February 1985.

Kinash RG and others: Inflammatory bowel disease: impact and patient characteristics, *Gastroenterol Nurs* 15(4):147, 1993.

Koku RV: Severity of low back pain: a comparison between participants who did and did not receive counseling, *AAOHN J* 40:84, February 1992.

Krishnan K, France R, Houpt J: Chronic low back pain and depression, *Psychosomatics* 26:299, February 1985.

Matussek P, Agerer D, Seibt G: Aggression in depressives and psoriatics, *Psychother Psychosom* 43:120, March 1985.

Rimon R, Laakso RL: Life stress and rheumatoid arthritis, *Psychother Psychosom* 43:38, January 1985.

Robinson L: Stress and anxiety, *Nurs Clin North Am* 25:935, December 1990.

Santonastaso R and others: Hypertension and neuroticism, *Psychother Psychosom* 41:7, January 1984.

Sarason I and others: Life events, social support, and illness, *Psychosom Med* 47:156, March/April 1985.

Starkman M, Appleblatt N: Functional upper airway obstruction: a possible somatization disorder, *Psychosomatics* 25:327, April 1984.

Traver GA, Leidy NK: Asthma and stress, *J Adv Med Surg Nurs* 1(4):25, 1989.

Weiner H: What the future holds for psychosomatic medicine, *Psychother Psychosom* 42(1-4):15, 1984.

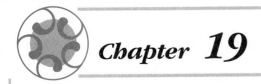

Chapter 19

Individuals with Substance Abuse and Dependence

Kem B. Louie

LEARNING OBJECTIVES

After studying this chapter, the student will be able to:

* Differentiate between substance abuse and substance dependence.

* Discuss the causative factors associated with substance abuse and dependence.

* Describe the effects of abuse of or dependence on narcotics, sedatives, hypnotics, central nervous system stimulants, hallucinogens, phencyclidine (PCP), and marijuana.

* Describe behaviors the nurse is most likely to observe when assessing an individual experiencing substance dependence.

* State examples of nursing diagnosis likely to be applicable to an individual experiencing substance dependence.

* Develop a hypothetical plan of nursing care for an individual experiencing substance dependence.

* State and explain nursing interventions likely to be effective with an individual who is substance dependent.

* Discuss the long-term treatment modalities for substance-dependent individuals.

KEY TERMS
Substance abuse
Substance dependence
Addictions nursing
Narcotics
Opiates
Withdrawal symptoms
Sedatives and hypnotics
Chronic alcoholics
Periodic, or cyclical, alcoholics
Barbiturates
Central nervous system stimulants
Cocaine
Crack
Amphetamines
Hallucinogens
Phencyclidine (PCP)
Marijuana
Self-help programs

Few human behaviors have consequences as far reaching as those of substance-dependent individuals. In addition to affecting their own physical, emotional, and social well-being, the behavior of substance-dependent individuals affects the well-being of their family and of society.

Substance abuse and **substance dependence** are major U.S. health problems (Figure 19-1). Not only do those affected require treatment for their habit, but they also are at significant risk of acquiring and transmitting human immunodeficiency virus (HIV) and hepatitis B through the use of contaminated needles and the practice of unprotected, indiscriminate sexual activity.

Substance abuse and dependence are also significant factors in the economic health of the United States. For example, industry has documented that alcoholism is one of the primary reasons for the loss of time and productivity both on the assembly line and in the executive suite.

Criminal activity is an integral aspect of drug dependence. "Hard" drugs must be procured from an illegal source, thereby contributing to the maintenance of organized crime. In addition, the price they command often causes individuals to resort to criminal activity to obtain sufficient funds to maintain their dependence. Even when drug-dependent individuals do not have to engage in criminal activity to support their dependence, they most certainly must spend money better used for other purposes. As a result, it is not unusual for their families to have inadequate food, clothing, and shelter. As the substance dependence increases, the source of legally gained income inevitably is cut off, usually because of these persons' inability to maintain their jobs.

Another complexity surrounding substance dependence is the inevitable involvement of the individual with both the legal and the health care systems. This overlap in social systems is not unique to these disorders, but the nature of the

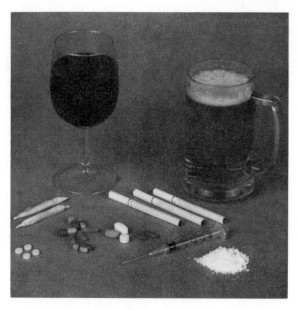

Figure 19-1

A wide variety of substances can be involved in substance abuse and dependence.

From Ray O, Ksir C: *Drugs, society, and human behavior,* ed 6, St Louis, 1993, Mosby–Year Book.

overlap is problematic, since the goals of the legal and health care systems are diametrically opposed. The goal of the legal system is to punish the offender, whereas the health care system views the individual as a person in need of help. This conflicting view of the same behavior developed partly because of lack of definitive information about the nature of substance dependence. Until research documents these behaviors as an illness or until society is willing to legalize dependence, the substance-dependent individual will remain caught between the divergent purposes of these two systems.

Caring for individuals with substance abuse and dependence has become a nursing specialty referred to as **addictions nursing.** The American Nurses Association has published standards that guide the nurse in caring for addictive clients and offers a national certification examination in the specialty. Two national nursing organizations devote their attention to addictions nursing, The National Nurses Society on Addictions and the Drug and Alcohol Nursing Association. Although the existence of this specialty is a testimony to an enlarging knowledge base and interest in this health problem, it is also a reflection of the increasing incidence and severity of the problem.

HISTORICAL PERSPECTIVE

The nontherapeutic use of mind-altering substances is as old as the history of humanity. The Old Testament gives an account of Noah becoming drunk on wine and apparently collapsing. The New Testament abounds with cautions against intemperance in many activities, including the drinking of alcoholic beverages. Thus it must be concluded that alcohol abuse was common in those days.

Historical reference to substance abuse is not limited to alcohol. Southwestern Plains Indians used hallucinogenic substances as an integral aspect of religious rituals. In the nineteenth century, cocaine was widely used throughout the civilized world, as was opium.

Not until the twentieth century, however, did the incidence of substance dependence become great enough to cause national concern. The Harrison Act of 1914 regulated drug traffic for the first time and provided for the licensing of certain groups such as physicians who could legally dispense these drugs for medicinal purposes. In the early 1920s the Volstead Act was passed, which made the sale of alcoholic beverages illegal. This law was ultimately repealed because it did little to curb the consumption of alcoholic beverages, but it did contribute to the development of crime syndicates that trafficked in the illegal manufacture and sale of liquor. The effect of the Harrison Act was similar to that of the Volstead Act; that is, addicts were forced to turn to illegal sources to obtain drugs. However, governmental response has not been the same. Rather than legalizing mind-altering drugs, as had been done with alcohol, stricter laws aimed at both the user and the supplier continue to be passed.

The number of alcohol-dependent persons in the United States has always been great. Alcoholism has existed in most ethnic groups at all socioeconomic levels. In contrast, before World War II, heroin addiction was most prevalent among Caucasians in the southern United States. Since the war the highest incidence of this type of drug dependence is found in northern urban areas among low-income African Americans and Hispanics.

The use of mind-altering drugs reached epidemic proportions in the 1960s and 1970s among lower-class and middle-class adolescents and young adults in urban and suburban areas throughout the entire United States. It appears that the level of drug usage among this group reached its peak in the 1970s. However, there has been a concomitant rise in alcohol use among adolescents and young adults. Epidemiological data recently reported by the National Institute of Mental Health indicate that alcohol abuse or dependence is the most frequent psychiatric disorder among males 18 to 65 years of age.

Of most recent concern is the increased use of cocaine. Before the 1980s cocaine was used primarily by those in the entertainment industry and young, upwardly mobile, middle-class, highly educated white males. Because of its current availability in the form of "crack," its price has dropped greatly, now making it within the economic reach of lower-income wage earners. Its availability, relatively low cost, and association with celebrities combine to make cocaine a fashionable drug.

SUBSTANCE ABUSE AND DEPENDENCE

When caring for individuals who use psychoactive substances, the nurse must differentiate between substance *abuse* and *substance dependence*. Many believe that substance dependence is determined solely by the presence of tolerance to the substance (the need for increasing amounts of a substance to produce the desired effect) and physiological symptoms when the substance is withdrawn. In addition to these criteria, however, substance dependence includes behaviors, thought processes, and other symptoms that indicate a lack of control of substance use despite its negative consequences. Substance abuse is a dysfunctional pattern of substance use for more than 1 month but does not meet the criteria for substance dependence.

The *Diagnostic and Statistical Manual of Mental Disorders* (third edition, revised) (DSM-III-R) differentiates between abuse of and dependence on psychoactive substances. The diagnostic criteria for substance dependence are:

A. At least three of the following:
1. Substance often taken in larger amounts or over a longer period than person intended
2. Persistent desire for substance or one or more unsuccessful efforts to cut down or control substance use
3. Much time spent in activities necessary to obtain substance (e.g., theft), taking sub-

stance (e.g., chain smoking), or recovering from its effects
4. Frequent intoxication or withdrawal symptoms when expected to fulfill major role obligations at work, school, or home (e.g., does not go to work because hung over, goes to school or work "high," intoxicated while taking care of his or her children) or when substance use is physically hazardous (e.g., drives when intoxicated)
5. Important social, occupational, or recreational activities given up or reduced because of substance use
6. Continued substance use despite knowledge of having a persistent or recurrent social, psychological, or physical problem that is caused or exacerbated by use of the substance (e.g., continues using heroin despite family arguments about it, cocaine-induced depression, worsening an ulcer by drinking)
7. Marked tolerance: need for increased amounts of the substance (i.e., at least a 50% increase) to achieve intoxication or desired effect or greatly diminished effect with continued use of the same amount

NOTE: The following criteria may not apply to cannabis, hallucinogens, or phencyclidine (PCP):
8. Characteristic withdrawal symptoms
9. Substance often taken to relieve or avoid withdrawal symptoms

B. Some symptoms of the disturbance have persisted for at least 1 month or have occurred repeatedly over a longer period.

The diagnostic criteria for substance abuse are:

A. At least one of the following:
1. Continued substance use despite knowledge of having a persistent or recurrent social, occupational, psychological, or physical problem that is caused or exacerbated by use of the psychoactive substance
2. Recurrent use in situations in which use

is physically hazardous (e.g., driving while intoxicated)

B. Some symptoms of the disturbance have persisted for at least 1 month or have occurred repeatedly over a longer period.

C. Person has never met the criteria for substance dependence for this substance.

It should be noted that the forthcoming DSM-IV proposes major revisions in the criteria related to substance abuse and dependence, not the least of which is changing the overall name of the category to "substance-related disorders" (see Appendix B). This change is proposed to enable inclusion of medication side effects as well as unintentional exposure to substances that affect the central nervous system and may lead to behavioral or cognitive disturbances. The criteria for abuse are also under discussion, particularly in regard to the 1-month duration requirement. Furthermore, the distinction between substance dependence and substance abuse will be sharpened by not repeating some or all of the criteria of substance abuse as criteria for substance dependence.

Both substance abuse and substance dependence are deleterious to the individual's physical, emotional, and social functioning and, as previously stated, often bring the person to the attention of the health care and legal systems.

CAUSATIVE FACTORS

Many theories have attempted to explain substance abuse and dependence. Research shows that multiple influences must be taken into consideration if these disorders are to be understood.

Biological factors

The role of biological factors in the development of substance abuse and dependence is not clear, although much research has been conducted in this area in regard to alcoholism. It has been demonstrated that the incidence of alcoholism varies significantly among ethnic groups and among families within these groups. Therefore, it is currently believed that there is probably a genetic predisposition to the development of this form of dependence. In addition, much current research is exploring the physiological factors that differentiate the alcoholic person from others who are able to drink alcohol without deleterious effects or a subsequent craving. One theory states some persons have a physiological inability to absorb and/or eliminate the substance. Another theory has postulated an allergic type of reaction among some people. Although there are fewer research studies concerning the influence of genetic and biochemical factors on the development of dependence on drugs other than alcohol, the idiosyncratic responses of some people to all other drugs are well known by clinicians.

Psychological factors

The factor contributing to substance abuse or dependence that has been explored most fully is the role of the person's personality. For example, it is believed that many persons who use depressant drugs such as alcohol, barbiturates, or heroin have not developed the ego defense mechanisms that would enable them to function as independent adults who can successfully cope with the stressor of daily living. Their use of these drugs enables them to blunt reality and withdraw from environmental and intrapsychic stressors.

In contrast, users of stimulant drugs such as amphetamines and cocaine are thought to have a personality bordering on grandiosity simultaneous with a need to defend consistently against fears of helplessness. The use of stimulant drugs allows such a person to feel active and potent in the face of an environment perceived as hostile and threatening.

Individuals who use hallucinogens and marijuana are believed to be struggling with tremendous amounts of repressed rage along with fears of annihilation and interpersonal isolation.

It is hypothesized that they attempt to cope with these feelings through the use of drugs that alter perception and cognition, often allowing them to feel "a cosmic unity."

Environmental factors

Environmental factors include the individual's family and the sociocultural environment in which the person lives.

Recently, much attention has been focused on the structure and rules of families of individuals who are substance dependent, particularly those who are alcohol dependent. The structure of such families has been found to be either *enmeshed,* where its members cannot function independent of each other, or *disengaged,* where there is little interdependence and family identity.

Regardless of their structure, all families have rules that set the guidelines for how they will function both within the family and with the environment. Sharon Wegscheider identifies three important characteristics of rules in the substance dependent family.

1. *Inhuman.* Rules often are unrealistic and impossible to keep. They encourage one to be dishonest and manipulative with others to avoid punishment or rejection. These rules also encourage one to be dishonest with oneself to avoid feelings of guilt.
2. *Rigid.* Rules make no allowance for differences in people or circumstances. They discourage change, seeing it as a potential threat to the status quo (especially that of the rule maker).
3. *Closed.* Certain areas of life are closed to communication. Information and feelings about these areas stay bottled up inside for each family member to handle alone.

Even this superficial discussion of the characteristics of the substance-dependent family makes clear the difficulty, if not impossibility, of a child in such a family being able to mature in a developmentally appropriate way. Thus one should not be surprised to learn that many substance-dependent persons come from families in which one or both parents were substance dependent.

The sociocultural environment of the substance-dependent individual is known to be a major determinant in the development and maintenance of the dependence. Societal norms that condone substance use and intoxication, peer group use of such substances, and the availability of licit and illicit drugs all combine to predict a high rate of substance dependence. When these factors exist in an environment fraught with multiple stressors, the likelihood of escaping substance abuse and dependence is minimal.

EFFECTS OF SUBSTANCE ABUSE AND DEPENDENCE

The DSM-III-R and the forthcoming DSM-IV classify the following substances as associated with both abuse and dependence: alcohol, amphetamines, caffeine, cannabis, cocaine, hallucinogens, inhalants, nicotine, opioids, phencyclidine (PCP), and sedatives, hypnotics, and anxiolytics. The following discussion categorizes most of these substances into six groups according to their actions and effects. Where applicable, the short-term treatment of the substance-dependent individual is described.

Narcotics

Narcotics are general depressants of the central nervous system and are used medically to relieve moderate and severe pain. Most narcotics are in the chemical class termed **opiates.** Morphine, heroin, and codeine are derivatives of opium; meperidine (Demerol) and methadone are synthetic substances. Although some opiate-dependent persons use morphine or meperidine, most do not have access to these drugs and use heroin, which is readily available on the streets of large cities.

These drugs are parenterally administered and produce a temporary state of well-being; troubles appear to be trifling and remote, and the person has a comfortable sense of complete relaxation. Individuals feel "normal," which means they feel as if their basic needs have been met. They feel sexually satisfied, full of food, free from anxiety and pain, and are not concerned with aggressive feelings. Whenever heroin-dependent individuals obtain an adequate dose, they may expose their addiction with an abnormal euphoria and contentment or even a sleepy languor. The pupils may show a telltale "pinpoint" constriction, and the arms and thighs usually are scarred or pigmented by the hypodermic needle. Other signs of narcotic intoxication include slurred speech, hypotension, dysphoria, apathy, psychomotor retardation, and impaired judgment.

Ever-increasing amounts are necessary to produce the desired effect, so the heroin user may require as much as 15 to 20 grains daily. Unfortunately, when the effects wear off and sufficient amounts are not immediately available, certain **withdrawal symptoms** promptly appear. Tears, sneezing, coryza, yawning, great irritability, and restlessness become quickly evident. Within 24 hours this is followed by abdominal cramps, vomiting, and diarrhea. To these distressing symptoms are added headache, sweating, and pains in the muscles and joints of the lower extremities. Finally, on the third day of abstinence the nervous irritability is so pronounced that the individual becomes hysterical, noisy, and threatening; the person frequently throws and destroys objects. Within a week, however, all these painful withdrawal reactions disappear.

Heroin dependence does not cause mental deterioration, but the treatment that addicts receive from society causes them to deteriorate socially. It is important to understand that the reality with which these individuals must cope contains few elements conducive to positive mental health. They become easy prey to drug pushers as early adolescents or sooner. Once "hooked," they must continue to live close to the source of drug supply, which means that the heroin-dependent individual is compelled to associate with the people who smuggle the drug into the country and the pushers who sell it. Few, if any, smugglers or pushers are themselves dependent on heroin. However, they actively support its use by others.

In addition to the heroin users found in large cities, a growing number of physicians and a lesser number of nurses are dependent on morphine and meperidine, which they illegally obtain from hospitals or fraudulently written prescriptions. State licensing authorities and professional organizations are actively involved not only in punishing these persons but also in facilitating their treatment and rehabilitation.

Withdrawal from opium derivatives has been made more humane through the use of methadone, which is a substitute for the opiate on which the individual is dependent. The use of methadone has been a somewhat controversial method of treating narcotic addiction. This is partly because methadone has been declared to be a narcotic by the Federal Bureau of Narcotics. However, some authorities believe that the use of methadone in treating heroin addicts holds the best hope for halting their criminal activities and for making them self-supporting citizens. It has been used most successfully with groups of heroin addicts in several large cities.

With methadone the individual loses the heroin dependency by becoming addicted to the "substitute," methadone. The user then requires regular doses of methadone daily.

This treatment has at least two advantages: (1) it is relatively inexpensive; an individual can be maintained on methadone for a few cents a day; and (2) individuals who are taking methadone do not lose their ability to function normally; they can usually hold a job and function as responsible citizens. Today most large cities have meth-

Table 19-1. Relationship between blood alcohol levels and behavior in a nontolerant drinker

BAL (mg/dl)	BAC	BEHAVIOR
5	1-2 drinks	Changes in mood and behavior; judgment is impaired.
10	5-6 drinks	Voluntary motor action becomes clumsy; legal level of intoxication in most states.
20	10-12 drinks	Function of entire motor area of the brain is depressed, causing staggering and ataxia; emotional lability is present.
30	15-18 drinks	Confusion; stupor
40	20-24 drinks	Coma
50	25-30 drinks	Death from respiratory depression

BAL, Blood alcohol level; *BAC*, blood alcohol accumulation *in excess of* alcohol metabolized.

adone clinics where several hundred individuals go to receive the daily dose of methadone. Most clinics require proof that individuals are not continuing to use heroin by requiring them to produce urine specimens free of the drug.

Sedatives and hypnotics

Sedatives and hypnotics are a category of abused drugs that includes alcohol, barbiturates, antipsychotic agents, and anxiolytic agents. Antipsychotic agents and anxiolytic agents are discussed in Chapter 10.

Alcohol dependence

Alcohol is a central nervous system depressant. The amount required to produce a demonstrable effect varies according to the interrelationship of such variables as the percentage of alcohol in the beverage, the tolerance the individual has developed to the substance, the person's physical and emotional state of health, and the nature of the environment in which the person is drinking. In addition, the amount and type of food in the stomach constitute a major factor that affects the rate of absorption. Hard liquor consumed by a person unaccustomed to alcohol who is emotionally upset, has not eaten all day, and is in the company of persons who are accepting of intoxication is certain to produce a very rapid effect (Table 19-1). The alcohol equiv-

---

ALCOHOL EQUIVALENCIES

Wine: 4 ounces equivalent to 12% alcohol
Beer: 12 ounces equivalent to 4% alcohol
Hard liquor: 1 ounce equivalent to 48% alcohol

---

alency in selected beverages is shown in the box above.

Once alcohol is absorbed into the bloodstream, it affects all body tissues, but its immediate effects are caused by its action on the brain. At a level of 0.05% alcohol in the blood, inhibitions are diminished and the individual is likely to say and do things that would be unacceptable if the person were sober. Interestingly, there is a societal norm that, to a point, excuses the behavior of an individual who has been drinking on the grounds that he or she has been drinking. This cyclical thinking is based on the belief that the behavior of a person when drunk is not a reflection of the person but rather a manifestation of the alcohol. The reality is that the impulses acted on emanate from the person, and the alcohol merely removes the barriers to their implementation.

At a level of 0.10% alcohol in the blood, motor and speech activity is impaired. For this reason

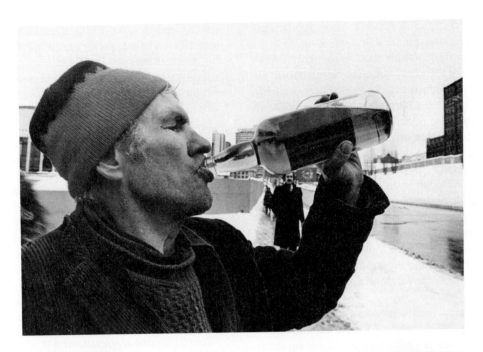

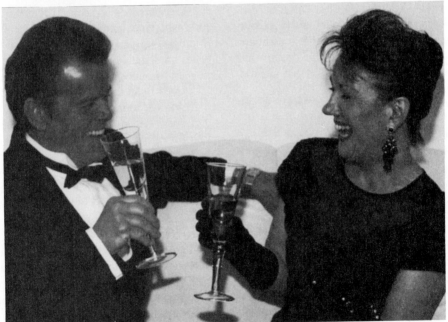

Figure 19-2

Alcohol dependence takes many forms, some not so easy to identify.

From Ray O, Ksir C: *Drugs, society, and human behavior,* ed 6, St Louis, 1993, Mosby–Year Book.

there is a continuing national campaign against driving a motor vehicle when drinking.

Alcohol dependence may take many forms (Figure 19-2). Individuals may be **chronic alcoholics,** which means they drink excessively and may be incapacitated most of the time. Other persons may be referred to as **periodic, or cyclical, alcoholics,** which means that they drink excessively during certain periods of their lives but during other periods may not drink at all. A third type of alcoholism is exhibited by individuals who drink large quantities of alcohol daily over a period of years. At first these persons may not seem to be seriously affected by this over-indulgence. Slowly and insidiously, however, physical, mental, and emotional deterioration occurs. Eventually they may be described as having alcoholic deterioration.

Short-term, immediate treatment of alcohol-dependent individuals is focused on withdrawing them from this substance and assisting them to attain or regain physical health. This is accomplished by symptomatic treatment of the anxiety, tremors, nausea, and diaphoresis that accompany withdrawal. Seizures and delirium tremens are serious, life-threatening conditions that may occur during detoxification.

Delirium tremens is an acute reaction to the withdrawal from a heavy and consistent intake of alcohol for several weeks without an adequate intake of food. In an individual who has been a chronic alcoholic for several years, delirium tremens may be precipitated by a head injury or a surgical procedure without the individual having consumed alcohol at the time of its appearance. Delirium tremens consists of confusion, excitement, and delirium. It is usually of relatively short duration and does not cause a profound or permanent change in the personality.

The delirium is preceded by loss of appetite, restlessness, and insomnia. Slight noises cause the patient to jerk with fear, and moving objects lead to great excitement and agitation. Gradually, consciousness becomes clouded, friends are no longer recognized, and shadows on the wall appear as insects or crawling animals. The person becomes terrified, picks imaginary threads off the bedclothing, and feels and sees nonexistent insects on the skin. There is a ceaseless fumbling and picking movement of fingers and hands. The person's face has an anxious or terrified expression, the eyes are bloodshot, the skin is moist with perspiration, the tongue and lips are tremorous, the pulse is rapid and weak, and there is always some elevation of temperature.

Anticonvulsant and sedative medications, along with high-potency vitamins and copious amounts of clear liquids, are employed during this phase of treatment, to both prevent and treat seizures and delirium tremens. Because of the serious physiological disequilibrium caused by withdrawal from alcohol, this procedure is best carried out in a hospital by staff who are knowledgeable about the varied problems involved.

Barbiturate dependence

Barbiturates are central nervous system depressants and include phenobarbital, pentobarbital (Nembutal), and secobarbital (Seconal). They are legally prescribed treatments for insomnia and epilepsy. Their effect is similar to that achieved by drinking alcohol. In some respects barbiturate dependence is more dangerous than dependence on alcohol because large numbers of pills can be and are taken at the same time by suicidal people, whereas it is unlikely that a sufficient amount of alcohol could be consumed at one time to result in death. In addition, the mental confusion caused by both alcohol and barbiturates often leads to these substances being used together, resulting in accidental death.

Early stages of barbiturate intoxication are manifested by muscular incoordination with ataxia, dizziness, nystagmus, slurred speech, and sluggish mentality. The person acquires many bruises and perhaps fractures by falling or stumbling against walls and furniture. In more profound barbiturate intoxication, there are varying degrees of stupor, speech is incoherent, memory is defective, and hallucinations may appear.

When aroused, the person is usually very irritable and resistive and has the symptoms of a person with delirium. Recovery may be slow and may leave in its wake a mild degree of permanent brain damage.

It is imperative that treatment of persons dependent on barbiturates begin with *gradual* withdrawal of the drug. Sudden, complete withdrawal is often fatal. Individuals who present themselves voluntarily for detoxification are also treated with a high-calorie, high-vitamin diet. Persons who are in a coma caused by barbiturate overdose must be treated aggressively with dialysis to lower the level of barbiturates in the blood.

Central nervous system stimulants

The most frequently abused drugs in the category of **central nervous system stimulants** are cocaine and crack and amphetamines.

Cocaine and crack

Cocaine was used for medical purposes in the late 1800s. It acts directly on the cerebral cortex and initially increases the sensation of mental and physical well-being (Figure 19-3).

Crack, a derivative of cocaine, was first seen in urban areas of the United States in the early 1980s. Unlike cocaine, crack is generally smoked rather than snorted or injected. Its use has become widespread throughout the United States, probably because its effects are more intense than those of cocaine and its price is lower.

Cocaine is absorbed very rapidly: 3 minutes when snorted, 15 seconds when injected, and 7 seconds when smoked. It metabolizes so quickly that users may take the drug every 20 to 30 minutes to maintain their high. Crack has an even shorter period of effect than cocaine; its high lasts only 5 to 7 minutes. The intensity of the euphoria created by crack, combined with the shortness

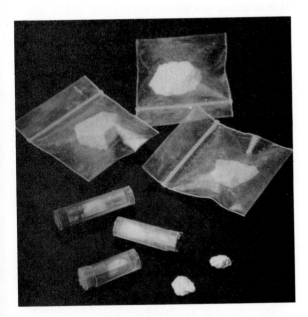
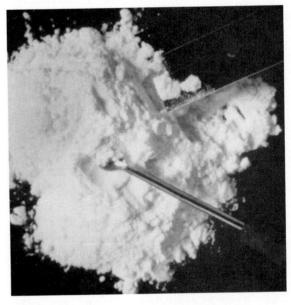

Figure 19-3
Crack cocaine and cocaine in powdered form.
From Ray O, Ksir C: *Drugs, society, and human behavior,* ed 6, St Louis, 1993, Mosby–Year Book.

of its duration, is largely responsible for the fast, intense dependency on this drug that users frequently report.

Signs of cocaine and crack use are tachycardia, dilated pupils, elevated blood pressure, insomnia, and anorexia. Behavioral changes include elation, grandiosity, impaired judgment, and even paranoid thinking.

Cocaine and crack are typically believed to be "safe" drugs because they do not produce definitive withdrawal syndromes. However, depression is common following withdrawal and may be severe enough to precipitate a suicidal attempt. This phenomenon is called *crashing* by its users. In 1983 the National Institute on Drug Abuse declared cocaine to be a "powerfully addictive" substance linked to cardiac arrests, seizures, and respiratory ailments. This agency has received reports of cocaine-related illnesses that have doubled since 1980. Cocaine-related deaths have tripled since that time, probably because of cocaine being "cut" with other substances by the dealer, and the user inadvertently overdosing by unknowingly purchasing cocaine that is more pure than that previously used.

Short-term treatment of cocaine and crack dependence is focused on treating any symptoms supportively. Long-term abstinence is difficult to achieve for the individual who has experienced the euphoria associated with the use of this drug unless the person develops other coping mechanisms and support systems.

Amphetamines

Numerous chemical compounds fall in the category of **amphetamines,** the most common of which are racemic amphetamine sulfate (Benzedrine) and methamphetamine (Desoxyn). In the past these drugs have been legitimately used in small doses under medical supervision to treat depression and curb appetite. Individuals who take these drugs solely to become "high" take from 6 to 200 times the daily dose usually prescribed by a physician. Intravenous amphetamines are called "speed" in street language.

The physiological effect of these drugs raises the blood pressure, sometimes to dangerous levels. Large doses have been known to cause immediate death, accounting for the saying among drug users that "speed kills."

Physical signs of amphetamine use include tachycardia, dilated pupils, elevated blood pressure, nausea and vomiting, and twitching. Behavioral signs include hostility, impaired judgment, impaired social and occupational functioning, euphoria, and increased energy.

Individuals who use amphetamines report these drugs increase their physical energy, sharpen their physical and sexual reactions, and increase their confidence. Thus a period of frantic activity results from the ingestion of large amounts of amphetamines. This is followed by a great letdown in which the fatigue and depression are so tremendous that the person is apt to seek release by taking the drug again. Chronic use of amphetamines can lead to a schizophrenic-like psychosis with paranoid features. This reaction is a result of the drug and is not related to the individual's premorbid personality. In addition, prolonged use at high dosages can lead to massive, irreversible brain damage that may result in death. The use of amphetamines today is not as great as it was in the 1970s, probably because of the drug's deserved reputation as highly dangerous.

Hallucinogens

Lysergic acid diethylamide (LSD, acid) is the most frequently abused of the **hallucinogens.** It was first used in research studies in an attempt to discover the cause of schizophrenia. Ingestion of reasonably small doses produces temporary hallucinations and other schizophrenic-like symptoms. The user experiences waves of color, and vibrations seem to pass through the head. Individuals report they have had an almost mystical experience in which the nature of emotional conflicts becomes clear.

Although little evidence indicates that the use of LSD causes physical dependence, it is dangerous for several reasons. First, this substance causes some individuals to believe they have supernatural powers, and more than one person has been killed in an attempt to fly. Second, although no hallucinogen withdrawal reaction occurs even after prolonged high-dose use, a panic reaction can occur, particularly in the first-time user. This reaction is referred to as a *bad trip* and may last as long as a week. In such instances, the user can be helped by being "talked down" by a trusted friend who remains with him and points out reality. Third, *flashbacks,* in which the user experiences hallucinations days or weeks after using a hallucinogen, can also occur.

Phencyclidine (PCP)

Phencyclidine (PCP) has historically been classified as a hallucinogen; however, it does not have hallucinogenic effects at low to moderate doses. Rather, low doses produce mild depression and then stimulation. High doses, however, can produce a schizophrenic-like psychosis with paranoid delusions and hallucinations.

PCP is also known as the *animal tranquilizer, angel dust,* or the *peace pill.* It comes in many forms, such as pills, capsules, and liquids, and is smoked, sniffed, swallowed, and injected. Physical signs of use include vertical or horizontal nystagmus, increased blood pressure and temperature, ataxia, muscle rigidity, seizure, blank stare, chronic jerking, and agitated movement. Psychological signs include belligerence, unpredictability, impulsiveness, impaired judgment and in severe cases, paranoia, hallucinations, and bizarre behaviors.

Marijuana

In the past, **marijuana** was an easily obtained and relatively inexpensive drug. It is a crude preparation from the whole *Cannabis sativa* plant, which grows wild in Mexico and is easily cultivated in the United States. It is usually absorbed into the body through the smoking of cigarettes called *reefers.* Hashish is prepared by scraping resin from the tops of the hemp plant.

The active ingredient in both marijuana and hashish is tetrahydrocannabinol, with hashish being much more potent.

Inhalation of marijuana causes a state of exhilaration or euphoria. Under its influence the user feels light in body, floating through space, and the general behavior is not unlike a mild mania. Marijuana is not an aphrodisiac, but it can lower inhibitions and intensify sexual pleasure. It seems to make many users temporarily passive, in contrast to alcohol, which frequently releases aggression. Marijuana affects the individual's sense of time but not necessarily motor and perceptual skills. Users become psychologically dependent on marijuana but may not become physically addicted as with morphine.

Signs of use include tachycardia, increased appetite, impaired motor ability, and talkativeness. Psychological signs include euphoria, intensification of perceptions, apathy, increased anxiety, and impaired judgment and memory.

Much attention has been given to marijuana by the government. Official arguments have been carried on in the press concerning the relative dangers of marijuana and the appropriate penalties that should be or should not be levied against people who use it. Unfortunately, there is a limited amount of research on which to base a scientific, unbiased judgment concerning the immediate dangers of smoking marijuana or the eventual outcome of long-term use of this drug. Many research findings have been contradictory. Certainly the present laws controlling its use are inequitable, as well as widely unenforceable.

NURSING CARE OF INDIVIDUALS WITH SUBSTANCE ABUSE AND DEPENDENCE

Nursing assessment

Although abuse of or dependence on each substance has its unique features, it is possible to cite some commalities about all persons with substance abuse or dependence. The following discussion presents behaviors as separate entities, but they are highly interrelated and are ad-

---

GENERAL ASSESSMENT QUESTIONS

1. What drug(s) did you take before coming to the hospital?
2. How did you take the drug(s) (e.g., intravenously, intramuscularly, orally, subcutaneously, smoking, intranasally)?
3. How much of the drug(s) did you take?
4. When did you last take the drug(s)?
5. How long have you been taking the drug(s)?
6. How often and how much do you take?
7. Under what circumstances do you take the drug(s)?

---

aptations to similar stressors. Further, behavior designed as an adaptation to one stressor often becomes a stressor itself in another dimension.

An integral aspect of the nursing assessment is the determination of the type of drug taken, its amount and frequency, the circumstances under which it is used, when it was last used, and what the individual's reactions are when the drug's use is discontinued (see the box above). It is important for the nurse to listen carefully to not only the words but also the defense mechanisms conveyed by the person's responses. Individuals' attitudes toward their dependence and the substances they are taking are often transmitted by their nonverbal behavior. For example, some persons may answer matter-of-factly, some may express great concern about their health and welfare, and still others may convey resentment about the nurse "prying" into their personal lives.

One widely used simple questionnaire* has been employed to assess the severity of alcohol use. This is referred to as the CAGE:

1. Have you ever felt you should *c*ut down on your drinking?
2. Have people *a*nnoyed you by criticizing your drinking?

---

*Ewing J: Detecting alcoholism: the CAGE questionnaire, *JAMA* 252(14):1905, 1984.

3. Have you ever felt bad or *g*uilty about your drinking?
4. Have you ever had a drink first thing in the morning to steady your nerves or get rid of a hangover (*e*yeopener)?

Two or three "yes" answers to these questions strongly suggest dependence on alcohol.

Health perception–health management

All physiological processes are affected or potentially affected by substance abuse and dependence. Examples of physiological alterations for each category of substance abuse are:

- Narcotics. Physical integrity is altered by the intravenous injection of the drug, leaving "track marks" and often causing local or systemic infections.
- Sedatives and hypnotics. Not only does malnutrition frequently occur, but gastric ulcers also may occur from large amounts of alcohol taken over long periods.
- Central nervous system stimulants. Because cocaine is often snorted, heavy users may have necrotic perforation of the nasal septum.
- Hallucinogens and PCP. Some evidence indicates that continued use of LSD and PCP creates chromosomal damage and teratogenicity (malformation of the fetus).
- Marijuana. Although many consider this drug to be among the safest, the fact that it is smoked contributes to decreased vital capacity and perhaps even lung cancer among heavy users.

CLINICAL EXAMPLE

Matthew's mother called the police and mobile crisis team because her son, 17, was locked in his room for 3 days. She suspected that he had been taking drugs with his friends. His mother reported that his personality changed, and he would not eat, bathe, or socialize with the family. Finally, when the nurse convinced Matthew to come to the hospital, the nurse assessed signs of drowsiness, hypotension, dysphoria, psycho-motor retardation, and impaired judgment. She immediately called the ambulance.

Nutritional-metabolic

Almost every individual who abuses or is dependent on a substance for any length of time has malnutrition. This in turn makes the person exceptionally susceptible to alterations in other physiological processes.

Activity-exercise

The motor behavior of a substance-dependent individual is always affected when the substance affects the central nervous system, as with opiates, alcohol, barbiturates, and amphetamines. In the person intoxicated with opioids, alcohol, and barbiturates, psychomotor retardation will be observed. Even small amounts of alcohol and low doses of barbiturates will produce incoordination and an unsteady gait in most users. Because of this, the individual often has bruises or fractures resulting from falls and bumping into furniture.

In contrast, intoxication with amphetamines results in psychomotor hyperactivity.

Self-care ultimately is affected in all individuals who are substance dependent. Hygiene and grooming become poor as the person's judgment becomes impaired.

CLINICAL EXAMPLE

Cassandra was taken to the hospital emergency room by an anonymous friend. On assessment, the nurse noticed that Cassandra's appearance was disheveled, her speech was impaired, she was talkative, and she was disoriented as to time and place. On further interviewing, Cassandra stated that she had not slept for 4 days. She complained that her "friend" had given her some sleeping pills to make her sleep. She denied taking any other drugs before coming to the hospital.

Recreation patterns are almost always altered in individuals who are substance dependent. In-dividuals who are dependent on large amounts of a substance must forgo recreational activities because all their time is spent obtaining the drug, using it, or engaging in activities to secure money to buy it.

Home maintenance is always altered when a person is dependent on a substance.

Sleep-rest

Sleep and arousal patterns are always impaired when the individual abuses or is dependent on substances affecting the central nervous system. Central nervous system depressants allow the person to fall into a stuporous sleep but cause a "rebound effect" about 4 hours later when the person awakens with a start, often with tachycardia. Central nervous system stimulants cause insomnia and initially are often taken to achieve this effect.

Cognitive-perceptual

Cognition processes are almost alwyas altered by substance abuse. Therefore, in the stage of acute intoxication, the nurse will observe alterations in decision making, judgment, memory, and thought processes. Whether these changes will remain after withdrawal from the substance depends on whether the drug has destroyed brain tissue. Long-term alcohol abusers, for example, show evidence of diminution of cognitive capacities even after they have been abstinent for years. The long-term effect of marijuana use on cognitive processes is the subject of much current research.

CLINICAL EXAMPLE

Lucas, a senior college student living off campus, was admitted to the college hospital because his history professor noticed that he was acting strangely in class. During the lecture, Lucas would stand up and go to the window and stare for several minutes; at other times he would sit by the door and lean the chair against the door until the period bell rang. He rarely spoke in class and handed in assignments in which he discussed an enemy of a foreign country coming to discredit him.

Alteration in attention is common in individuals who use drugs that affect the central nervous system. Central nervous system depressants cause inattention, whereas stimulants cause hyperalertness.

Alterations in sensory perception are always present in individuals who use hallucinogens. They are also present in individuals with delirium tremens after withdrawal from large quantities of alcohol imbibed over long periods.

Self-perception/self-concept

There is much debate about whether a poor self-concept contributes to substance dependence. Regardless of the eventual answer to this question, continued substance abuse and dependence undoubtedly lead to altered self-esteem.

Feeling states are always altered during the stage of acute intoxication, and this alteration is the conscious goal of initial substance use. As previously stated, individuals use narcotics to create a feeling of "normalcy," sedative hypnotics to create a feeling of calm, and central nervous system stimulants to create a feeling of euphoria. Withdrawal from any substance often creates anxiety, often to the degree of panic. Furthermore, during those periods when they are not using the drug, many individuals experience guilt, sadness, and shame about their behavior when they were "high."

CLINICAL EXAMPLE

During an Alcoholics Anonymous (AA) meeting, Janson, 54, stood and began to tell the group the effects of his long-term drinking on his family. He sounded remorseful and occasionally cried openly as he talked about not seeing his children or grandchildren. He admitted that when he was drinking, he was "immune" to the feelings of loss and problems in his life.

Role-relationship

Interpersonal processes are always affected in the domains of impulse control, family processes, role performance, and social interaction.

Impulse control is impaired because dependent individuals have no choice but to go to any length to obtain the substance if they are to avoid withdrawal symptoms. This may mean that they engage in behaviors such as lying, stealing, physical aggression, or prostitution even though these behaviors may be otherwise abhorrent to them. Furthermore, when acutely intoxicated with a substance that affects the central nervous system, individuals become accident prone and a potential danger to themselves and others.

As previously explained, family processes are always altered. Since the family operates as a system, the existence of a substance-dependent member precipitates responsive family adaptation that hinder the development of family members and the family as a unit.

The substance-dependent individual ultimately has severe alterations in role performance, often losing a job or failing out of school.

Sexuality-reproductive

Sexuality is frequently altered, especially with abuse of substances that affect the central nervous system. Social interaction with individuals who do not use the substance on which the individual is dependent is often curtailed, and social isolation or withdrawal frequently occurs.

Coping–stress tolerance

All persons with substance abuse and dependence demonstrate difficulty in coping with the stressors of daily living. Their use of substances often began as a dysfunctional means of coping. As with most dysfunctional adaptations, substance use quickly becomes a stressor in and of itself and further impairs the individual's coping ability, thereby contributing to a self-defeating cycle of behavior.

Value-belief

Unquestionably individuals who are substance dependent feel powerless over their addiction and hopeless about release from the vicious cycle of obtaining the drug, taking the drug, experiencing its effect, coming down from the effect, obtaining the drug, and so on. They often report that life has lost all meaning other than that related to the drug.

CLINICAL EXAMPLE

Manuel, 26, has been in drug detoxication for several days. He has been to this hospital three times before in the last year. All the nurses on the unit know him. One day he said to the nurse, "I guess I'm doomed to be like this for the rest of my life."

NURSE: Tell me more about this.

MANUEL: I'll never get better. I keep coming back to this place.

NURSE: You sound hopeless about your disease.

MANUEL: Look at what I've done to my parents and wife. I even stole from and lied to them. I don't know if I can ever face them again.

NURSE: You can't change what has happened in the past, but you can begin to change what happens to your future. It's important to learn more about your disease and cope with the cravings for the drug. We'll help you.

Nursing diagnosis

As with all nursing diagnoses, the nursing diagnoses for the individual with substance abuse or dependence are based on the themes identified during the assessment phase of the nursing process.

Accepted NANDA nursing diagnoses that may be specifically applicable to the individual with substance abuse and dependence include:

Altered health maintenance
Noncompliance (specify)
High risk for infection
High risk for injury
Altered protection
Altered nutrition: less than body requirements
Impaired skin integrity
Constipation
Diarrhea
Altered patterns of urinary elimination
Activity intolerance
Impaired physical mobility
Self-care deficit, bathing/hygiene; dressing/ grooming
Diversional activity deficit
Impaired home maintenance management
Decreased cardiac output
Altered (specify type) tissue perfusion
Sleep pattern disturbance
Knowledge deficit (specify)
Altered thought processes
Decisional conflict (specify)
Sensory/perceptual alterations
Fear
Anxiety
Hopelessness
Powerlessness
Body image disturbance
Personal identity disturbance
Self-esteem disturbance; situational low self-esteem; chronic low self-esteem
Anticipatory grieving
Dysfunctional grieving
Altered role performance
Impaired social interaction
Altered family processes
Altered parenting
High risk for violence: self-directed or directed at others
Sexual dysfunction
Altered sexuality patterns
Rape-trauma syndrome
Ineffective individual coping
Defensive coping
Ineffective denial
Posttrauma response
Ineffective family coping: compromised
Ineffective family coping: disabling
Spiritual distress

To develop a nursing diagnosis that fulfills its function of providing direction for planning nursing care, the nurse is encouraged to postulate and state etiological or antecedent factors and connect the two phrases by using the term "related to." For example:

Altered role performance related to inability to work because of dependence on heroin.

Planning and implementing nursing care

The plan for nursing care is derived from the nursing diagnoses and includes the objectives of the care, the nursing interventions, and outcome criteria. To be effective, the plan needs to be highly individualized. The suggestions that follow should be seen as general guidelines to be used if they are appropriate to the client's needs.

In general, the objectives of all nursing care for the individual with substance abuse or dependence should relate to assisting the client to regain physiological homeokinesis, to increase self-esteem, to develop functional methods of coping with stress, and to remain drug free.

Until recently, the nurse was likely to be in a position to give care to an individual with substance abuse or dependence only when the person was admitted to an acute care hospital because of serious physiological alterations caused either by drug abuse or dependence or by another unrelated illness. There is an increasing awareness, however, that some persons with a severe mental illness, particularly young adult, chronically ill clients, present themselves as substance-dependent individuals, when in reality their substance dependence is an adaptation to the symptoms of their mental illness. Consequently, these individuals are now being treated simultaneously for their drug dependence and their mental illness in psychiatric units of general hospitals or in psychiatric hospitals. They are often referred to as *multidisabled* or *mentally ill chemical abusers (MICAs)*, and psychiatric nursing is assuming an increasing responsibility for their care. It is also important to understand that individuals may be dependent on more than one substance, a condition referred to as *polysubstance addiction.*

Since the client's nursing diagnoses are often interrelated, stemming as they do from similar etiologies or antecedents, the student should see that the appropriate nursing interventions are also interrelated. In other words, by intervening in one dimension, the nurse will also affect other dimensions.

Health perception–health management

When clients are intoxicated or being withdrawn from a substance, meeting their physical needs is of paramount importance. Every body system is likely to be in a greater or lesser state of disequilibrium, and in some instances the client may be in danger of dying. It is important that the nurse be particularly alert to the client's level of consciousness, the maintenance of a patent airway, adequate fluid intake and output, and prevention of injury.

Once clients are drug free, the nurse will find that they probably will have some residual physiological alterations resulting from their substance dependence. As previously stated, malnutrition is common among all substance abusers. In addition, other problems may be specific to the effects of the drug that was abused or to its mode of transmission, such as skin infections in the opiate-dependent individual and peripheral neuropathy in the alcohol-dependent person. The nurse needs to address these problems as she or he would with any person who exhibited the same alterations.

Nurses need to monitor the somatic therapies that may be prescribed to control the substance use. For example, disulfiram (Antabuse) has been used in the treatment of alcoholism. Disulfiram inhibits the intake of alcohol by producing unpleasant physical reactions such as facial flushing, tachycardia, respiratory distress, drop in blood pressure, and nausea and vomiting. These reactions usually occur within 30 minutes after drinking and last up to an hour. Disulfiram is taken daily. Substances and foods containing alcohol can also produce these adverse reactions in clients taking disulfiram. Examples of such frequently used substances and foods are mouthwashes, after-shave lotions, cough medicines, and food sauces and

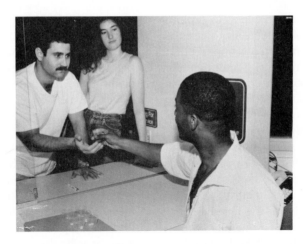

Figure 19-4
Methadone maintenance programs require the clients to show up each day to receive the methadone. This makes it easier to keep track of the clients and to counsel them on a regular basis.
From Ray O, Ksir C: *Drugs, society, and human behavior,* ed 6, St Louis, 1993, Mosby–Year Book.

flavor extracts that contain alcohol. Naltrexone (Trexan) is similar to disulfiram in use with those dependent on narcotics. The success of these antagonists depends on the person taking them daily.

For persons dependent on heroin, methadone (Dolophine) maintenance is the somatic treatment of choice (Figure 19-4). This drug blocks the craving for and withdrawal symptoms from heroin and enables the person to carry on normal activities of living. However, methadone can also produce dependence and withdrawal symptoms.

Cognitive-perceptual

Nurses should include health teaching about the disease and its progression in their plan of care. This information is designed to educate the client about the effects of the substance on the mind and other body systems, as well as its effect on the unborn. Clients should also be taught that recovery from substance dependence is a long-term process and that relapse is part of the disease's cycle. They should be helped to identify

and use various outpatient services that offer group, family, and marital counseling, in addition to their use of **self-help programs.** Research has shown that individuals dealing with substance abuse and dependency benefit from group therapy and should be encouraged to participate in formal and self-help groups.

Self-perception/self-concept

The substance-dependent person is an individual with very low self-esteem. Thus the nurse is most therapeutic when focusing on the client's strengths, acknowledging them, and helping the person build on them. For example, having the client participate in decision making about activities and providing opportunities for success can be important interventions if the nurse also acknowledges the client's wise judgments and achievements. The client also needs to be helped to see that one achievement can lead to another and that each is not an isolated event.

Substance-dependent clients who no longer have access to drugs inevitably will express great anxiety. It is helpful if the nurse takes their feelings seriously and encourages clients to explore their source. For example, clients may share the fact that sitting in a room with a group of other people makes them "nervous." Although the nurse may find this difficult to believe because they appear to be confident and competent, the nurse needs to understand that their use of drugs is a powerful indicator that they do feel insecure without the blunting or stimulating effect of the drug. Therefore it is helpful to explore with clients their worst fears about what may happen in the group and then assist them to problem solve a functional solution if the fears become reality.

Anger is another feeling often displayed by individuals undergoing treatment for substance abuse or dependence. Since it is often very anxiety producing for substance-dependent clients to express anger, their ability to do so is often indicative of increasing ego strength. To the extent that the anger is reality based, it is therapeutic for the nurse to acknowledge this feeling and help in discovering productive outlets. However, sometimes clients use their anger about real or fantasized wrongs that they have experienced in the past as a means of avoiding dealing with the present or planning for the future. In this situation the nurse can be most therapeutic by listening in a matter-of-fact manner, but then insisting that the client get on with the task at hand. The tendency for substance-dependent clients to ruminate about problems in their past is the basis for the famous Serenity Prayer used so successfully by Alcoholics Anonymous.

Role-relationship

It is important for the nurse to appreciate fully that substance-dependent clients are likely to have difficulty controlling their impulses. Understanding this, however, does not mean that the nurse should condone unacceptable behavior. Early in the treatment regimen, clients need to be confronted in a nonjudgmental nonpunitive way with the fact that they will be held responsible for their behavior. Therefore the consequences of behavior, such as lying, taking drugs, or being verbally or physically assaultive, need to be made clear. It is imperative that all staff behave toward the client in a consistent manner when and if these infractions occur.

Various behaviors are exhibited when interacting with individuals with substance use. These include denial, projection, rationalization, manipulation, and hostility.

Clients need to be helped to plan realistically for a future life without drugs. The first step in this process is to help them explore what drugs meant and to identify and grieve about the losses they will experience without the drugs. These losses may be very concrete, such as friends and activities, or they may be more abstract, such as a way of life. After the grieving process has taken place, practical issues such as where they are going to live, what type of work they want to prepare for, and how they are going to develop a social network with people who do not use drugs are topics that need to be addressed.

The client's family is in need of as much help as the client. Not only do they have many issues to deal with about events in the past, but they must also adjust to changes in the client. The nurse can be most helpful to the family by ensuring that they become involved in group counseling, either through the mental health facility or with the appropriate self-help organization.

LONG-TERM TREATMENT OF SUBSTANCE-DEPENDENT INDIVIDUALS

Although most communities have medical facilities for treating individuals with substance dependence, the rate of relapse is very high. Therefore some authorities believe that a more realistic approach to the problem of substance dependence would be to supply dependent individuals with a minimum weekly supply of the substance on which they are dependent, such as occurs in methadone maintenance programs in large cities. It is argued that this practice would make the illegal traffic in drugs unprofitable and would aid in diminishing the crimes that persons now commit to obtain money to buy drugs. Ideally, it would also then be possible for substance-dependent individuals to purchase adequate food and therefore maintain their physical health instead of denying themselves food to purchase the substance.

Mental health professionals have had less long-term success in treating substance-dependent individuals than have lay organizations. The oldest and most successful of these organizations is Alcoholics Anonymous (AA). AA was founded in 1935 by two alcoholic persons and usually admits to membership only individuals who have a desire to stop drinking. It has had a dramatic development and today numbers more than 1 million members throughout the world. AA offers alcoholic persons answers to their emotional needs because it uses psychological principles that have been recognized as being effective in helping troubled people. AA also has affiliated groups. One is for spouses (Al-Anon), one for children (Ala-Teen), and another for adult children of alcoholics.

Because membership is limited to individuals who themselves have been unable to control the problem of alcohol, members have much sympathy for, patience with, and understanding for each other. Through the program they are able to meet alcoholics' dependency needs by seeking them out, encouraging them, helping them find jobs, accompanying them to meetings of the organization, and helping them develop a sense of personal value and worth. Members are encouraged to admit that they are powerless over alcohol and in need of help from a power greater than themselves. They search out their own past errors and, having admitted them to another human being, undertake to make amends for them. They strive to follow a simple code of living that eventually becomes a philosophy of life. The organizational meetings include testimonials by the members concerning their struggles with alcohol and their eventual triumph.

AA offers an experience in group participation and the use of group support. This organization is able to assist its members to develop a new emotional orientation toward life and to begin to meet the problems of life without the aid of alcohol. Many physicians refer alcoholic patients to this organization for help. Most social agencies work closely with AA, and it is generally accepted as the most helpful approach to the problem of alcoholism available at this time.

As with the treatment of alcohol-dependent persons, the most effective long-term treatment for drug-dependent individuals is conducted by self-help groups. These include Narcotics Anonymous (NA), Chemical Dependency Anonymous (CDA), and Cocaine Anonymous (CA).

Residential self-help programs have been particularly successful in the rehabilitation of drug-dependent individuals. These residential centers are found in many large cities. Their treatment program is based on the concept of a *therapeutic community* (TC), which seeks to alter the personality of the affected individual because of the belief that substance abuse is a symptom of an immature personality. The goals of these residential communities include abstinence from drugs and the development of skills for employment. These programs are usually under the direction of a professional who has training and experience specific to the rehabilitation of drug-dependent individuals. However, most of the therapy and work required to maintain the residence is done by the drug-dependent individuals who are there to be helped or by those who have been helped and stay on as employees. Several group sessions are held each week, during which members of the group are supportive of each other but are also very straightforward in demanding that the group members face their rationalizations, evasions, personal problems, and social deceptions. If members return to drug use, they are expected to leave. Residents generally stay at least 15 months.

Most self-help groups base their treatment on the philosophy of the Twelve Steps, originally developed by AA (see the box on p. 360).

THE TWELVE STEPS OF ALCOHOLICS ANONYMOUS

1. We admitted we were powerless over alcohol—that our lives had become unmanageable.
2. Came to believe that a power greater than ourselves could restore us to sanity.
3. Made a decision to turn our will and our lives over to the care of God *as we understood Him*.
4. Made a searching and fearless moral inventory of ourselves.
5. Admitted to God, to ourselves, and to another human being the exact nature of our wrongs.
6. Were entirely ready to have God remove all these defects of character.
7. Humbly asked Him to remove our shortcomings.
8. Made a list of all persons we had harmed, and became willing to make amends to them all.
9. Made direct amends to such people whenever possible, except when to do so would injure them or others.
10. Continued to take personal inventory, and when we were wrong, we promptly admitted it.
11. Sought through prayer and meditation to improve our conscious contact with God *as we understood Him,* praying only for knowledge of His will and the power to carry that out.
12. Having had a spiritual awakening as the result of these steps, we tried to carry His message to alcoholics, and to practice these principles in all our affairs.

The Twelve Steps are reprinted with permission of Alcoholics Anonymous World Services, Inc. Permission to reprint this material does not mean that AA has reviewed or approved the contents of this publication. AA is a program of recovery from alcoholism *only*—use of the Twelve Steps in connection with programs and activities which are patterned after AA, but which address other problems, does not imply otherwise.

KEY INTERVENTIONS FOR CLIENTS WITH SUBSTANCE ABUSE AND DEPENDENCE

Meet the physical needs of clients during detoxification; this intervention is of paramount importance.

Address the residual physiological alterations resulting from substance dependence in the same manner as these needs would be met in any person.

Monitor the effects of the somatic therapies that may be prescribed to control the substance use.

Teach clients about the disease and its progression.

Focus on the client's strengths and help the client build on them.

Help clients problem solve functional solutions to dilemmas they fear.

Encourage clients to focus on the present and the future, not on the past.

Behave toward clients in a consistent manner, confronting them in a nonjudgmental, nonpunitive manner if they break the rules of the treatment setting.

Assist the client's family by encouraging them to become involved in group counseling.

NURSING CARE PLAN: *A Heroin-Dependent Individual*

CASE FORMULATION

David S. is a 24-year-old, single man who was admitted to a long-term residential drug rehabilitation program after a 2-week inpatient stay on a detoxification unit for withdrawal from heroin. David began using marijuana and then heroin when he was a junior in high school because his 14-year-old girlfriend refused to date him any longer. About the same time, David was sent by his mother, who lived in New York City, to attend high

NURSING CARE PLAN: *A Heroin-Dependent Individual— cont'd*

school in a distant southern city because his parents were getting a divorce.

According to David, marijuana made him feel excited, stimulated, and happy. Everything seemed more pleasant, and he enjoyed his daydreams. He was also sexually stimulated by the drug. About the same time, he tried taking barbituates, which made him sleepy. Because he did not enjoy their effect, he did not continue them. He got drunk a few times, but alcohol failed to produce the calmness and contentment he was seeking. Since marijuana did not completely satisfy him either, he was convinced that his willpower would be great enough to allow him to stop using this drug when he wanted to be free of it.

David first took heroin in the vein. He described feeling a "flash," which was accompanied by a flush of blood from the abdomen to the head and a feeling of happiness. Although the "flash" passed away, a constant feeling of euphoria remained. For the first time in his life he experienced a feeling of deep contentment. He said, "It didn't affect my intellect, only my emotions. I was happy and content." From that time on he took heroin to assist him in facing any situation that caused him to be tense or anxious. Heroin helped him feel independent of his mother and reduced his nervousness when he was out with a girl. Although heroin gave him a feeling of contentment, it lessened his sexual desire and made it impossible for him to reach a sexual climax.

After David discovered the contentment heroin could achieve for him, he became involved in crimes to support his drug habit.

As his need for larger and larger quantities of heroin grew, making his habit more costly, his crimes became more frequent and more serious. His mother repeatedly intervened to keep him out of jail by paying his fines. He entered several colleges but because of his drug habit was never able to stay in any of them for more than a semester.

Finally David tried to withdraw himself from heroin. He thought he could achieve this by himself, since he had been withdrawn twice before in treatment centers. He was not able to accomplish his goal and finally at 24 years of age signed himself into a detoxification unit in the hope of stopping the drug so that he could return to college. He had set for himself the goal of becoming an engineer.

Following the 2-week detoxification program, staff members recommended to David that he admit himself to a long-term residential treatment setting because of the chronic nature of his difficulties and his past inability to remain abstinent when confronted by stressful life events.

The residential drug rehabilitation program was staffed by a variety of professional and nonprofessional staff, including recovered drug addicts. The staff worked with David to develop a plan of care designed to meet his individual needs and enhance his strengths. On admission to the center, David was drug free. He appeared undernourished but was in no acute physical distress. He initially gave evidence of being highly motivated and tested in the superior range on a standardized intelligence test.

During the admission interview, David re-

Continued.

NURSING CARE PLAN: *A Heroin-Dependent Individual— cont'd*

counted the following information about his early childhood. He stated that his parents were married when his mother was 16 years old. David was their first child, and he recalled his mother often reminding him that his birth had been traumatic for her. During David's formative years, his father suffered from tuberculosis and spent many months in a sanitarium. David remembered that when he was 3 and 4 years old his mother fondled his genitals when she bathed him. As he grew older, she allowed him to observe her dressing and bathing but scolded him if he showed interest in her body.

Nursing Assessment

David's history reveals several factors that potentially contributed to his dependence on heroin for a sense of well-being. He described the feelings of happiness, contentment, relief of anxiety, and independence that he experienced when using heroin.

David's relationship with his mother was highly ambivalent and conflictive. From the time he was a child, he had been given the message that he was unwanted and unloved. Because of her own difficulties in adjustment, David's mother was unable to provide him with a healthy environment in which to develop and grow. Her sexually provocative behaviors contributed to David's poor psychosexual adjustment and his anxieties in relation to intimacy with women. David's attempts to separate from his mother were unsuccessful. Her continual interventions on his behalf with the police enabled him to continue his substance dependence while maintaining his unhealthy, dependent rela-

tionship with her. The absence of a healthy male role model further hindered David's ability to develop effective adaptations to stress. He seemed to rely solely on drugs for a sense of well-being and autonomy and used drugs to deal with all anxiety-provoking situations.

David failed to develop a healthy sense of self as an autonomous male individual. His dependence on drugs may have been a substitute for the dependence he experienced in relation to his rejecting and controlling mother. The adaptation was dysfunctional in that his use of drugs further impeded his ability to negotiate the adolescent tasks of separation and identity development.

David appeared undernourished, probably because of his use of funds to purchase heroin rather than food. His work history was poor, as was his school performance, and he had begun to rely on stealing to purchase heroin. David's strengths included his superior intelligence and his apparent motivation to remain free of drugs and to pursue a career. His willingness to commit himself to a long-term rehabilitation center indicated his emerging recognition of the severity of his drug dependence and his desire for change.

Nursing Diagnosis

Based on the nursing assessment that included prior knowledge of the family dynamics and an understanding of the dynamics underlying substance abuse and dependence, the nurse formulated the following nursing diagnoses for David S:

Altered nutrition: less than body require-

NURSING CARE PLAN: *A Heroin-Dependent Individual— cont'd*

ments related to inadequate food and fluid intake

Ineffective individual coping related to long-term reliance on drugs to cope with stressful life events

Impaired social interaction related to fear of rejection and psychosexual conflicts

Planning and Implementing Nursing Care

The nursing care plan for David S. is summarized in the box on pp. 365 and 366. The team working with David consisted of a variety of professional and nonprofessional members and included a primary nurse, the team psychiatrist, a psychiatric social worker, and an occupational therapist. In addition, David attended self-help group meetings daily. These meetings were held each evening at the center and were attended by several persons recovering from drug dependence, one of whom served as David's sponsor.

The staff members assigned to David were mature individuals experienced in the treatment of clients with substance dependence. They approached David in a hopeful, caring, and supportive fashion, while clearly maintaining boundaries of separateness and setting firm limits. The initial task of treatment was to assist David to recognize and accept his heroin addiction as a problem, thereby breaking through the massive defense of denial common to drug-dependent individuals. Despite David's high motivation to be drug free, the treatment team expected that David eventually would express ambivalence in relation to treatment, and they would need to help him remain

abstinent at that time. Finally, treatment would focus on assisting David to develop alternative coping methods to handle stressful life events and uncomfortable feelings to prevent a return to reliance on drugs as a coping style.

The treatment approach consisted of a variety of modalities, including group therapy, peer groups, milieu therapy, peer pressure, recreational and expressive-creative therapies, and assistance with developing social and vocational skills. A contract developed by David and the team outlined mutual expectations for treatment participation. In addition, David was expected to do his share of housekeeping and meal preparation as outlined by the community in weekly meetings. David agreed to the plan as written and was given his final copy of the contract. He agreed to remain in the program for 1 year; to remain drug free, as evidenced by daily urine screens; and to follow the contract as written. David was assigned a primary nurse whose plan was to establish a supportive but firm relationship, to develop a climate of acceptance that allowed for the expression of feelings, and to facilitate David's full participation in the program as outlined. Violation of the treatment plan would constitute grounds for immediate review and potential discharge.

Evaluation

David's participation and progress were reviewed by all staff members with David present on a biweekly basis. Although he made steady progress, his course of treatment was not without difficulty. After 2 months at the center, it was thought that

Continued.

NURSING CARE PLAN: *A Heroin-Dependent Individual— cont'd*

David was ready to handle an all-day pass to visit with his mother. David had verbalized the hope that he could use some of his new knowledge and behaviors and that the meeting would go well. On David's return, his urine drug screen revealed that he had used marijuana while on pass, despite his earlier denial of any drug use. He began to challenge staff when confronted and vehemently denied that the action had any meaning, stating, "It doesn't mean anything . . . it wasn't heroin, just pot. What's the big deal?" David was confronted by his peers in group therapy the following day and became withdrawn, sullen, and nonverbal for several weeks. He then began to discuss his fears related to a "life without drugs" with his primary nurse, who encouraged him to discuss and explore these issues in the various groups he attended. David responded to this suggestion by accusing the nurse of being rejecting, just like his mother. The nurse remained accepting of these feelings and encouraged David to discuss them. Gradually he began to use groups and peers for increased support and became particularly close to a group of men close to his age. They relied on one another for support and encouragement.

Each new anxiety-producing circumstance David confronted led to a desire to return to drug use. As he began to explore career avenues, his anxiety again increased, as did the desire to rely on drugs. David feared each new step toward an independent and drug-free existence. He often expressed the feeling that others were "forcing" him to quit drugs and was frequently reminded by peers that he had voluntarily chosen to make a commitment to treatment.

David slowly continued to progress toward recovery. He gradually developed an interest in pottery and became quite skilled. He began to expand his support network and develop new relationships. He became particularly helpful with individuals new to the program. In addition, he began to discuss and explore his angry but dependent feelings toward his mother. He began to attend a local university part time to pursue his interest in engineering and was permitted more time away from the center in an effort to encourage independent living and confront stress while support was available.

As the time of David's discharge drew near, many separation issues arose. David's fears about living independently emerged in full force. He angrily stated that he felt as if he was being "thrown out." He expressed the wish to remain longer. David was assisted in coping with these feelings by peers and staff. He was encouraged to continue his involvement with support groups in the community and contracted to volunteer at the center once a week. At the time of discharge, staff members were hopeful that David had made much progress and would continue to make gains with available supports, meetings with his sponsor, and weekly visits to his therapist. He had not made much progress in the area of heterosexual relationships and continued to be quite anxious and fearful when he contemplated dating and intimacy. It was hoped that David would begin to explore this issue in the future with his therapist.

NURSING CARE PLAN FOR DAVID S.

Nursing diagnosis	Objective (rationale)	Nursing interventions	Outcome criteria
Altered nutrition: less than body requirements related to inadequate food and fluid intake	Client's nutritional status will improve. (Optimum nutrition is necessary for physiological homeokinesis and to prevent residual physiological alterations.)	Monitor client's intake, encouraging three well-balanced meals each day. Supplement daily meals with high-calorie nutritional snacks between meals.	Within 1 week, client gains 5 pounds. Within 1 month, client shows evidence of adequate nutrition in hair, skin, eyes, and mucous membranes.
Ineffective individual coping related to long-term reliance on drugs to cope with stressful life events	Client will abstain from drug use. (Total abstinence from drugs is fundamental to rehabilitation.)	Convey a caring but firm attitude. Conduct daily urine screens for drugs. Encourage daily participation in self-help groups. Encourage frequent meetings with sponsor. Discuss drug cravings. Offer positive appraisals for abstinence.	Within 2 weeks, client: Obtains urine for drug screens without reminder and remains drug free. Attends self-help group meetings daily without reminder. Identifies alternative actions to take to diminish drug cravings.
	Client will recognize and accept his drug addiction as a problem. (Denial is common among substance-dependent individuals. Rehabilitation cannot begin until denial is overcome.)	Convey hope and support while confronting emerging evidence of the use of denial. Encourage participation in self-help groups, peer groups, and community discussion.	Within 2 weeks, client: Willingly attends self-help groups and peer groups and meets with sponsor daily without reminder. Initiates discussions of behaviors related to addiction and negative impact of these behaviors on life goals.
	Client will develop alternative coping methods to deal with stressful life events and uncomfortable feelings. (Unless functional coping methods are learned, chance of relapse is great.)	Accept expressions of fear related to loss of heroin as a coping method. Assist with exploration of new coping styles. Encourage and monitor attendence of biweekly group therapy. Encourage participation in expressive activities (e.g., art, music, poetry).	Within 1 month, client: Begins to discuss ways to deal with uncomfortable feelings. Plans and begins creative project. Attends group therapy without reminder.

Continued.

NURSING CARE PLAN FOR DAVID S.—cont'd

Nursing diagnosis	Objective/rationale	Nursing interventions	Outcome criteria
	Client will develop and follow through with career and educational plans. (Concrete plans for the future build self-esteem and help prevent relapse.)	Discuss educational and career interests, conveying hope and support. Offer positive appraisals for success. Refer to vocational counselor.	Within 1 month, client: Initiates discussion related to career plan. Meets with vocational counselor.
Impaired social interaction related to fear of rejection and psychosexual conflicts	Client will develop sense of trust in close relationships and belief that identity can be simultaneously maintained. (Ability to relate comfortably with others is essential to mental health.)	Establish trusting relationship in daily meetings, conveying support and acceptance of client as individual with value.	Within 2 weeks, client initiates conversation in meetings with primary nurse.
	Client will explore and discuss anxieties related to intimate relationships with women. (Establishing mature heterosexual relationships is a developmental task of young adulthood.)	Encourage autonomous and healthy behaviors and independent decision making. Encourage discussion by use of reflective listening, conveying acceptance and support.	Within 2 weeks, client identifies feelings and fears related to intimacy.

KEY POINTS

1. Substance abuse and dependence can be explained only through the understanding of multiple interacting and overlapping biological, psychological, physiological, and environmental factors.

2. Intravenous drug use with contaminated needles increases the risk of the individual becoming infected with human immunodeficiency virus (HIV) or hepatitis B.

3. An alcohol-dependent individual may drink excessively all the time, may drink to excess only periodically, or may drink large quantities of alcohol daily over a period of years.

4. Delirium tremens is an acute reaction to the withdrawal from a heavy, consistent intake of alcohol and must be treated medically.

5. Barbiturates are central nervous system depressants that have an effect very similar to that of alcohol. Dependence can be dangerous because of the possibility of a lethal overdose. Withdrawal should never be abrupt.

6. Inhalation of marijuana causes a state of exhilaration or euphoria. Many research findings about this drug are contradictory.

7. Hallucinogens may cause individuals to believe they have supernatural powers and to attempt such feats as flying.

8. Assessment of the substance-dependent individual usually reveals biopsychosocial, economic, and cognitive problems.

9. The objectives of nursing care of individuals with substance abuse or dependence should include

assisting them to regain physiological well-being, to increase their self-esteem, to develop functional methods of coping, and to remain drug free.

10. Nurses are most therapuetic when they focus on clients' strengths and help them see that their achievements can build on each other and that their self-esteem can be raised.

11. Although no single effective means of long-term treatment of substance-dependent individuals has been developed, therapeutic communities (TCs) and self-help groups such as Alcoholics Anonymous (AA) have been most successful in the process of recovery.

SUGGESTED SOURCES OF ADDITIONAL INFORMATION

Adams FE: Drug dependency in hospital patients, *Am J Nurs* 88:477, April 1988.

Arneson SW, Schultz M, Triplett JL: Nurses' knowledge of the impact of parental alcoholism on children, *Arch Psychiatr Nurs* 1:251, August 1987.

Bean-Bayog M: Alcoholism as a cause of psychopathology, *Hosp Community Psychiatry* 39:352, April 1988.

Bell K: Identifying the substance abuser in clinical practice, *Orthop Nurs* 11:29, March/April 1992.

Bingham A, Bargar J: Children of alcoholic families, *J Psychosoc Nurs Ment Health Serv* 23(12):13, 1985.

Busch D, McBride AB, Benaventura L: Chemical dependency in women: the link to OB/GYN problems, *J Psychosoc Nurs Ment Health Serv* 24(4):26, 1986.

Cadoret RJ and others: An adoption study of genetic and environmental factors in drug abuse, *Arch Gen Psychiatry* 43:1131, December 1986.

Caroselli-Karinja M: Drug abuse and the elderly, *J Psychosoc Nurs Ment Health Serv* 23(6):25, 1985.

Compton P: Drug abuse: a self-care deficit, *J Psychosoc Nurs Ment Health Serv* 27(3):22, 1989.

Eells MAW: Interventions with alcoholics and their families, *Nurs Clin North Am* 21:493, September 1986.

Eells MAW: Strategies for promotion of avoiding harmful substances, *Nurs Clin North Am* 26:915, December 1991.

Ellison Hough ES: Alcoholism: prevention and treatment, *J Psychosoc Nurs Ment Health Serv* 27(1):15, 1989.

Green P: The chemically dependent nurse, *Nurs Clin North Am* 24:81, March 1989.

Haack MR: Collaborative investigation of adult children of alcoholics with anxiety, *Arch Psychiatr Nurs* 4:62, February 1990.

Jack LW: Use of milieu as a problem-solving strategy in addiction treatment, *Nurs Clin North Am* 24:69, March 1989.

Khantzian EJ: The self-medication hypothesis of addictive disorders: focus of heroin and cocaine dependence, *Am J Psychiatry* 142:1259, November 1985.

McKelvy MJ, Kane JSA, Kellison K: Substance abuse and mental illness: double trouble, *J Psychosoc Nurs Ment Health Serv* 25(1):20, 1987.

McMahon J, Jones BT: The change process in alcoholics: client motivation and denial in the treatment of alcoholism within the context of contemporary nursing, *J Adv Nurs* 17:173, 1992.

Montgomery P, Johnson B: The stress of marriage to an alcoholic, *J Psychosoc Nurs* 30(10):13, 1992.

Nighorn S: Narcissistic deficits in drug abusers: a self-psychological approach, *J Psychosoc Nurs Ment Health Serv* 26(9):22, 1988.

Nubel AS, Solomon LZ: Addicted adolescent girls: familial interpersonal relationships, *J Psychosoc Nurs Ment Health Serv* 26(1):32, 1988.

O'Brien CP, Woody GE, McLellan T: Psychiatric disorders in opioid-dependent patients, *J Clin Psychiatry* 45:9, December 1984.

Sullivan EJ: A descriptive study of nurses recovering from chemical dependency. *Arch Psychiatr Nurs* 1:194, June 1987.

Trevelyan J: The forgotten addicts, *Nurs Times* 84:16, April 1988.

Vandegaer F: Cocaine: the deadliest addiction, *Nursing '89* 19:72, February 1989.

Williams E: Strategies for intervention, *Nurs Clin North Am* 24:95, March 1989.

Wing DM, Hammer-Higgins P: Determinants of denial: a study of alcoholics, *J Psychosoc Nurs* 31(2):13, 1993.

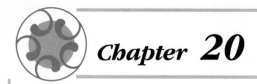

Chapter 20

Individuals with Personality Disorders

LEARNING OBJECTIVES
After studying this chapter, the student will be able to:
• Describe the characteristics exhibited by a person with the medical diagnosis of personality disorder.

• Discuss the causative factors associated with personality disorders.

• Describe behaviors the nurse is most likely to observe in an adult with borderline personality disorder.

• State examples of nursing diagnoses likely to be applicable to an adult with borderline personality disorder.

• Discuss nursing interventions likely to be effective with an adult with borderline personality disorder.

• Describe behaviors the nurse is most likely to observe in an adult with antisocial personality disorder.

• State examples of nursing diagnoses likely to be applicable to an adult with antisocial personality disorder.

• Discuss nursing interventions likely to be effective with an adult with antisocial personality disorder.

• Develop a hypothetical plan of nursing care for an adult with antisocial personality disorder.

KEY TERMS
Personality traits
Borderline personality disorder
Antisocial personality disorder
Separation-individuation
Impaired impulse control
Rescue fantasy
Vocational therapy

Personality has been defined as *the aggregate of the physical and mental qualities of the individual as these interact in characteristic fashion with the environment*. When an individual's personality is characterized by an identifiable trait or style that is relatively enduring regardless of the circumstances, that individual may be seen as "eccentric," or "odd," or "different." For example, some persons are suspicious in most situations in which they find themselves, others overreact with great emotion to everyday events, and still others are fearful most of the time. For many people, these personality traits do not cause personal distress or interfere with their ability to live satisfying and satisfactory lives. Some persons, however, are distressed by the way in which they characteristically relate to the world around them but are unable to alter their behavior. In other instances, individuals may see nothing unusual about their behavior, but others find it objectionable. Such persons may have a personality disorder even though they do not exhibit the flagrant symptoms lay persons usually associate with mental illness.

Although nurses often come in contact with individuals with personality disorders in work and social settings, they are unlikely to be in the position of providing care to these persons, who rarely seek treatment for this disorder alone. However, two exceptions exist. Individuals with borderline personality disorder and those with antisocial personality disorder may require hospitalization for varying periods of time. Therefore this chapter focuses on the care of individuals with these personality disorders.

HISTORICAL PERSPECTIVE

Although individuals with borderline personality disorder undoubtedly have existed throughout history, this disorder was not officially considered to be a distinct syndrome until 1980, when this diagnosis first appeared in the *Diagnostic and Statistical Manual of Mental Disorders* (DSM-III). This does not mean to say that

borderline personality disorder had been unknown until 1980. In fact, one of the foremost authorities on treating persons with borderline personality disorder, Dr. Otto Kernberg, has been writing about this syndrome since the 1960s. However, since the official recognition of borderline personality disorder, an abundance of both professional and lay literature has addressed the characteristics, dynamics, and interventions associated with this disorder.

In contrast, the phenomenon of antisocial personality disorder has been well known for years, although such individuals were labeled *sociopaths* or *psychopaths* in the past. Although this terminology is no longer used, the characteristics and numbers of these persons remain the same as they have throughout history.

PERSONALITY DISORDERS

Personality traits are those characteristics of individuals that make them unique and form the basis for the way they perceive the world and how they relate to others. Individuals with a personality disorder exhibit an extreme manifestation of a personality trait. For example, if shyness interferes with a person's ability to live a satisfying and satisfactory life, this person would be considered to have a schizoid personality disorder.

The DSM-III groups personality disorders into three clusters. Cluster A includes paranoid, schizoid, and schizotypal personality disorders. People with these disorders often appear odd or eccentric. Cluster B includes antisocial, borderline, histrionic, and narcissistic personality disorders. People with these disorders often appear dramatic, emotional, or erratic. Cluster C includes avoidant, dependent, obsessive-compulsive, and passive-aggressive personality disorders. People with these disorders often appear anxious or fearful.

Because persons with borderline personality disorder and those with antisocial personality disorder are likely to require psychiatric treatment, these disorders are discussed in this chapter.

Borderline personality disorder

For reasons that are not known, the vast majority of individuals with **borderline personality disorder** are women. Some authorities believe that this disorder is a precursor to dissociative disorders, particularly multiple personality disorder, which is seen almost exclusively in women.

Individuals with borderline personality disorder have not developed an integrated sense of self. Even though they are chronological adults, they are unable to define who they are and what values and goals undergird their lives. For example, they are likely to vacillate widely among career choices, values, and goals for their life, first making one set of decisions and then shifting to another set that is in marked contrast to the first. This inability to develop an integrated sense of self results in erratic behavior and feelings of "emptiness," which is often expressed as boredom.

Not surprisingly, individuals with borderline personality disorder have a deep fear of being alone because they look to others to fill the void in their sense of self. Consequently, they are continuously establishing intense relationships, each of which initially is seen as the answer to their problems. Unfortunately, these relationships are doomed to fail because individuals with borderline personality disorder seem to be unable to view themselves and others realistically as human beings with strengths and limitations. Rather, persons are seen as being totally good or totally bad. This phenomenon is based on the primitive defense mechanism of "splitting." It is not unusual for the very same person who is beloved to become the object of intense hatred less than a week later because he or she was found deficient in meeting the individual's inordinate needs. For example, if the newly found friend arrives 5 minutes late for a date, the individual with borderline personality disorder

might construe this as evidence that her friend does not really care about her. This perception of interpersonal interactions leads to much overt and covert manipulation by the individual with borderline personality disorder.

The third prominent characteristic of individuals with borderline personality disorder is extreme shifts in mood over a very short time. When they are experiencing stress, especially that related to real or perceived abandonment, these individuals are likely to respond with massive anxiety, depression, or anger. Although the nature of this reaction may be understandable, the extent of it is out of proportion to the stressor. What is even more surprising is that within hours or a few days the person's mood may change to one of cheer and pleasure, often associated with having "found a new friend."

During periods of depression and anxiety, these persons often make suicidal gestures, characteristically scratching or gouging their wrists and arms. It is not clear whether this behavior is an attempt to gain attention, an effort to inflict pain to confirm the existence of self, or both. During periods of anger they tend to provoke fights and may injure themselves and others. They also engage in real and symbolic self-destructive, impulsive behaviors such as casual sex, shopping sprees, substance abuse, and binging.

Antisocial personality disorder

Individuals with **antisocial personality disorder** are persons who have a long history of dysfunctional behavior in the areas of interpersonal relationships and occupational endeavors. In addition, they often have a criminal record, may be dependent on alcohol or drugs, and frequently engage in sexually deviant behavior. What is so outstanding about these persons, however, is not their history or even their behavior, but rather the initial impression they make. Even when their past is known, such individuals easily impress strangers with their articulate expression, their ability to rationalize or justify their behavior, their fantasized exploits, and their general appearance. The casual acquaintance quickly succumbs to this charisma and becomes a staunch supporter.

Behind this effective facade of charm is a personality incapable of valuing other people. Rather, these persons view others as objects to be manipulated to achieve their purposes. These individuals are characterized by a total lack of responsibility and an inability to conform to even the minimum moral and legal standards of society if these conflict with the fulfillment of their desires. They possess poor judgment and insight, do not profit by experience or punishment, and are notoriously unreliable. They consciously fabricate stories to impress the listener and have an uncanny ability to rationalize contradictions in their stories. In addition, they seem incapable of experiencing guilt or remorse for their behavior, although they will express these feelings if they believe it will be to their advantage to do so.

For reasons that are unknown, this personality disorder occurs almost exclusively in men. In addition, these persons are always of at least average intelligence, with many having superior intellectual abilities. Because of their criminal behavior, many of these persons are found in jails and prisons. It is unlikely, however, that the professional criminal has an antisocial personality. A successful life of crime requires long-range, careful planning. This is impossible for individuals with an antisocial personality because their behavior is characterized by impulsiveness and a low tolerance for frustration.

CAUSATIVE FACTORS

The causative factors of personality disorders are essentially unknown. However, since many behaviors of these individuals would be considered normal at a much earlier stage of personality development, some authorities believe that the basis of these disorders lies in the individual's arrested psychosexual development. Even if future research confirms this hypothesis, questions still remain about what factors contribute to fix-

ation at an earlier stage of psychosexual development.

Many authorities believe that the fundamental problem of individuals with borderline personality disorder is their earlier inability to resolve the **separation-individuation** process in infancy. During early infancy the infant and the mothering one have a symbiotic relationship whereby they are emotionally fused. This stage of development is an extension of the physical symbiosis experienced when the infant was in utero. By the age of 5 months, however, infants have developed sufficiently to be able to begin the process of separating from their mothering one and embark on the long process of establishing their own identity as separate, distinct human beings. This is a gradual process that takes years to achieve, although success in the stages of infancy and early childhood is necessary to provide the foundation on which the tasks of later childhood and adolescence can be built. For example, one of the earliest signs of the separation process is when infants visually and tactilely explore the mothering one's face and can recognize her among a group of adults, thereby indicating that they are beginning to differentiate her from themselves and others. If this does not occur, in later stages of development the child is unlikely to be able to leave the mothering one comfortably even for short periods.

A major goal of the separation-individuation process is the development of a unified sense of self in which the total personality is integrated. Although this is not fully achieved until late adolescence or early adulthood, the beginnings of a unified self-concept are apparent in healthy children by age 3. For reasons that are unknown, individuals with borderline personality disorder have been unable to develop this unified, integrated self-concept and continue to use the primitive defense mechanism of splitting, whereby they view themselves and others as all good or all bad.

Studies of the histories of individuals with antisocial personality disorder reveal that they were emotionally impulsive and maladjusted children. Adjustment difficulties before age 15 are one criterion of this diagnosis. Some authorities believe that careful history taking would indicate antisocial behavior before age 12 in most, if not all, individuals who develop antisocial personality disorder as adults. These adjustment difficulties include poor school performance related to frequent truancy; petty crimes, including thefts and arson; and a uniform lack of satisfactory relationships with family, peers, and authority figures.

These individuals have apparently failed to develop a socialized superego. The personality appears to be dominated by the primitive demands of the id. The ego has failed to establish a mature identity or to evolve socially useful adaptations and controls. In some ways these individuals have failed to make a positive identification with parents or parental substitutes who could have provided the love, security, recognition, and respect that children require if they are to develop into emotionally healthy adults. Failure to make a positive identification and to develop socially acceptable controls on their behavior may have their origin in parent-child relationships.

Social scientists who have conducted longitudinal studies of these individuals report that they frequently come from home environments in which there is only one parent, who is likely to be alcohol or drug dependent, who has an antisocial personality, or both. As a result, the child has little or no supervision, and the rules of conduct that are established are enforced inconsistently. The child is, in essence, left to fend for himself or herself, often on the streets of large cities.

Although these familial factors are present often enough to be noteworthy, it is important to understand that not every child who is a product of such a background develops an antisocial personality disorder. Furthermore, some adults who have antisocial personality disorder do not have this family background. Therefore it must be concluded that other, as yet unknown, factors are necessary for the development of antisocial personality disorder.

NURSING CARE OF INDIVIDUALS WITH BORDERLINE PERSONALITY DISORDER
Nursing assessment

For purposes of clarity, typical behaviors of persons with borderline personality disorder are discussed by categories. Although behaviors in each category are presented as separate entities, they are highly interrelated and are adaptations to similar stressors. Further, behavior designed as an adaptation to one stressor often becomes a stressor itself in another dimension. Therefore, nursing care directed at altering one behavior will inevitably have an effect on others.

Health perception–health management

Physiological processes are not necessarily altered in clients with borderline personality disorder. However, this condition does not provide immunity to physiological alterations, so a complete physical examination must be completed and any physiological problems addressed.

Because of the client's self-destructive behavior, the nurse should be particularly alert for signs of wound infection and indications of malnourishment.

Nutritional-metabolic

Many clients with borderline personality disorder have alterations in eating patterns, often binging and purging, with the resultant sequelae. See Chapter 21 for a discussion of this dysfunctional adaptation.

Activity-exercise

Although motor behavior is usually not altered, the individual with borderline personality disorder who is ill enough to require psychiatric treatment will invariably display impulsivity, which may be exhibited through motor behavior. This is especially likely when clients feel angry because of some real or imagined slight, at which time they may lash out at others, the environment, or themselves. Inexperienced nurses typically view the client's impulsive motor behavior as unpredictable, since they have not yet learned to appreciate fully the depth of reaction these clients experience in response to untoward events and people who do not do exactly the "right" thing at the right time. For example, one client spontaneously assaulted an aide who announced that a planned unit picnic had to be canceled because of thunderstorms.

Recreation patterns may be antisocial and involve substance abuse and sexual promiscuity. Individuals with borderline personality disorder have great difficulty being alone, so they seek activities that involve other people. However, they also have an inability to delay gratification, so they are likely to become impatient and irritable when involved in recreational activities that are characterized by rules and competition, as is true of many games.

Self-care in regard to grooming and hygiene may or may not altered. Home maintenance management is not necessarily affected.

Cognitive-perceptual

Cognitive processes are often altered in regard to decision making and judgment. As previously discussed, these clients have a diffused identity and thus are unable to make decisions based on long-term goals and deeply held values. Their poor judgment is evidenced by the spontaneity of their decisions without reference to long-term consequences. Although delusions are not present, their thought processes indicate a highly personalized interpretation of others' actions. For example, the previously mentioned client who assaulted the aide after he canceled the picnic exclaimed, "How could he have done that to me?"

Self-perception/self-concept

Perhaps the most fundamental problem of clients with borderline personality disorder is their undeveloped self-concept. As previously discussed, these individuals have not developed a sense of self and therefore appear to "try on" self-concepts, often based on the identity of the individual who is currently idealized. Therefore the nurse will observe a great deal of mimicking behavior, reminiscent of the normal behavior of children 3 to 6 years old.

Altered feeling states and feeling processes are prime characteristics of clients with borderline personality disorder. These persons experience an extreme depth of emotion, especially anger, anxiety, elation, and sadness in response to what others see as relatively trivial events. As previously discussed, these extreme emotions are accompanied by mood swings, which are almost always precipitated by an external factor. For example, it is not unusual for one nurse to report to another that the client is exceptionally depressed, only for the second nurse to discover the client in the day room laughing and joking with others.

Role-relationship

Impaired impulse control is another major characteristic of clients with borderline personality disorder. Their impulsivity and feelings of emptiness and boredom, combined with their rage at themselves and others, often result in physical assaults on the environment, others, and themselves. Suicidal or self-destructive acts are common in hospitalized clients and are likely to be the factors that made hospitalization necessary.

CLINICAL EXAMPLE

Meredith, age 22, is well known to the mental health system of the city in which she lives. One evening she called the mental health "hot line" and said she was going to kill herself by slashing her wrists. Although she was crying, her loud voice conveyed more anger than sadness. The nurse on duty instructed Meredith to go to the emergency room of the hospital. When she arrived, the nurse immediately saw that Meredith's left forearm was oozing serosanguineous fluid. Meredith reported that she had "peeled the skin off" with a razor blade. She did not seem concerned about her arm. In fact, she seemed much more calm than she had sounded over the telephone.

The client with borderline personality disorder becomes involved in intense but superficial interpersonal relationships. As previously discussed, these relationships are always short lived because of the client's tendency to view others as all good or all bad and consequently to idealize or devalue others. Therefore the client's interpersonal experience is turbulent.

Of particular note is that the client's behavior seriously strains family relationships. It is not unusual for the client to consciously or unconsciously relate to one family member as a savior and to another as the source of all the difficulties. One can easily see how this situation can result in one family member being pitted against another.

Role performance is seriously altered, and the client is likely to have a long history of failure in both school and work situations. One should understand, however, that clients are characteristically unable to appreciate the part they played in creating these failures. Rather, they will convincingly relate long, involved stores about how they were victims of others' inadequacies.

Sexuality-reproductive

In an effort to help themselves feel "whole," individuals with a borderline personality disorder are likely to engage in frequent sexual activity, often with serial partners. Therefore the nurse needs to assess for the presence of sexually transmitted diseases and to ascertain whether the client practices birth control. Their sexual activity places these clients at high risk for rape and other forms of sexually related violence.

CLINICAL EXAMPLE

Nancy, age 30, has been hospitalized more than 40 times since she was 15 for treatment of bor-

derline personality disorder. She is now an outpatient at the local mental health clinic. She appeared at the clinic this week with numerous bruises over her body and face and reported she had been assaulted by a man she met at the state fair. Further investigation revealed that Nancy was picked up by this man, had sex with him, and then tried to take money from his wallet "in payment for her services." When the man saw what she was doing, he beat her up and left her behind one of the game booths in the arcade. Because of her history of sexual promiscuity, Nancy had semiannual tests for human immunodeficiency virus (HIV). She had always tested negative for the virus. Four months after this event, Nancy's routine HIV blood test returned positive.

Coping–stress tolerance

Individuals with borderline personality disorder give much evidence of being unable to cope in a functional manner with the stressors of everyday life. They have a tendency to personalize events, which interferes with reality testing and problem solving, both of which are necessary to develop functional coping mechanisms.

Value-belief

Closely related to the client's identity diffusion is the client's unclear value system. Because the client has not been able to develop a value system to guide behavior, it is not unusual for the client to engage in antisocial behavior such as sexual promiscuity but then feel great remorse about these actions.

Nursing diagnosis

As with all nursing diagnoses, the nursing diagnoses for the individual with borderline personality disorder are based on the themes identified during the assessment phase of the nursing process.

Accepted NANDA nursing diagnoses that may be specifically applicable to the individual with a borderline personality disorder include:

High risk for infection

High risk for injury

Diversional activity deficit

Altered thought processes

Decisional conflict (specify)

Fear

Anxiety

Personal identity disturbance

Self-esteem disturbance; situational low self-esteem; chronic low self-esteem

High risk for self-mutilation

Altered role performance

Impaired social interaction

Altered family processes

High risk for violence: self-directed or directed at others

Rape-trauma syndrome

Ineffective individual coping

To develop a nursing diagnosis that fulfills its function of providing direction for planning nursing care, the nurse is encouraged to postulate and state etiological or antecedent factors and connect the two phrases by using the term "related to." For example:

Personal identity disturbance related to unresolved separation-individuation process

Planning and implementing nursing care

The plan for nursing care is derived from the nursing diagnoses and includes the objectives of the care, the nursing interventions, and outcome criteria. To be effective, the plan needs to be highly individualized. The suggestions that follow should be seen as general guidelines to be used if they are appropriate to the client's needs.

In general, the objectives of all nursing care for the individual with borderline personality disorder should relate to helping the client learn to develop an integrated sense of self and a realistic perception of others and to control impulsive behaviors.

Since the client's nursing diagnoses are often interrelated, stemming as they do from similar etiologies or antecedents, the student should see that the appropriate nursing interventions are also interrelated. In other words, by intervening in one dimension, the nurse will also affect other dimensions.

Activity-exercise

Prevention is the key to helping the client deal with impulsive motor behavior. Rather than viewing the client's behavior as unpredictable, the nurse is encouraged to understand that clients often experience an extreme amount of rage over which they have little control. Clients' inability to control what they feel does not mean they cannot learn to control their behavior. Rather than focusing on the inappropriateness of the anger, the nurse can be most helpful to clients by teaching them socially acceptable ways of discharging this emotion. For example, clients can learn to punch a pillow rather than hitting another person when they feel as if they will explode with anger.

Cognitive-perceptual

Because clients with borderline personality disorder are in contact with reality and their memory is not affected, a written contract between the nurse and the client has proved to be a very useful tool. This contract is developed by the client and the nurse together, specifies the goals to be achieved, and delineates the behaviors and actions in which both the client and the nurse will engage. For example, the contract may specify that the client will keep a journal of those situations that cause anger and that the client will not act on this anger but rather approach the assigned nurse to discuss the situation. The nurse's responsibility would be to inform the client of when the nurse will be available to discuss the journal and then meticulously adhere to that time frame.

Self-perception/self-concept

Learning to develop personally and socially acceptable outlets for the client's emotions is one of the greatest challenges that face the nurse and the client. Often the nurse initially must help clients to identify and label the emotion they are feeling. For example, clients with borderline personality disorder often confuse boredom and sadness. Unless clients can be helped to learn the words that describe their feelings, they will not be able to talk about these emotions to others and will be more likely to act them out. Once clients can identify the emotions they are experiencing, they can be helped to learn how to identify the themes and patterns that precipitate various feelings. For example, even though it may be obvious to the staff, it may come as a surprise to the client that every time she has a visit from her mother she responds with sadness and a desire to mutilate herself. Once the precipitants of emotions are identified, it becomes possible for the client to learn functional coping mechanisms through such techniques as role playing and problem solving.

As previously stated, the goal of all nursing care for the client with borderline personality disorder includes assisting the client to develop an integrated sense of self and perception of others. The nurse can be most helpful in assisting clients to achieve this goal by relating to them with meticulous consistency, demonstrating acceptance of them as individuals with value and worth regardless of behavior, and helping them to view themselves and others in a realistic light by discussing the reality of situations with them. This takes much time, patience, and commitment on the nurse's part.

Role-relationship

Because clients use the defense mechanism of splitting, thereby seeing everything and everyone as all good or all bad, the staff needs to be keenly alert to preventing the dissension that occurs among staff when clients tell their "favorite" nurse how badly they are treated by another nurse. Only by developing an in-depth understanding of the dynamics underlying the behavior of clients with borderline personality disorder and a heightened sense of self-awareness can

nurses hope to avoid the pitfall of believing that only they understand the client or that only they can be of help to the client. This is necessary not only to prevent the client from manipulating the staff by pitting one against the other, but also to present a unified approach so that the client will have the opportunity to experience consistent limit setting and learn that it is possible for the staff to care about the client while still enforcing the rules.

Ironically, the more the staff is successful in enforcing uniform limits on the clients' behavior, the greater the initial likelihood that clients will attempt to mutilate themselves or otherwise act out. This behavior should be seen as testing. Although the staff has the responsibility to protect the client at all times, they should resist the temptation to focus on the acting-out behavior but rather should continue to focus on the feelings that precipitated the behavior. For example, one client approached the nurse carrying a light bulb, which she smashed on the counter once she got the nurse's attention. The client then stated that she was going to cut her wrist.

KEY INTERVENTIONS FOR CLIENTS WITH BORDERLINE PERSONALITY DISORDER

Develop a behavioral contract with the client, including goals and the behaviors and actions of both the nurse and the client. Meticulously adhere to the contract's terms.

Help clients identify and label the emotions they are feeling.

Help the client learn to identify themes and patterns that precipitate various feeling states.

Help the client learn functional coping mechanisms.

Relate to the client with acceptance and consistency.

Help clients "reality test" by discussing the reality of situations with them.

Do not succumb to "splitting" behaviors. All staff must present a unified approach to the client.

While ensuring client safety, focus on the client's feelings, not on acting-out, self-mutilative behavior.

Because the nurse knew this client well, she made no attempt to get the jagged glass from her and did not comment about it. Rather, the nurse asked the client what she was feeling and was not surprised when the client placed the glass on the counter a few minutes into the discussion.

NURSING CARE OF INDIVIDUALS WITH ANTISOCIAL PERSONALITY DISORDER
Nursing assessment
Health perception—health management

Physiological processes are not altered by the personality disorder itself but are almost always altered secondary to the individual's lifestyle. For example, there are likely to be physiological sequelae to substance abuse, sexual promiscuity, homelessness, inadequate nutrition, and physical aggression. In addition, the person with an antisocial personality disorder is unlikely to engage in health-seeking behaviors. Therefore the individual should have a complete physical examination on admission to a mental health facility.

Activity-exercise

Motor behavior of an individual with antisocial personality disorder is not necessarily altered. However, recreation patterns are likely to consist of activities that are antisocial. For example, substance abuse and prostitution are common.

A combination of lack of material resources and little motivation often leads to self-care alterations in grooming and hygiene. Therefore the individual with antisocial personality disorder may be unclean and unkempt. In other instances, however, the person may present quite the opposite picture.

Home maintenance management is greatly impaired in that persons with antisocial personality disorder are not concerned about such aspects as home or community. They are satisfied if they have a bed to sleep in and are not necessarily appreciative or even understanding of the efforts of a wife or parent in the unlikely event that such a person might attempt to maintain a comfortable, clean environment.

Cognitive-perceptual

Although cognitive process are not altered in and of themselves, the individual with antisocial personality disorder consistently uses judgment and makes decisions that reflect a total lack of concern for the rights of others or the rules of society. The person is concerned only about short-term gratification of needs and is willing to risk almost any consequence to meet these needs. As a result, the individual often has a long history of arrests, often for petty thievery, vandalism, and vagrancy.

Self-perception/self-concept

Despite much evidence to the contrary, persons with antisocial personality disorder view themselves in the most positive light while seeing others as inadequate. A testimony to this alteration in perception processes is their ability to explain convincingly their history on the basis of deficiencies in others or unfortunate circumstances over which they had no control.

Individuals with antisocial personality disorder are incapable of experiencing any depth of emotion, despite the feeling tone they convey often being appropriate to the situation. It is this fact that inexperienced nurses initially find so confusing. In reality, these persons have learned appropriate emotional responses as a means of influencing others' reactions. Because they are actually incapable of feeling anxiety, guilt, fear, or remorse, threats of retribution are useless in motivating them to change their antisocial behavior.

Role-relationship

Individuals with antisocial personality disorder have a long history of impaired interpersonal relationships. Because they have engaged in many antisocial acts and because they ultimately alienate everyone with whom they come in contact, they experience social isolation. When individuals whose friendships the person has cultivated realize how they were manipulated, their anger may be so great that the physical safety of the person with antisocial personality disorder may be in jeopardy. For this reason these persons are transferred from unit to unit if they are hospitalized for a long time. Those who are serving prison terms require periodic transfers to maintain their safety.

Of almost diagnostic significance is the nurse's reaction to the person. Despite all the nurse may know about the person, this individual is able to "con" the inexperienced nurse into defending and supporting antisocial actions and believing that she or he alone can help the client. These feelings are termed **rescue fantasy**, and nurses, who are inclined to be nurturing, are particularly vulnerable to the development of this phenomenon.

The individual's role performance is seriously compromised. It is likely that these individuals never finished high school, although they may speak as if they have great knowledge. If they ever had a job, it is unlikely that they were able to hold it for very long.

CLINICAL EXAMPLE

Ralph, age 35, is a handsome man of average build who smiles frequently. He was sentenced to the state psychiatric forensic hospital by a judge who had found him guilty of raping an elderly woman in her home. During the admission procedure the nurse found it almost impossible to believe that this good-looking, articulate individual could have committed such a crime. Ralph assured the nurse that he was innocent. He maintained not only that he was innocent of raping Mrs. Thomason, but also that he was her only source of help and that by detaining him, the judge was doing a great disservice to Mrs. Thomason. He explained that Mrs.

Thomason was 78 years old and demented and that he did yardwork and other handyman projects for her. In fact, he continued, if it had not been for him, Mrs. Thomason would have been unable to stay in her home. With his being in the hospital, Ralph doubted Mrs. Thomason would be able to manage for very long. In any event, he expressed confidence that this "mix-up" would be straightened out once his lawyer had the time to interview Mrs. Thomason and her physician. In the meantime, he suggested that he might develop a class for clients who needed to learn English, since he had a bachelor's degree in teaching English as a second language.

Sexuality-reproductive

Individuals with antisocial personality disorder are likely to be sexually promiscuous. Many are easily able to attract a sexual partner because of their charming manner. However, their sexual activity is devoid of any feeling for their partner and often is merely a means to relieve physiological tension. Clients should be assessed for sexually transmitted diseases and birth control practices.

Coping–stress tolerance

The individual with antisocial personality disorder is particularly unable to cope with stress. As previously stated, these persons engage in almost any activity, no matter how antisocial and no matter what the consequences, to relieve stress.

Value-belief

A prominent characteristic of individuals with antisocial personality disorder is that their values are in conflict with the social order. As previously stated, they will go to any length to gratify their needs, regardless of the consequences or who is hurt in the process. At the same time, they seem incapable of internalizing values that are socially acceptable.

Nursing diagnosis

Accepted NANDA nursing diagnoses that may be specifically applicable to the individual with antisocial personality disorder include:

Altered health maintenance

High risk for injury

Self-care deficit, bathing/hygiene; dressing/ grooming

Diversional activity deficit

Impaired home maintenance management

Altered thought processes

Personal identity disturbance

Altered role performance

Social isolation

Impaired social interaction

Altered family processes

Altered sexuality patterns

Ineffective individual coping

To develop a nursing diagnosis that fulfills its function of providing direction for planning nursing care, the nurse is encouraged to postulate and state etiological or antecedent factors and connect the two phrases by using the term "related to." For example:

Impaired social interaction related to manipulation of others

Planning and implementing nursing care

The plan for nursing care is derived from the nursing diagnoses and includes the objectives of the care, the nursing interventions, and outcome criteria. To be effective, the plan needs to be highly individualized. The suggestions that follow should be seen as general guidelines to be used if they are appropriate to the client's needs.

In general, the objectives of all nursing care for the individual with antisocial personality disorder should relate to assisting the client to alter behavior so that it does not infringe on the rights of others and to be accountable for actions.

Since the client's nursing diagnoses are often interrelated, stemming as they do from similar etiologies or antecedents, the student should see that the appropriate nursing interventions are also interrelated. In other words, by intervening in one dimension, the nurse will also affect other dimensions.

Activity-exercise

Individuals with antisocial personality disorder need a variety of challenging activities throughout the day. They are likely to plead for special privileges, but the nurse should be cautious about granting such requests. As with all other clients, they should be rewarded for acceptable behavior. If possible, these individuals should be placed in situations in which they can obtain socially acceptable satisfactions. Thus, success in some type of **vocational therapy** is ideal. It is essential to insist these clients fulfill the responsibilities expected of them, since they are likely to cooperate only at their own convenience.

Because individuals with antisocial personality disorder lack a well-developed social conscience, they usually function poorly in group activities. However, insofar as possible, it is suggested that they be helped to accept a role in some of the available group functions.

Role-relationship

Some persons believe that an individual who behaves in an antisocial way is a criminal and therefore should not be treated within the health care system. Others believe that little, if anything, is wrong with these persons and therefore they do not require treatment. Both these extreme attitudes can prove detrimental to the individual who engages in antisocial acts and to society.

Although the current trend is to keep as many individuals as possible out of institutions, many authorities still believe that persons with antisocial personality disorder require hospitalization if they are to be treated with any hope of success. The institution should provide a friendly, accepting, humane environment, where firm, reasonable, consistent, and enforceable limits and controls are placed on behavior. A permissive atmosphere is usually not helpful for these individuals. They need to be helped to develop a socialized superego, and such growth may be fostered by an organized, structured, controlled environment.

The treatment goals should include helping them to accept and use more socially approved attitudes and standards in their relationships with other people. To achieve this, they must be helped to trust other people. It is hoped that this can be achieved through the development of a therapeutic relationship with one of the members of the professional treatment team. Since the psychiatrist is usually the ultimate authority in the treatment team, it would probably be helpful if the therapeutic relationship could be developed with a psychiatrist who could provide the necessary discipline.

The treatment goals can be promoted through a system of rewards and prohibitions, with socially acceptable behavior being rewarded with privileges and less acceptable behavior being responded to by the withholding of privileges.

If their behavior has developed out of negative social and cultural influences, these clients should be helped to seek a more acceptable social situation. They should be encouraged not to return to the same environment.

Because clients with antisocial personality disorder are often attractive, intelligent, and interesting conversationalists, they easily gain control of the situation by manipulating others. It is helpful to remember that although these individuals are usually clever in manipulating others, they frequently use extremely poor judgment. They are likely to be troublemakers among other clients and have been known to organize psychotic individuals for the purpose of accomplishing their antisocial plans.

Although nurses can be most effective if they use a helpful, friendly approach when dealing with the individual who exhibits antisocial behaviors, they also need to be constantly alert to the possibility of the client attempting to gain control of the situation. The clinical team should identify approaches they believe will be most effective in dealing with such individuals and should list the responsibilities that they will be expected to fulfill. When these decisions have been made, it is of primary importance for all hospital personnel to be consistent in carrying them out and in holding the individual to fulfilling these obligations.

These individuals do not profit by being scolded or lectured. Such an approach is never helpful and will serve only to arouse angry feelings. Since it is thought these individuals learn little from experience, punishing them accomplishes nothing. Limits must be set on their behavior, since they frequently indulge in temper tantrums or destructive activities to achieve their objectives.

When these clients engage in antisocial behavior, it is important to treat them in such a manner that they know the staff want to help them even though they cannot be allowed to continue the behavior they are exhibiting.

Because of the personality characteristics that result in behavior that is superficially pleasing,

---

KEY INTERVENTIONS FOR CLIENTS WITH ANTISOCIAL PERSONALITY DISORDER

Keep the client busy with activities that have the potential for resulting in socially acceptable outcomes, such as vocational therapy.

Develop an environment where firm, reasonable, consistent, and enforceable limits and controls are set on behavior.

Plan for the development of a therapeutic relationship with an experienced mental health professional who has authority in the situation.

Reward socially acceptable behavior with privileges; withhold privileges when client engages in socially unacceptable behavior.

Be alert to manipulation of staff and other clients.

staff misjudge persons with antisocial personality more often than any others with whom they come in contact. Inexperienced staff are likely to think that a perfectly normal person is being detained for treatment without justification; in this case a more experienced health professional must be consulted for clarification.

NURSING CARE PLAN: *An Individual with Antisocial Behavior*

CASE FORMULATION

James Baxter is a 30-year-old, unmarried man who was admitted to the state psychiatric hospital after being arrested for vagrancy and following children as they walked to school in the morning. He is the oldest child of a woman who divorced his father after many episodes of abuse to both her and James. Shortly after leaving her husband, James's mother took him and his two younger siblings to live in a rooming house, the only accommodations she could afford. Within a week she was befriended by another tenant, an unemployed, alcohol-dependent man 20 years her senior. This man moved in with the Baxters, ostensibly to save money, and within a month convinced Mrs. Baxter to move with him to the rural area in which he had been reared. Even though they had no financial resources, they were successful in renting a rundown shack on several acres of land. This property was owned by an absentee landlord. It was in this environment that James remained until he was 15 years old.

On moving to the rural community, the family was befriended by well-meaning members of the local church. However, James was unable to curb his antisocial behavior, which included truancy, killing and dismembering a cat, setting small fires in the bedrooms of the home, and stealing money from Sunday school offerings. Amazingly, he was never held back in school even though he was functionally illiterate. In fact, his teachers routinely appeared at the home on Christmas Eve with many gifts for all the children. When his mother asked to have him repeat a grade, the school authorities stated their belief that such an action would hinder the progress the teachers thought he was making.

James became involved with the law for the first time at age 12, when he volunteered to solicit money for a church benevolence. He was successful in collecting $70, which he spent on candy, cigarettes, and arcade games.

The minister of the church brought legal charges against James, who was placed on 1 year's probation in the custody of his mother, although Mrs. Baxter was incapable of controlling him.

When James was 15 years old, the landlord evicted the family from their home because they had not paid rent for the past 3 years. The landlord indicated he would have been willing to wait for the rent if they had maintained the house and land. However, since the house was in a state of extreme disrepair and the acreage was strewn with garbage and machine parts, he believed he had no choice

Continued.

NURSING CARE PLAN: *An Individual with Antisocial Behavior—cont'd*

but to evict them. The social service agency to whom the family was well known found them an apartment in a community 20 miles away. On the trip to this apartment the family stopped in a public rest area. James ran out of the back door of the restroom and hitchhiked 400 miles to a large metropolitan area. His mother never notified the police that he was missing, and they have not seen each other since that time.

On arriving in the city, James quickly became prey to a "pimp" who fed, housed, and clothed him in return for his services as a prostitute for businessmen whose sexual preference was young boys. He was so endearing that several businessmen gave him money and personal gifts, in addition to the fee they paid for his services. When his pimp discovered this extra source of income, he was so enraged that he almost beat James to death.

James fled this situation and since then has been drifting in the "skid row" section of another large city. He has a lengthy criminal record for petty crimes and has been committed to a psychiatric hospital four times.

On admission, James appeared malnourished but was in no acute physical distress. The mental status examination indicated no psychosis or organic disturbance. He stated he was following the children to protect them from predators.

Nursing Assessment

This case history demonstrates rather clearly many of the characteristics of an individual with antisocial personality disorder. As a young child, James was severely abused by his father and probably a witness to this man's abuse of his mother. It is not unreasonable to assume that he adapted to his fear through repression. James's mother seemed incapable of providing the support or structure necessary for a child to develop in a mentally healthy way. Her becoming involved with an older, unemployed, alcohol-dependent man indicates her poor judgment.

James's childhood behavior indicates a wide range of antisocial behaviors. Significantly, despite these behaviors and his lack of academic achievement, there is evidence James was well liked by his teachers. Also significantly, his first known act of stealing occurred in defiance of the church that had befriended him and his family.

This man failed to develop a socialized superego. Thus his behavior was dominated by instinctual demands, he failed to develop a constructive identity, and he had not incorporated socially useful controls. As with other individuals who are said to possess antisocial behaviors, he seemed incapable of conforming to social or legal standards. Even though he was previously treated at several psychiatric hospitals, he did not profit by this experience or by his encounters with the law.

Despite his dirty clothing and malnourished physique, the nurse found him quite charming and convincing in his explanations of his behavior.

Nursing Diagnosis

The assessment data, including present behavior, past experiences, and an under-

NURSING CARE PLAN: *An Individual with Antisocial Behavior—cont'd*

standing of the underlying dynamics, led to the development of the following nursing diagnoses for James Baxter:

Altered nutrition: less than body requirements related to inadequate food and fluid intake

Ineffective individual coping related to lack of impulse control

Planning and Implementing Nursing Care

The plan of nursing care developed for James Baxter is summarized in the box on pp. 384 and 385. It should be noted that no psychotropic medications were prescribed.

The team psychiatrist assumed primary responsibility for James's treatment in the belief that this client would respond best to the member of the team who had the most authority.

The nursing staff who gave care to James were mature, experienced individuals. They strove to develop a friendly, accepting, humane environment while at the same time establishing firm, consistent, reasonable, and enforceable controls. Because they had previous experience working with clients with antisocial personality disorder, they were alert to James's manipulative behavior and were not fooled by his charm.

James was assigned a single room to prevent his influencing other clients in private. A schedule of activities, which included occupational therapy, recreational therapy, and reading classes, was developed. A plan of specified rewards and withholding of privileges was designed to accompany each ac-

tivity and was implemented depending on James's participation. A copy of this schedule and reward structure in the form of a contract was given to James. He and the psychiatrist both signed it. This contract specified that no excuses would be accepted as reasons for James's lack of attendance at the scheduled activities.

Evaluation

The contract specifying James's behavior was reviewed by all staff and rigidly adhered to. He showed little difficulty in fulfilling the terms of the contract and therefore received a number of rewards. For example, he was allowed to stay in the day room and watch the television until midnight for each activity he attended and participated in for a week. This resulted in his staying up late for four nights a week.

An unanticipated negative outcome of James's treatment was that he bragged to other clients about how special he was, as evidenced by his private room and television privileges. Three weeks after admission, he found his room ransacked and his few personal belongings gone or destroyed. Another client quickly admitted he had done this to "teach him a lesson." James was very distraught and apparently fearful about this event, and several nursing staff members freely sympathized with him.

At this point, a team conference was called to evaluate James's progress and current status. The absolute necessity of pointing out the part James played in this incident was stressed. His apparent distress and fear were viewed as ungenuine and as an attempt at

Continued.

NURSING CARE PLAN: *An Individual with Antisocial Behavior—cont'd*

manipulation. In addition, the contract was revised to make it more stringent. It was the team's consensus that the only real progress James had made in 3 weeks was a return to a sound nutritional status.

James remained in the hospital for another 3 weeks before he was discharged to a transitional living situation. Although his presence on the unit created identifiable tension, some staff were sad to see him leave. His behavior on the unit had become more acceptable, but the staff had little hope he would be able to maintain this level of functioning in the community.

NURSING CARE PLAN FOR JAMES BAXTER

Nursing diagnosis	Objective (rationale)	Nursing interventions	Outcome criteria
Altered nutrition: less than body requirements related to inadequate food and fluid intake	Client's nutritional status will improve. (Optimum nutrition is essential for physiological homeokinesis.)	Make sure client eats three well-balanced meals each day as served in cafeteria. Supplement meals with high-calorie, nutritionally sound snacks (e.g., milk shake) three times a day until 20 pounds have been gained.	Within 1 week, client gains 5 pounds. Within 1 month, client's hair, skin, eyes, and mucous membranes show evidence of adequate nutrition.
Ineffective individual coping related to lack of impulse control	Client will learn impulse control through behavior modification techniques. (An increase in impulse control is basic to the development of functional coping mechanisms; since internal controls are absent, external controls are likely to be most effective in learning impulse control.)	Assign to a single room. Plan schedule of activities designed to increase number of skills. Enforce client's participation in scheduled activities by rewards and withholding privileges as specified in contract.	Within 2 weeks, client attends and participates in three of the four scheduled daily activities spontaneously and without complaint.
		Do not allow staff to be drawn into client's manipulation (e.g., all requests for privileges must be made directly to Dr. F.; all decisions about nursing care to be made by Ms. R.).	Within 1 month, client gives evidence of attempting to gain rewards by altering behavior.

NURSING CARE PLAN FOR JAMES BAXTER—cont'd

Nursing diagnosis	Objective (rationale)	Nursing interventions	Outcome criteria
	Client will develop an increased sense of accountability for own actions. (If client is able to learn that he, too, is harmed by his socially unacceptable behavior, he may be able to alter such behavior.)	As situation arises, teach client socially acceptable behaviors and consequences to himself and others of ignoring these. For example, stealing another client's property hurts both persons. Enforce rewards and withholding privileges as outlined in contract with meticulous consistency.	Within 1 month, client cites consequences to himself and others of his behavior.

KEY POINTS

1. Individuals with a personality disorder exhibit an extreme manifestation of a personality trait.

2. Individuals with borderline personality disorder have not developed an integrated sense of self and therefore alternately see themselves and others as all good or all bad, depending on the situation.

3. It is believed that a major factor in the development of borderline personality disorder is the person's earlier inability to establish the self as separate and distinct from the mothering one.

4. Assessment of the individual with borderline personality disorder characteristically reveals impulsivity; antisocial recreation patterns; fear of being alone; extreme depth of emotions accompanied by mood swings; physical assaults on the environment, others, and self; intense but superficial interpersonal relationships; and an unclear value system.

5. The objectives of all nursing care for the individual with borderline personality disorder relate to helping the client learn to develop an integrated sense of self and a realistic perception of others and to control impulsive behaviors.

6. Individuals with antisocial personality disorder are incapable of valuing other people and manipulate them to achieve their own purposes.

7. It is believed that persons with antisocial personality disorder have failed as children to make a positive identification with parents or parent substitutes.

8. Assessment of the individual with antisocial personality disorder characteristically reveals lack of concern for the rights of others and rules of society, lack of impulse control, inability to experience any depth of emotion, social isolation, a positive perception of self and a negative perception of others, and values in conflict with the social order.

9. The objectives of all nursing care for clients with antisocial personality disorder relate to assisting them to alter their behavior so that it does not infringe on the rights of others and to be accountable for their own actions.

SUGGESTED SOURCES OF ADDITIONAL INFORMATION

Ashton E: The narcissistic personality disorder: the great cover-up—a challenge to the counsellor, *Can J Psychiatr Nurs* 14, April-June 1990.

Brobyn LL, Goren S, Lego S: The borderline patient: systemic versus psychoanalytic approach, *Arch Psychiatr Nurs* 1:172, June 1987.

Burrow S: The deliberate self-harming behaviour of patients within a British special hospital, *J Adv Nurs* 17(2):138, 1992.

DuBrul T: Separation-individuation roller coaster in the therapy of a borderline patient, *Perspect Psychiatr Care* 25(3,4):10, 1989.

Frosch JP: The treatment of antisocial and borderline personality disorders, *Hosp Community Psychiatry* 34(3):243, 1983.

Gallop R: The patient is splitting: everyone knows and nothing changes, *J Psychosoc Nurs Ment Health Serv* 23(4):6, 1985.

Gallop R: Escaping borderline stereotypes, *J Psychosoc Nurs Ment Health Serv* 26(2):16, 1988.

Gallop R: Self-destructive and impulsive behavior in the patient with a borderline personality disorder: rethinking hospital treatment and management, *Arch Psychiatr Nurs* 6:178, June 1992.

Gallop R and others: How nursing staff respond to the label "borderline personality disorder," *Hosp Community Psychiatry* 40:815, August 1989.

Hartman D, Boerger MJ: Families of borderline clients: opening the door to therapeutic interaction, *Perspect Psychiatr Care* 25(3,4):15, 1989.

Hickey BA: The borderline experience: subjective impressions, *J Psychosoc Nurs Ment Health Serv* 23(4):24, 1985.

Kaplan CA: The challenge of working with patients diagnosed as having a borderline personality disorder, *Nurs Clin North Am* 21:429, September 1986.

Kernberg O, Haran C: Interview: milieu treatment with borderline patients: the nurse's role, *J Psychosoc Nurs Ment Health Serv* 22(4):29, 1984.

Lion JR, editor: *Personality disorder: diagnosis and management,* Baltimore, 1974, Williams & Wilkins.

Martin SL, Burchinal MR: Young women's antisocial behavior and the later emotional and behavioral health of their children, *Am J Public Health* 82:1007, July 1992.

McEnany GW, Tescher BE: Contracting for care: one nursing approach to the hospitalized borderline patient, *J Psychosoc Nurs Ment Health Serv* 23(4):11, 1985.

Miller FT and others: Psychotic symptoms in patients with borderline personality disorder and concurrent axis I disorder, *Hosp Community Psychiatry* 44:59, January 1993.

Nehls N: Group therapy for people with borderline personality disorder: interventions associated with positive outcomes, *Issues Ment Health Nurs* 13:255, 1992.

O'Brien P, Caldwell C, Transeau G: Destroyers: written treatment contracts can help cure self-destructive behaviors of the borderline patient, *J Psychosoc Nurs Ment Health Serv* 23(4):19, 1985.

Pelletier LR, Kane JJ: Strategies for handling manipulative patients, *Nursing '89,* May 1989, p 81.

Piccinio S: The nursing care challenge: borderline patients, *J Psychosoc Nurs* 28(4):22, 1990.

Reid WH: The antisocial personality: a review, *Hosp Community Psychiatry* 36(8):831, 1985.

Rowe J: The student nurse and the borderline patient, *Issues Ment Health Nurs* 6:311, 1984.

Simmons D: Gender issues and borderline personality disorder: why do females dominate the diagnosis? *Arch Psychiatr Nurs* 6:219, August 1992.

Thompson JE: Finding the borderline's border: can Martha Rogers help? *Perspect Psychiatr Care* 26(4):7, 1990.

Wester JM: Rethinking inpatient treatment of borderline clients, *Perspect Psychiatr Care* 27(2):17, 1991.

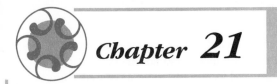

Chapter 21

Populations at Risk

children and adolescents

Beatrice C. Yorker

CHAPTER OUTLINE

Historical perspective
Disorders beginning in infancy or childhood
  Developmental disorders
  Disruptive behavior disorders
  Anxiety disorders
Guidelines for meeting the needs of children with
  emotional disturbances
  Child abuse
Disorders beginning in adolescence
  Eating disorders: anorexia nervosa and bulimia
    nervosa
  Adolescent suicide

LEARNING OBJECTIVES

*After studying this chapter, the student will be
able to:*

- Define the diagnosis of mental retardation.

- Describe the behaviors exhibited by a child with
the diagnosis of pervasive developmental disorder.

- Discuss the ways in which an academic skills disorder or motor skills disorder might interfere with
a child's development.

- Describe the characteristics of two types of disruptive behavior disorder in children.

- Differentiate between separation anxiety disorder
and overanxious disorder in children.

- State general guidelines for meeting the needs of
children with emotional disturbances.

- Describe the dynamics of violence and abuse in
families.

- State general guidelines for meeting the needs of
survivors of family violence.

- Describe the characteristics of an adolescent with
the eating disorders of anorexia nervosa and bulimia nervosa.

- State general guidelines for meeting the needs of
an adolescent with anorexia nervosa or bulimia
nervosa.

- Describe the characteristics of a suicidal adolescent.

- State general guidelines for meeting the needs of
an adolescent who is suicidal.

- Develop a hypothetical plan of nursing care for an
adolescent who is suicidal.

KEY TERMS

Therapeutic foster care
Mental retardation
Psychometric tests
Intelligence quotient (IQ)
Residential care
Down syndrome
Mainstreamed
Pervasive developmental disorders
Autistic disorder
Facilitated communication
Academic skills disorders
Motor skills disorders
Attention-deficit hyperactivity disorder
Conduct disorder
Separation anxiety disorder
Overanxious disorder
Hyperactive
Play therapy
Child abuse
Adolescence
Anorexia nervosa
Bulimia nervosa
Adolescent suicide

There probably is no other group for which the title "populations at risk" is more appropriate than the group represented by the children and adolescents of the United States. About one third of the nation's population is under 18 years of age, and it is estimated that 17% to 22% of this group has a mental disorder. Furthermore, many authorities forecast that the incidence and prevalence of mental disorders and dysfunctional behavior among this population will increase over the next two decades. Despite this dire situation, there is a gross shortage of health care professionals who are educationally and experientially prepared to address these problems. The seriousness of this situation can be appreciated if one remembers that the children and youth of a society are that society's future.

The identification and treatment of mental disorders of children and adolescents are recognized as an area of specialization in both medicine and nursing. Nurses who work in child and adolescent mental health care settings combine approaches of pediatric, psychiatric, and developmental specialties. Thus this topic deserves more attention than can possibly be provided in one chapter of a textbook devoted primarily to the field of adult psychiatric nursing. Nevertheless, this chapter is included to present a brief overview of the field in the hope that all students will become sensitized to the emotional needs of children and adolescents and their families and that some will become interested in pursuing further preparation in this rewarding subspecialty.

HISTORICAL PERSPECTIVE

Interest in the prevention and treatment of emotional disorders of children and adolescents did not develop until recently. Before 1920 many authorities believed that mental illness was limited to adults. The occasional emotionally disturbed child who came to the attention of physicians was thought to be a clinical curiosity. This view reflected limited knowledge about the nature of childhood and adolescence.

Several factors led to an increased interest in childhood and adolescence as stages of development distinct from adulthood. In preindustrial societies the progression from childhood to adulthood was rapid and accompanied by limited choices. Children were taught to take over the tasks and chores required to meet the family's basic needs. Formal education was limited for the vast majority of children. However, the emergence of the industrial society created numerous social changes that postponed the age at which the passage into adulthood occurred. Since industrialization and expanding technology required increased education and training to prepare for a productive adulthood, the stage of adolescence was delineated as a transitional period between childhood and adulthood during which this specialized training should occur. Therefore, the student role set adolescents apart as a distinct and separate population.

The post–World War II baby boom created a very large subgroup of adolescents in the 1960s and 1970s. A distinct adolescent culture emerged, and interest in its unique development and distinct problems led to a more careful examination of this age group.

The nurse's role in the treatment of emotionally disturbed children and adolescents has traditionally been minimal, often limited to the provision of physical care and the administration of medications. However, as more nurses pursued graduate education in psychiatric nursing through funds made available by the National Mental Health Act of 1946, the therapeutic potential of nurses in the care of children and youth became evident. In 1954 the first graduate program in child psychiatric nursing was opened at Boston University. Although many such programs exist today, there are fewer graduates than necessary to provide the required leadership in the prevention and treatment of emotional disorders of children and adolescents. The career opportunities in child and adolescent psychiatric nursing include inpatient, residential, or outpatient settings; schools; **therapeutic foster care;** homeless shelters; pediatric hospitals; and many other innovative care settings. Nurses who work with children must have a basic understanding of developmental needs and must be comfortable engaging in play, games, nurturing, and age-appropriate, therapeutic modalities.

DISORDERS BEGINNING IN INFANCY OR CHILDHOOD

This discussion is limited to those disorders that usually have their onset during infancy or childhood. However, it should be noted that the major mental disorders of adulthood, such as depression and schizophrenia, may begin during childhood and adolescence.

Developmental disorders
Mental retardation

Since mental retardation is not a mental illness, its relevance to psychiatric nursing is often questioned. However, the individual with mental retardation is three to four times more likely than others to develop a mental disorder, the treatment of which must take into account the individual's intellectual limitations. Therefore, it is important for the psychiatric nurse to have an understanding of what is meant by mental retardation. Additionally, a sizable portion of public and private sector health care is devoted to this population.

The term **mental retardation** is used to describe a condition in which a general delay occurs in the individual's intellectual and social development during the early years of life. If the person's development is normal by age 18, mental retardation is not an appropriate diagnosis.

The diagnosis of mental retardation is made only after a multifaceted assessment of the individual. This includes a study of the person's physical, social, cultural, educational, vocational,

and emotional capacities. However, the determination of mental retardation leans heavily on the results of a battery of **psychometric tests** from which a definitive score is derived. This score represents the individual's mental age. Although authorities continue to call attention to the limitations and weaknesses of the several psychological tests currently in use, intelligence testing continues to be one of the major tools in categorizing individuals in relation to intellectual functioning. Such categorization is useful for many practical reasons, especially in planning educational programs.

A score called the **intelligence quotient (IQ)** is calculated by use of a formula in which the mental age (MA) is divided by the chronological age (CA) and multiplied by 100. Therefore the formula is:

$$IQ = \frac{MA}{CA} \times 100$$

Obviously an IQ cannot be determined in infancy, and the diagnosis of mental retardation is not made in many individuals until they reach school age. However, the existence of characteristic physical features or severe physical impairment in many profoundly and severely retarded individuals sometimes allows this diagnosis to be made at birth or shortly thereafter.

The *Diagnostic and Statistical Manual of Mental Disorders* (DSM-III-R) categorizes mental retardation into four degrees of severity:

Degree of severity	IQ
Mild	50-55 to approximately 70
Moderate	35-40 to 50-55
Severe	20-25 to 35-40
Profound	Below 20 or 25

Most individuals with an IQ below 20 or 25 are incapable of benefitting from educational programs on even the simplest level. In addition, complex physical problems often coexist with profound retardation. Some individuals who are severely mentally retarded can learn to talk and be trained in basic hygiene skills, although it may take years of effort for them to achieve these skills. Many persons with profound and severe mental retardation require intensive **residential care.** Facilities that provide care for this population may include units ranging from intensive care units, where care is given to those with tracheostomies, central venous lines, and other highly technological treatments, through units where less restrictive care is provided, such as supervised outings and communication and skills training. Fortunately, persons with profound or severe mental retardation account for only about 5% of all individuals who are mentally retarded.

Individuals who exhibit moderate mental retardation can learn to talk and eventually master the skills necessary to take care of themselves. Although they will always require supervision for their own safety and protection, by adulthood it is possible for them to function well in familiar settings, perhaps even becoming employed in unskilled jobs.

Individuals who are mildly mentally retarded account for the largest proportion of mentally retarded persons. These individuals may not be distinguishable from others until childhood. These persons benefit from educational programs that emphasize concrete academic skills, social adjustment, and vocational preparation. Many become gainfully employed at jobs that require simple repetitive tasks and can live independently if supportive services are available.

Although the cause of mental retardation is unknown in approximately 75% of the individuals so diagnosed, certain hereditary and perinatal factors are known to result in impaired intellectual capacity. For example, a genetic abnormality within chromosome 21 results in **Down syndrome** (Figure 21-1); maternal alcohol or drug use during pregnancy may result in prenatal damage reflected by mental retardation; and postnatal head injury or ingestion of

toxins such as lead often leads to mental retardation.

The care of mentally retarded individuals in the United States has undergone a dramatic revolution over the last two decades. Legislation and government funding have enabled all but the most profoundly retarded to live at home and to attend local schools where an individualized program of study to meet their specific needs is designed by specialists in special education. This program may call for classes separate from those attended by nonretarded children, it may require that the child be **mainstreamed** with all other children, or it may dictate a combination of both types of learning experiences. As adults, most persons with mental retardation are able to live in the community, either independently or in group home situations where appropriate supervision is provided.

CLINICAL EXAMPLE

Lisa is a 24-year-old woman who has an IQ of 40. She had normal intelligence until she was 3 years old and had a massive head injury from an automobile accident. After Lisa recovered from the accident, she no longer could talk, feed herself, or use the toilet. In general, she required the care associated with an infant. Her large extended family devoted much time to caring for her and stimulating her to attempt tasks appropriate for the next developmental stage. Lisa began to say simple words at age 10, began feeding herself at age 12, and was successfully toilet trained at age 16. From ages 6 to 21 Lisa was transported by the local school district to a special education class, where she had the services of physical therapists, occupational therapists, and special education teachers. By age 21, Lisa was able to communicate sufficiently to make her needs known. She was also able to feed herself and bathe and dress with supervision. Her aging parents placed her in a local residential care facility, where she spends 4 hours a day punching holes in manuscripts before they are placed in loose-leaf binders. Lisa's parents visit

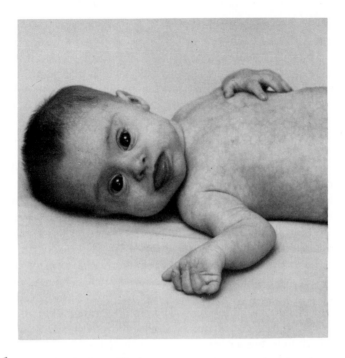

Figure 21-1
Down syndrome in infant.
From Whaley LF, Wong DL: *Nursing care of infants and children,* ed 4, St Louis, 1991, Mosby–Year Book.

weekly and comment that their daughter appears happy and proud of her achievements.

Pervasive developmental disorders

Until recently the illnesses known as **pervasive developmental disorders** were thought to be psychoses of infancy and childhood and have had the diagnostic labels of atypical development, symbiotic psychosis, or childhood schizophrenia. A pervasive developmental disorder of infancy or childhood is a condition in which the individual's entire development is severely and profoundly impaired, particularly in developmentally appropriate social interaction, communication and imaginative activity, and range of activities and interests. In addition, abnormalities often are seen in cognitive skills; posture and motor behavior; responses to sensory input; eating, drinking, and sleeping patterns;

and mood. Self-injurious behaviors typically occur. The most severe form of pervasive developmental disorder is autistic disorder.

Autistic disorder is often recognized by the end of the first year of age and usually by 3 years of age. It occurs much more often in boys than girls and may be misdiagnosed as mental retardation. Children with this disorder seem to be living in a world of their own and show little or no ability to relate to other human beings, including their mother. They appear not to recognize their mother as different from other people. They do not communicate in any meaningful way, and although they may use words, they do so in a highly personalized manner that only family members are likely to understand. Many of these children are obsessively attached to some inanimate object such as a doll or teddy bear, which they may play with for hours. In addition, they are likely to become very upset and have temper tantrums if their environment is altered in any way. Many engage in self-destructive motor behaviors such as head banging and biting their own limbs. Interestingly, they frequently twirl around at an amazing speed without becoming dizzy and seem to enjoy music.

The cause of autistic disorder is not known. The earlier belief that parental rejection was the major causative factor has not been supported by research. The prevailing view of autism is that it is a neurobiological disorder with complex and interacting causes. Autism involves several marked brain abnormalities and possible genetic and neurotransmitter (or neurochemical) abnormalities.

Promising treatments are emerging, and nurses are very involved in studying innovative therapies. For example, **facilitated communication** allows an autistic child to use a computerized letterboard to spell words. Some children whose speech was profoundly disturbed or absent have been able to demonstrate their intelligence and academic capabilities in this way. Physical therapy and movement are incorporated into educational programs for autistic children. A new and unresearched treatment involves *hearing conditioning* and seems to benefit those autistic children who experience painful reactions to sound.

Specific developmental disorders

Unlike pervasive developmental disorders that affect the individual's entire being, various developmental disorders are specific to impaired development in a particular area. Among these are academic skills disorders and motor skills disorder. Even though treatment of children with these disorders usually occurs within the school system, they are mentioned here because their existence often impacts the child's self-esteem and affects the family system, perhaps bringing them to the attention of the mental health system. For example, children who are not able to read

at grade level are in danger of being held back in school, thereby separating them from peers and impeding successful completion of other developmental tasks. On the other hand, if children are promoted into the next grade without being able to adequately deal with the academic demands of that grade, they are likely to develop feelings of inadequacy brought on by continual failure.

The **academic skills disorders** include impairment in arithmetic skills, expressive writing skills, reading skills, articulation (pronunciation) skills, expressive language skills, or language comprehension. For a child to be diagnosed with one of these disorders, it must be demonstrated that there is no physiological basis for their existence, such as mental retardation or a congenital anatomical abnormality. With the specialized help now available in all public schools, almost all children who have these disorders can be greatly helped.

Motor skills disorder is characterized by impairment in motor coordination not explained by a physical disorder such as cerebral palsy. Although the clumsiness exhibited by a child with this disorder greatly interferes with the ability to function effectively, much help is available through the special education programs in the public schools.

Disruptive behavior disorders

Of great concern is the disruptive behavior disorders, which are characterized by behavior that is socially disruptive and usually very distressing to the individuals with whom the child associates.

Attention-deficit hyperactivity disorder is diagnosed in children who are overactive, both physically and verbally. These children are unusually distractible and therefore unable to concentrate on any one task or to sit still. These characteristics result in their being unable to complete tasks, follow directions, or respond appropriately in social situations. For example, they frequently interrupt others, often with comments that are extraneous to the topic. Being around these children has been described as being in the middle of a whirlwind. As a result of their behavior, they often alienate others and do poorly in school. Consequently, their initial problems are likely to be compounded by low self-esteem.

Children with a **conduct disorder,** or oppositional defiant disorder, display a pattern of behavior that is antisocial. This almost always involves physical aggression toward others and purposeful defiance of rules, deliberately damaging or destroying property, truancy, lying, stealing, sexual offenses, and the abuse of drugs. As with adults with antisocial personality disorder, these children apparently feel no remorse or guilt over their behavior and therefore are very difficult to treat.

Anxiety disorders

Although all children display signs of anxiety on occasion, some children experience anxiety continuously or with predictability in specific situations. For example, children with **separation anxiety disorder** have extreme anxiety when they are actually or potentially separated from significant adults, usually their mother. They often display "clinging" behavior, experience an upset stomach or headache, and understandably refuse to go to school or to stay overnight at a friend's house. This disorder greatly interferes with their successfully achieving the developmental tasks appropriate for their age.

Some children are not anxious about a particular event but rather experience generalized anxiety continuously. When this anxiety is maintained for more than 6 months, they may warrant the diagnosis of **overanxious disorder.** Children with this disorder worry about everything that is occurring both to them and to others in their family. For example, an elementary school child may be distraught about having to participate in a school concert, or an older child may express fear that the father will be laid off from work after reading in the newspaper about lay-

offs in another company. Furthermore, these children are particularly adept at conjuring up tragedies that might befall them or their family. One 10-year-old child who developed the symptoms of this disorder when his mother took a job outside the home expressed fear about her being killed in an automobile accident, his burning the house down when he turned the oven on as instructed to prewarm it for dinner, and the house being burglarized while it was empty during the day. Clinicians are aware that the sources of anxiety disorders may also involve the parents. Children who resist going to school may be meeting a parent's unconcious needs. Treatment should involve the family and can be behavioral or insight oriented; medication may be used as well.

GUIDELINES FOR MEETING THE NEEDS OF CHILDREN WITH EMOTIONAL DISTURBANCES

Providing therapeutic care for disturbed children is one of the greatest challenges a nurse can face. However, it is one that must be met, since the nurse is most likely to have both initial and sustained contact with these children in residential and community mental health treatment centers. The behavior of children with emotional problems is frequently more baffling and more difficult to understand than the behavior of adults who have a mental illness. If the care provided for disturbed children is to be therapeutic, it must be based on the child's individual needs. The nurse, as with all other individuals working with disturbed children, will find it necessary to study the child and the symptoms displayed to identify immediate needs and to respond to them in a realistic and helpful way. In so doing, an attempt is made to offer the child experiences that can correct, in some measure, the negative experiences that may have been experienced in the past.

As the nurse understands that the behaviors the child exhibits are symptoms of more basic problems, the nurse will learn to be sensitive in responding to the disturbed behavior. Unquestionably the disturbed behavior requires a response; however, if this becomes the primary focus of intervention, one runs the risk of reinforcing the behavior with the result that it may not only continue but actually worsen. Rather, the goal should be an attempt to discover the nature of the underlying problem, and the intervention should be directed toward its resolution, not merely toward the obliteration of the symptom. For example, it is known that attempts to stop a child from nail biting are generally unsuccessful when this behavior is the sole focus of concern. To intervene on a level more basic than the presenting symptom, the nurse needs to work collaboratively with other professionals involved in the child's care, such as the primary therapist, the pediatrician, and the social worker.

Since many of these children are highly sensitive to their environment and the people who are a part of it, nurses need to examine their feelings, attitudes, and behaviors in an attempt to understand their own reactions to the child. In this way they can modify their behavior for the child's benefit.

Disturbed children require attention and guidance in the same areas of personal care that mothers usually provide. Thus the adult working with disturbed children will need to be involved actively in the child's bathing, toileting, feeding, dressing, and play activities. In addition, these children require organization and supervision in a variety of play activities, protection from potentially dangerous situations, and at times appropriate limit setting. As with normal children, each disturbed child is unique and occasionally needs special understanding and attention. It is a demanding task to respond as a wise adult to all the situations that may arise from the activities of daily living. The cooperation of all involved in the situation is required to assist such children to express their needs and find satisfying ways of meeting them.

Sometimes disturbed children, as with all children, need to be held, cuddled, rocked, or comforted. Such an activity is clearly within the nurse's role and necessitates much knowledge, sensitivity, and mature judgment to realize when and how much of such gratification is therapeutic for each child.

When admission to a treatment center is recommended for disturbed children, it is done in the hope that the milieu of the center will provide greater opportunities for ego development than can be provided elsewhere. Thus the goal for the treatment of every child is to develop a climate that will encourage adaptive aspects of the child's ego that in turn encourage experimentation with new methods for coping with the environment and for developing more effective ways of interacting with people.

Disturbed children are frequently unclear about simple aspects of reality and need to have repeated clarification about these confusions. Thus the nurse-child interactions should logically focus on the reality of the situation, with emphasis placed on verbal communication about reality matters.

Inappropriate response to environmental stimuli is a frequent problem for the disturbed child. The nurse needs to help the child recognize more appropriate responses to stimuli. Opportunities should be provided for the child to test and use these new responses.

Consistency in dealing with any child is of major importance and is especially necessary in providing care for disturbed children. When several people are involved in providing care for children, consistency is difficult to achieve but is nonetheless important. Ensuring a consistent approach depends on adequate communication among all people involved. Thus frequent staff meetings involving all the adults who come in contact with the child are essential. Every adult involved must understand what approach is being made to each child, why it has been adopted, and what it is expected to achieve. Repeated clarification of the treatment goals for each child is essential. Each staff member must have frequent opportunities to share with the group personal experiences in caring for the child. Thus all will be equally aware of the child's progress, and inconsistencies in the treatment approach can be eliminated.

Establishing and enforcing reasonable limits for children are an important responsibility of all staff members. Sometimes disturbed children become **hyperactive** and exhibit destructive behavior. Occasionally they might become physically out of control and threaten others' safety. It may be necessary to restrain these children to avoid injury to themselves or to others. Most agencies have policies for restrictive interventions such as time-out, locked seclusion, various forms of physical restraint, or medication. Although policies may vary, the general legal guidelines state that the only indications for the use of seclusion or restraint are to:

1. Prevent imminent harm to self or others.
2. Protect the therapeutic environment from damage.

It is never legally permissible to use seclusion or restraint as punishment or for staff convenience.

The nurse frequently has an opportunity to talk with the parents of disturbed children. A nurse is an available professional person to whom parents can turn to share their concerns or to ask advice about some aspect of behavior the child has developed. The nurse's interest in their child and willingness to listen to their fears and doubts are therapeutic for the parents.

Another important nursing function that cannot be overemphasized is providing anticipatory guidance to families to prepare them for the behaviors that can be expected as the child progresses through each developmental stage. Many parents, particularly mothers, feel most comfortable in sharing their concerns with a nurse. Appropriate reassurances and instruction can be of inestimable value in helping parents to provide acceptance and guidance for an emotionally disturbed child. In addition, appropriate antici-

patory guidance of parents may play an important role in the prevention of behavioral disturbances caused by unrealistic expectations of children who are basically healthy.

Play therapy is almost universally employed in the treatment of children with emotional problems. Its use is based on the knowledge that play is the medium through which children normally express themselves. Therapists use play as a means of gaining insight into children's unconscious feelings and attitudes about their lives. Play therapy has the additional function of enabling some children to work through some of the problems they are experiencing. The therapy room is furnished with a variety of toys and other equipment with which the child may choose to play. The therapist remains in the playroom with the child and spends time in becoming acquainted with the child and in developing a relationship of trust. The therapist observes the child carefully and listens attentively. If the therapist and the child have developed a trusting relationship, the therapist may ask the child to tell something about the meaning of the play in which he or she is engaging. Usually a complete dollhouse and a family of dolls are part of the equipment in a play therapy room. This equipment is purposefully included because the way the child plays with the family of dolls provides insights into the relationships the child is experiencing with family members. Since the child's emotional life revolves around family members, these insights are significant.

When children are questioned about spanking or punishing one of the child dolls excessively, one learns much about the punishment the child has experienced or fantasizes that he or she should have experienced. Children sometimes try to destroy an offending child doll or one of the adult members of the doll family. When asked to talk about these occurrences, the child may explain some unconscious fear or feelings toward a sibling or a parent. Thus, play therapy helps the therapist and the child to communicate with one another. Even when the child is essentially nonverbal, much can be learned from observing the child at play.

It is important that the form of play therapy chosen be appropriate to the developmental level at which the child is functioning. For example, finger painting and other forms of artwork may be used in therapy. This type of activity may appeal more to some children than does playing with toys. This is especially true with an older child. Much can be learned from the child's choice of color, the topic featured in the artwork, and the story the child may tell about the painting when it has been completed.

Child abuse

Over the past 20 years the emotional consequences of **child abuse** have become much clearer as a result of research and treatment in the area of family violence. Although the exact numbers of abused children are difficult to obtain, clinicians are aware that an alarming number of children treated in hospitals and clinics show signs of abuse. Abuse can be verbal, physical, emotional, and sexual. Neglect is also a form of abuse. Nursing views child abuse as a multifaceted issue involving social forces, parental factors, and vulnerability of the child. Abuse and violence tend to be transgenerational, or present from generation to generation in a family. Stress, poverty, and lack of social support seem to be particularly damaging to families at risk for abuse.

Child abuse has been recognized as a social problem only over the past century, although maltreatment of children has been recorded throughout history. In 1974 the Child Abuse Prevention and Treatment Act was passed. This means that in every state, nurses and other professionals who interact with children are required to report abuse. Nurses may worry about reporting abuse if they have no proof. Proof of abuse is not necessary. Nurses must report even *suspected* abuse. The child protection agency is responsible for making a determination of whether child abuse occurred. Nurses should re-

member that signs of child abuse may be cries for help, similar to the clues a person who is suicidal may give.

Intervention for child abuse must include making all reasonable attempts to support the parent or parents and preserve the family. Social services have learned that removing a child from a primary attachment figure can have devastating emotional consequences. Many abused or neglected children fear loss of their parents or their home more than they fear the abuse. Even abusive parents love their children and do not intend to harm them. Stressors, lack of effective parenting skills, and childhood experiences of violence are common reasons parents abuse. Parents do not generally abuse their children out of true disregard for them. It is important, therefore, for nurses to remember that reporting child abuse does not necessarily mean that the child will be removed from the home. Reporting child abuse does ensure that a thorough evaluation of the child's safety will be conducted and that a variety of support services may be offered.

Guidelines for meeting the needs of victims of abuse

Many child and adolescent inpatients have a history of significant physical and/or sexual abuse. The emotional consequences of abuse may be compounded by multiple placements in foster care. One of the goals of a therapeutic milieu is to provide safe, consistent nurturance for children. This is critical for children with a history of abuse. The abused child or adolescent may exhibit any or all of the following characteristics:

- Inability or difficulty establishing relationships
- Mistrust of caregivers
- Extreme physically aggressive behavior toward others
- Withdrawal
- Night terrors
- Excessive clinging to caregivers or nursing staff

- Sexual acting out
- Abuse of younger children
- Other socially deviant or illegal behavior (e.g., running away, prostitution, drug and alcohol abuse)

Examples of nursing interventions that can be helpful with children or adolescents with a history of abuse include the following:

1. Provide several uninterrupted periods of interaction between the nurse and the child each day. Allow the child to set the agenda, and let the child know when and for how long to expect these interactions. This provides a consistent, accepting relationship.

2. Encourage the child to take responsibility for his or her damaging behavior. Express understanding for their frustration, but point out that just as they do not like being treated badly, they cannot use their own previous experiences of abuse or violence to justify mistreating others.

3. Be aware of the child's unique history of abuse and plan treatment accordingly. For example, a child who was often locked up in a closet would be reinjured by the experience of being locked in a seclusion room. A child who was tied to the bed and molested would have an extreme panic reaction to being placed in leather restraints that immobilize both arms and both legs to the four corners of a hospital bed. A child whose mother was beaten at night might be very fearful of the dark or of noises at night.

4. Group treatment with other survivors of abuse is being implemented in many child and adolescent treatment facilities. A skilled clinician who is trained in treatment of abuse should colead these groups with members of the nursing staff. Confidentiality is very important in these groups.

Treatment is long and often difficult but has the potential of stopping the transgenerational cycle of abuse. Nurses play a key role in identifying child abuse and family violence and often take leadership positions in addressing the factors that contribute to the emotional consequences of abuse.

DISORDERS BEGINNING IN ADOLESCENCE

Adolescence is the term used to describe the period of life between the ages of 12 and 18. This period spans the developmental phase between childhood and adulthood that is marked by intense biological, cognitive, intrapsychic, and interpersonal changes. One of the major tasks of adolescence is separation from the family as a means of establishing an independent identity and assuming an adult role in society. This struggle for independence is often awkward and at times stormy as the individual experiences confusion and fear regarding the ability to master the tasks of this stage. The adolescent wrestles with the desire to stay close to protective parental figures and the simultaneous desire for freedom and autonomy. This ambivalence is often manifested by continual conflicts between the adolescent and the parents.

The adolescent is engaged in an intrapsychic struggle in an attempt to establish a new psychological equilibrium. In addition, the individual is exerting much effort to control new desires and impulses that result from biological maturation. The outcome of these struggles is largely determined by the success with which earlier developmental tasks have been achieved.

Today's adolescent confronts this critical developmental period during a time of great stress generated by the highly complex society in which we live. The stresses of contemporary Western culture may contribute to the distress, alienation, loneliness, and despair that at times characterize the adolescent experience. The number and severity of emotional problems of adolescents continue to increase. Adolescent suicide has been described as an epidemic in the United States; the rate has tripled in the last 20 years. Self-destructive behaviors such as drug abuse, alcoholism, eating disorders, and sexual promiscuity are also on the rise.

Adolescents may develop many of the mental disorders described earlier in this chapter as beginning in childhood and infancy. Major mental illnesses such as schizophrenia may also first develop during adolescence. However, nurses should be aware of the unfortunate trend of medicalizing many developmentally appropriate but difficult aspects of adolescence (e.g., intense reliance on a peer group for approval, anger, or withdrawal directed toward authority figures; adopting dress and styles that may offend adults; emotional highs and lows). Some serious emotional problems that typically develop during adolescence deserve special attention, that is, eating disorders and adolescent suicide.

Eating disorders: anorexia nervosa and bulimia nervosa

The incidence and awareness of the eating disorders known as anorexia nervosa and bulimia nervosa have risen dramatically in recent

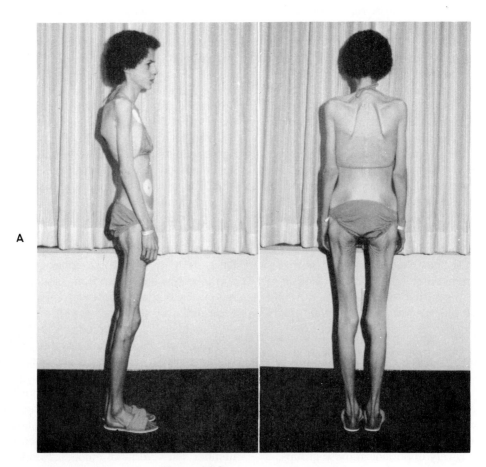

Figure 21-2

A, Anorectic woman before treatment.

years. Both disorders usually begin in adolescence and young adulthood and primarily affect females. Although much has been written on eating disorders in recent years in both professional and popular literature, authorities disagree about the cause and treatment of these disorders.

Anorexia nervosa is the term used to describe a disorder characterized by extreme weight loss, behavior designed to effect weight loss, an intense fear of fat, a distorted body image, and peculiar patterns of eating and handling food (Figure 21-2). The term *anorexia* is a misnomer in that it means loss of appetite. However, the anorectic person rarely experiences loss of appetite until late in the illness.

The individual with anorexia nervosa usually comes to the attention of the health care system after a drastic reduction in weight. Therefore she has an emaciated appearance. She has drastically reduced her total food intake, most specifically those foods containing carbohydrates. The person has ritualistic and bizarre eating habits, such as hiding and hoarding foods, collecting recipes, dawdling and methodically rearranging food on

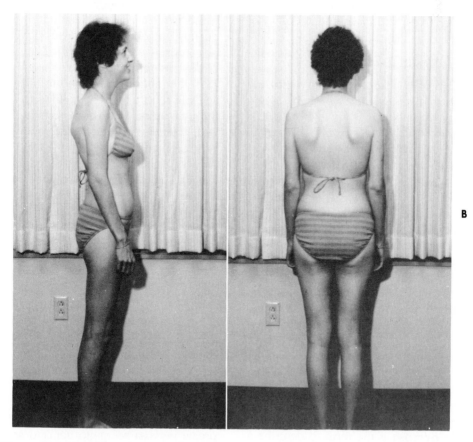

Figure 21-2, cont'd
B, Same woman after *gradual* refeeding, nutritional management, and psychological therapy.
From Williams SR: *Nutrition and diet therapy*, ed 7, St Louis, 1993, Mosby–Year Book.

the plate, and refusing to eat with family or in public. These individuals have an intense fear of becoming fat, despite their often emaciated appearance. Symptoms of depression are often evident, such as sleep disturbances, crying spells, and suicidal ideation. These persons usually have amenorrhea and a lack of interest in sexual activity. They often engage in excessive exercising and are preoccupied with food and weight loss. Physical signs include hypothermia, bradycardia, dependent edema, dehydration, hypotension, and lanugo, a fine downy hair covering the body. Laboratory tests reveal electrolyte imbalances, including hypokalemic alkalosis secondary to self-induced vomiting and laxative abuse. These individuals are often withdrawn and socially isolated.

CLINICAL EXAMPLE

Bernadette is a 20-year-old straight-A nursing student who collapsed one day when leaving class. When the instructor ran to her side, it appeared that Bernadette was not breathing. The instructor immediately began administering CPR, and Bernadette began breathing on her own almost immediately. When the rescue squad arrived minutes later, the instructor helped Bernadette onto the stretcher. When grabbing her arms, the instructor was shocked to realize that they were pencil thin, camouflaged by several sweat shirts. When she looked at Bernadette's legs, the instructor became aware that Bernadette also was wearing several sets of sweat pants. When she discussed this event with other faculty, they all recalled incidents when Bernadette had appealed to them to increase her grade from 92 to 93 or from 95 to 96 even though she would have received an A regardless of the point value. Therefore, they all had quickly agreed to her request and thought no more about it.

Bulimia nervosa is the term to describe a disorder marked by episodic, uncontrolled, and rapid consumption of food over a short time (binge eating), inconspicuous eating during a binge, and termination of the binge by abdominal pain, sleep, social interruption, or self-induced vomiting. The bulimic individual makes repeated attempts to lose weight by severe dieting, fasting, laxative abuse, or self-induced vomiting. She is aware that her eating behaviors are abnormal and is plagued by self-deprecating thoughts and depressed moods.

The individual with bulimia nervosa often appears healthier than the client with anorexia nervosa because the behavior is generally less incapacitating. This person is usually of normal body weight or slightly overweight but may report frequent fluctuations in weight. Whereas the individual with anorexia nervosa is often shy and withdrawn, the client with bulimia nervosa is frequently outgoing. The individual will often report low self-esteem and self-loathing, symptoms of depression, and a fear of losing control. The person is able to describe the binge episodes and will report frequent attempts to lose weight through fasting or severely restricted diets, laxative abuse, or self-induced vomiting. The individual usually has an excessive fear of fat and a preoccupation with weight and weight loss. Physical signs usually relate to the behaviors of self-induced vomiting and laxative abuse and include electrolyte imbalances, cardiac irregularities, edema, dehydration, swollen salivary glands, broken blood vessels in the eyes, tooth decay from erosion of the enamel, broken nails and scars on the knuckles from self-induced vomiting, and general gastrointestinal distress. The individual with bulimic behaviors often describes a loss of control. If the binge-purge behaviors are excessive, the person becomes socially isolated and dominated by these behaviors. Family relationships are often strained and disturbed, and both the individual and the family feel helpless, angry, and rejected.

An understanding of bulimia nervosa and anorexia nervosa seems to demand an openness to numerous views because the study of these disorders is relatively new and the causative factors are likely to be many.

Social theorists point to the dramatic rise in the incidence of these disturbances in recent years. Some relate this rise to societal pressures to be thin, to the changing role of women and the conflicting messages given to females, and to the absence of a clear set of values and norms that guided the behavior of adolescents of previous generations. Still others believe that these disorders are biological in origin or that a biological predisposition exists.

Some theorists propose a behavioral perspective and suggest that these behaviors are learned patterns. Others use a psychodynamic framework and suggest that these behaviors reflect a developmental arrest in the very early years of childhood around issues of trust, autonomy, and separation-individuation. Family theorists propose that the behaviors take place within the context of disturbed family relationships, faulty communication, and lack of boundaries between family members. Recent research notes an association between incest and the development of sexual abuse and eating disorders.

A general consensus exists among experts that an appropriate model for the treatment of persons with these disorders must integrate biological, psychological, and social perspectives. These disorders manifest themselves in disturbances in all subsystems. The symptoms are physiological, psychological, and social. Appropriate interventions clearly must address the whole person, and a plan of nursing care must be individualized to meet the client's needs.

Guidelines for meeting the needs of adolescents with eating disorders

Individuals with eating disorders pose specific challenges to professionals, who often feel frustrated and helpless in their efforts to nurture those who reject their attempts. Food and eating are quite symbolic in this culture, often representing love and nurturance. Individuals with eating disorders have conflicts that specifically focus on these symbols, and their behaviors may be viewed by some as rejecting and hostile. In caring for clients with such disorders, one must keep in mind the powerful sense of ineffectiveness that seems to grip them and work toward building a relationship of collaboration and trust.

Numerous treatment modalities have evolved to treat clients with anorectic and bulimic behaviors. The nursing care plan should be developed in collaboration with the client in an effort to capitalize on strengths as well as to intervene in dysfunctional behaviors. The meanings of the behaviors must be understood if a therapeutic plan is to be developed. Although diverse opinions exist as to the most appropriate method of treatment, the general consensus is that consistency and agreement among the health care workers must exist for treatment to be effective. Thus, collaboration and communication within the team are imperative for the effective care of these clients.

Immediate interventions and short-term goals generally focus on a restoration of normal nutritional status because complications of malnourishment may be serious and eventually lead to death. The various inpatient treatment programs are derived from several models, including those based on behavioral interventions in which positive reinforcements are used to reward weight gain and/or stabilization and an appropriate intake of a balanced daily diet. During this phase of treatment, it is imperative that staff offer support and consistency. An attitude of firm caring has been found helpful. In addition, treatment must address such potentially dangerous behaviors as suicidal gestures and other acting-out behaviors that sometimes exist.

Long-term goals and interventions are aimed at the underlying issues as previously discussed, as well as the establishment of more functional coping mechanisms and healthy relationships. In an attempt to help the individual develop a sense of autonomy, the nurse might help the client plan and test new independent behaviors. The client with an eating disorder often possesses a sense of ineffectiveness. The nurse might assist the individual to identify and express these feelings and then facilitate situations in which the client might achieve a sense of mastery and success. Some treatment units offer art and poetry therapy, which gives the client the chance to express feelings while simultaneously experiencing a sense of achievement when projects are completed.

Group therapies and support groups are often used to assist individuals to improve social skills and reduce the social isolation they experience. These groups also encourage autonomous and independent behavior in a population that is struggling to separate from family and achieve identity. Group cohesiveness and activities often facilitate this process.

Family therapy is often employed with clients and their families to try to alleviate family stress and achieve effective communication and healthy relationships. The nurse also might individually encourage the client to identify family stressors and recognize the dysfunctional behaviors previously used to cope with stress.

Educational groups are used in the treatment of these individuals. Information is provided about healthy nutrition, the physical consequences of anorectic and bulimic behaviors, and the social pressures exerted on women of today to remain unhealthily thin. In addition to providing information, it is likely that such groups facilitate sharing and help these individuals to recognize that they are not alone in their struggles.

Psychotherapy with a qualified individual is aimed at helping the individual to discover the underlying causes of the problems and the source of the anorectic and bulimic symptoms. In addition, some psychopharmacological agents have been shown to be helpful in the treatment of these disorders.

Nurses who work with individuals who have anorexia nervosa or bulimia nervosa can tell many stories about the challenges and frustrations they confront. The client is ambivalent, confused, and in conflict about the task of separation and often manifests this conflict through anger directed at the nurse. In addition, the individual often rejects the nurse's efforts to nurture. Nursing is a predominantly female profession, faced with the same issues that all women in our society are confronting. Thus the nurse may tend to identify with the female experiencing an eating disorder. This is especially true of young nurses who have only recently made the passage into adulthood. On the other hand, the very nature of the profession puts the nurse in an ideal position to develop new insights about the feminine nature of eating disturbances. Therefore, nursing is in the position to make many contributions to the understanding of these individuals.

Adolescent suicide

Suicide is one of the major causes of death for persons between the ages of 10 and 24. The adolescent suicide rate has increased rapidly in the last two decades. It is frightening to realize that authorities believe that the real incidence of **adolescent suicide** is even greater than the statistics indicate.

Authorities on adolescent development are defining this problem as catastrophic and epidemic. Understanding of and knowledge about adolescent suicide remain limited, and experts are struggling to define methods of prevention and intervention. Much of what was said in Chapter 16 about the individual contemplating suicide applies to the suicidal adolescent as well. However, certain factors are unique to the adolescent population.

Although the shocking rise in the incidence of adolescent suicide is recognized, the causes of such behavior are not clearly understood. Studies of adolescent suicide behavior indicate individual, familial, and sociocultural issues as factors influencing this behavior.

Some studies indicate a familial tendency toward suicidal behavior, which possibly is learned. Major psychiatric disorders such as depression and schizophrenia seem to be linked to suicidal attempts in some adolescents. An impulsive personality trait has also been identified in some adolescents who have attempted or committed suicide. It has also been suggested that adolescents do not have a clear, realistic sense of death or of the finality of the act of suicide. Therefore, suicidal behavior may be an effort to express anger or hostility toward loved ones or to make others feel sorry for real or imagined offenses.

Confusion over emerging sexual impulses and gender identity typically occurs during adolescence, and suicide may represent an effort to resolve such conflicts. Substance abuse has also been linked to teenage suicide.

In terms of family dynamics, several factors seem to relate to suicidal behaviors. Such factors include broken homes, family disorganization, overly strict parental discipline, lack of communication, and suicidal behavior in family members.

Much attention has been focused recently on the sociocultural factors that contribute to suicidal behavior in adolescence. The dramatic rise in incidence points to the influence of social change. Various researchers note that violence has become acceptable in our society and that the adolescent has become numb to violence. In addition, authorities point to increased family mobility and rootlessness, which lead to a sense of alienation and loneliness at a time when group affiliation is vital. Social isolation often precedes a suicidal act.

Other authorities discuss the prevailing stress found in our Western culture as a factor contributing to the incidence of adolescent suicide. In addition, adolescents in our society do not really have a place; they are neither child nor adult. They are often segregated into educational institutions where strong relationships with adults are lacking at a time when guidance and support are required.

It is also believed that the media have, at times, sensationalized or romanticized the act of suicide. Such idealization of the act may contribute toward suicide among those already contemplating the act. For example, epidemics of suicide have been reported in certain schools, reflecting the communicable nature of the behavior. If suicide is glorified or seen as a plausible method of coping with the life crises of adolescence, the number of suicides is likely to increase.

Although studies of suicidal behavior in adolescents indicate that it is determined by numerous and diverse individual, familial, and social factors, one factor is almost always present. This central issue is a sense of *invisibility*—a feeling that one is not recognized or appreciated and a belief that one has very little impact on the world around him or her.

Characteristics of the suicidal adolescent

It is believed that many adolescents contemplating suicide give clues to their plans and intentions. Some of these clues and behaviors are identified in Chapter 16. The nurse must be sensitive to such clues, which include preoccupation with themes of death, the expression of suicidal ideas, and the giving away of valued possessions. For example, one adolescent boy worked part time for years to buy a sports car. The day before he attempted suicide, he offered the car to his older brother.

Changes in sleeping patterns are often noted. The suicidal adolescent sleeps either too much or too little. Changes in eating patterns and resultant weight gain or loss may occur. The person typically withdraws from family and friends. The individual often has changes in school performance, including lower grades and truancy. Extreme fluctuations in mood, such as outbursts of anger alternating with crying spells, often occur. Finally, drug or alcohol abuse is often found in suicidal adolescents.

A previous suicidal attempt increases the likelihood of a later attempt. In addition, the recent suicide of a friend or family member increases the probability that the adolescent will act on suicidal impulses.

Although clues to suicide are often given by the potentially suicidal adolescent, the nurse must be cautioned that the absence of clues does not eliminate the possibility of suicidal behavior. If any suspicion of suicidal ideas is present, it is much better to risk confronting these than to ignore this potential problem.

CLINICAL EXAMPLE

Martin, 16 years old, was an excellent student in a private school, had few friends, and spent his time writing poetry. His parents were successful professionals. They had long ago adjusted to Martin seeming to be different from other boys his age and therefore were surprised when Martin announced he wanted to have a newspaper delivery route. When they questioned Martin about the reason for this decision, he stated that he thought he was an increasing financial burden to them and wanted to "begin earning my own way." Martin's parents tried to reassure him that he was not a burden, financially or otherwise, but were pleased that he wanted to do something other than write poetry. On the seventh day of his job, Martin jumped in the lake near his home and drowned.

Guidelines for meeting the needs of an adolescent who is suicidal

The nurse caring for the suicidal adolescent should be familiar with the principles outlined in Chapter 16 on the care of the suicidal adult. An environment that facilitates a sense of worthiness and conveys a caring attitude is vital. The suicidal adolescent should have opportunities to participate safely in activities that enhance a sense of mastery and self-esteem. The individual must be safe and secure while able to engage in adolescent group activities. The therapeutic relationship offers the opportunity for the suicidal adolescent to express and explore feelings in a climate of empathy and concern.

In the event of a successful adolescent suicide, the nurse must deal with the anguish of many affected individuals. At times the nurse may be able to offer assistance to family members, school counselors, and others involved. It has been said that the true victims of suicide are the survivors. Surviving family members experience intense remorse and feelings of guilt. In addition, such a crisis will magnify any existing problems in marital and family relationships. The principles of crisis intervention, as outlined in Chapter 24, are useful in such situations. Siblings must be observed carefully because suicide in one family member may precipitate such behavior in others.

The nurse may also be consulted by school officials concerned about the potential epidemic nature of the problem. Education that focuses on the realistic aspects of death and the impact of the behavior on loved ones is often enormously beneficial. Peers must be helped through the grieving process and the stages of shock and denial, developing awareness, and eventual acceptance.

It is imperative that the nurse be concerned with the prevention of adolescent suicidal behavior. Since nurses function in varied settings, they have many opportunities for involvement in this aspect of care. Research indicates that early recognition of the warning signs is vital. Once again, education seems to be a valuable tool. The nurse may be asked to collaborate with school officials and other professionals in providing education about suicide, as well as assistance for adolescents in coping with stress and depression.

Experiences that offer the adolescent opportunities to develop a sense of belonging and mastery might be the best way to prevent suicidal behavior. Recreational activities and centers, clubs, and church groups may help prevent the desperate sense of loneliness and alienation that contributes to all the disturbances of adolescents. Ongoing adult involvement in the lives of adolescents enhances the probability of successful resolution of this developmental phase, and nurses have a responsibility to provide some of this involvement.

NURSING CARE PLAN: *A Suicidal Adolescent*

CASE FORMULATION

Jennie Burns, 15 years old, was referred to the community mental health center by the school counselor with the approval of her mother after having been treated for taking 15 aspirins. She came to the center willingly and described herself as unhappy, upset, and without friends. The school counselor was concerned about Jennie, who had entered the school as a new student only a few months earlier. Her concern focused on the following problems: Jennie had made no friends, was receiving failing grades, was absent from school almost half the time, and was involved in almost no school clubs or extracurricular activities. She made the referral after learning of Jennie's suicidal gesture.

Jennie talked freely to the nurse at the mental health center and stated she could not study because she did not sleep well at night. She described nightmares that frightened her and kept her awake, the content of which featured an older man who molested her sexually.

In discussing her family, she spoke of the frequent fights between herself and her mother over her mother's drinking and her mother's boyfriend. About a year ago Jennie's mother and father had separated, and they were in the process of getting a divorce when she came to the clinic. After her parents separated, Jennie's father moved to another city and rarely found time to come back and visit with his three children, of whom Jennie was the oldest. She blamed her mother for the separation and the move from their old neighborhood and the school she had attended all her life.

Jennie's two brothers had become her responsibility since her mother's interest in her boyfriend had increased. Thus she was expected to supervise her younger brothers, prepare their meals, and do the laundry. With this amount of work expected of her, Jennie stated she was too tired to attend school more than half the time. Jennie's brothers did not follow her directions and resented her attempts to supervise them. Thus, conflict among the children was present in this family, with no adult to act as a buffer in such conflicts. Jennie felt unloved and unwanted.

Her mother's boyfriend was a large, middle-aged taxi driver who often teased Jennie. She told the nurse that she disliked him intensely and stated that she was afraid of him. In addition, she did not want anyone taking her father's place in the home because she loved her father very much.

Jennie was somewhat smaller in stature than most girls her age. Her breasts had not yet begun to develop, and she was extremely anxious about this fact. She viewed her flat-chested appearance as a serious defect that made her different from other girls. Also, she had not yet begun to menstruate, which increased her belief that she was different and lacking in feminine appeal. Unfortunately, Jennie was not physically attractive because her hair was dull and unkempt and her complexion sallow.

Jennie's mother was invited to come to the clinic to discuss the treatment plans for her daughter. She found it difficult to arrange a convenient time because she held a part-time job. However, she finally kept the appointment and gave much of the same in-

Continued.

NURSING CARE PLAN: *A Suicidal Adolescent—cont'd*

formation about the family situation as did Jennie. However, Jennie's mother stated that the conflict among the children was caused by Jennie's attempt to boss her brothers. She believed that Jennie's resentment of her boyfriend was the cause of many of their disagreements and declared that her dates were none of her daughter's business. According to her mother, Jennie was her father's favorite child, but he did not deserve her devotion.

Jennie's developmental history, as related by her mother, was uneventful except that Jennie had been enuretic until age 9. This problem reappeared after the separation of the parents and was present even now. Her mother also reported that Jennie had responded to discipline by having temper tantrums. These began when she was being toilet trained and continued until she was 9. Although she no longer had what could be described as temper tantrums, she did fly into rages. These rages seemed to be related to the mother's boyfriend and the approaching divorce. The mother stated that because of her job and home responsibilities, she had not been able to work with the school counselor.

Nursing Assessment

Jennie appeared to be experiencing difficulties in resolving the tasks of normal adolescent development, since several factors impinged on her life. Such factors included the loss of a close relationship with her father, a recent move, increased responsibilities at home, family conflicts, a perceived lack of attention and love, and the recent presence of her mother's boyfriend, whom Jennie feared and resented. All these factors might have contributed to the difficulties in adjustment that Jennie was experiencing, which culminated in a suicidal gesture. Adolescence is a time when the individual experiences ambivalent feelings toward the parents, which include a desire for love and affection along with a seemingly conflicting desire for autonomy and emancipation from the parents. The loss of her father at such a time might have made Jennie feel abandoned and guilty. In addition, her mother did not appear able to provide the love and support required during this period. Jennie might be blaming her mother for the loss of her father.

Jennie moved at a time when peer relationships and group involvement are important, and she found it necessary to enter a strange school and develop new relationships, something she had always found difficult. Her responsibilities at home might have prevented her from performing well at school, establishing successful relationships with peers, and engaging in extracurricular activities, which are all potential sources of self-esteem for adolescents. Jennie had not developed the physical characteristics of a woman and felt different and unloved.

Jennie's mother might have been poorly equipped to offer Jennie the love and support she needed for the successful resolution of earlier developmental tasks. The presence of enuresis and temper tantrums in childhood might have indicated the anger and frustration that Jennie felt toward her mother in early years and an effort to gain control and autonomy. The reappearance of enuresis when Jennie's father left home might represent the revival of these previous childhood feelings toward her mother be-

NURSING CARE PLAN: *A Suicidal Adolescent—cont'd*

cause Jennie now blamed her for the loss of her father.

Jennie's behavior disturbances reflected the difficulties she was experiencing with the tasks of adolescent development. Her rages might have reflected feelings of rejection and were directed toward her mother for saddling Jennie with home responsibilities, withholding love, and introducing an unwanted man into the home. The increase in Jennie's nightmares might relate to the introduction into the family of her mother's new boyfriend. Her social isolation might indicate feelings of low self-esteem and a fear of competition and failure. These feelings of inadequacy seem to have been reinforced by Jennie's slow sexual development.

Nursing Diagnosis

Based on the nursing assessment that included prior knowledge of the family dynamics and an understanding of the dynamics underlying adolescence, the nurse formulated the following nursing diagnoses specific to Jennie's emotional response:

  High risk for violence: self-directed related to anger at mother

  Impaired social interaction related to low self-esteem and fear of competition and failure.

  Altered role performance related to disturbed family relationships

  Self-care deficit, bathing/hygiene; dressing/grooming related to poor body image and feelings of worthlessness

Planning and Implementing Nursing Care

The plan for nursing care for Jennie is summarized in the box on pp. 408 and 409.

Jennie was admitted to a residential treatment setting for adolescents with behavior disturbances, where many opportunities for corrective experiences were available. After her needs were assessed and the nursing diagnoses were formulated, a plan of care was developed. An appointment was made for a physical examination to determine any specific cause of her slow sexual development. The examination revealed no significant findings.

A trusting therapeutic relationship was established with Jennie's primary nurse, who treated Jennie with respect and dignity and listened carefully to whatever she said. Her opinions were accepted, and the nurse avoided judging and moralizing.

The nurse attempted to convey a firm, caring attitude. She encouraged Jennie to function independently by establishing fair and reasonable limits while also praising autonomous behaviors, encouraging participation in extracurricular activities, and including Jennie in decisions regarding her care and treatment.

It was thought that Jennie's problems at school were a partial reflection of her problems at home. Continued efforts were made to involve Jennie's mother in treatment, although her resistance indicated that Jennie might have to learn to accept her mother's limitations and develop independent coping skills to deal with family stress.

Finally, Jennie was encouraged to participate in age-appropriate activities in an effort to assist her to develop healthy peer relationships and a sense of belonging.

Evaluation

Evaluation of the plan of nursing care and

Continued.

NURSING CARE PLAN: *A Suicidal Adolescent—cont'd*

its implementation was based on the outcome criteria developed in the planning phase.

Jennie made steady progress in the residential treatment setting, where ample opportunities were provided for healthy relationships and corrective experiences with both adults and peers. Her rages disappeared, and verbal hostility diminished. A tutor assisted Jennie to focus on school work, and improvement was noted. It seemed that her external controls improved, and her self-esteem was enhanced.

Discharge to outpatient services was recommended, where Jennie would continue in psychotherapy with a clinical nurse specialist.

NURSING CARE PLAN FOR JENNIE BURNS

Nursing diagnosis	Objective (rationale)	Nursing interventions	Outcome criteria
High risk for violence: self-directed related to anger at mother	Client will direct anger and hostility into socially acceptable activities. (Safe, age-appropriate activities are healthy outlets for anger and lead to decreased need to direct anger inward.)	Encourage participation in age-appropriate expressive and physical activities, such as sports, art, music, and physical exercise. Comment positively on successful participation.	Within 1 month, client: Reports absence of suicidal ideation. Spontaneously and independently participates in alternative activities.
	Client will explore feelings. (Increased self-awareness is necessary to prevent future suicidal feelings.)	Use reflection to encourage expression of feelings. Convey acceptance of angry feelings. Convey interest. Encourage problem solving.	Within 1 month, client: Spontaneously verbally expresses feelings of anger. Shows evidence of problem-solving behaviors.
Impaired social interaction related to low self-esteem and fear of competition and failure	Client will become involved in age-appropriate occupational and recreational activities. (Successful participation in age-appropriate occupational and recreational activities leads to increased self-esteem and social support.)	Encourage participation in activities, such as clubs, church groups, and recreational and occupational therapies. Accept feelings of frustration. Comment positively on successful participation.	Within 2 weeks, client: Spontaneously involves self in one group activity weekly. Reports success in one activity.

NURSING CARE PLAN FOR JENNIE BURNS—cont'd

Nursing diagnosis	Objective (rationale)	Nursing interventions	Outcome criteria
	Client will become involved in adolescent group therapy. (Group therapy is highly effective in assisting adolescents to explore their feelings and develop functional adaptations.)	Refer to group therapy. Encourage biweekly attendance. Comment positively on attendance and involvement. Accept expressions of frustration and fear.	Within 2 weeks, client: Attends group therapy biweekly. Spontaneously expresses her feelings.
Altered role performance related to disturbed family relationships	Client will express interest in school subjects and assignments. (Success in school leads to increased self-esteem and allows for the development of skills necessary for effective functioning in the future.)	Discuss school topics with client and encourage and reinforce interests; offer positive appraisals for success. Suggest and encourage involvement in extracurricular activities. View the family as a system.	Within 1 month, client: Reports interest in one school topic. Earns improved school grades. Identifies family stressors and demonstrates efforts to problem solve.
	Client will identify family stressors and engage in problem-solving techniques. (An ability to identify stressors and the development of effective, functional adaptations enable the adolescent to achieve control and hope.)	Recognize that as client's behavior alters, the system will enter disequilibrium. Assist with identification of stressors in family.	
Self-care deficit, bathing/ hygiene, dressing/ grooming related to poor body image and feelings of worthlessness	Client will exhibit improved hygiene and grooming. (Improved hygiene and grooming are likely to elicit positive reflected appraisals, thereby increasing self-esteem; they are also one indication of increased self-esteem.)	Encourage client to engage in daily routines of hygiene and grooming. Offer compliments for improved appearance.	Within 2 weeks, client shows interest in grooming, such as combing hair and wearing age-appropriate dress.

KEY POINTS

1. Although mental retardation is not a mental illness, the individual who is mentally retarded is much more likely than others to develop a mental illness.

2. The cause of mental retardation is unknown; however, some hereditary and perinatal factors are known to result in impaired intellectual capacity.

3. A *pervasive developmental disorder* of infancy or childhood is a condition in which the individual's entire development is severely and profoundly impaired.

4. Two types of specific developmental disorders, those specific to impaired development in a particular area, are *academic skills disorders* and *motor skills disorder*.

5. Children with *disruptive behavior disorders* display behavior that is socially disruptive and distressing to those with whom the child associates.

6. Children with *anxiety disorders* display anxiety continuously or predictably in specific situations.

7. Disturbed children need attention and guidance in the same areas of personal and emotional care that mothers usually provide.

8. Consistency in dealing with a disturbed child is especially important when several people are providing care in a hospital setting.

9. The nurse's goal in treating disturbed children should be an attempt to discover the nature of the underlying problem. Intervention should be directed toward resolving the problem, not merely alleviating the symptoms.

10. It is important that play therapy, which enables the therapist and the child to communicate with one another, be appropriate to the developmental level at which the child is functioning.

11. The nurse is therapeutic in dealing with the parents of a disturbed child by listening to their fears and doubts and by providing anticipatory guidance.

12. Abuse and violence tend to be transgenerational, or present from generation to generation in a family.

13. As a result of the 1974 Child Abuse Prevention and Treatment Act, nurses and other professionals who interact with children are required to report actual or suspected abuse.

14. Safe, consistent nurturing in a therapeutic milieu is critical for children with a history of abuse.

15. Treatment of children who have been abused is long and often difficult but has the potential of interrupting the transgenerational cycle of abuse.

16. *Anorexia nervosa* is a disorder occurring most often in adolescents and is characterized by extreme weight loss, behavior directed toward weight loss, and intense fear of fat, distorted body image, and peculiar ways of handling food.

17. *Bulimia nervosa* is a disorder usually occurring in adolescence and is marked by episodic, uncontrollable, and rapid consumption of food over short periods (binge eating) and termination of the binge by abdominal pain, sleep, social interruption, or self-induced vomiting.

18. Appropriate treatment for anorexia nervosa and bulimia nervosa must address the whole person, and a plan of nursing care must be individualized to meet the client's needs.

19. Immediate short-term goals for the individual with an eating disorder usually focus on a restoration of normal nutritional status, whereas long-term goals aim toward the establishment of more functional coping mechanisms and healthy relationships.

20. Therapies for the individual with an eating disorder include group therapy and support groups, family therapy, educational groups, and psychotherapy.

21. Suicide among adolescents in the United States has greatly increased in the last two decades; it is believed that the rising incidence may reflect sociocultural factors and stressors.

22. One central issue related to adolescent suicide is a sense of invisibility—a feeling that one is not recognized or appreciated and a belief that one has very little impact on the world around him or her.

23. Adolescents contemplating suicide often give clues to their plans and intentions: being preoccupied with themes of death, expressing suicidal ideas, and giving away valued possessions.

24. The nurse is therapeutic when providing opportunities for the adolescent who is suicidal to develop a sense of worthiness, belonging, mastery, self-esteem, safety, and security.

SUGGESTED SOURCES OF ADDITIONAL INFORMATION

Barlow DJ: Therapeutic holding: effective intervention with the aggressive child, *J Psychosoc Nurs Ment Health Serv* 27:10, January 1989.

Campbell J, Humphreys J: *Nursing care of survivors of family violence,* St Louis, 1993, Mosby–Year Book.

Carbrary JA: Trends in adolescent psychiatric hospitalization, *J Child Adolesc Psychiatr Ment Health Nurs* 4:68, April-June 1991.

Cerrato PL: Nutritionist on call: helping food addicts kick the habit, *RN* 50:75, August 1987.

Clunn P: *Child psychiatric nursing,* St Louis, 1991, Mosby–Year Book.

Deering CG: Developing a therapeutic alliance with the anorexia nervosa client, *J Psychosoc Nurs Ment Health Serv* 25:10, March 1987.

Dippel NM, Becknal BK: Bulimia, *J Psychosoc Nurs Ment Health Serv* 25:12, September 1987.

Dworkin RH and others: Social competence and positive and negative symptoms: a longitudinal study of children and adolescents at risk for schizophrenia and affective disorder, *Am J Psychiatry* 148:1182, September 1991.

Edmands MS: Overcoming eating disorders: a group experience, *J Psychosoc Nurs Ment Health Serv* 24:19, August 1986.

Federation S: Sexual abuse: treatment modalities for the younger child, *J Psychosoc Nurs Ment Health Serv* 24:21, July 1986.

Friesen BJ, Koroloff NM: Family-centered services: implications for mental health administration and research, *J Ment Health Administration* 17:13, Spring 1990.

Geary MC: A review of treatment models for eating disorders: toward a holistic nursing model, *Holistic Nurs Pract* 3:39, November 1988.

Harnett NE: Conduct disorder in childhood and adolescence: an update, *J Child Adolesc Psychiatr Ment Health Nurs* 2:74, April-June, 1989.

Hogarth CR: *Adolescent psychiatric nursing,* St Louis, 1991, Mosby–Year Book.

Hubbard GB: Perceived life changes for children and adolescents following disclosure of father-daughter incest, *J Child Adolesc Psychiatr Ment Health Nurs* 2:78, April-June 1989.

Jacobson J: Speculations on the role of transitional objects in eating disorders, *Arch Psychiatr Nurs* 2:110, April 1988.

Jaffe ES: Working with troubled teens, *RN* 58, February 1991.

Lilly GE, Sanders JB: Nursing management of anorexic adolescents, *J Psychosoc Nurs Ment Health Serv* 25:30, November 1987.

McBride AB: Coming of age: child psychiatric nursing, *Arch Psychiatr Nurs* 2:57, April 1988.

Miles MW: Bulimia nervosa and gender identity: symbols of a culture, *Holistic Nurs Pract* 3:56, November 1988.

Morris PA: The prevalence of children with a history of sexual abuse hospitalized in the psychiatric setting, *J Child Adolesc Psychiatr Ment Health Nurs* 4:49, April-June 1991.

Oehler JM, Burns MJ: Anorexia, bulimia, and sexuality: case study of an adolescent inpatient group, *Arch Psychiatr Nurs* 1:163, June 1987.

Opie ND: Improving nursing care services for children and adolescents with severe emotional disorders, *J Child Adolesc Psychiatr Ment Health Nurs* 2:14, January-March 1989.

Pothier MS: Kaleidoscope of excellence, *J Child Adolesc Psychiatr Ment Health Nurs* 5:38, October-December 1992.

Pothier PC: Child mental health problems and policy, *Arch Psychiatr Nurs* 2:165, June 1988.

Puskar KR: Difficulties with teens: can nursing consultation help? *J Child Adolesc Psychiatr Ment Health Nurs* 5:34, July-September 1992.

Puskar K and others: Suicidal and nonsuicidal coping methods of adolescents, *Perspect Psychiatr Care* 28:15, April-June 1992.

Riley EA: Codependency and the eating-disorder client, *Nurs Clin North Am* 26:765, September 1991.

Rosenfield S: Family influence on eating behavior and attitudes in eating disorders: a review of the literature, *Holistic Nurs Pract* 3:46, November 1988.

Rubin RL: Assisting adolescents toward mental health, *Nurs Clin North Am* 21:439, September 1986.

Valente S: Adolescent suicide: assessment and intervention, *J Child Adolesc Psychiatr Ment Health Nurs* 2:34, January-March 1989.

West P, Evans C: *Psychiatric and mental health nursing with children and adolescents,* Gaithersburg, Md, 1992, Aspen.

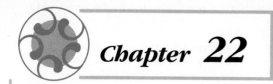

Chapter *22*

Populations at Risk
elderly persons

LEARNING OBJECTIVES

After studying this chapter, the student will be able to:

* Discuss three social factors that affect the ability of elderly persons to achieve ego integrity successfully.

* Discuss life review, loneliness, and loss and grief as manifested by elderly persons.

* Describe nursing interventions designed to prevent or alter depression, suspiciousness, and dementia in elderly persons.

* Discuss the causative factors associated with Alzheimer's disease.

* Describe the behaviors exhibited by a person with Alzheimer's disease.

* State general guidelines for meeting the needs of an individual with Alzheimer's disease.

* Develop a hypothetical plan of nursing care for an individual with Alzheimer's disease.

KEY TERMS

Alzheimer's disease
Powerlessness
Life review
Loneliness
Major interpersonal loss
Depression
Suspiciousness
Dementia
Reality orientation
Psychomotor agitation
Confabulation

Old age is an integral part of the life cycle, not one stage separated from the rest of life. Unfortunately, the United States is a youth-oriented society, and elderly persons are viewed as a homogeneous group to which predominantly negative characteristics are ascribed. For example, a common but erroneous belief is that once a person has reached the arbitrarily established age of retirement, he or she becomes at best, useless, or at worst, a burden to the family and to society. It is also believed that individuals over 65 or 70 years of age inevitably become forgetful and confused. Although elderly persons share much in common with each other, as do persons in any other developmental stage, they are also individuals who continue to adapt in the ways they have learned in earlier years. Elderly individuals have the potential to continue to learn and develop. Survival with esteem, not mere physical survival, is the goal of the aged person (Figure 22-1).

HISTORICAL PERSPECTIVE

Throughout history an occasional individual always has lived to reach the age of 80, 90, or

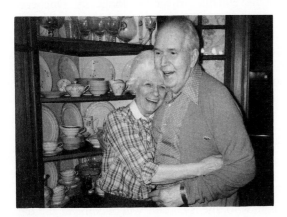

Figure 22-1

Elderly individuals with high self-esteem.

From Burke MM, Walsh MB: *Gerontologic nursing: care of the frail elderly,* St Louis, 1992, Mosby–Year Book.

even 100. However, never before has the life expectancy of the average individual been as long as it currently is. Until the twentieth century, it was the unusual individual who lived beyond 50 years of age. Many women died in childbirth; the general population was vulnerable to epidemics of respiratory infections and other communicable diseases; and few effective treatments existed for such life-threatening illnesses as cancer and cardiovascular disease. In addition, occupational hazards took their toll, and the death rate from accidents was high. These factors, combined with few preventive measures, resulted in what is now seen as a short life expectancy. Therefore, illnesses associated with old age were rarely experienced and poorly understood.

Because of the increased life expectancy and effective treatment of illness and injuries, the number of persons 65 years of age or older is larger than ever before. It is projected that more than 13% of the total population will be over age 65 by the year 2005, representing a 60% increase in this age group from 1980. As the number of people who live longer increases, a concomitant increase occurs in the health care needs of this population, including mental health needs. Until recently, it was assumed that a person who lived long enough would eventually become "senile" and that the symptoms of confusion and regression associated with this diagnosis were inevitable outcomes of the aging process. As the number of persons in this age group increases, this assumption can no longer be made without being validated by research.

Research about mental disorders of elderly persons has led to the identification of **Alzheimer's disease,** which is discussed in depth in this chapter. It was first discovered in 1906 by a German neurologist, Alois Alzheimer. Dr. Alzheimer treated a 51-year-old woman who exhibited all the symptoms associated with senility of elderly individuals. He became curious about her symptoms in light of her young age. After her death, he examined her brain and discovered that parts of it contained clumps of twisted nerve cell fibers that he called "neurofibrillary tangles." Although he did not understand what caused these abnormal nerve cell configurations, he believed their existence created the patient's behavior. Alzheimer's disease was assumed to be rare and to affect only relatively young persons, leading to it being called a "presenile dementia."

With the advent of the electron microscope in the 1960s, scientists discovered the same neurofibrillary tangles in elderly persons diagnosed as having senile dementia. Thus, it is now concluded that Alzheimer's disease is not rare or confined to the relatively young, but rather accounts for more than 50% of the cases of dementia in aged persons.

THE AGING PROCESS

No exact definition of old age exists. It is a developmental stage defined by complex physiological, psychological, and sociological factors. It has been defined by some gerontologists as the period marked by the relinquishing of mid-life roles (career, parenting) and the view of oneself as being elderly.

The elderly population is a diverse group. Elderly persons have as many individual differences as do those in earlier developmental stages. The negative stereotyping that has been applied to elderly individuals is called *ageism,* a term representing the discriminatory practices against the elderly in our culture. The stereotype that describes all elderly persons as irritable, forgetful, rigid, regressed, and confused is a distorted and limited view. Most elderly individuals can be healthy and productive and continue to learn and develop when they are allowed to do so (Figure 22-2).

CLINICAL EXAMPLE

Mrs. Hilda Gustafson, 83 years old, has been widowed for 15 years. Her parents had been quite wealthy and believed their children should be educated to make a contribution to society. Therefore, they enrolled Hilda in a private teachers' college after she finished high school. Hilda did very well in college, both academically and socially. She became engaged to marry a young man who was also preparing to become a teacher. After graduation, Hilda had no difficulty securing a position, which was to begin in the fall. During the summer between her graduation and when she would begin work, Hilda and a girlfriend traveled across the United States to have a last "fling." During this vacation, Hilda met a seaman with whom she fell madly in love. Although she and this man spent every moment together, Hilda believed this relationship had no future, and she returned home at the scheduled time. As planned, she began her new job, married, had two children, and became a major leader in her community over the next 40 years. She had no further contact with her "summer love." When Hilda's husband died, she was 68 years old. She responded to her loneliness by immersing herself even further into community activities. By the time she was 78, however, she found herself less enthusiastic about her activities and confessed to her children that she was "bored and embarrassed" by the many awards she was receiving. She suspected that she was being honored not for her achievements but for her longevity. One evening, on a sudden impulse, she called operator assistance in the city she had visited during the summer of 1932 and gave the name of her lover. Three persons were listed with that name. On the first try, Hilda located this gentleman and made arrangements to fly there the next weekend. They found themselves to be very compatible and for the last 5 years have spent 6 months of each year living in his home and 6 months living in hers. With a twinkle in her eye, Hilda says she is not willing to remarry because she does not want the burden of caring for this man who, she is certain, will become ill and die before she will.

Although elderly persons are individuals with diverse needs and strengths, they share some commonalities, as do persons in other devel-

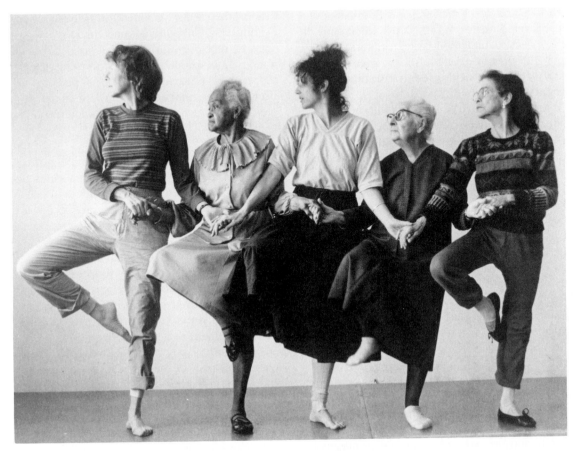

Figure 22-2
The elderly can continue to learn new things and develop new interests, such as modern dance.
From Burke MM, Walsh MB: *Gerontologic nursing: care of the frail elderly,* St Louis, 1992, Mosby–Year Book.

opmental stages. Physiological changes often occur as a result of normal aging, but the rate of change varies with each individual and with each organ system. These changes include increasing perceptual difficulties, diminished psychomotor abilities, and memory deficits that are reflected by difficulty in recall. However, these physiological changes appear to create little difficulty in the achievement of life goals for most elderly persons. In contrast, social and psychological changes profoundly affect the aged person.

Social factors

Although aged persons are beset by the same social problems as young people, their options for dealing with such problems are more limited. One example is economic inflation, during which the value of savings and pensions is eroded and few opportunities exist for employment, even if an older person were able to secure and hold a job. In our society, elderly persons as a group are poor. In certain groups, that is, Native Americans and African Americans, more than 75% of elderly persons live below the poverty level. Poverty not only deprives persons of the means to fulfill their basic needs adequately, but it also deprives them of a powerful social tool. It takes money to look one's best and to attend many social functions.

Another example of a social phenomenon that affects elderly persons is the change from small, stable communities to large, mobile urban centers. This change affects people of all ages and often results in a feeling of **powerlessness.** Older persons in particular can be left without family to help cope with the bureaucracies necessary for survival in a complex society. The result often is a sense of alienation and worthlessness.

The accelerating rate of social change, as well as technological change, has subjected human beings to an unprecedented need to adapt. The ability of elderly persons to make effective adaptations is dramatically impeded by a society that puts no value on age. Simple cultures value older persons because this group passes on the legends of the culture. In contrast, in an industrialized society, mythology that remains important is written down, printed, and sold. Therefore, in a society characterized by the nuclear family and printed and electronic communication media, no role exists for the elderly. In a society such as this, Erikson's psychosocial task of aging, the achievement of ego integrity versus despair, might be difficult to achieve, especially since the negative attitudes of society toward aging often have been internalized by elderly persons themselves.

Psychological factors

As a result of normal aging, the individual's characteristic personality often becomes more prominent. Thus the suspicious individual may become even more so in old age. Habitual ways of behaving continue, as do social skills, verbal skills, judgment, and comprehension.

Elderly persons exhibit several characteristic behaviors while confronting the tasks of aging.

The nurse caring for elderly individuals in any setting can offer assistance and enhance this process by recognizing the normal tasks and facilitating their resolution. The following experiences and behaviors of elderly persons are frequently encountered by the nurse, and suggestions are included for possible interventions.

Life review

Life review is the process of thinking about the meaning of one's life. Most authorities believe that life review is a nearly universal occurrence as older persons face the prospect of impending death. On the one hand, life review facilitates achieving closure to one's life. On the other hand, it leads to personal growth by bringing unresolved crises to consciousness, allowing them to be talked about at length in such a way as to facilitate their resolution.

The life review process involves reminiscence—remembering the significant events, people, and places in the past that helped to shape and provide meaning to the individual's life. When individuals are engaged in life review, they find this an all-engrossing task. They have little interest in the events of the present, whereas the events of the past are recalled and recounted in minute detail.

Because all elderly people probably reminisce, whether alone or with another person, it is vital that the nurse facilitate this process as a means of providing interpersonal feedback. Furthermore, planning for nursing intervention will become more individualized to the client's needs if the life review process is used both as an aspect of assessment and as a means for intervention. At the very least, the nurse giving care to an elderly person must allow time to listen actively to reminiscences and provide appropriate feedback.

Loneliness

More than any other group, aged persons often experience **loneliness.** Moustakos observes:

Elderly citizens in our society are particularly affected by the social and cultural changes and by the separation, urbanization, alienation, and automation in modern living. There is no longer a place for old age, no feeling of organic belonging, no reverence or respect or regard for the wisdom and talent of the ancient. Our elderly citizens so often have feelings of uselessness, so often experience life as utterly futile.

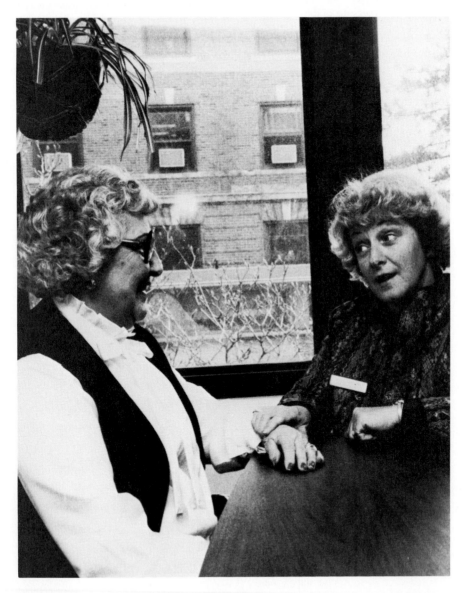

Figure 22-3
Nurses can reach out to help combat loneliness in the elderly.
From Gress LD, Bahr RT: *The aging person: a holistic perspective,* St Louis, 1984, Mosby–Year Book.

Old age is fertile soil for loneliness and the fear of a lonely old age far outweighs the fear of death in the thinking of many people. Loss of friends and death of contemporaries are realities. The mourning and deep sense of loss are inevitable, but the resounding and lasting depression which results and the emptiness and hopelessness are all a measure of the basic loneliness and anxiety of our time.*

To combat the loneliness of elderly persons, nurses need to reach out consistently to the older person. Five minutes daily for 5 days is a louder message of concern and caring than is 20 to 30 minutes once in a while. Attempts to involve the older person in a relationship must be persistent.

---

*Moustakos C: *Loneliness,* Englewood Cliffs, NJ, 1961, Prentice-Hall.

Nurses need to be aware of their own feelings of loneliness that may be triggered by the loneliness they sense in the older person. Younger nurses in late adolescence often experience profound loneliness as they seek their own identity and thus often want to move away from others who are experiencing loneliness. Therefore the withdrawal of the older person may evoke a mutual feeling of withdrawal in the nurse. Nurses must be conscious of their own feelings and aware of their needs when they are tempted to withdraw from the older person.

Loss and grief

When a **major interpersonal loss** occurs, physical changes that the individual had not been previously aware of are often brought to aware-

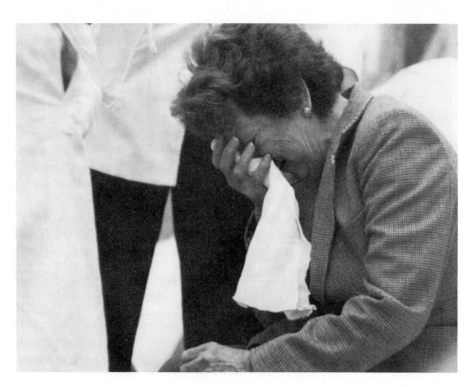

Figure 22-4
Grief helps to resolve the pain associated with a major interpersonal loss.
From Payne WA, Hahn DB: *Understanding your health,* ed 3, St Louis, 1992, Mosby–Year Book.

ness and perceived as losses. This phenomenon, in turn, intensifies the significance of the interpersonal loss. For example, it is not unusual to hear an elderly woman remark, "If my husband had died 10 years ago, I could have managed this house by myself, but now I'm not physically able to keep the place up."

The need to grieve for losses may not be seen as necessary by the older person, and grief may be avoided because of the pain associated with this process. Many aged persons develop physical problems rather than grieving, thereby directing their attention and the attention of others away from the loss and its attendant emotions to the somatic concerns. Consequently, the crisis associated with the loss is not resolved.

Older persons' limited energy level and reluctance to experience pain and resentment allow them to deal with these feelings only for short periods. The nurse must observe for signs that the older person has had enough for now, but the willingness to return again and again to the painful area both by the nurse and by the older person is necessary for the resolution of the crisis. One 89-year-old man who had experienced a major illness was talking about the loss of his mother when he was 7 years old. He paused and said, "There are losses that everyone expects as they go through life and those you get through. However, there are losses that you feel that, in some way, you caused or that it was your fault, and those are much harder to bear. And the worst losses are those that refresh old wounds—they bring the pain of other losses to the surface. These are very hard losses to bear."

The nurse can be most effective in helping the elderly person resolve grief about a major interpersonal loss by:

1. Assisting the person to accept the pain of the loss by validating that it is appropriate to feel pain over losses.
2. Encouraging the expression of sorrow and sense of loss by commenting on nonverbal communications, such as a shaky voice or teary eyes.
3. Facilitating the expression of hostility by viewing it as a sign of the older person's feeling of vulnerability.
4. Facilitating the expression of guilt. When the person says, "If only I had done . . .," it is helpful if the nurse restates this comment by saying, "I sense you blame yourself for . . .." Only if the person is able to acknowledge that he or she feels guilty can the reality of the situation be explored.
5. Assisting the older person to talk about the person who has died. Asking questions about how they met and the experiences they shared is most facilitative of helping the bereaved person to relive meaningful experiences.

The process of grieving over a major interpersonal loss may take as long as 2 years for elderly persons. Signs that individuals are beginning to resolve their grief in a healthy way include indications that they are beginning to see themselves as separate from the deceased person. The most common indicator of this differentiation is a movement away from talking about "we" to referring to "I." In addition, the healthy resolution of grief is evidenced by behaviors indicating adaptations to an environment that acknowledges the absence of the deceased person. For example, the widow who disposes of her husband's clothing to use his closet for storing her sewing materials has made a constructive environmental adaptation that acknowledges her husband's death. Finally, the person who is successfully resolving grief over a major loss is able to form new relationships that are mutually satisfying and rewarding.

BEHAVIOR DISTURBANCES OF ELDERLY PERSONS

As with younger individuals, elderly persons have widely varying needs and strengths. Most elderly persons are able to lead active, productive lives and continue to develop and learn during this developmental period. A person who has successfully completed earlier developmental tasks has a higher possibility of successfully completing the task of aging, and a helpful and supportive environment certainly contributes to its successful resolution. Nevertheless, difficulties sometimes arise.

Depression

Depression is a major health problem among the elderly, but often its symptoms are ignored or misdiagnosed. Some physiological symptoms of depression—constipation, slow movements, and insomnia—are erroneously expected as signs of aging so they tend to be ignored. Apathy and lack of interest in the environment, both characteristics of depression, often are stereotypically viewed as characteristic of the aging process. Finally, cognitive changes such as memory loss may lead to a diagnosis of dementia rather than depression.

The frequency of depression in elderly persons is growing. The severity and the number of depressions in aged persons have increased, and a close relationship exists between physical illness and depression. The nurse who helps older persons maintain and sustain an interest in controlling factors that keep them healthy, such as diet and exercise, helps to prevent depression.

Suicide prevention is an important aspect of nursing care when working with depressed elderly persons (see Chapter 16). Nurses must be aware that some elderly, physically ill persons are unwilling to see any alternative except death. Fears about of the process of dying, experiencing unremitting pain, being alone, and not being in control of their lives are frequently cited factors in the choice of suicide as means of coping. Common life-threatening behaviors of older people are refusal of medication, failure to follow the prescribed medical regimen, and refusal to eat or drink. Overt suicidal attempts by the elderly are more likely to be successful than in other age groups.

The current controversy about assisted suicide for persons who have a terminal illness, many of whom are elderly, raises many professional, ethical, and legal issues about which the nurse should become knowledgeable.

Developing a therapeutic relationship with depressed elderly persons will allow them to begin to express and explore feelings and reestablish a sense of self-worth. The individual must feel safe and secure, and the environment should convey empathy and concern. In addition to intervening therapeutically on an individual basis with the elderly depressed person, group activities are often very useful in helping to alleviate depression. Reminiscence groups, remotivation groups, and other quasisocial, task-oriented groups have been successfully used by nursing personnel in helping the depressed older person. Traditional individual and group psychotherapy, once reserved for younger adults, is now considered an appropriate and effective intervention for some elderly persons who are depressed.

Suspiciousness

Extreme **suspiciousness** or outright paranoia can be encountered in older persons, particularly in those who were not trusting in their earlier years. When this personality structure is compounded by the hearing and sight losses that accompany aging, the person is likely to misinterpret others and the environment and conclude that the world and the people in it are hostile. All persons experience instances in which they are the object of hostility or discrimination, but suspicious elderly persons overgeneralize these isolated events so that their view of the environment becomes consistent with their preconceived ideas of persecution. The necessity for change that accompanies relocation sets a fertile stage for the onset of a paranoid reaction in elderly persons.

CLINICAL EXAMPLE

Mrs. Daniels, a 75-year-old widow, had lived by herself in the inner-city apartment she shared with her husband until his death 5 years ago.

Mrs Daniels's daughters, who live in the suburbs, became increasingly concerned about their mother's safety in the inner city. They prevailed on her to move and finally, after 6 months, were able to convince her that she would be better off living in a newly constructed apartment complex for senior citizens in a better section of the city. Shortly after she moved, Mrs. Daniels began to suspect that people were stealing her belongings. She also began hearing voices that told her they were going to "get her" in retaliation for the way she had behaved when she was a child. Mrs. Daniels told her daughters about these experiences. The communtiy mental health nurse was called in to assess the situation.

Appropriate goals when working with older persons who are exhibiting unwarranted suspiciousness include reducing their anxiety level by establishing a relationship with them, helping them to restructure the environment to maximize their sense of control, and minimizing sight and hearing deficits by the use of prosthetic devices or by adapting the environment to accommodate the sensory loss. Throughout all these interventions, the nurse's consistent presence and availability are of inestimable value in helping the aged person give up feelings of suspiciousness.

Dementia

Dementia is an organic mental disorder characterized by impairments in short-term and long-term memory, abstract thinking, and judgment, accompanied by personality change. These impairments and personality change must significantly interfere with the individual's work, usual social activities, or relationships to warrant the medical diagnosis of dementia. Dementia may be reversible or progressive, depending on the specific organic cause. For example, brain tumors and hypothyroidism are the cause of some dementias. In these clients the mental symptoms are alleviated when the underlying cause is treated. Unfortunately, more than 50%

of individuals with dementia have Alzheimer's disease, which at this point cannot be prevented or cured. Therefore the dementia associated with this illness is irreversible and progressive.

Research indicates that the diagnosis of dementia is often misapplied to those with depression and dysfunctional adaptations to the normal process of aging interacting with the inordinate stressors experienced by elderly persons. Thus, it is essential that the assessment of elderly individuals manifesting the symptoms of dementia be multidimensional and include psychosocial and environmental factors as well as biophysiological aspects.

Individuals with dementia are in obvious need of intervention. Initially, nurses might attempt to orient the person by introducing themselves and proceeding in the least threatening manner to elicit only the information needed to help with the immediate problem. For instance, the nurse might say, "My name is Miss Jones. You seem afraid of something on the wall, Mrs. Smith. Would you tell me what is frightening you?" Hospitalization for any reason is a time of high risk for increased confusion and therefore an appropriate time for the nurse to begin preventive intervention. All persons need to know what is going to happen to them when they are hospitalized, but when a person with dementia is hospitalized, knowledge and support are critical to the prevention of confusion and to keeping the person accessible to intervention when confusion does occur. Demands placed on all elderly persons who are hospitalized should be kept to a minimum. This is particularly true for those with dementia. Young technologists need to learn that radiographs, blood tests, and other tests cannot be hurried because this creates a situation in which the client feels highly anxious, incompetent, and out of control.

All staff members should be aware of basic strategies of care. For example, individuals should be approached slowly to avoid startling them. They should be called by name at all times, and nurses should use their own names often.

Elderly persons who close their eyes often are not asleep. The nurse needs to get as near as possible to keep eye contact at the person's level. Touch contact should be initiated carefully and gently, perhaps by taking the individual's hand at first. If the client pulls away, attempts to establish touch contact should be made later.

All unnecessary stimuli should be closed out when the nurse is trying to engage the individual in conversation. If the person is frightened, someone should stay with the client. In this regard a family member could be very helpful if this person understands what is expected and receives some positive reinforcement.

Basic **reality orientation** is very helpful and should be part of the therapeutic relationship from the beginning. For instance, the nurse might say, "You are in the hospital for your broken hip, and in a few minutes we're going to help you sit in a chair where you can watch the *Today Show*." It is important to keep the routine in the hospital as near to the usual lifestyle as possible. The more the lifestyle is changed, the greater the risk of confusion. Medications, especially those for control and sedation, should be used with caution. It is not unusual for the physician to order the initial dose at one-third the usual adult dose. Even though the amount of medication given may be small, it is imperative that the nurse systematically and frequently monitor the client's response to these medications.

Whatever the person is able to do alone should be encouraged and help given only to ensure success with the task. Food should be placed so that the person can see it and smell it. The elderly person with dementia often needs to be told what the food is. If the client is not eating well, high-calorie drinks offered frequently help to maintain nutrition. The nurse should encourage the family to help with nutritional problems because they may know and be able to supply some favorite foods.

Family members may be very helpful if they are taught how to deal with the individual with dementia. For example, the family should be made aware that is it not helpful to withhold information from the person. Sometimes family members and staff members think they are sparing the client's feelings. In reality, the person almost always knows that something is amiss but does not know how to deal with mixed* communication and thus becomes confused, often acting bewildered. When the dementia is advanced, individuals need to know what day it is, where and when the meals are served, where the bathroom is, and what time of day it is, morning, afternoon, or evening.

It is inspiring to see a nurse model creative care of an elderly person with dementia. Often, nurses must use their whole being to explore the meaning of the client's behavior and to respond in a way that is helpful and dignified to the person. Modeling excellence in terms of caring for aged persons with dementia is the best way to teach staff and families.

Alzheimer's disease

Alzheimer's disease is a degenerative brain disease, causing a dementia that is progressive and irreversible. This illness accounts for more than 50% of all persons with dementia and represents the fourth leading cause of death among elderly persons. It is estimated that by the year 2030, more than 2 million persons will be afflicted with this disease.

Alzheimer's disease most often occurs after age 65 but may occur as early as age 40. Its course from onset to death ranges from 2 to 20 years, with the usual course being 5 years. Previously, it was referred to as presenile dementia when it occurred in individuals under age 65 and as senile dementia in those 65 and older. These terms and the age distinctions they imply are no longer used.

When it was known as senile dementia, the dementia associated with Alzheimer's disease was thought to be an inevitable consequence of the aging process that resulted from impaired blood circulation to the brain. Today it is known that such is not the case. Although the cause of Alzheimer's disease is not known, biopsy of brain tissue reveals characteristic neurofibrillary tangles and neuritic plaques, both of which contain abnormal proteins. Study of the molecular biology of Alzheimer's disease has identified the precursor to these abnormal proteins, the amyloid precursor protein, which is believed to cause neuronal death. The characteristically reduced levels of the neurotransmitter acetylcholine found in the brains of persons with Alzheimer's disease are likely to result from this loss of neurons. Other biochemical research points to the possibility of a virus or environmental toxins as necessary but not sufficient factors to cause Alzheimer's disease.

It is known that genetics play a role in transmission of Alzheimer's disease. From 10% to 30% of all persons with Alzheimer's disease develop the illness at a relatively early age. These persons come from families in whom it has been demonstrated that 50% of the children or siblings of the person also develop the disease. Furthermore, almost all persons with Down syndrome are likely to develop Alzheimer's disease if they live past age 40. It is well documented that Down syndrome is a genetic disorder involving an extra copy of chromosome 21. The gene for the amyloid precursor protein has also been located on chromosome 21. Therefore, much current research on Alzheimer's disease involves attempting to discover a possible connection between Alzheimer's disease and chromosome 21, although to date a gene that could be responsible for Alzheimer's disease has not been identified. Currently, both the public and the private sectors in the United States are committed to uncovering the cause of Alzheimer's disease through research.

Characteristics of the individual with Alzheimer's disease

Alzheimer's disease is devastating for the person and family alike. Its onset is insidious, and a uniformly progressive deterioration follows.

Early signs include loss of memory, difficulty with language, poor attention span, and personality changes. Later, poor judgment, confusion, agitation, incontinence, and severe personality changes are evident. Finally, the individual is no longer able to walk or to control elemental functions and gradually sinks into coma and death.

The motor behavior of an individual with Alzheimer's disease is always affected. In the early stages of the illness, the person is likely to have activity intolerance because of reduced energy. **Psychomotor agitation** typically occurs as the illness progresses, and in later stages, gait is impaired because of increased neurological involvement. Ultimately the person becomes bedridden.

Self-care is greatly altered. Initially, individuals may not care for themselves because of their memory deficit. For example, they may forget to brush their teeth or eat lunch, although they are still capable of engaging in both these activities. Later in the course of the illness, the individual not only may forget to carry out activities of daily living, but also may be unable to do so when reminded.

For reasons that are not known, sleep patterns are affected by Alzheimer's disease. It is not unusual for the individual with this illness to awaken during the night and roam about the house, not realizing it is still nighttime. Even more potentially dangerous is the likelihood that the person will go outdoors and wander away, perhaps inadequately dressed for the weather.

Since Alzheimer's disease stems from a progressive brain degeneration, the cognitive processes of decision making, judgment, knowledge, learning, memory, and thought processes all are greatly affected. In fact, alterations in cognitive processes are the first sign of the illness, particularly alterations in memory. In the early stage of the illness, the individual and those close to him or her are aware of the loss of memory, particularly for short-term events. Many persons try to adapt to this memory loss by writing innumerable notes to themselves, the location of which they may also forget.

Understandably, individuals with Alzheimer's disease are unable to care for their home in a purposeful, sustained manner. Furthermore, their environment may indirectly pose many threats to their safety. For example, they may set their house on fire because they forgot to turn off the gas burner, which ignited a nearby pot-holder.

In the early stage of the illness, individuals are aware of their deterioration and are likely to experience a severe depression. Anger also is often expressed because of frustration at not being able to remember the names of people or to identify common objects. Mood swings are common in the later stages of the disease.

Interpersonal processes are always affected. Families of the affected individual must witness the deterioration of their loved one, who gradually does not recognize them and who eventually behaves as a total stranger. Unfortunately, the frustration experienced by family members sometimes leads to their verbally and even physically abusing the individual with Alzheimer's disease. Any abuse often goes unreported because the individual is fearful of doing so or does not remember its occurrence.

Because of their memory deficit, persons with Alzheimer's disease often confabulate. **Confabulation** is the unconscious "filling in" of memory gaps by imaginary and often complex experiences, which are recounted in a detailed and plausible way as though they were factual.

Since the individual and family are aware of the progressive deterioration, social isolation and withdrawal often occur early in the illness as a means of protecting everyone from embarrassment. Unfortunately, early social isolation seems to enhance mental deterioration.

The individual with Alzheimer's disease has great difficulty concentrating on any one thing and therefore is easily distracted. Until memory and awareness completely fail, the person must struggle with the feelings associated with diminished self-esteem. Unfortunately, this is often a losing battle, since others, friends and strangers alike, are likely to treat the individual in a condescending, derisive manner.

For the length of time individuals remain aware of their deterioration, they experience profound helplessness, hopelessness, and powerlessness. These feelings form the bašis for depression and low self-esteem. Individuals who have had a well-defined spiritual life in earlier years also often express spiritual despair and distress.

In the final stages of the illness, all physiological processes are altered. Incontinence, abnormal reflexes, and seizures are common terminal symptoms. Throughout the entire course of their illness, individuals with Alzheimer's disease are unusually subject to infection and injury, probably secondary to other factors such as poor hygiene and nutrition and memory loss.

Guidelines for meeting the needs of the individual with Alzheimer's disease

Clients with Alzeimer's disease need to be encouraged and helped to perform as many activities of daily living as they can. The longer they can feed, bathe, and dress themselves, the more the deterioration can be slowed. Since assisting and reminding the client require much time and patience, nurses often find it easier and quicker to do these tasks for the client. This practice is deleterious to the client's well-being and should be avoided if at all possible.

Interventions for sleeplessness include warm baths, soft music, warm milk, light exercise, and a small amount of wine. When the individual is agitated, it is important to be aware of safety factors. At times, small doses of antipsychotic agents are used for acutely disturbed states and extreme restlessness. Care must be taken in the administration of these medications because of the prolongation of drug elimination in elderly persons.

The nurse can help delay cognitive deterioration through communication techniques and sensory stimulation. The therapeutic relationship can provide a forum for the discussion of feelings, opinions, and the facilitation of daily life decisions. In the early stages of the disease, both individual and group techniques can be used. Group discussions can focus on stimulating topics and encourage active participation. Creative therapies are useful, including art, creative writing, and poetry. Later in the disease process, more individual approaches are indicated.

Encouraging life review is a frequently employed therapeutic tool. By assisting the individual to reminisce, long-term memory is stimulated, and the opportunity to resolve earlier life crises is made available.

Memory impairment can be impeded through the use of environmental aids and clues. One family used signs to remind their relative of routine tasks and safety factors. Simple lists may also be of assistance in the early phase. Precautions can be taken to ensure environmental safety, such as installing gates, rearranging furniture, and removing dangerous objects.

The client with symptoms of the later stages of Alzheimer's disease is assisted by many of the interventions discussed earlier in this chapter. Clear and consistent communication is employed. The individual is approached calmly and always addressed by name. Basic reality orientation is helpful.

In the course of the disease process, the client may become quite agitated and combative. The nurse must be prepared to intervene and to accept these behaviors nonjudgmentally. The nurse must continue to afford the individual the respect and dignity that she or he would show to any client.

The families of persons with Alzheimer's disease are in desperate need of assistance and support. Efforts should be made to maximize their strengths, allow for the expression of feelings, provide education, and mobilize social supports. The nurse can help the family to prepare for the time when the institutionalization of their loved one may be necessary. The Alzheimer's Disease and Related Disorders Association (ADRDA) is an organization with more than 100 chapters in the United States that has much to offer persons with Alzheimer's disease and their families. These services include hot lines, self-help groups, and respite care programs. The nurse can educate the family about this organization and other local services.

The nurse caring for the client with Alzheimer's disease must be aware that the disease is progressive and irreversible. Individuals will eventually become bedridden and helpless, and it will be necessary to meet their most basic needs.

NURSING CARE PLAN: *An Individual with Alzheimer's Disease*

CASE FORMULATION

Mr. Chall is a prominent 65-year-old attorney who was admitted to the hospital for a diagnostic workup. He had been experiencing memory loss, which had seriously affected his professional performance until he had felt forced to take a leave of absence. He admitted that he had been attempting to disguise these problems for some time but lately had been finding these attempts more and more difficult. He described finding himself standing in the middle of a room at home having no idea why he was there or how he got there.

In addition, Mr. Chall was finding it more and more difficult to conduct conversations

Continued.

NURSING CARE PLAN: *An Individual with Alzheimer's Disease—cont'd*

and found himself practicing and rehearsing. He described having to think carefully about every word he said. He reported feeling depressed and wishing to withdraw from social interactions.

Although Mr. Chall was known for his pleasant personality, his wife reported recent disturbing changes. He had begun losing his temper at his wife and daughters at the slightest provocation. The family felt that they had to "walk on eggs" when he was nearby.

Mr. Chall had always been most meticulous about his personal hygiene and grooming. Recently, however, he had begun to find routine tasks more difficult. His wife noted that his grooming was often poor. At times he dressed in the same suit for several days in a row, and his shirts and ties were spotted with food stains. Such behavior was highly unusual for such a meticulous man.

Both Mr. Chall and his family were extremely concerned. After a thorough assessment and diagnostic workup, he and his family were informed that he had Alzheimer's disease. On hearing the diagnosis, Mr. Chall became deeply disturbed and manifested further evidence of withdrawal behaviors. The family was devastated and turned to the staff for support and assistance.

Nursing Assessment

Mr. Chall appeared to be experiencing many of the behaviors manifested by individuals in the early stages of Alzheimer's disease. Fading memory was evident, as were attempts to mask this symptom. Mr. Chall was experiencing difficulties with language and

some trouble with the performance of the routine tasks of daily living. These symptoms were impairing his work and social life.

Personality changes were among Mr. Chall's predominant symptoms. Abrupt temper tantrums were noted by the family members, despite a previously pleasant personality. Mr. Chall reported feelings of depression and a desire to withdraw from social interactions.

As a result of Mr. Chall's behaviors, the family was experiencing a very difficult time. Both Mr. Chall and his family were further devastated when the diagnosis of Alzheimer's disease was learned.

Nursing Diagnosis

The assessment data, including present behavior, past life experiences, and an understanding of the underlying physiology, led to the development of the following nursing diagnoses for Mr. Chall:

Altered thought processes related to memory impairment and cognitive deterioration

Impaired verbal communication related to organic brain disease

Self-care deficit, bathing/hygiene related to cognitive deterioration

Ineffective individual coping related to awareness of cognitive deterioration and diminished sense of self-worth

Altered family processes related to impairment of family member

Planning and Implementing Nursing Care

The plan of nursing care for Mr. Chall is

NURSING CARE PLAN: *An Individual with Alzheimer's Disease—cont'd*

summarized on pp. 428 and 429. Interventions were based on the present behaviors. However, the progressive nature of this disorder was kept in mind and appropriate revisions were made as changes in Mr. Chall's status occurred. It was decided that Mr. Chall would remain in the hospital for 1 week, allowing time for the family to prepare to offer the needed support and assistance. Long-term plans were postponed for the present, although the potential inevitability of placement in a long-term care facility was recognized.

A therapeutic relationship was established by Mr. Chall's primary nurse, who treated him with respect and dignity and approached him in a clear, consistent manner on a regular basis. Mr. Chall was encouraged to communicate his feelings and his interests to the nurse, who listened in a caring, supportive, and interested manner. Mr. Chall was encouraged to review his life's achievements and memories, as well as to discuss his present-day concerns and ideas. Participation in a discussion group was encouraged, where stimulating topics were explored. In addition, Mr. Chall was encouraged to participate in creative therapies, such as art and creative writing.

The nurse assisted Mr. Chall to develop memory aids to help him to recall daily tasks and routines. He developed lists and reminders to help him structure his daily activities.

A daily routine was planned to assist Mr. Chall with bathing and hygiene. Clothes were laid out the night before, with the assistance of the nurse when necessary.

Finally, the nurse directed some of her energy toward the needs of the family, who felt devastated as a result of Mr. Chall's deterioration and poor prognosis. Education was provided, along with support and assistance with crisis resolution. The family was referred to the local chapter of ADRDA, an organization that could provide much support and assistance in planning for the future.

Evaluation

Evaluation of the plan of nursing care and its implementation was based on the outcome criteria developed.

Mr. Chall showed some improvement while in the inpatient setting. He reported that he felt less depressed, although he continued to feel embarrassed and fearful of social interactions. However, he was able to discuss the feelings related to the loss of his health and continued his efforts to communicate with others. Mr. Chall found the memory aids extremely helpful as reminders for the tasks of the day and felt more control over his actions as a result. He continued to experience changes in mood, including mild temper tantrums.

The family became involved in the local chapter of ADRDA and reported that they were receiving much assistance from this organization. Although unable to make long-term plans, they received many helpful suggestions about how to best provide for Mr. Chall's needs when he returned home. The nursing staff believed that the family continued to experience denial related to Mr. Chall's prognosis but that with the support

Continued.

NURSING CARE PLAN: *An Individual with Alzheimer's Disease—cont'd*

of the services they had engaged, they would eventually come to terms with the inevitability of Mr. Chall's deterioration and death. At the time of Mr. Chall's discharge, the family appeared able to receive him warmly into the home for the present. They were advised to use the recommended support services as they took on the physical and emotional task of caring for their loved one.

NURSING CARE PLAN FOR MR. CHALL

Nursing diagnosis	Objective (rationale)	Nursing interventions	Outcome criteria
Altered thought processes related to memory impairment and cognitive deterioration	Client will maintain environmental contact and interaction. (Continuing environmental contact and interaction may impede cognitive deterioration.)	Establish therapeutic relationship with client. Interact with client in clear, consistent manner. Assist with development of memory aids (signs, lists). Provide reality orientation and sensory stimulation. Ensure client safety.	Within 1 week, client: Lists routine daily tasks. Develops appropriate memory aids.
Impaired verbal communication related to organic brain disease	Client will maintain communication with others. (Communication with others helps maintain relationships, facilitates life review, and may impede cognitive deterioration.)	Accept and respect client's attempts to communicate. Encourage discussion of life review and present-day events. Encourage participation in group discussion. Facilitate family discussions and interactions.	Within 1 week, client: Spontaneously discusses daily events with nurse. Actively participates in group discussions.
Self-care deficit, bathing/hygiene related to cognitive deterioration	Client will perform tasks of bathing and dressing. (Self-care increases self-esteem and may impede cognitive deterioration.)	Establish and implement bathing and dressing routine. Encourage client to perform own hygiene as able. Assist with dressing as necessary.	Within 1 week, client: Follows the established bathing and dressing routine. Accepts assistance as needed.

NURSING CARE PLAN FOR MR. CHALL—cont'd

Nursing diagnosis	Objective (rationale)	Nursing interventions	Outcome criteria
Ineffective individual coping related to awareness of cognitive deterioration and diminished sense of self-worth	Client will verbally express his feelings and problems. (Verbal expression of feelings and problems allows for reality testing and reassurance and may prevent depression.)	Meet regularly to allow client opportunity for ventilation. Convey empathy and support. Use reflective listening techniques to facilitate conversation. Sit in silence and offer acceptance if the client does not wish to talk.	Within 1 week, client spontaneously discusses feelings and recent losses with nurse.
Altered family processes related to impairment of family member	Family will cope with present crisis and prepare for and accept prognosis. (Alzheimer's disease can precipitate a family crisis, which can be addressed through education, support, and problem solving.)	Meet with family members three times weekly. Offer education and refer to local support services. Offer support and encourage expression of feelings. Facilitate problem solving.	Within 1 week, family discusses present and future plans for care of Mr. Chall.

KEY POINTS

1. Elderly persons have as many individual differences as persons in earlier stages of life. In addition, elderly individuals in our society have commonalities of experience.

2. Social factors that impair the ability of elderly persons to achieve ego integrity successfully include poverty, social mobility, and social change.

3. Life review is a nearly universal occurrence in older persons as they face the prospect of impending death.

4. Nurses need to be aware of their own feelings of loneliness that may be triggered by the loneliness they sense in the older person.

5. The need to grieve over losses may not be seen as necessary by the older person and may be avoided because of the pain associated with this process.

6. In addition to the nurse's intervening on an individual basis with the elderly depressed person, group activities are also very useful in helping to alleviate depression.

7. The nurse's consistent presence and availability are of great value in helping the aged person give up feelings of suspiciousness.

8. Dementia is an organic mental disorder characterized by impairments in short-term and long-term memory, abstract thinking, and judgment accompanied by personality change.

9. When a person with dementia is hospitalized, knowledge of how to intervene therapeutically is critical to the prevention of confusion and to keeping the person accessible to intervention when confusion occurs.

10. Alzheimer's disease is an irreversible progressive and degenerative dementia that accounts for more than 50% of all the dementias of old age.

11. The primary cause of Alzheimer's disease is not known, although biochemical and genetic factors

have been identified as contributing to the disease.

12. Individuals with Alzheimer's disease characteristically display an intolerance for activity; self-care deficits; altered sleep patterns; memory loss; depression, anger, and mood swings; progressive deterioration, leading to social isolation and withdrawal; and ultimate alteration of all physiological processes.

13. Appropriate nursing interventions for persons with Alzheimer's disease address the cognitive deterioration and include communication techniques and sensory and environmental stimulation. The family must be offered the support and education needed to care for their loved one, to develop future plans, and to work through the grieving process.

SUGGESTED SOURCES OF ADDITIONAL INFORMATION

Abraham IL and others: Therapeutic group work with depressed elderly, *Nurs Clin North Am* 26:635, September 1991.

Batt LJ: Managing delirium: implications for geropsychiatric nurses, *J Psychosoc Nurs Ment Health Serv* 27:22, May 1989.

Beadleson-Baird M, Lara LL: Reminiscing: nursing actions for the acutely ill geriatric patient, *Issues Ment Health Nurs* 9(1):83, 1988.

Chesla CA: Parent's illness models of schizophrenia, *Arch Psychiatr Nurs* 3:218, August 1989.

Clary C, Dever A, Schweizer E: Psychiatric inpatients' knowledge of medication at hospital discharge, *Hosp Community Psychiatry* 43:140, February 1992.

Farran CJ, Keane-Hagerty E: Communicating effectively with dementia patients, *J Psychosoc Nurs Ment Health Serv* 27:13, May 1989.

Feil N: Validation therapy . . . with late onset demented populations, *Geriatr Nurs* 13:129, May/June 1992.

Fishman S: Relationships among an older adult's life review, ego integrity, and death anxiety, *Int Psychogeriatr* 4(suppl 2), 1992.

Fishman SK: Health professionals' attitudes toward older people, *Dent Clin North Am* 33:7, January 1989.

Given CW, Collins CE, Given BA: Sources of stress among families caring for relatives with Alzheimer's disease, *Nurs Clin North Am* 23:69, March 1988.

Haldeman K, Gafner G: Are elderly alcoholics discriminated against? *J Psychosoc Nurs Ment Health Serv* 28:6, May 1990.

Hall GR: Care of the patient with Alzheimer's disease living at home, *Nurs Clin North Am* 23:31, March 1988.

Hall GR, Buckwalter KC: From almshouse to dedicated unit: care of institutionalized elderly with behavioral problems, *Arch Psychiatr Nurs* 4:3, February 1990.

Harvis KA, Rabins PV: Dementia: helping family caregivers cope, *J Psychosoc Nurs Ment Health Serv* 27:6, May 1989.

Hong CS: Doubly disadvantaged... people with a mental handicap in need of reality orientation, *Nurs Times* 85:69, August 1989.

Kolcaba K, Miller CA: Geropharmacology treatment: behavioral problems extend nursing responsibility, *J Gerontol Nurs* 15:29, May 1989.

Kozlak J, Thobaben M: Treating the mentally ill at home, *Perspect Psychiatr Care* 28:31, April-June 1992.

Kurlowicz LH: Social factors and depression in late life, *Arch Psychiatr Nurs* 7:30, February 1993.

Lindblom L and others: Chemical abuse: an intervention program for the elderly, *J Gerontol Nurs* 18:6, April 1992.

Maas M: Management of patients with Alzheimer's disease in long-term care facilities, *Nurs Clin North Am* 23:57, March 1988.

Marion TR, Stefanik-Campisi C: The elderly alcoholic: identification of factors that influence the giving and receiving of help, *Perspect Psychiatr Care* 25:32, March/April 1989.

Masters JC, O'Grady M: Normal pressure hydrocephalus: a potentially reversible form of dementia, *J Psychosoc Nurs Ment Health Serv* 30:25, June 1992.

Mayers K, Griffin M: The play project: use of stimulus objects with demented patients, *J Gerontol Nurs* 16:32 January 1990.

Morency CR: Mental status change in the elderly: recognizing and treating delirium, *J Prof Nurs* 6:356, November/December 1990.

Roberts BL and Algase DL: Victims of Alzheimer's disease and the environment, *Nurs Clin North Am* 23:83, March 1988.

Scharnhorst S: AIDS dementia complex in the elderly: diagnosis and management, *Nurs Pract* 17:37, August 1992.

Skinner PV, Jordan D: Home management of the patient with Alzheimer's disease, *Home Health Care Nurs* 7:23, January/February 1989.

Stevens GL, Baldwin BA: Optimizing mental health in the nursing home setting, *J Psychosoc Nurs Mental Health Serv* 26:27, October 1988.

Tillman-Jones TK: How to work with elderly patients on a general psychiatric unit, *J Psychosoc Nurs Ment Health Serv* 28:27, May 1990.

Travis SS, Moore SR: Nursing and medical care of primary dementia patients in a community hospital setting, *Appl Nurs Res* 4:14, February 1991.

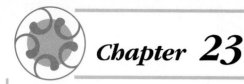

Chapter 23

Populations at Risk

persons with a physical illness

LEARNING OBJECTIVES

After studying this chapter, the student will be able to:

- State general guidelines for meeting the emotional needs of persons who have a physical illness.

- Describe common emotional reactions precipitated by the use of mechanical devices in treating persons with a physical illness.

- Describe common emotional reactions precipitated by organ transplants.

- Describe common emotional reactions precipitated by the loss of a body part.

- Describe common emotional reactions precipitated by cardiac surgery.

- Describe common emotional reactions precipitated by an untoward obstetrical experience.

- Describe common emotional reactions precipitated by an abortion.

- Describe common emotional reactions of individuals with acquired immunodeficiency syndrome (AIDS).

- Discuss the emotional aspects of death and dying as described by Kübler-Ross.

- Develop a hypothetical plan of nursing care for an individual who is dying.

KEY TERMS

Psychiatric liaison nurse

Body image

AIDS

Thanatology

Denial

Anger

Bargaining

Depression

Acceptance

Many individuals who have a physical illness are in a state of crisis precipitated by the nature of their illness, its treatment, or both. Consequently, nursing has a tremendous opportunity to promote the mental health of many persons if nursing will reclaim its heritage of meeting the emotional needs of persons with a physical illness. Unfortunately, all too often the emotional needs of these individuals are given little attention, and student nurses frequently look to their psychiatric nursing experience to provide them with direction in giving more comprehensive care to individuals who have a physical illness. Therefore this chapter is devoted to helping the nurse develop an understanding of some common emotional needs of the individual with a physical illness, although no situation in this chapter can be discussed in depth.

HISTORICAL PERSPECTIVE

Before the current advances in the medical and nursing sciences, nurses could do little to assist individuals who had a physical illness other than helping them meet their most basic physical needs. However, the time-honored nursing actions of bathing and feeding clients certainly must have met many of their emotional needs as well.

As medical science developed, physicians delegated to nurses procedures they no longer had time to perform. An example of such a procedure is the assessment of vital signs. Some nurse authors believe that as an occupation, nursing eagerly embraced these delegated technical procedures in an attempt to gain higher status by mimicking physicians. Whether this interpretation is true or not, current nursing care of persons with a physical illness is characterized by the execution of an increasing number of highly technical procedures, often to the neglect of attempts to meet the person's emotional needs. It is not unusual for a client to report that the most understanding person encountered while in the hospital was an aide or housekeeper.

Growing dissatisfaction with nursing care has been the subject of numerous studies. These studies indicate that only a few complaints are related to physical care. Most dissatisfaction relates to the failure of professional nurses to establish satisfying interpersonal relationships with individuals receiving their services. The nurse is frequently said to lack warmth, to fail to give individuals a feeling of being important, to fail to listen empathically to the concerns of individuals being cared for, or to fail to ask enough questions to gather the necessary data to make wise decisions about the individual's needs.

The use of the **psychiatric liaison nurse,** a relatively recent resource, can immeasurably enhance achieving the goal of meeting the emotional needs of clients with a physical illness. The subspecialty of psychiatric liaison nursing was developed in the 1970s and requires preparation at the master's degree level. Psychiatric liaison nurses have particular expertise in developing nursing interventions based on their assessment of the responses of physically ill individuals who have emotional responses seen as problematic by the nurses who care for them. Therefore, many activities of the liaison nurse focus on consultation with the nursing staff and working with the client's family and significant others, as well as working with the client.

GUIDELINES FOR MEETING THE EMOTIONAL NEEDS OF PERSONS WHO HAVE A PHYSICAL ILLNESS

Individuals who have a physical illness experience a variety of feelings, which may include intense anxiety, hostility, depression, elation, fear, anger, and sorrow. These are the same feelings that may be expressed by persons who have a mental illness. Perhaps one of the few differentiations that can be made between the reactions of these two groups is the presumed ability of individuals with a physical illness to maintain conscious control of their behavior and to use better judgment than individuals who have a mental illness. However, even these expected differences are not always observed.

It is often difficult and more challenging to recognize and cope with the emotional needs of persons with a physical illness than it is to address effectively the emotional needs of persons who have a mental illness. Because part of the problem of persons with a mental illness is their lack of emotional control, they sometimes express needs openly and directly. These individuals' needs may be difficult to understand, but their existence is obvious. Because they are said to have a mental illness, the nurse realizes that part of the task is to help them cope with their emotional problems. In contrast, individuals with a physical illness usually attempt to control their feelings and to solve their own problems, and nurses frequently expect them to do so. Nurses sometimes fail to recognize that in addition to these clients' need for physical care, persons who have a physical illness need the same acceptance, understanding, and concern as those who have a mental illness.

Good physical care is always the first place to start in meeting the emotional needs of persons who have a physical illness. The nurse can demonstrate a caring attitude about the individual by an unhurried approach; by attentive, perceptive listening; and by anticipation of physical needs. It is also important that the nurse not respond to the client's anger with an angry response. Nurses will not be tempted to respond angrily if they understand the frustration and fear that are the bases for the client's outburst. Likewise, nurses must not attempt to minimize the client's concerns by using hollow phrases such as, "Tomorrow will be a better day."

The very occurrence of a physical illness serious enough to warrant hospitalization interrupts the normal lifestyle of the individual and family. As a result, some degree of stress is produced, to which the individual and family may or may not be able to adapt successfully. In addition, any physical illness for which hospitalization is necessary forces the individual to assume a dependent role that may be disturbing. Although society's view of masculinity and femininity is becoming less stereotyped, a dependent role is still seen as particularly problematic for men, who are often expected to portray an image of strength and independence and who may see physical illness as an expression of weakness. Inability to accept the forced dependency required in many hospitals is one reason for the uncooperative behavior of some individuals.

The modern hospital is a highly organized creation of a mechanized world. Regardless of the nature of the illness that brings individuals to the hospital, they are expected to submit to a variety of procedures without always understanding what these tests are or why they are being done. Clients often believe such procedures are being performed without their consent or without their having been given any explanation. Many procedures that seem commonplace to health professionals, such as enemas, catheterizations, and intravenous infusions, may be viewed by clients as intrusions into their bodies. Not only may individuals have no understanding of the reasons for the procedure, but they may also believe that they have lost control over their bodies. At the same time, clients frequently are covertly given the message that they should be thankful for these procedures. This conflict may result in an increase in their anxiety level, which, paradoxically, decreases the effectiveness of the procedure itself. Therefore, it is imperative for their physical and emotional well-being that the nurse provide clients with an opportunity to explore their feelings about the procedure and give them an appropriate explanation of its nature.

Although clients may have signed an operative permit, they are not likely to realize that this may cover a variety of tests and procedures before the actual surgery is performed. The physician may have explained the preoperative tests, but the anxiety level of many individuals is so high that they are unable to comprehend what the physician is saying. Even when individuals are able to concentrate on the physician's words, they do not always understand the full meaning of them, and the preoperative procedures may still come as a shocking surprise. It is not difficult to understand that newly admitted surgical clients may be frightened and think they have lost their identities. Such a situation could be eased if nurses understood the importance of giving reassurance, if they could identify the basis for any anxiety, and if they were skillful in giving emotional support. Sometimes reassurance requires only a few minutes of time spent listening, answering questions, and recognizing that the individual is a unique human being reaching out for understanding and help.

Sometimes the results of hospital procedures, especially surgical procedures, precipitate an emotional crisis. Such a crisis is overwhelming for a person who has already developed the feeling of being lost, forgotten, and reduced to a childlike state of dependence in the hospital. These feelings may actually impede recovery and may cause an extremely traumatizing experience.

Self-help groups

The nurse should make an effort to become aware of the increasing number of community-based organizations designed to provide information and support to individuals and their families who have experienced certain medical or surgical procedures or the death of a family member. For example, there are ostomy clubs throughout the United States whose members are people who have had ileostomies or colostomies and who meet regularly to discuss the ways in which they have solved the problems they encounter. In some parts of the United States, similar groups are available for persons who have undergone mastectomies, laryngectomies, abortions, or myocardial infarcts. By being aware of the availability of these organizations in the community, the nurse will be able to inform others of them. Although these clubs are not designed to substitute for medical supervi-

sion, the value of the support and understanding that can be gained from persons who have had similar experiences is inestimable in helping individuals and families to regain or attain a state of positive mental health.

Emotional reactions precipitated by use of mechanical devices

Advances in biomedical science have provided several life-sustaining devices that make it possible to prolong the lives of many individuals who otherwise would be doomed to death. One of the most frequently used is the hemodialysis machine.

The hemodialysis machine may produce a profound emotional response. Individuals who must rely on such a machine recognize how dependent they are on the device for life itself. They also become aware that their activities are circumscribed by the need to be attached to the machine for 8 to 10 hours, two or three times each week. This schedule interferes with work, ability to make a living, social life, and family life.

Individuals who must rely on mechanical devices often believe that they have lost control of their bodies and of their destinies. This may lead to a loss of confidence and self-esteem. Such losses result in behavior that requires emotional support and understanding.

Dependency on a mechanical device to sustain life creates anxiety in almost all individuals. It causes many to feel dehumanized and to be concerned about the maintenance of their personal autonomy. In addition, the individual may be resentful and angry or may be depressed and respond by being tearful, uninterested in surroundings, and uncommunicative. On the other hand, the individual may express anger and frustration at the situation by speaking sharply to nurses or family members. Such clients may express fear by demanding constant attention and that the nurse remain with them at all times. They may express disturbed emotional feelings by being critical of the hospital or clinic where they must go for the dialysis. They may fear that the

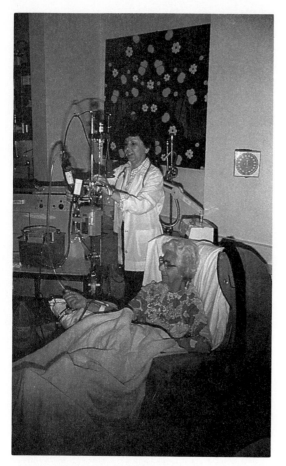

Figure 23-1

Hemodialysis delivery system

From Lewis SM, Collier IC: *Medical-surgical nursing: assessment and management of clinical problems,* ed 3, St Louis, 1993, Mosby–Year Book.

device will fail to function properly and thus end their life abruptly.

Because the hemodialysis machine must be attached to the individual so often, a permanent arteriovenous shunt is implanted in an arm or leg to provide access to an artery or vein. Individuals with these shunts have been known to tear them out, losing much blood. This action is usually considered a suicidal gesture; the rate of suicide among individuals who resent their dependence on hemodialysis machines is high.

Family members have been taught to operate portable dialysis machines and thus free the individual from constantly returning to a hospital or clinic to have the blood cleansed. However, this practice makes it necessary to teach a family member to operate the machine and requires that this person be available when the treatments are scheduled. This amount of dependence on another person is also cause for hostility and resentment among some individuals and has not provided the solution to the time-consuming dialysis procedure as originally intended.

In summary, the currently available life-saving biomedical devices are capable of improving the individual's physical health but do not always improve emotional health. Specifically, clients who must rely on hemodialysis machines are chronic worriers. They worry about all the daily problems of living that confront everyone. They require nurses who are skilled in understanding that their behavior is sometimes an expression of anger, fear, and depression brought on by their resentment of being dependent for life on a mechanical device and being unable to control the situation. They require much reassurance and emotional support.

Emotional reactions precipitated by organ transplants

Organ transplants are viewed by medical scientists as providing a viable alternative for individuals with seriously damaged organs, especially hearts and kidneys. As increasingly effective drugs are developed to combat the problem of tissue rejection, the number and type of organ transplants increase.

Almost from the initiation of organ transplant surgery, it was recognized that providing an organ for an individual from the body of another could be an emotionally disturbing experience for both the person donating the organ and the recipient. Thus, psychiatric evaluation of the donor and recipient was begun soon after some of the earliest kidney transplants were performed. Since there were more individuals awaiting transplant surgery than appropriate organs available, it was possible to choose the organ recipients carefully. Those who were thought to be able to accept an organ from another individual without being emotionally disturbed were chosen. Likewise, donors were stable individuals before agreeing to supply an organ for another. One mother who donated a kidney to a son was heard to shout at him, "What do you expect from me? Wasn't it enough that I gave you life? Do you also demand a part of my body?"

Organ transplant procedures are long, involved surgical techniques. Individuals who are the focus of such procedures are aware of their physical condition and that they have a serious illness. They realize that without a transplant, their lives would end within a short time and that the only hope for the future lies in the replacement of the damaged organ. Thus, they are willing to undergo the procedure, even though they recognize the seriousness of the situation and the possibility that the organ may be rejected. These individuals are understandably fearful of what the future will bring. Although many recipients of such surgery have been able to cope successfully with their anxieties and fears, some have responded with full-blown psychiatric reactions. Few situations exist in which an individual is placed under so much stress as when undergoing an organ transplant. Nurses working with these individuals need to be sensitive to their emotional responses, to be realistically reassuring, and to provide as much emotional support as they require. The individual should be encouraged to discuss concerns and fears about death, dependency on others, and loss of self-esteem.

That an individual who was close to death would grieve over the loss of a useless body part comes as a surprise to many nurses. Nevertheless, this often occurs, and to be helpful, the nurse must assist the individual with the grieving process. In general, the nurse needs to express concern for the individual and interest in his or her future welfare.

Emotional reactions precipitated by loss of a body part

Every person has a mental image of his or her own body that is called the **body image.** This body image may be realistic, or it may be part of individuals' wish-fulfilling fantasy about themselves. To a large extent, an individual functions within the boundaries of this unconscious image. A young man once said in a hopeless voice, "I can never marry. What woman would want a man with one short leg?" This man's body image was so misshapen and ugly that he was scornful of it. Because he could not accept his own body, he was convinced that no one else could. He was especially convinced that no woman could want him as a marriage partner. Although he was reasonably attractive, his reaction to all aspects of life was in keeping with this attitude of being worthless and of having an unacceptable body.

Some people maintain an unrealistic image of themselves that was realistic at an earlier period in their lives. For example, one may hear a large, matronly woman ask a saleswoman for a size 12 dress. Without making a comment, the understanding clerk brings out the required large size and helps the customer try on the garment.

Surgical removal of a breast or the uterus is among the most emotionally disturbing surgical procedures that women must face. It is unfortunate that many nurses have not been helped to understand the meaning these experiences have for some women and have not been assisted in helping with the feelings precipitated by such surgical procedures.

Although people respond in highly individual, unique ways to the same surgical procedures, almost all women unconsciously believe that they have been mutilated by a breast amputation or the removal of the uterus. If given an opportunity after such a surgical procedure, many women express feelings about not being a whole woman or about being of less value to the world than they were before the procedure. They may express fears about losing the acceptance of their sexual partners.

Many women pass through a period of mourning for the lost part of the body. Nurses need to understand the realistic reasons that underlie the frequent tears shed by women hospitalized on a gynecological unit of the hospital and should accept this as an expression of a normal emotional response about an extremely upsetting experience. Crying is probably one of the most helpful ways of expressing grief. Unfortunately, some women cannot cry about this type of problem. Instead, they may repress their feelings of despair and sadness and respond in other ways that may be more difficult for the nurse to understand and cope with. After breast surgery, one woman turned her face to the wall, refused to see any visitors, and requested that even her husband be excluded from the room.

Sadness and mourning may be expressed in a reaction that appears to an observer as an outburst of anger. The individual may respond as does a child when something of value is taken away. This response may be an expression of underlying depression, but the external reaction is one of anger at having lost something that was highly valued. Another frequent response to such a surgical loss is the woman's unconscious feeling that she is being punished for some real or fantasized transgression that may have occurred years before. This feeling may lead the woman to respond as if she were unworthy of attention from friends or relatives.

The possible reasons for the many emotional reactions to breast amputation and hysterectomy are as varied as the women who require these procedures. The important point for the nurse to remember is that these experiences are difficult for women to accept; that individuals respond to them in highly individual ways, depending on their life situation and personality; and that the nurse needs to demonstrate an understanding and caring attitude about the woman and her feelings.

Women are not the only people who are unable to accept an altered body image. All individuals who submit to disfiguring surgery of any type have a variety of fears that focus on their concern about being acceptable to other people, especially their sexual partners. Procedures involving amputation of a leg or disfiguring facial surgery are especially difficult for individuals to accept. However, it has been noted that people are able to accept body mutilation more readily when the location is such that it is evident to everyone. This phenomenon may result from the belief that something obvious must be recognized and talked about. Some individuals refrain from mentioning a problem that is hidden under clothing. They are therefore burdened with a tremendous amount of unresolved sensitivity for years. Perhaps the much joked-about American habit of discussing one's surgery and exhibiting the surgical scar at social gatherings has some psychologically healing attributes. It is therapeutic to help individuals discuss their feelings about their surgical procedures.

Nurses should avoid censuring individuals who blame the surgeon for their disfigured bodies. It is a natural human response to relieve anxiety by blaming someone else for an unhappy situation that the individual cannot control with usual defenses.

CLINICAL EXAMPLE

Mr. Carson was hospitalized for plastic reconstruction of a thumb that was lost in an accident involving high-voltage electricity. After several skin grafts and months of repeated hospitalizations, he was disturbed when he saw the reconstructed thumb. It was many times larger than a normal thumb and was covered with short hair because the skin graft had been taken from his thigh. Mr. Carson had expected a normal-looking thumb and had looked forward to having a functioning hand as a reward for the frequent boring hospitalizations. He was bitterly disappointed and disgusted at the appearance of the thumb. He remarked to the nurse, "Look at that! It's obscene. I am going to sign myself out of this hospital and have my own doctor cut this thing off." The nurse reported this reaction to the head nurse, who said, "He should be ashamed of himself for criticizing his doctor, who is the best plastic surgeon in this part of the country. The doctor has worked terribly hard on that thumb." Mr. Carson did leave the hospital against medical advice. He was angry and disappointed and never returned for subsequent surgeries.

A colostomy is another emotionally disturbing experience for individuals. In our culture the emphasis placed on cleanliness and fastidiousness in personal hygiene creates a serious conflict for those who find it medically necessary to resort to a colostomy. Cultural attitudes toward toileting, which are taught early in a child's life, sometimes cause the adult to rebel at the thought of caring for a colostomy. Probably no surgical procedure has the potential for presenting individuals with more emotional and social problems than does a colostomy. Although thousands of individuals have been able to adjust successfully to colostomies, the nurse should not forget that the person who is just beginning to cope with the problems presented by the loss of normal bowel function has many hurdles ahead. Individuals who have undergone a colostomy worry about their acceptability to their friends and their sexual partners. Persons who have received support in working through their feelings about their colostomies report that they have been able to maintain satisfying sexual relations. Unfortunately, others find that it becomes emotionally impossible for them to do so.

It is helpful if individuals with colostomies are encouraged to express their feelings, attitudes, and questions about their condition. Individuals are not helped by nurses who insist on the light, gay approach and refuse to involve themselves in serious conversation about these problems. The person with a colostomy deserves a nurse who will give the situation thoughtful, empathic, realistic consideration.

Such procedures as colostomies are performed only when they are necessary to save the individual's life. The nurse cannot alter the problems that such a procedure presents but can help individuals to talk about the problem, to accept the reality of this situation, and to learn all they can about the condition so they can handle it as effectively as possible.

CLINICAL EXAMPLE

Mr. Bell was a fastidious man who understood English poorly. He entered the hospital with a diagnosis of far-advanced carcinoma of the rectum. He had suffered a great deal before coming to the hospital and was grateful when surgery relieved the pain. A colostomy opening was established. His physical recovery was rapid. When Mr. Bell was discharged, he left many gifts for the hospital staff. In every way he appeared to be happy and grateful. The surgeon had attempted to explain the seriousness of the problem before surgery, and the nurses believed that Mr. Bell understood the nature of his surgery and the need for a permanent colostomy. One week after discharge, he returned to the surgical clinic and requested admission to the hospital to have the colostomy opening closed. Again the surgeon explained the nature of the procedure and the permanent character of the surgery. Mr. Bell left the clinic without appearing to be upset. The next day the newspapers carried a notice of his suicide.

The problems experienced by Mr. Bell undoubtedly grew out of his inability to understand the English language and his attitude toward the importance of physical cleanliness. Although his response to the colostomy was unusual, many individuals will admit that in the beginning of their experience with a colostomy, they occasionally wondered if life was worthwhile under such circumstances. Of particular significance in this situation was Mr. Bell's lack of expression of any negative feelings. If the health care personnel truly understood and appreciated the enormous emotional significance of a colostomy, they would have viewed Mr. Bell's behavior as an untoward response and could have intervened in a way that might have prevented the suicide.

Surgical procedures on the male genitourinary tract sometimes cause severe emotional conflicts. Occasionally such surgery precipitates a psychotic reaction.

CLINICAL EXAMPLE

Mr. Anderson was a middle-aged gentleman who was a devoted church member. He was admitted to a surgical unit because of symptoms of prostatic hypertrophy. A successful procedure was performed to relieve the distressing symptoms. Within 1 or 2 days, he was complaining of suggestive pictures on the walls of his room, which he said the hospital authorities had placed there to torment him. The nurses were confused by these complaints because no pictures were hanging in his room. Mr. Anderson told the psychiatrist who was called to talk with him that the annoying pictures were of young nude women. He stated that a man of his principles should not be surrounded by such lewd art.

The psychiatrist concluded that Mr. Anderson was not able to accept that a man of his social standing would indulge in such an active fantasy life dealing with sexual material. To relieve his own anxiety about his unconscious sexual longings, which were dramatically brought to light by his complaint about the nude pictures, he unconsciously used the mechanism of projection. It was more acceptable to him and safer to his self-esteem to blame the hospital for hanging pictures of nude women around the room than to accept the explanation that the pictures represented his own fantasies.

This unusual reaction was undoubtedly precipitated by the surgical procedure, but it would not be accurate to say that the procedure caused the response. During most of Mr. Anderson's life, he probably had exerted great emotional energy to repress unacceptable sexual thoughts. The

emotional crisis presented by the surgical experience, combined with the effects of the anesthesia, was apparently enough to make it impossible for him to continue to repress his unacceptable thoughts.

Emotional reactions precipitated by cardiac surgery

Individuals respond to life-threatening situations uniquely, depending on the coping mechanisms they have developed and the attitude of personal security they maintain. In view of this, it is difficult, if not impossible, to predict how a specific individual will respond to any surgical procedure, especially one that is potentially as dangerous as cardiac surgery.

No matter how well the individual appears to be anticipating the procedure, the nurse must realize that cardiac surgery is a major crisis and that the person is struggling to control feelings of anxiety and fear. The person cannot avoid being concerned about the possibility of death and the separation from family and friends.

Individuals who have accepted that they must undergo cardiac surgery have come to this decision after months or years of cardiac symptomatology. They may have been semi-invalids because of these symptoms, or the surgery may have been planned in the hope of preventing future invalidism. Thus the individual's fear of the outcome of the procedure is coupled with anticipation of great improvement in health in the immediate future.

The nurse assigned to the individual before cardiac surgery should be prepared to anticipate any number of reactions, depending on the individual's personality. The client may deny the seriousness of the situation and avoid discussing it. This attitude probably suggests that the person finds it difficult to bear the burden and thus copes by avoiding the topic. A different person may discuss fears, may become tearful, and by identifying many personal needs, may insist that the nurse stay in the room. A third individual may appear to be angry and sarcastic and may be critical of the way the nurse performs the necessary nursing procedures. Each of these individuals deserves a calm, empathic nurse who is a good listener and who understands that the individual's emotional response is his or her way of coping with a crisis situation. The nurse should encourage the person to express feelings and concerns and should respond to questions in an honest, straightforward manner without alarming the client. Such individuals deserve to be assured that they will be cared for by a team of physicians and nurses who are knowledgeable, skillful, and deeply interested in their welfare and comfort.

After the surgical procedure, clients will be helpless and dependent for a short time. As they become aware of their dependence on others and on mechanical devices, they may respond in a variety of ways. They may be depressed and hopeless or angry and sarcastic. The postsurgical response depends to a large extent on the coping mechanisms the individual has used in the past.

Just as during the preoperative period, these clients require a quiet, calm, reassuring nurse who listens carefully to their comments and encourages them to express their anxieties and concerns. Reassurance is essential for these individuals, as is focusing on the reality of the improvement they are making.

Emotional reactions precipitated by an untoward obstetrical experience

Many nurses choose to work in obstetrics because the obstetrical unit is said to be a happy place. In talking about their work, obstetrical nurses frequently emphasize the great happiness of mothers and fathers when a new baby is born. Much happiness is present among new parents, but nurses should not overlook that a few new mothers are emotionally distressed and in great need of understanding and reassurance because they have delivered imperfect babies or their babies have failed to survive. Women who deliver imperfect babies may be as troubled as mothers whose babies are stillborn.

Production of perfect babies has traditionally been thought to be one of the most important tasks performed by women. When a woman fails in this effort, she sometimes wonders about her effectiveness and her intrinsic value. Therfore, mothers of imperfectly formed babies or premature infants are frequently distressed by doubts concerning their own adequacy as women and by guilt about their responsibility for the existence of the problem. Some nurses may be surprised to learn that almost all mothers whose babies are born prematurely or congenitally imperfect respond with questions that reflect concern about themselves. They ask questions such as, "What did I do to cause this?" or "Why has this happened to me?" Since the cause of prematurity and many congenital imperfections is not always understood, scientific explanations of these events often cannot be given. Even when scientific explanations are available, they do little to remove the personal sense of failure these mothers often feel.

Guilt causes people to feel uncomfortable. When a mother feels guilty about her baby's imperfections, she may reject it outright or may spend the rest of her life punishing herself for failing to give her child a perfect body. This punishment might take the form of slavishly serving the child in an attempt to make up in every possible way for the child's poor start in life. This reaction is one of the disguised forms that rejection may take.

As in many other situations, the nurse cannot alter the reality of the difficult situation but can encourage the mother to talk about her feelings. If the mother can be helped to discuss some of these feelings, she may feel less guilty and may be able to eliminate some emotion about the problem so that constructive steps can be taken and solutions planned.

Some women who have set high achievement goals for themselves find it particularly difficult to accept an imperfect baby.

CLINICAL EXAMPLE

Dr. Keller was an English professor from a large midwestern university. She became pregnant for the first time at age 40. She and her husband were moderately happy about this new development in their lives. However, they were sorry to have to give up their plans for a sabbatical leave and a trip abroad. When the baby boy was born, he had a bilateral cleft lip (harelip) and a cleft palate. When the nurse brought the baby to his mother, she looked at him and said, "That can't possibly be my child," The nurse assured Dr. Keller that it was her little boy. She said to the nurse, "Don't bring that baby in here again. I won't have a baby that looks like that!" In 2 days, Dr. Keller was discharged from the hospital without asking to see her baby again. The father arranged for a nurse to help him take his son to a distant city, where he had an appointment with a famous surgeon who specialized in repairing cleft lips. Within a few weeks, Dr. Keller began to experience overwhelming feelings of anxiety and guilt for which she saw no cause. These feelings became so intense that she sought professional help. Through psychotherapy, this mother eventually was able to understand the highly personalized meaning that the birth of her imperfect baby had for her.

Emotional reactions precipitated by abortion

Few situations in a woman's life have such a potential for producing a variety of emotional responses as does abortion. The woman's response is highly individual and depends on many factors. Some of these factors include her religious beliefs and cultural background. Some religious groups are explicit in their teaching against abortion, whereas others are more inclined to leave such a decision to the woman and her physician. Some cultures emphasize the relationship between a woman's intrinsic value to society and her ability to produce children; others place more importance on the quality of life that can be provided for the mother and child. Another factor is the woman's relationship with the father. If the relationship is a stable one and the man agrees that abortion is a wise decision, the woman's reaction may be less emotionally distressing than if he wishes her to maintain the pregnancy. If the pregnancy is unwanted because of the circumstances surrounding conception (e.g., rape) or if the fetus has been identified as being seriously defective, the opportunity for abortion may be greeted with relief.

Some individuals may be convinced that they have discarded the early religious instructions that they received and the attitudes taught within the family about such controversial questions as abortion. However, these attitudes are difficult to discard and may greatly influence the woman's emotional response even though they are not recognized consciously.

Many women are able to accept an abortion without experiencing any untoward emotional reaction. However, certain individuals may express feelings of serious personal loss, deep regret, shame, guilt, a loss of self-esteem, and sadness. Such individuals may have difficulty sleeping, experience a loss of appetite, exhibit a lack of interest in their home and work, express resentment toward the man involved, and cry frequently.

Unless the nurse visits the home or works with women in a clinic situation, little opportunity exists to be helpful to these individuals, since abortion is usually completed within a few hours and usually does not require overnight hospitalization.

If opportunities are available, it is helpful to encourage the woman to discuss her feelings and how she perceives the situation. In certain individuals an abortion may precipitate a crisis. In this case the person should be treated as any other individual who is overwhelmed by a problem of daily living.

Women anticipating an abortion should have an opportunity to examine the situation with the help of a nurse therapist. Because abortion is irreversible, alternatives should be thoroughly explored before a choice is made.

Emotional reactions of individuals with acquired immunodeficiency syndrome (AIDS)

No other illness in recent memory has evoked the type and amount of widespread reaction seen in response to the disease of **AIDS.** At this point, no cure exists for AIDS, it is associated with a lifestyle stigmatized by society, and it is increasing in incidence. Therefore the client, his or her social group, the family, and society all are profoundly affected by this illness.

The professional literature abounds with current information about the comprehensive care of the client with AIDS; the student is referred to these articles for specifics. In general, however, it is necessary for all nurses to understand that the diagnosis of AIDS, in itself, precipitates a situational crisis of catastrophic proportion. Because many of these persons acquired this illness secondary to a lifestyle stigmatized by society, that is, homosexual or bisexual behavior or intravenous drug use, they are confronted not only with the loss of health and likely death but also with the potential losses of a job and financial security, housing, sexual activity, and social acceptance. If nurses are to be truly helpful to the person with AIDS, they must examine their own beliefs, value system, and fears so that they do not inadvertently contribute to the all-too-frequent discrimination experienced by these persons. Furthermore, the nurse needs to develop the ability to differentiate between the individual's emotional responses to the illness and the responses to others' reactions if the nurse is to provide individualized care (Figure 23-2).

The first stage of the crisis is characterized by denial alternating with overwhelming anxiety, anger, and acute emotional turmoil. To appreciate fully this normal response, the nurse needs

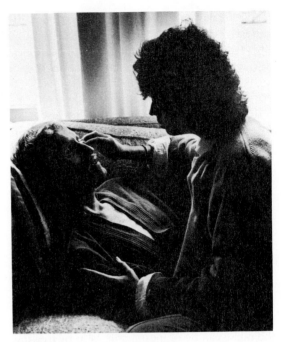

Figure 23-2

Compassionate support.

From Hood GH, Dincher JR: *Total patient care,* ed 8, St Louis, 1992, Mosby–Year Book.

to understand that many of these individuals are at a point in their life when they are just beginning to actualize their future. The diagnosis of AIDS represents a death sentence that creates a massive assault on their total stability. Therefore, denial is accurately interpreted as a healthy defense mechanism that should be supported unless doing so increases danger to the client. Concomitant with denial is these persons' inability to understand or remember what they are being told, including instructions. Therefore the nurse is most helpful when writing down information the individual must have, such as names and telephone numbers of referrals.

In marked contrast to denial, some persons newly diagnosed with AIDS express a temporary sense of relief when told of their diagnosis, since they had experienced symptoms before seeking medical help and had privately feared this diagnosis, Therefore the confirmation of this dreaded diagnosis makes public what was a private terror and enables discussion about it.

As the illness progresses and individuals experience physiological symptoms that greatly interfere with the ability to function, they are likely to become very depressed, perhaps even suicidal. Once again, this response is understandable in that they are experiencing some very real losses about which they must grieve. In addition to the losses resulting from the illness itself, it is unfortunately not unusual for individuals with AIDS to find themselves rejected by family and friends, to be at risk for eviction and loss of employment, and to be the object of many other forms of social ostracism. This societal response often precipitates feelings of isolation, guilt, anger, and low self-esteem.

When providing care for clients with AIDS, the nurse can be of inestimable help by treating them with the same skill, sensitivity, and respect as the nurse would extend to any other client who has a serious illness. This means making frequent contact, encouraging these persons to talk about their feelings and listening nonjudgmentally, reaching out to touch them, and limiting use of isolation precautions only to those necessary. The specter of a patient with AIDS lying in a private room having contact only when necessary with a fully gowned, gloved, and masked nurse is truly frightening.

If possible, another helpful intervention is to assist persons with AIDS to become involved in a support group where the reality basis for their responses can be validated and where they can receive assistance in planning to meet their needs.

In the final phase of the illness, the individual is likely to accept the diagnosis and simultaneously attempt to live each day constructively within the limits imposed by the physical debility while also preparing for death. The nurse needs to be aware, however, that each instance of opportunistic infection and each news bulletin about a new medication thrusts the person into another crisis. Many patients with AIDS report that one of the most difficult aspects of living with their illness is the "roller coaster" of emotions that they experience as hope vacillates with despair.

As persons with AIDS receive more effective symptomatic care and live longer, many develop dementia related to the invasion of the virus into the central nervous system. Thus the patient may display symptoms of cognitive impairment and psychomotor retardation or agitation. Some become blatantly psychotic. Therefore, it is likely that an increasing number of patients with AIDS will be seen in psychiatric units or psychiatric hospitals.

Emotional aspects of death and dying

No discussion of the emotional needs of persons who have a physical illness would be complete without addressing the needs of the individual who is dying. With the development of complex medical technology, the ability to prolong life has increased. This ability has raised questions about the quality of life and in the opinion of some has contributed to the unconsciously held belief that death occurs only as a result of the failure of the individual or the health care team to "try hard enough."

It is important for all health care personnel to understand that death is an inevitability and that dying persons have a right to be treated humanely. It is not humane to surround dying persons by machines and technicians so that the family cannot even reach them. The opposite often occurs as well; that is, the person with a terminal illness is figuratively abandoned. Individuals in this situation are often relegated to rooms farthest away from the nurse's station, receive only cursory attention from medical and nursing staff, and may have few visitors.

The nurse must be concerned about remedying both these extreme situations. Nursing, more than any other health care profession, has the opportunity and the obligation to assist the dying person and family to achieve a satisfactory resolution of this last phase of life. To fulfill this responsibility, the nurse needs to develop an understanding of the emotional needs of the person who has a terminal illness.

Dr. Elisabeth Kübler-Ross, a pioneer in **thanatology** (the study of death), has studied the responses of hundreds of persons with a terminal illness. Her subjects included persons of all ages, socioeconomic levels, and cultural backgrounds. These persons also represented a wide variety of illnesses and injuries, both acute and chronic. Regardless of their differences, Kübler-Ross found that all dying persons progress through a similar process of emotional response. Her formulation, which is probably familiar to most nurses, delineates five stages of dying.

Denial is the initial response caused by the person not being able to deal emotionally with the reality of impending death. To deal with the intense anxiety that this news engenders, the person used the ego defense of denial. As a result, persons in this stage often express the belief that a mistake has been made in laboratory reports or that the physician is incompetent. As in dealing with any person who is using the defense of denial, nurses are most helpful if they understand that this defense is operative because the individual has sustained a massive emotional assault that he or she cannot handle directly without endangering the integrity of the personality. Consequently, the wise nurse intervenes in a manner that allows the individual to maintain this defense while simultaneously not avoiding the reality of the situation. For example, the nurse would not encourage a person in this stage of the dying process to make plans for the funeral, but the nurse would encourage the person to take medications as they were prescribed. Because the reality of the situation is such that the individual soon becomes sicker, the length of this stage is relatively short in individuals who are mentally healthy. Illnesses that initially do not have symptoms that cause incapacitation, such as chronic lymphocytic leukemia, may en-

able even mentally healthy persons to cling to the denial of their dying.

Anger characterizes the second stage of the dying process. During this stage, individuals often believe they are victims of fate, circumstances, medical incompetence, or a vengeful God. Their thoughts and verbalizations center around the question, "Why me?" They fear the dependency their illness creates and often resent their family and the health care workers who try to be of help. Since feeling and expressing anger are not acceptable to many people, some dying persons may express their anger in covert rather than overt ways. Most nurses recognize the anger and underlying anxiety in individuals with a terminal illness who complain about everything and everyone. Only the sensitive, insightful nurse recognizes the same dynamics in the individual who expresses anger in passive ways, such as "forgetting" to take medication and then asking the nurse what to do.

Bargaining is the third stage of the dying process characterized by the individual attempting to gain more time by trading off "good" behavior. Most often, dying individuals bargain with supernatural powers: God, fate, or whatever higher Being they believe can effect a change in their condition. Bargaining takes the form of, "If you (let me live until Christmas) then I (will bequeath half of my money to the church)." The behavior that the person "trades off" is highly individualized and is probably related to earlier unresolved conflicts. The bargaining stage is helpful to the dying person in that it temporarily eases the anxiety and enables the person to deal with the pain and dependence that may accompany the illness.

The **depression** stage follows bargaining. Depression begins when the reality of the situation can no longer be ignored and the uselessness of denial, anger, and bargaining is apparent. The depression that the individual feels is a response to an overwhelming sense of anticipated loss, the loss of his or her entire world. At this stage, dying persons look and act depressed and often have no need to talk with others about how they feel. They must use their energy to confront the fact that what is done is done and what is undone will remain so. Because they are depressed, persons in this stage of dying make few demands. Consequently, their behavior is often misinterpreted as "cooperative."

Acceptance is the final stage of the dying process when individuals have come to peace with themselves about their death being imminent. Acceptance is characterized by an affective void; the person is neither happy nor depressed. Interests, even in personal care, narrow. During this time, only those persons who are most significant to the person are able to elicit a positive response. The presence of others is merely tolerated. This does not mean, however, that the dying person cannot receive comfort from the nursing interventions of a warm, caring nurse. It does mean that the most effective interventions are likely to be nonverbal in the form of physical comfort measures delivered in a competent, compassionate way.

Understanding the emotional needs of the dying person is of value to the nurse only if this knowledge is combined with self-awareness. Since death and dying are not viewed by our culture as natural phenomena, nurses, as with most people, have been taught since early childhood to avoid the subject. This cultural attitude may be compounded by the nurse's own developmental stage. The developmental stages of adulthood and middle age are the stages most nurses are in and may prove to be particularly problematic in regard to the issues of death and dying. The stage of adulthood, especially early adulthood, is a time when people view all things as being possible. As a result, the nurse in this stage may be prone to view the person with a terminal illness as representative of the failure of the health care team. Nurses dealing with the developmental tasks of middle age may be actively dealing with the awareness of their own mortality reinforced by the declining health of their parents. The person with a terminal illness may represent the nurses' vulnerability to the prospect of their own death.

In either instance, the nurse may feel anxious and guilt ridden and avoid dealing with these feelings by avoiding the patient. When the person cannot be avoided, the nurse avoids the reality of the situation by assuming a false air of cheerfulness, by changing the subject when the person or family start to talk about death, or by not answering the client's questions. Other nurses may respond angrily to dying persons, as if their dying were their fault. This counterproductive response seems especially justifiable to the nurse when the dying person's poor health habits, such as smoking, have obviously contributed to the terminal illness. Only if nurses can be helped to explore and confront their own feelings about the dying process will they be able to give the skilled, compassionate care the dying person deserves.

NURSING CARE PLAN: *An Individual Who Is Dying*

CASE FORMULATION

Mrs. Harper, a 78-year-old widow, has chronic lymphocytic leukemia, the treatment of which now requires her to go to the hospital monthly for blood transfusions.

Mrs. Harper lived in her mother's home until she married at age 25. She and her new husband had wanted to marry earlier, but Mrs. Harper was needed at home to help care for her father, who was ill and ultimately

NURSING CARE PLAN: *An Individual Who Is Dying—cont'd*

died of cancer. Mrs. Harper was an executive secretary. Despite her marriage and no economic need to do so, she worked continuously until her retirement at age 62. She and Mr. Harper had two daughters, the first when Mrs. Harper was 30 and the second 10 years later. Mrs. Harper responded to the birth of her second daughter by becoming seriously depressed for 2 years. Although she was still able to work during this time, she was completely unable to care for the children or the house. As a result, her widowed mother moved in with the Harpers to care for the family and the home. Ten years later, her mother had a stroke and required much care until she died. Both daughters studied professions and are now working and living with their families in other states.

When the Harpers retired, they sold the family home and bought a much smaller home in another area of the United States that had been Mr. Harper's boyhood home. Although Mrs. Harper knew no one in the community, she agreed to the move to placate Mr. Harper, a domineering and demanding person. Five years after the move, Mr. Harper died after a lengthy illness related to complications of diabetes. Throughout his illness, Mrs. Harper devoted herself exclusively to meeting his needs, even to the extent of staying in the hospital around the clock for weeks on end.

After Mr. Harper's death the daughters were worried about how Mrs. Harper would manage by herself. As a result, they telephoned her every other day and were often worried, since she was seldom home. Finally, the older daughter asked her mother where she went so frequently. Mrs. Harper responded by saying that she was not about to answer for her whereabouts, since this was the first time in her life that she was free of responsibility and could do as she wished. For the next 8 years, Mrs. Harper lived comfortably and happily, associating frequently with the many friends she made and visiting her daughters on holidays.

Mrs. Harper discovered that she had chronic lymphocytic leukemia 2 years ago as a result of bloodwork that she had done at a community health clinic that offered free screening examinations and laboratory tests to senior citizens. The results of her bloodwork were mailed to her by certified mail accompanied by a letter strongly urging her to consult her physician. Even though her physician's tests confirmed the diagnosis and she was referred to an oncologist for treatment, Mrs. Harper confided in her daughters that she never felt better and that she was sure there was some sort of mix-up, probably in the laboratory. Despite her denial of her illness, she kept her appointments with the physician and conscientiously took the prescribed medication.

Within 18 months, Mrs. Harper became increasingly tired and resistant to the effects of the chemotherapy. As a result, she now requires blood transfusions along with medication.

One month ago, Mrs. Harper spent a week with her older daughter to attend the high-school graduation of one of her granddaughters. Several other family members also were house guests for the occasion, including Mrs. Harper's younger daughter and her 8-year-old daughter. This child was very active and talkative, probably because of fatigue and boredom, since no other children were present. Mrs. Harper alarmed and surprised

Continued.

NURSING CARE PLAN: *An Individual Who Is Dying—cont'd*

everyone by responding to the child and her mother with thinly concealed rage, frequently yelling at the child to behave herself and telling her daughter that she was not any better a mother than she had been a child.

When Mrs. Harper arrived for her transfusion this morning, the nurse asked how she was feeling. Although the nurse was undoubtedly inquiring about her physical health, this question precipitated an outpouring of anger about how "bad" her young granddaughter was and how her own daughter did not know how to control the situation.

Nursing Assessment

Mrs. Harper's background and her current illness give many clues as to why she may be reacting the way she is. Although her early family history of living with her parents and not marrying until she fulfilled her responsibilities to care for her dying father is not unusual for a woman of her age, her working continuously outside the home as an executive secretary was an exception for a woman of her generation. Therefore, Mrs. Harper likely was meeting a need for independence while simultaneously attempting to behave dutifully in the manner appropriate for a women at that time. When she gave birth to a second child at age 40, she may have perceived this event as a potential loss of independence to which she responded with depression. The ego strength of this woman and the importance of her job as a coping mechanism are attested to by her being able to continue work despite her depression. It also appears that she suppressed many of her needs for independence after she retired, as evidenced by her willingness to move to a strange area and to care for her husband devotedly during his long illness. However, once these responsibilities were met, she asserted her strong need for independence, as evidenced by her response to her children's questions about her activities.

Mrs. Harper's response of denial to the news that she had a life-threatening illness is congruent with what is known about the first stage of dying. This response is particularly common when the illness does not cause major symptoms or dysfunction. Since she complied with the physician's treatment regimen, it was possible to support her denial and thereby allow her to adjust gradually to the inevitability of failing health. However, once the medication became ineffective and transfusions were necessary, it was no longer possible for Mrs. Harper to deny the gravity of her situation and, most important, her impending loss of independence. Therefore the nurse assessed Mrs. Harper's anger at her 8-year-old granddaughter as being displaced rage about her own feelings of loss of control, characteristic of the second stage of the dying process. It is also interesting to note that Mrs. Harper's anger extended to the child's mother, whose birth 40 years earlier had precipitated Mrs. Harper's depression. It is likely that she was now outwardly expressing the anger that she had turned inward for so many years.

Nursing Diagnosis

Based on the nursing assessment, which included prior knowledge of the family dynamics and an understanding of the dynam-

NURSING CARE PLAN: *An Individual Who Is Dying—cont'd*

ics underlying the dying process, the nurse formulated the following nursing diagnosis specific to Mrs. Harper's emotional response:

Anxiety related to impending loss of independence caused by illness

Planning and Implementing Nursing Care

A sample nursing care plan for Mrs. Harper is found in the table that follows.

The nurse's immediate objective was to allow and encourage Mrs. Harper to talk about her feelings, which might enable her to see that the anger she felt toward her granddaughter's and daughter's behavior was a displacement of her own rage about having a terminal illness. The nurse also knew it was important to take this time if Mrs. Harper were to have an emotionally corrective experience by being able to express her anger about the birth of her second daughter. The nurse was careful to respond to Mrs. Harper in an accepting, empathic way, even though many people might not understand how one could be currently angry about an event that happened 40 years ago and a situation that was yet to occur.

Since the nurse was not surprised or frightened by Mrs. Harper, as was her family, she was able to implement this approach effectively.

Evaluation

Mrs. Harper talked so long about her feelings that the transfusion had to be rescheduled for later in the week. Although she gave no evidence that she understood the relationship between her current anger and the impending loss of independence caused by her illness, she did express the insight that she had always been "furious" with her younger daughter because Mrs. Harper thought she was too old to deal with a baby when she became pregnant.

The nurse made sure that she would be on duty when Mrs. Harper came for her next appointment so they could continue their discussion during the transfusion. She also noted on the care plan the necessity to contact the daughters about Mrs. Harper's future care, with the goal of helping them explore ways in which they could assist their mother to remain as independent as possible for as long as possible.

NURSING CARE PLAN FOR MRS. HARPER

Nursing diagnosis	Objective (rationale)	Nursing interventions	Outcome criteria
Anxiety related to impending loss of independence due to illness	Client sees her anger as stemming from her impending loss of independence and repressed rage at younger daughter. (Identifying source of anger	Listen in an accepting, empathic way. Reflect back client's content and tone. Encourage client to make all decisions that are possible.	Within 1 month, client verbalizes relationship of her anger to impending loss of independence and repressed rage at younger daughter.

Continued.

NURSING CARE PLAN FOR MRS. HARPER—cont'd

Nursing diagnosis	Objective (rationale)	Nursing interventions	Outcome criteria
	often alleviates anxiety and creates opportunity for reality testing.)	Contact daughters to plan for continuing independence of client for as long as possible.	Within 6 months, client begins to grieve loss of independence. Client continues to schedule appointments and comply with medical instructions indefinitely. Within 2 weeks, client's daughters will confer with nurse.

KEY POINTS

1. As medical science developed, physicians delegated to nurses procedures they no longer had time to perform.

2. A psychiatric liaison nurse can help achieve the goal of meeting the emotional needs of patients who are physically ill.

3. Good physical care is always the first place to start in meeting the emotional needs of persons who have a physical illness.

4. Any physical illness that requires hospitalization forces the individual to assume a dependent role that may be disturbing.

5. Individuals who must rely on mechanical devices often feel that they have lost control of their bodies and of their destinies.

6. Providing an organ for an individual from the body of another could be an emotionally disturbing experience for both the person donating the organ and the recipient.

7. Every person has a mental image of his or her own body that is called the body image.

8. All individuals who submit to disfiguring surgery of any type fear that they will not be accepted by other people, especially their sexual partners.

9. Individuals respond to life-threatening situations uniquely, depending on the coping mechanisms they have developed.

10. Women who have set high achievement goals for themselves may find it difficult to accept an imperfect baby.

11. Few situations in a woman's life have such a potential for producing a variety of emotional responses as does abortion.

12. The client with AIDS, the client's social group and family, and society all are profoundly affected by this illness.

13. It is important for all health care personnel to understand that death is an inevitability and that dying persons have a right to be treated humanely.

14. The five stages of dying include denial, anger, bargaining, depression, and finally acceptance.

SUGGESTED SOURCES OF ADDITIONAL INFORMATION

Artinian B: Bending expectations for marital role performance of dialysis patients, *Fam Community Health* 12(4):47, 1990.

Bernstein SB: Breaking the vicious circle of noncompliance, *Nursing '89* 19:74, January 1989.

Boccellari AA, Dilley JW: Management and residential placement problems of patients with HIV-related cognitive impairment, *Hosp Community Psychiatry* 43:32, January 1992.

Breault AJ, Polifroni EC: Caring for people with AIDS: nurses' attitudes and feelings, *J Adv Nurs* 17:21, 1992.

Broadhurst C: Adjusting to amputation, *Nurs Times* 85(43):55, 1989.

Brockopp DY and others: The dying patient: a comparative study of nurse caregiver characteristics, *Death Studies* 15:245, 1991.

Butler MJ: Family transformation: Parse's theory in practice, *Nurs Sci Q* 68, 1988.

Cancer nursing: learning to cope with an artificial limb, *Nursing* 4(17):16, 1990.

Carmack BJ: Balancing engagement/detachment in AIDS-related multiple losses, *Image* 24:9, Spring 1992.

Carr EW: Psychosocial issues of AIDS patients in hospice: case studies, *Hospice J* 5(3-4):135, 1989.

Cassem EH: Depression and anxiety secondary to medical illness, *Psychiatr Clin North Am* 13:597, December 1990.

Christenson JL: Chronic pain: dynamics and treatment strategies, *Perspect Psychiatr Care* 29:13, January-March 1993.

Cohen SM and others: Another look at psychologic complications of hysterectomy, *Image* 21(1):51, 1989.

Feather BL, Wainstock JM: Perceptions of postmastectomy patients. Part II: Social support and attitudes towards mastectomy, *Cancer Nurs* 12(5):301, 1989.

Flaskerud JH: AIDS: psychosocial aspects, *J Psychosoc Nurs Ment Health Serv* 25:8, December 1987.

Grabbe LL, Brown LB: Identifying neurologic complications of AIDS, *Nursing '89* 19:66, May 1989.

Grant SM: The hospitalized AIDS patient and the psychiatric liaison nurse, *Arch Psychiatr Nurs* 2:35, February 1988.

Hall JM, Stevens PE: AIDS: a guide to suicide assessment, *Arch Psychiatr Nurs* 1:115, April 1988.

Hart CA: The role of psychiatric consultation liaison nurses in ethical decisions to remove life-sustaining treatments, *Arch Psychiatr Nurs* 4:370, December 1990.

Henderson KJ: Dying, God, & anger: comforting through spiritual care, *J Psychosoc Nurs Ment Health Serv* 27(5):17, 1989.

Hospice techniques: preparing for the death of a loved one, *Am J Hospice Palliative Care* 14, July/August 1992.

Hough EE and others: Family response to mother's chronic illness: case studies of well and poorly adjusted families, *West J Nurs Res* 13(5):568, 1991.

Icenhour ML, Calvert H: EBV: managing the physiological and psychosocial implications of the Epstein-Barr virus, *J Psychosoc Nurs* 27(4):20, 1989.

Kübler-Ross E: *Questions and answers on death and dying,* New York, 1974, Macmillan.

Leidy NK and others: Psychophysiological processes of stress in chronic physical illness: a theoretical perspective, *J Adv Nurs* 15:478, 1990.

MacNeil-Zimberg M: Helping cancer patients cope, *J Psychosoc Nurs Health Serv* 23:31, June 1985.

McCain NL, Gramling LF: Living with dying: coping with HIV disease, *Issues Ment Health Nurs* 13(3):271, 1992.

Meisenhelder JB, LaCharite CL: Fear of contagion: a stress response to acquired immunodeficiency syndrome, *Adv Nurs Sci* 11(2):29, 1989.

Morrow BR and others: Dying with dignity: hospice care on the unit, *J Psychosoc Nurs Ment Health Serv* 27(11):10, 1989.

Newell R: Body-image disturbance: cognitive behavioural formulation and intervention, *J Adv Nurs* 16:1400, 1991.

Novotny MP: Psychosocial issues affecting rehabilitation, *Phys Med Rehabil Clin North Am* 2:373, May 1991.

Pheifer WG, Houseman C: Bereavement and AIDS: a framework for intervention, *J Psychosoc Nurs Ment Health Serv* 26:21, October 1988.

Regan-Kubinski MJ, Sharts-Engel N: The HIV-infected woman: illness cognition assessment, *J Psychosoc Nurs Ment Health Serv* 30(2):11, 1992.

Uzark K, Crowley D: Family stresses after pediatric heart transplantation, *Prog Cardiovasc Nurs* 4:23, January-March 1989.

Valente SM, Saunders JM: Dealing with serious depression in cancer patients, *Nursing '89* 19:44, February 1989.

van Servellen G and others: Coping with a crisis: evaluating psychological risks of patients with AIDS, *J Psychosoc Nurs Ment Health Serv* 27(12):16, 1989.

Wallace B, Herbert CC: Managing the psychosocial problems associated with replantation surgery, *Crit Care Nurs Q* 13(1):55, 1990.

White NE and others: Coping, social support, and adaptation to chronic illness, *West J Nurs Res* 14(2):211, 1992.

Whyte DA: A family nursing approach to the care of a child with a chronic illness, *J Adv Nurs* 17:317, 1992.

Worth C: Handle with care, *Am J Nurs* 89:196, February 1989.

Wright LK: Life threatening illness, *J Psychosoc Nurs Ment Health Serv* 23(9):6, 1985.

Section Five

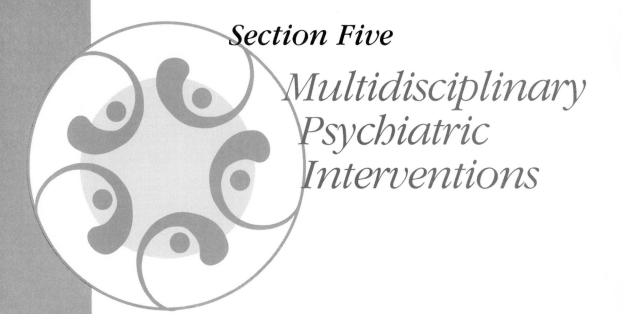

Multidisciplinary Psychiatric Interventions

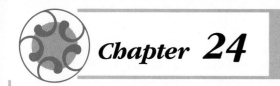

Chapter 24

Crisis Theory and Intervention

LEARNING OBJECTIVES
After studying this chapter, the student will be able to:

- Define the term *crisis*.

- Differentiate between developmental and situational crises.

- Discuss the characteristics of a crisis state.

- Discuss the sequential phases of a crisis state.

- State the goal of crisis intervention.

- Discuss in sequence the steps of crisis intervention.

KEY TERMS
Crisis intervention
Crisis
Developmental events
Situational events
Developmental crises
Anticipatory guidance
Situational crises
Denial
Increased tension
Disorganization
Attempts to reorganize
Attempt to escape the problem
Local reorganization
General reorganization
Unsuccessful resolution
Pseudoresolution
Successful resolution

Crisis intervention is a subject of interest to all health professionals. It is a technique that is used successfully by persons with a variety of backgrounds to aid individuals and families in understanding and effectively coping with the intense emotions that characterize a crisis state. Once clients are able to deal with their emotions, they often are able to make appropriate decisions regarding behavior that may be required for resolution of the problems that surround the crisis. Although the responsibility for crisis intervention does not fall into the province of any one health care discipline, a discussion of it is included in this text because nurses are often in the position to engage in this technique or to counsel other health care professionals in its use. Furthermore, psychiatric nurses are expected to have particular expertise in understanding and managing emotional problems and are often viewed by their colleagues as consultants in crisis states.

HISTORICAL PERSPECTIVE

As with many other contemporary innovations in American psychiatry, crisis theory and intervention had their foundation in the experiences of the military during World War II. During that war, more psychiatric casualties occurred than physical ones, even after an attempt had been made to screen out those persons with a history of mental illness. Many casualties were precipitated by the soldier's experiences in combat. Psychiatrists in the medical corps, led by Dr. William Menninger, treated some of these soldiers close to the front, primarily because of a shortage of personnel and the inaccessibility of other treatment settings. Much to the surprise of all, those who received immediate, reality-oriented, supportive intervention and who were returned to combat as soon as possible fared better emotionally than did their counterparts who were evacuated to treatment centers and treated with psychoanalytically oriented interventions.

After the war the techniques used so successfully were applied with equal success to civilians who were victims of disasters. Perhaps the most famous of these was the fire in 1942 at the Cocoanut Grove, a nightclub in Boston. The emotional reactions of the survivors of this disaster were studied in depth over a period of years by Eric Lindemann. His findings about the symptoms and management of acute grief remain the classic work in the field.

Despite its use earlier, crisis intervention did not become a recognized treatment modality until the 1960s. During that time, Gerald Caplan made numerous contributions to the literature on the subject and was instrumental in developing a theory to explain the manifestations of a crisis in essentially healthy people and postulating intervention techniques. Since that time, numerous others from all health care disciplines have contributed to the growing body of knowledge about the subject.

DEFINITION OF CRISIS

The term **crisis** is often used by lay persons to describe a situation or a feeling state. It is not unusual to hear an individual say about an event, "It was a crisis." If the event referred to was a turning point in a situation, the use of the term is correct according to the dictionary definition of the word. When referring to a feeling state, persons often report that they are in a crisis when they are very upset. Almost always, this is an incorrect use of the word according to its technical definition.

Mental health authorities define a crisis as *a state of disequilibrium resulting from the interaction of an event with the individual's or family's coping mechanisms, which are inadequate to meet the demands of the situation, combined with the individual's or family's perception of the meaning of the event*. Therefore a crisis refers to an interactional process among these three variables that is reflected in the feeling state of the individual or family. Although anxiety usually underlies the feeling state, the individual may feel depression, anger, fear, or any other of a wide range of emotions. However, the emotion is not unique to a crisis, and neither is the event. Rather, the meaning of the event to the individual or family and their inability to cope with it produce the crisis. Therefore, not every person who is anxious, depressed, angry, or fearful is in a crisis, and a traumatic event does not necessarily produce a crisis in those whom it affects.

Health professionals are greatly interested in crisis intervention for several reasons. First, more people are voluntarily seeking mental health care for problems that are not necessarily indicative of long-standing dysfunction. In the past, because of the social stigma associated with mental illness, mental health counsel was sought only if the person was severely disturbed and exhibiting bizarre symptoms such as hallucinations or delusions. Although more stigma still is associated with mental illness than with physical illness, society is gradually becoming more accepting of the value of mental health treatment, so more people voluntarily seek help for less severe problems. These problems are often individual or familial crises.

Second, as professionals have gained more experience in dealing with persons in a crisis, they have realized that former unresolved crises often emerge to consciousness in conjunction with the present crisis. Therefore, intervention can be directed toward both the present and the past situations, providing a unique opportunity to help the client resolve long-standing problems in a relatively short time.

Finally, crisis intervention is of great interest to mental health professionals because it provides a specific opportunity to prevent mental illness and to promote mental health. Prevention of mental illness is achieved by helping clients to use already established coping mechanisms they have successfully used in the past or by assisting them to develop new, healthy defenses. If this can be achieved, the necessity for the client to resort to dysfunctional coping patterns can be avoided.

Promotion of mental health through crisis in-tervention has been documented by researchers who have engaged in follow-up studies of individuals and families who have experienced crises. It has been demonstrated that three possible outcomes of a crisis state exist: (1) the client may reintegrate at a lower or less healthy level of functioning than the one before the crisis; (2) the client may reintegrate at the same level of functioning as previously, probably as a result of completely repressing the crisis situation and its attendant emotions; or (3) the client may reintegrate at a higher, healthier level of functioning than the level before the crisis experience. This last possible outcome was a startling realization at the time it was first described because the goal had always been prevention of mental illness. The idea that people could actually grow and benefit from an emotionally traumatic experience opened vast potential for increasing the level of mental health in a large population. Some authorities see a crisis as a catalyst that disturbs previous habits, evokes new responses, and becomes a major factor in charting new developments. Therefore the challenge that a crisis provokes may bring forth new coping mechanisms that serve to strengthen the individual's adaptive capacity and thereby, in general, to raise his or her level of mental health.*

Research studies have further documented that, although any one of the three outcomes can occur with or without skilled intervention, resolution of the crisis resulting in a lower level of functioning or the same level of functioning is more likely to occur without intervention, and resolution of the crisis resulting in a higher level of functioning is more likely to occur with intervention. Consequently, to promote mental health and prevent mental illness, an increasing number of communities have established crisis intervention centers. These centers may take the form of mental health emergency rooms, suicide

---

*Rapaport L: The state of crisis: some theoretical considerations. In Pared HJ, editor: *Crisis intervention: selected readings,* New York, 1965, Family Service Association of America.

prevention clinics, family guidance clinics, or telephone crisis services. Whatever the name, these centers are always staffed by personnel skilled in crisis intervention.

TYPES OF CRISES

Two types of events may precipitate a crisis state: developmental and situational events. **Developmental events** are situations that naturally occur during the lifetime of an individual and the family, for example, the birth of a child. Therefore, developmental events are predictable. **Situational events,** on the other hand, do not inevitably occur to all individuals or families and therefore are unexpected. An example of a situational event is an automobile accident.

One should understand, however, that very few events inevitably produce a crisis state in all persons. If the student reviews the definition of crisis, it will be clear that the nature of the event is only one factor in the production of a crisis. In addition to the event, the other two necessary factors are the personalized meaning of the event to the individual and family and the nature and extent of their coping mechanisms. These must interact in such a way as to produce a state of disequilibrium. For example, a hysterectomy may be well received by a 50-year-old unmarried career woman who sublimates her maternal needs through the children of friends and relatives and whose emotional energy is directed toward her profession. Another 50-year-old woman experiencing the same surgical procedure may be plunged into a state of crisis because her identity unconsciously has been formed around her role as mother and homemaker, and the hysterectomy marks the end of her childbearing years, thus threatening her sense of self. To take this example one step further, the same career woman may enter a state of disequilibrium or crisis if she loses her job or retires, whereas the homemaker might respond to a loss of her outside job with an inner sense of relief.

Developmental crises

Developmental crises are well documented. The student will remember that each stage of development has its own developmental task, the achievement of which requires the individual to emphasize certain behaviors and to minimize others. Consequently, the family as a unit is called on to adjust and adapt to the changes experienced by each of its members. Although these changes in individuals are most pronounced during infancy and early childhood, they occur throughout the entire life cycle. Therefore, any family unit is likely to have members who represent at least two different developmental stages. Many families have members who may be experiencing one of five or six different developmental stages, each stage having its own needs and manifestations. When this is the case, family disequilibrium typically occurs because behaviors that meet the needs of one or more of its members may be in direct opposition to the needs of other members. Although technically not a developmental crisis, an increasingly common example of such a situation is the phenomenon of adult children who return to the home of their parents to live after having been away for a few years. This phenomenon is occurring more often today, related in part to problems in the society at large. A scarcity of jobs makes it difficult, if not impossible, for some young adults to become economically independent. Nevertheless, the young adult is developmentally ready to work on establishing independence but is in a position of dependence on the parents. On the other hand, the parents are developmentally ready to address their generativity needs by engaging in community activities, not by nurturing a family. One can readily appreciate the nature and extent of the family disequilibrium that may result from this situation.

Developmental crises are characterized by their predictability. For example, behavioral scientists know that a young married couple will have new demands placed on them when their first child is born. No matter how eagerly they may anticipate this event, many young parents react with depression and frustration when the infant's dependency needs cause them to alter their previous spontaneous lifestyle. During mid-life this couple may go through an anxiety-laden period when they question the value of the direction they have taken in their marriage, family, and work. Finally, the same couple might become depressed and frustrated once again when they find that their long-anticipated freedom from responsibility for childrearing is limited by the financial and physical limitations of old age. Although the transition from one developmental phase to another is always fraught with a certain degree of increased individual and familial tension, these transitional periods can be prevented from becoming crises through the use of anticipatory guidance.

Anticipatory guidance is primarily an educative process that helps prepare the individual and family for behavioral changes likely to occur in the near future. This process has been greatly aided by the proliferation of information about behavior during each developmental phase now available in newspapers, magazines, and paperback books. Therefore, many families successfully engage in their own anticipatory guidance without requiring the assistance of health care professionals.

Public health nurses are in a unique position to provide anticipatory guidance. As they visit families in their homes, they have the opportunity to assess the entire family situation, even though they might be present to give care to only one member. For example, the nurse might counsel the mother of a 2-year-old in regard to the meaning of his negativistic behavior while visiting the home to administer a parenteral diuretic to the grandmother. The opportunities for anticipatory guidance by nurses are not limited to home visits. The nurse is in a position to assess the family dynamics when a member is hospitalized for a physical illness and visitors seek out the nurse to ask advice covertly about their problems rather than those of the client. The astute nurse will recognize these clues and respond in a helpful way.

Situational crises

Situational crises cannot be as accurately predicted as developmental crises. Situational events that can precipitate a state of crisis include such major catastrophes as the unexpected death of a family member in an accident, the loss of a home through fire or flood, and sudden widespread economic depression, as occurred in the 1930s. The event does not have to be as catastrophic as these to precipitate a state of crisis. Any event, no matter how minor or even how desired it may superficially appear, may combine with the individual's or family's perception of it to produce a situation that is believed to be *hazardous* to the system's equilibrium. If the event is perceived as hazardous, and if the individual or family does not have adequate coping mechanisms available to ward off such a threat, a state of crisis will ensue. Although most people would understand why a family might enter into a state of crisis after their home was burned in a fire that killed their infant daughter, few lay people would understand why a family might enter a state of crisis after the father receives a major promotion to the position for which he has been striving for many years. In this example, the promotion might represent a threat to a satisfying lifestyle, a change in social class and social group, and increased responsibility for all family members. Therefore, although the family would undoubtedly gain many things they desire and have worked for, to do so they must give up the familiarity of their former life. They may not have immediately available the coping mechanisms necessary to make a smooth adjustment.

Whether the type of event that precipitated the crisis is developmental or situational, the characteristics of the crisis state remain essentially the same.

CHARACTERISTICS OF A CRISIS STATE

A crisis state is not an illness but rather an upset in the system's steady state. Although the behaviors displayed by those experiencing the crisis may vary, massive free-floating anxiety is at the basis of these behaviors. The anxiety may be perceived as such, or it may take the form of depression or anger at various points in the crisis state. Since great amounts of anxiety cannot be sustained by the human being without serious damage to the personality organization, individuals consciously and unconsciously actively seek to reorganize their personality in such a way that they rid themselves of this unbearable emotion. Therefore, *a state of crisis is self-limiting,* usually from 4 to 6 weeks in length. It is almost always resolved in this time frame, although not always in the healthiest way. If new, more adequate coping mechanisms are not developed within this period, the individual is likely to repress the events and emotions surrounding the crisis to avoid the further personality disorganization that would result from a prolonged, high level of anxiety. Thus a pseudoresolution to the state of crisis is achieved.

As previously discussed, a crisis state seems to be a response to an event, whether developmental or situational, that is perceived as hazardous. Consequently, a crisis state is highly individualized, and an event that may precipitate a crisis in one individual or family may not necessarily have the same effect on another individual or family. Hazardous events are further categorized into three groups: (1) those that represent a *threat* to fundamental instinctual needs or to the person's sense of integrity, (2) those that represent a real or perceived *loss,* and (3) those that represent a *challenge.*

Another characteristic of the crisis state is that *it rarely affects an individual without also affecting those significant others who comprise the individual's social support system.* In most instances, this system is the family group. Therefore, it is usually inappropriate to view an individual as being in a state of crisis without also

taking into consideration that it is highly likely the family is also in a state of crisis. This point has numerous implications for intervention. Any resolution to the crisis achieved by an individual in isolation from a previously established social system may be short lived if it is not workable within the system as a whole.

Because of the mobility of the U.S. population and the subsequent demise of the large, extended family, many persons have developed support systems that are not limited to and may not even include family members. Therefore, it is important to recognize that friends and neighbors may serve as significant others to an individual, even though these persons may not be relatives in the traditional sense. This social pattern is increasingly seen in older persons whose spouses have died and whose married children live far away. In all instances the individual being counseled should be the one who defines his or her significant social system, not the crisis counselor, who may be misled into making assumptions based on traditional societal patterns.

PHASES OF A CRISIS STATE

Whether an individual or a family is in a state of crisis, the crisis seems to run through a series of definable, although overlapping, phases.

The initial phase is **denial,** which usually lasts for a period of hours. Denial is a defense mechanism that the mind unconsciously employs to protect itself from the sudden assault of intense anxiety. Denial is evident when a 55-year-old executive calmly returns to his usual business activities after being informed by the corporate president that he has been fired. In most mentally healthy persons, the reality of the situation quickly becomes apparent and leads into the next phase of crisis, characterized by increased tension.

During the phase of **increased tension,** the persons involved make valiant efforts to continue their activities of daily living but do so while attempting to cope with ever-increasing amounts of anxiety. During this phase, therefore, the individual or family remains functional, although those who know them can easily see indications of increased tension in the form of hyperactivity or psychomotor retardation. A common example of this phase is seen in persons who are successfully making funeral arrangements for a loved one who has just died unexpectedly. The phase of increased tension is followed by disorganization.

During the phase of **disorganization,** those in a crisis seem to "fall apart." They can no longer continue with activities of daily living, become obsessively preoccupied with the event, and may remember earlier events they thought they had forgotten and that, unknown to them, have a symbolic link to the current situation. During this phase, persons are consciously flooded by great anxiety and fear they may be "losing their mind." Being in a state of crisis may or may not be apparent to them. If it is not, as is often the case, persons usually become highly anxious about their anxiety, thereby compounding the problem. Therefore it is during this phase that most persons seek professional help, if this has not been done earlier.

The next phase of a crisis is characterized by **attempts to reorganize.** With or without assistance, the individual or family attempts to bring previously used coping mechanisms to bear on the current situation. At this point the mechanisms used are likely to be short range and directed specifically at the immediate problem. For example, the homemaker who has not been able to mobilize sufficient energy to wash the dishes for the last 3 days may wheel the portable television into the kitchen in an attempt to divert her mind sufficiently to get through the increasingly large stack of dirty dishes. The mental mechanism this woman is using is suppression. If attempts at reorganization are successful at this point, they tend to build on one another and lead to general reorganization, the ultimate goal of crisis resolution. The affected persons grad-

ually resume their normal activities of daily living, becoming anxious and depressed only when specific stimuli are present to remind them of the crisis situation. The attempt at reorganization lasts for weeks, if successful.

A phase characterized by an **attempt to escape the problem** occurs within days if initial attempts to reorganize are unsuccessful. Without appropriate intervention, blaming typically occurs during this phase. The persons involved tend to "escape the problem" by projecting responsibility for its existence onto other people, societal institutions, or a supernatural phenomenon such as God or fate. Blaming behaviors, at the very least, create increased tension in a system already overwhelmed by stress and at worst lead to actions that ultimately compound rather than relieve the problem. For example, the husband who blames his wife's lack of supervision for their son's juvenile delinquency may initiate divorce proceedings only to find himself totally alone and still highly anxious a year later when the divorce becomes final. A couple who blame the rigid narrow-mindedness of the community in which they live for their failure to be accepted into the local country club may decide to move to a distant state only to find that they have left behind their primary support system, their co-workers. A highly religious man in this phase of crisis may officially leave his church as a means of publicly rejecting the God whom he blames for his problems. In so doing, he may also cut himself off from the human social system whose support he has used in the past and could benefit from now.

Regardless of whether the persons involved in the crisis resort to blaming behaviors or whether they attempt to escape the problem by consciously pretending it does not exist (as opposed to denial, which is an unconscious defense mechanism), this phase rarely results in a successful resolution to the crisis.

After failing at attempts to escape the problem, the individual or family moves into the phase of **local reorganization.** This phase has characteristics similar to the phase "attempts to reorganize" previously described.

After the local reorganization phase, the final phase of **general reorganization** occurs. It may take up to a year before new patterns of behavior are sufficiently well integrated into the individual's personality organization or the family's interactional structure and communication system to withstand additional stress on the system. However, the acute phase of the crisis is usually over within the 6-week period previously mentioned.

Unsuccessful resolution of a crisis state occurs when, during any phase, the individual or family adopts pathological means of adaptation, which serve to obscure and compound the crisis. This is most likely to occur when the individual's ego strength is already weakened or when the family has been using dysfunctional adaptations before the crisis. The outlook is particularly dim when skilled intervention is not sought or available and the persons involved resume functioning on a level lower than the one at which they had previously been functioning.

Pseudoresolution occurs when the crisis is repressed and the individual or family have learned nothing from the experience, returning to their former level of functioning. Although all may appear well, these people have missed a valuable opportunity to increase their repertoire of adaptive responses. Furthermore, future crises are likely to be compounded by the reemergence of the conflicts surrounding the previously unresolved repressed one. See Figure 24-1 for a schematic representation of the processes leading to successful, unsuccessful, or pseudoresolution of a crisis state.

TECHNIQUES OF CRISIS INTERVENTION

The goal of crisis intervention is to assist individuals to seek new and useful adaptive mechanisms within the context of their social support system. By so doing, the crisis counselor helps involved persons to reorganize their individual personalities and their social system on a higher level of functioning than that previously experienced. If this goal is achieved, these persons are better able to deal successfully with future developmental and situational events that inevitably will occur within their lifetimes.

It is important to note that many people in a state of crisis are not aware of this fact. They may come to or telephone a crisis intervention center with vague, diffuse complaints such as, "I can't sleep," "I'm afraid I'm losing my mind," or "I'm afraid that something dreadful is going to happen." On the other hand, friends or relatives may bring a person for treatment, stating that he is "not behaving like himself."

The initial step in intervention is to take the time to assess the situation thoroughly. Direct questions are appropriate, since the individual or family is likely to be in the phase of disorganization, during which it is very difficult for them to focus their thoughts and feelings. In addition to collecting identifying data, it is important to ask specifically who else is involved in the problem.

The next step is to define the event. The persons involved may state initially that nothing unusual has occurred. If they respond in this way, it is not because they are lying, but rather because they are truly unaware of the significance of the event in their lives. To elicit this information, it is helpful to ask persons to review in detail what has occurred in their lives over the past 2 weeks. If this account indicates nothing unusual, even with specific questioning, the interviewer asks clients to go back 1 week further. Rarely is it necessary to go back further than 4 weeks. In the course of the narrative, the precipitating event will probably become clear to the interviewer and sometimes to the client as well. If the client is still unaware of the hazardous event, the interviewer can repeat back the situation identified from the narrative and suggest that many people would find this situation troublesome. This intervention almost always elicits a surprised emotional response from the client.

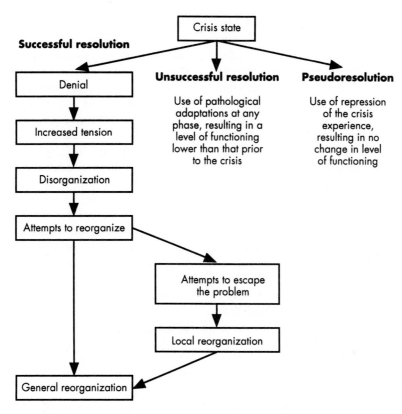

Figure 24-1

Processes leading to resolution of a crisis state. Successful resolution of such a state follows a series of phases before culminating in the ultimate goal of general reorganization. The initial four phases are experienced by all persons. Some persons may then move directly from attempts to reorganize to general reorganization. Others may need to take a temporary detour and attempt to escape the problem. When this attempt fails, they proceed to local reorganization, eventually reaching the goal of general reorganization. Successful resolution results in functioning at a level higher than that before the crisis.

CLINICAL EXAMPLE

Mrs. Curry received a regularly scheduled monthly visit from the public health nurse. Instead of finding her in the kitchen cleaning up after breakfast as usual, the nurse found Mrs. Curry sitting on the living room couch, still in her nightgown and robe, crying and wringing her hands. The nurse sat down next to her and asked what was wrong. Mrs. Curry replied, "I don't know. I don't know. I just feel awful, as if something horrible is happening to me. Please

help me." The nurse then asked if something unusual had happened since her last visit. Mrs. Curry replied, "No, nothing, except I am going crazy." The nurse asked Mrs. Curry to tell her how the days had been for her starting 2 weeks ago. Although Mrs. Curry protested mildly at having to go through the last 2 weeks in such detail, she complied with gentle questioning from the nurse. The nurse was not surprised to hear that Mrs. Curry's mother-in-law had moved into the home 6 days ago. After 1 or 2 days of settling-in activities, the mother-in-law requested to cook the meals "for my son" so that she would feel useful. Mrs. Curry stated that she felt resentful about turning over the meal preparation to her husband's mother but in turn felt guilty about her reaction, since she would now have more free time. As a result, she dismissed her feelings as "unreasonable," agreed to her mother-in-law's request, and made arrangements to go clothes shopping with a friend late the following afternoon. When the following afternoon arrived, Mrs. Curry could not meet her friend because she was immobilized by anxiety, the source of which was unknown to her. Since that time she had been relatively sleepless and decreasingly involved in the household activities. This narrative was related by Mrs. Curry matter-of-factly and with no particular emotion until the nurse said, "Many people find that when a new member of the family moves in, there is a major adjustment to make. I wonder if that's what could be troubling you?" At that point, Mrs. Curry began to sob but stopped wringing her hands.

Once the event and those involved have been identified, they are helped to develop a plan for coping with the crisis situation. To be effective in this step, the crisis counselor needs to explore with the clients the resources that are available and known to them and to suggest resources available in the community about which they might not know. Most mentally healthy people have numerous interpersonal, social, and community resources available to them but may need help to identify the appropriate ones to use and from which to accept aid. For clients to benefit from this step, they need to be encouraged to make as many arrangements for help as possible by themselves. However, since high levels of anxiety often interfere with cognitive comprehension and retention of information, it is important to write out information. For example, if it is decided that the clients could benefit from a talk with a representative of a social service agency,

the name and telephone number of the agency and a suggested day and time for the clients to call for an appointment should be clearly written down.

These steps in crisis intervention are designed to help the clients achieve a correct cognitive perception of the situation, which is enhanced by the counselor seeking the facts surrounding the situation and helping the clients keep the problem in their consciousness.

Another vital aspect of crisis intervention is assisting the clients in managing their feelings. To achieve this goal, the clients need to develop an awareness of their feelings. Appropriate verbalization of them, assisted by the reflection of the crisis counselor, leads to desensitization and mastery of the feelings that seem overwhelming. In helping clients deal with their feelings, it is important not to give them false reassurance, although it is helpful to tell them that they are likely to feel better in 1 or 2 months despite this perhaps seeming impossible at this point. As previously stated, it is also important not to encourage them to blame others. If the counselor falls into this trap, the result is to support the clients' natural avoidance of looking at their own behavior, thereby decreasing their opportunities to develop more mature patterns of coping.

All these steps are usually gone through in the initial contact with persons in a crisis. Such an interview may take longer than the traditional 50-minute therapy hour. Since the best results in crisis situations seem to be achieved through intensive but short-term intervention, it is advisable to spend as much time as necessary, as often as necessary, with the clients without engendering unwarranted dependency. At the end of the first visit, the crisis counselor makes a specific appointment to see the clients again, preferably in a few days but no longer than a week later. In the meantime, the clients should know how they can contact the counselor and should be encouraged to do so if they think it is necessary.

Often the knowledge that help is readily available is sufficient to enable the clients to manage without a telephone call until the next appointment.

During subsequent contacts the clients are assisted to go through the same steps again. In addition, the plan made in the previous session needs to be evaluated in terms of its effectiveness. If it seems to be working, the plan should be reinforced by supporting the clients' efforts at implementation. If the plan is not working or if new factors have altered the situation, the plan needs to be revised accordingly, but always with the mutual agreement of those involved.

In summary, crisis intervention is designed to help essentially healthy persons who are in a state of disequilibrium to help themselves. This goal is facilitated by assisting them to achieve correct cognitive perception of the situation and to gain effective management of their emotions. **Successful resolution** of crisis situations results in clients developing a larger repertoire of adaptive mechanisms, which in turn enables them to function on a level higher than the level on which they were functioning before the crisis state. In this way, effective crisis intervention prevents mental illness and promotes mental health.

KEY POINTS

1. Because society is more accepting of mental health treatment, more people voluntarily seek help for problems that are not indicative of long-standing dysfunction.

2. After a crisis, an individual may reintegrate at a lower level of functioning, at the same level, or at a higher, healthier level than before the crisis.

3. Events that may precipitate crises are developmental (predictable) or situational (unexpected).

4. Developmental crises can be prevented through anticipatory guidance, which helps prepare the individual and family for behavioral changes likely to occur in the near future.

5. A crisis state is not seen as an illness but rather as an upset in the steady state of the system, in which massive free-floating anxiety occurs.

6. A state of crisis is self-limiting, usually from 4 to 6 weeks' duration.

7. A crisis state seems to be a response to an event perceived as hazardous—a threat, a loss, or a challenge.

8. A crisis state affecting an individual usually also affects the significant others who constitute the social support system.

9. The first four phases of a crisis state are experienced by all persons: denial, increased tension, disorganization, and attempts to reorganize.

10. An attempt to escape the problem occurs if initial attempts to reorganize are unsuccessful. Failure to escape is followed by local reorganization and, finally, general reorganization.

11. Unsuccessful resolution of a crisis state occurs when pathological adaptations are used at any phase of the crisis state. Pseudoresolution occurs when the crisis experience is repressed and leads to no change in the level of functioning.

12. The goal of crisis intervention is to assist the individual to seek new and useful adaptive mechanisms within the context of the social support system.

13. An effective plan for coping with the crisis situation must include awareness of available resources.

14. To manage their feelings successfully, clients need to develop an awareness of them.

SUGGESTED SOURCES OF ADDITIONAL INFORMATION

Aguilera DC: *Crisis intervention: theory and methodology,* ed 6, St Louis, 1990, Mosby–Year Book.

Britton JG, Mattson-Melcher DM: The crisis home: sheltering patients in emotional crisis, *J Psychosoc Nurs Ment Health Serv* 23:18, December 1985.

Crisis intervention, *Adv Nurs Sci* 6, 1984.

Gaston S: Death and midlife crisis, *J Psychosoc Nurs Ment Health Serv* 18:31, January 1980.

Harrison DF: Nurses and disasters, *J Psychosoc Nurs Ment Health Serv* 19:34, December 1981.

Hatch C, Schut L: Description of a crisis-oriented psychiatric home visiting service, *J Psychosoc Nurs Ment Health Serv* 18:31, April 1980.

Hayes G and others: After disaster: a crisis support team at work, *Am J Nurs* 90:61, February 1990.

Mishel MH and others: Uncertainty in illness theory: a replication of the mediating effects of mastery and coping, *Nurs Res* 40:236, July/August 1991.

Mitchell CE: Identifying the hazard: the key to crisis intervention, *Am J Nurs* 77:1194, 1977.

Murphy S: After Mount St. Helens: disaster stress research, *J Psychosoc Nurs Ment Health Serv* 22:8, July 1984.

Norman E: PTSD: the victims who survived, *Am J Nurs* 82:1696, 1982.

Parad HJ, editor: *Crisis intervention: selected readings,* New York, 1965, Family Service Association of America.

Sheehy G: *Passages: predictable crises of adult life,* New York, 1976, EP Dutton.

Webster DC: Solution-focused approaches in psychiatric/mental health nursing, *Perspect Psychiatr Care* 26(4):17, 1990.

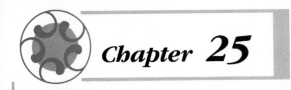

Chapter 25

Group Theory and Intervention

Power and control phase
Working phase
Group cohesiveness
Termination phase
Psychodrama
Abreaction
Catharsis
Transactional analysis
Gestalt therapy
Facilitators

CHAPTER OUTLINE
Historical perspective
Characteristics of groups
Group therapy
   Considerations in establishing a therapy group
   Characteristics of group therapy
   Group development
   The leader's role
Socialization groups: a remotivation technique
Psychodrama
Transactional analysis
Gestalt therapy
Selection of a therapeutic group
Growth and self-actualization groups

LEARNING OBJECTIVES
After studying this chapter, the student will be able to:

* Discuss the characteristics of groups.

* State the goal of a therapeutic group.

* Discuss the developmental phases of a therapeutic group.

* State examples of the role of the leader in each phase of group development.

* Discuss the characteristics of socialization groups.

* Describe psychodrama, transactional analysis, and gestalt therapy as group interventions.

KEY TERMS
Group association
Subgroups
Role
Norms
Attractiveness
Preaffiliation phase

Human beings spend most of their time in group situations. They live, work, play, learn, and worship in groups. **Group association** is a prominent part of everyone's life because human beings are inherently social and because in complex, technological societies, individuals are interdependent and must rely on each other for services. Therefore the nature of our humanness and the nature of the society in which we live dictate the necessity for a social structure organized around groups.

The individual's first experience with groups occurs in infancy when he or she is incorporated into the family, a specialized type of natural group. The second major group situation most people experience is school. Significant group associations continue throughout the entire life span. Despite the pervasiveness of groups in our society, however, few persons give any thought to the nature and function of groups.

HISTORICAL PERSPECTIVE

Interestingly, the intervention known as group therapy did not originate within the mental health care delivery system. Rather, it began in 1905 as a technique to assist patients with tuberculosis to learn about their illness and to receive emotional support from each other. The success of these groups soon led to their use with patients who had "nervous disorders." Not until World War II did group therapy became a standard intervention for the treatment of persons diagnosed with a mental illness.

During World War II, many members of the civilian population and many Armed Forces personnel required psychiatric help. It became obvious that the traditional treatment methods at that time could not provide the help required by the large population of individuals who had a mental illness. To make maximum use of psychiatrically trained personnel, a plan was initiated through which patients were encouraged to talk out their problems in groups. As psychiatrists worked with this method and developed an ef-

fective technique that could be taught to others, it became apparent not only that group therapy was a more efficient means by which relatively few personnel could treat many, but also, more importantly, that this mode of therapy had effects that could not be achieved through individual, one-to-one therapy. Some theorists believe one reason for this positive effect is that groups tend to simulate the familial situation; the leaders are seen in the role of parent figures and group members are seen as siblings. Therefore, it becomes possible for persons who have had difficulty in their early family relationships to work experientially through many problems as a result of their interaction with other group members. Group members also find support and reassurance in the realization that others have problems similar to theirs. Consequently, group intervention is seen as the treatment of choice for some individuals.

CHARACTERISTICS OF GROUPS

A group is not a mere collection of individuals. Rather, a group is an identifiable system composed of three or more individuals who engage in certain tasks to achieve a common goal. Furthermore, to be a group, the members must relate to each other, usually around the tasks and goals of the group. The individuals who ride the elevator in a skyscraper office building to reach their offices may share the common goal of going to work, but they rarely relate to each other about this goal. Therefore, they would not be considered a group. If, however, the elevator stalled between floors and its occupants expressed their fears to each other, offered each other emotional support, made plans to get themselves out of their predicament, or otherwise began relating to each other, they would quickly become a group in the technical sense of the word.

As identifiable systems, groups share certain characteristics regardless of their differences in size, task, or goal. Since nursing care is often rendered in group situations, it is important for the nurse to develop an understanding of these characteristics.

Groups can be composed of as few as three or as many as 20 members. The upper limit of membership size is determined by the number of individuals who can easily relate to each other at the same time. In most group situations, it is not possible for more than 20 people to meet this criterion, and even then difficulty is encountered. When a group is larger than the number of individuals who can comfortably relate to one another simultaneously, **subgroups** are formed. For example, the 100-member senior class at the local high school cannot possibly function as a total group but is likely to be an aggregate of subgroups. Groups that are very small (three or four members) also are not likely to be the most effective, since insufficient membership may exist to fulfill all the roles necessary for the achievement of the group's goal.

All groups have goals, which may be multiple or single. Multiple goals may have equivalent importance, or they may be prioritized according to their value. Group members may or may not be equally aware of and supportive of the group's goals. However, the group's effectiveness is strongly related to the degree to which the members are aware of and supportive of the goals. When the goals have been achieved, the group either disbands or determines new goals. Natural groups, such as families, tend to remain as groups by redefining their goals. Groups that have been formed around a single goal tend to disband after achievement of that goal. An example of such a group is the previously mentioned high-school senior class. The graduating seniors typically feel a strong group association and promise to maintain contact with each other after graduation, but because the group has achieved its goal and disbands, the group members rarely follow through on their promise.

A group is a system and, as such, functions in a manner designed to maintain its equilibrium. Therefore the behavior of any one member affects and is affected by all other group members

and must be seen as reflective of group behavior. Learning to view group behavior from a holistic perspective, rather than as a summation of individual interactions, is a difficult task for most students. A frequently used example that may be helpful in this regard is a symphony orchestra. If the listener attends to only the notes played by each individual, the person will have a distorted impression of how the finished piece sounds, since each musician contributes only a part of what is necessary to the completed piece. However, when a listener attends to the contributions of all the musicians put together, a synchronized, harmonious piece is heard. This example not only illustrates the concept that the whole is different from and greater than the sum of its parts, but also implies that each part is necessary and of great value. In a group, individuals have great value, but the result of their interactions is a product that can be best appreciated only when viewed from a group perspective.

The interactional behavior of the group's members has a great effect on the group's ability to achieve its goal. The term used to designate the behavior of group members is **role.** A role is the characteristic behavioral pattern employed by a group member and is determined by the personality of the individual and the needs of the group. At any point in time, the group has a need to address the tasks necessary to achieve its goal, while simultaneously maintaining its existence. Addressing the task is achieved through roles that have a content orientation, and group maintenance is achieved through roles that have a process orientation.

The *content* of a group is the overt verbal exchange, whereas the *process* is the underlying meaning the content has to the group, not to the individual. For example, Mr. Jones might say, "I'm not sure how to proceed." If Mr. Jones is viewed as an individual rather than as a group member, the content of his statement could lead one to believe that he feels insecure, a somewhat negative assessment. If this same content is viewed within the context of a group, it would be more appropriate to interpret the process as a need of the group for orientation and Mr. Jones as fulfilling the role of orienter. This interpretation not only conveys a positive tone, but also is more accurate than the individually based one.

The roles assumed by group members relate to either the content or to the process of the group. Task-oriented or content-oriented roles, as suggested by Robert Bales,* include coordinator, orienter, recorder, observer and commentator, opinion seeker or giver, elaborater, information seeker or giver, and initiator. Roles related to group maintenance or a process orientation include energizer, encourager, dominator, aggressor, compromiser, blocker, harmonizer, and rejecter.

These lists of roles are not intended to reflect all the possible roles a group member could assume. However, they do represent the most frequently seen behaviors of group members, and they also illustrate the reciprocal nature of content and process interactions (e.g., information seeker or giver, encourager or blocker).

Since human beings have numerous experiences in many groups, by the time they reach adulthood most have developed a large repertoire of group behaviors. Therefore any one individual may assume different roles in different groups and different roles at different times in the same group, dependent in part on the group's needs. Consequently, it is impossible to predict with complete assurance the role any individual will assume in a group. Furthermore, since the behavior of any group member affects and is affected by all other group members, it is not unusual for an individual to behave in a group in a way that is quite different from how he or she behaves when relating to only one other individual.

To function effectively, groups develop rules

or **norms** that govern their operation. Some norms may be externally imposed, but the norms with the most meaning are those that have emerged from within the group. For example, group members are much more likely not to smoke if that norm was established by the group rather than by the superintendent of the building in which they meet. Norms are sometimes fully known to all members and therefore can be explicitly stated. Other norms are not consciously formulated by the group but rather have evolved as a result of the group's experience. Whether the group norms are explicit or implicit, their purpose is to influence the group's behavior. Since implicit norms cannot be overtly conveyed, individuals who join an established group may be in a precarious position because they may unknowingly violate an implicit norm and receive a negative, nonverbal reaction from the others. The violation of implicit group norms is the basis of many social faux pas. The power of implicit norms is attested to by the excruciating embarrassment experienced by the person who has committed a social error, even when the reality of the error does not warrant such a reaction.

Another characteristic of groups is that each group has a unique identity, while at the same time sharing much in common with all other groups. The student will recognize this characteristic as also being true of individuals. The uniqueness of each group is based on the specific interactional combination of its size, its goals and the tasks designed to achieve its goals, the roles its members characteristically assume, and the norms the members establish to govern its operation. On the other hand, all groups share enough in common that an individual is able to apply what has been learned in previous group associations to new group experiences. When a group is first formed, its members tend to behave in the ways they found to be successful in previous groups. As the group develops its own unique characteristics, its members modify their behavior to a greater or lesser degree to adapt

*Bales R: *Interaction process analysis: a method for the study of small groups,* Reading, Mass, 1950, Addison-Wesley.

to the group's uniqueness, thereby further enlarging their repertoire of group behaviors.

The unique identity of a group is often recognized by both members and nonmembers. The student should be familiar with the "in-group, out-group" phenomenon, in which two superficially identical groups are valued very differently by their members. The group term for the value placed on a group by both its members and nonmembers is **attractiveness.** An in-group is seen as being attractive, an out-group unattractive. The group's degree of attractiveness is determined to a large extent by its unique identity; the mere altering of a few members, goals, or norms does not succeed in altering the group's identity or resultant attractiveness.

Finally, all groups, as with individuals, go through predictable developmental phases. However, the time at which the group moves from one phase to another is not as uniform as with individual development. Rather, the speed of group development is determined by several factors unique to the group, such as the anticipated duration of the group's life, the developmental strengths and weaknesses of its members, the importance the group places on its goal, the relevance of its norms to its goals, and the group's attractiveness. In addition, groups may skip developmental phases for a variety of reasons. However, all groups must go through beginning and ending phases. These and the intermediate phases of group development are described in conjunction with the discussion of group therapy in this chapter.

GROUP THERAPY

Considerations in establishing a therapy group

Group psychotherapists differ in their approach when establishing a therapeutic group. Questions involving the size of the membership, the frequency of meetings, and the characteristics of the participants must be decided. As might be expected, authorities answer these questions according to their personal treatment philosophies.

Some group psychotherapists insist on a balanced group, which means that only individuals of the same age, sex, and diagnostic category should be included. Others do not believe that a balanced group is necessary or even conducive to the best possible group interaction. Another consideration is whether to include persons with different levels of intelligence or verbal skills. Since group therapy depends on effective communication skills, this may be an important consideration.

Certainly a decision must be made as to the group's size. Most authorities agree that a group should not be larger than 10, but many group leaders prefer a group no larger than six. They also agree that the membership of a group should be stable.

A definite place in which to hold the group meeting must be identified. It should be quiet, comfortable, and private. The frequency and time of meeting must be decided, as well as the date when group meetings will begin and end. When these decisions have been made and the group has come together for the first time, these norms should be shared with the members so that they will understand the nature of the contract they have with each other and with the group leader.

Some group leaders prefer to talk with potential group members before the actual group meetings begin. In this way, each individual is acquainted with the nature of the sessions before the first meeting.

Characteristics of group therapy

The therapeutic group, as with other groups, has a specific goal. It differs from a social group because its goal is to assist individuals to alter their behavioral patterns and to develop new and more effective ways of dealing with the stressors of daily living. To achieve this goal, individuals meet together regularly for a stated period to express their ideas, feelings, and concerns; to

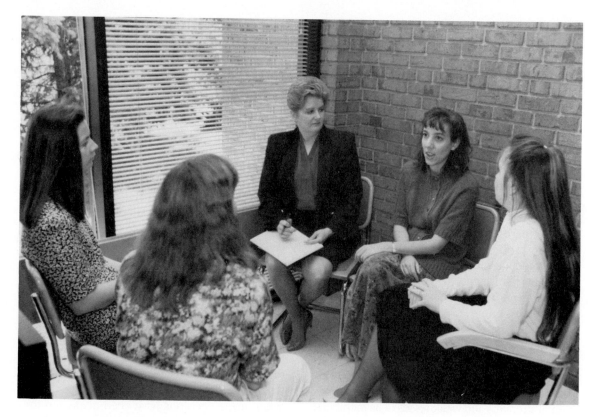

Figure 25-1
Group therapy.

examine their current ways of behaving; and to develop new patterns of behavior.

The group leader works to develop among the group members a sense of trust in her or him as an individual and as a group leader. The leader avoids being critical or judgmental of the behavior of individual group members and relies on group action to control unacceptable behavior. The group leader strives to convey to the group members an acceptance of them as individuals and respect for them as people. The leader avoids exerting undue control over the group or being the authority in the situation.

For a group to have maximum therapeutic effect, it is essential that members learn to know and trust not only the leader but also each other. Therefore, this becomes an important goal, the achievement of which is facilitated by the leader when she or he refers questions to the group, encourages participation from all members, and shows acceptance and respect for each individual. By engaging in these behaviors, the leader acts as a role model for the members. The inexperienced group leader will be surprised at how quickly the group members learn to act toward each other in the manner suggested by the leader's behavior.

Group development

Every group, as with every individual, progresses through several developmental phases.

The first developmental phase of a group is the **preaffiliation phase** or *becoming acquainted phase*. During this time, group members behave toward each other as strangers and are obviously distrustful of each other and of the leader. Their expectations of the group activity are, of necessity, determined by experiences they have had in other groups. Although members are likely to be overtly polite to each other, their behavior also indicates an approach-avoidance dilemma. That is, most members are eager to become involved with each other but simultaneously fear the risks that such involvement may entail. During this stage the leader is most effective when she or he provides structure, protects members from embarrassment by not allowing them to prematurely reveal highly personal information, and gently invites trust.

The second developmental period is the **power and control phase** of experiencing intragroup conflict. Unavoidably, conflict will emerge during this time, since the members are in the process of establishing their positions in the group relative to the positions of other members and the leader. Often, group members look at the leader for sanction or condemnation of another member. If leaders fall into this trap, they are likely to find the group critical of them because of their decision. In this instance, it is always wise to deflect the question about a member's behavior back to the group by a comment such as, "I wonder what the rest of you think about Mr. Jones's question?" During this second phase of group development, the group attempts to formalize relationships through the establishment of explicit norms. These attempts should be supported as long as they do not infringe on the rights or safety of one or more members. Throughout the group process, the leader has the responsibility of protecting the safety of individuals and property, but the necessity for doing so becomes greatest during this second phase of group development. During the second phase, group sessions may seem nonproductive in that the members alternate competitive, aggressive behavior with apathetic withdrawal. Interrelated with this phenomenon is the great danger of membership dropout.

If the leader can help the group safely navigate through this phase, characteristics of the third phase will emerge. This is called the **working phase** or the *phase of intimacy and differentiation*. During this phase the group's work is achieved. It is a period of relatively high communication in which members appropriately share personal feelings and concerns about emotional problems.

During the group's working phase, the members' sense of belonging, or **group cohesiveness,** is at its highest. When a group is cohesive, its members tend to feel emotionally close to one another, and individuals respond well to advice offered by other members. Consequently, during this period an opportunity exists for emotional reeducation and relearning. The members discover through the reactions of the other group members that there are many different reactions to their feelings and behavior. They come to realize how universal their problems are and that they are not as unique in their difficulties as they may have believed.

The last developmental phase is precipitated by the approaching time for the group to conclude its meetings. Thus it is the **termination phase** and may require several meetings to work through the feelings of the group members. The goal of the termination phase is to help group members integrate what they have learned about themselves and the behavioral changes they have made so that they can use these in the future. If the termination phase is not handled skillfully, not only will this goal not be achieved, but the group members may also leave the group feeling that the only thing to be gained by group association is more emotional pain. During this period the members relive previous periods when they experienced personal loss of someone very close to them. They may express feelings of being abandoned, rejected, or forsaken. The expression of these feelings provides an excellent opportunity to help individual group members deal with these feelings and work through them.

Four phases of group development have been described. However, these phases overlap one another, and only the first and the last are seen in all groups. Groups that meet for only a few sessions or groups whose members have great difficulty in trusting others are not likely to be able to move through the phase of experiencing intragroup conflict and the working phase. Consequently, the termination phase will not be as meaningful and therefore not as difficult as when the group has traveled successfully through all developmental phases.

The leader's role

The group leader is the key to a successful group therapy experience. Leaders need to be aware of their own behavior and its effect on others. The effectiveness of the preaffiliation phase for the group largely depends on how the leader orients the members to the group process, to each other, and to the leader. The phase of experiencing intragroup conflict can be successfully resolved if the group leader is able to be supportive to the members and successfully establishes a feeling of acceptance and respect for all. As the group moves into the working phase, the leader is able to involve the less verbal members by redirecting questions to them or by asking them for their perceptions of a situation. The leader sometimes provides essential factual information that is important to the resolution of an issue. On occasion the leader may help members learn what others think about their behavior or their responses. The leader assists members in exploring situations they bring to the group from the outside and helps them to think through and test out more appropriate ways of responding.

As the group develops, the leader will be confronted with a variety of specific problems in group interaction that will necessitate intervention. Problems such as members' silence, monopolizing behavior, tardiness, and acting out typically occur and require the leader's skill if the group session is to be effective. It is beyond the scope of this text to discuss these problems and possible appropriate interventions, but the student should be aware that excellent references are available that provide specific direction. However, the most effective group leaders are able to vary their style of intervention based on their assessment of the group's needs.

Skillful termination of a group requires first and foremost that leaders recognize their own feelings of loss. If they recognize their feelings, they are less likely to act them out by doing such things as "forgetting" the final meeting, acting punitively to members who express a sense of loss, or promising members that they will maintain contact when this is not possible or desired. The skillful group leader will understand that the anger at her or him and other members typically expressed during this phase is a reflection of the severity of the loss the members are experiencing. The leader will not respond to anger with anger but will help the group members to acknowledge their sadness about the disbanding of the group.

Finally, the skillful group leader will help the group members to identify what they have gained through their association. If they identify these gains, the members will be able to take away something concrete that helps to offset the emotional loss.

Many group therapists believe that it is most beneficial to the group if two staff members act as co-therapists. In this situation, one therapist is able to concentrate on the content being expressed while the other therapist focuses primarily on the group process. Although the co-therapists may change their function from one group session to another, it is believed that co-leaders who are experienced and comfortable with each other can view the group more comprehensively and therefore provide the group

with helpful direction in regard to both content and process.

SOCIALIZATION GROUPS: A REMOTIVATION TECHNIQUE

Psychiatric hospitals are frequently heavily populated with clients who appear to have lost interest in reality, to have lost a sense of personal value, and who seem to be unaware of other persons with whom they come in daily contact. Group interaction is one of the most successful ways of stimulating these people to rekindle their interest in their surroundings.

The nurse may be the only person who is available or interested in developing some form of group experience that will encourage these individuals to begin to communicate with each other and with the staff. The primary goal of these group activities is to facilitate socialization and is most easily achieved by focusing on a task. If several persons come together as a group and carry on an activity for a few sessions, the initial attempt has been successful.

The focus of the group activity depends almost entirely on the individuals to be included as members. Their age, educational backgrounds, and physical health will greatly influence the choice of activities that can be suggested.

Some individuals might be interested in a current events discussion group. Others who show no interest in reading the newspaper or listening to television news reports would not be interested in such a group activity. Some might be interested in forming a poetry reading group, whereas others would abhor such an activity. Some might enjoy sewing or knitting while they visit together; others would not.

In view of this wide variation in personal abilities and taste, the first rule to follow in initiating any recreational or motivational activity is to be well acquainted with the individuals who will form the group membership. The leader will find that it is wise to encourage the members to participate in selecting the focus for the group meetings. Although the leader will formulate some tentative plans for the first meeting, these need to be flexible and easily changed in case the members have other suggestions.

The leader will find that at first many persons will be reluctant to participate. Some individuals may require more than one friendly invitation to attend. Some who have lost interest in reality carry on an active fantasy life. Any group activity must compete with these fantasies for the individual's attention and enjoyment. Thus the leader should offer the group members refreshments during the initial group meetings. As the group becomes cohesive, the members' interest in the group activity may become great enough to overshadow the food as the major enjoyment of the meeting.

The leader should vary the focus of the group activity from time to time to maintain the interest of the group members. As the members become acquainted with one another, they themselves will suggest changes in the focus or the format of the meeting.

The following are some concrete suggestions for planning an effective socialization group experience*:

1. Develop a flexible plan that provides for change and spontaneity.
2. Encourage all group members to participate in planning.
3. Keep the plan practical and within achievable limits.
4. Initiate activities that group members are able to handle.
5. Provide something specific such as refreshments that will give each group member some tangible satisfaction.
6. Avoid monotony by varying the focus of group activity.
7. Maintain consistency in the feeling tone of

---

*Brown M, Fowler GR: *Psychodynamic nursing—a biosocial orientation,* ed 4, Philadelphia, 1972, Saunders.

each meeting so that group members' expectations will be fulfilled.

PSYCHODRAMA

Another type of therapeutic experience sometimes provided for a group of clients is called **psychodrama.** This technique was developed by J.L. Moreno, a psychiatrist who began working with emotionally disturbed individuals in a theater in Vienna as early as 1941. Psychodrama is usually conducted by a leader who has been especially prepared to direct this type of activity. Although a variety of methods may be used, one of the more frequent techniques places the leader on a stage in front of an audience of clients and staff members. The leader identifies a situation in which interpersonal conflict is involved, then invites members of the audience to come to the stage to act out this human relations problem.

When members of the audience agree to accept parts in the drama, they are told the essential facts about the roles they are to play. The chosen situation frequently focuses on a conversation with the significant members of a family. In the role of an actor, individuals are given a specially selected part that affords them an opportunity to express their inner conflicts freely as a situation is acted out with other performers who symbolize or represent persons who are the real objects of the individuals' love or hate. For example, a son who normally represses his hostility toward his father may freely express it as an actor and may even reveal its basis. On the other hand, if he is induced to take the father role, he may then be more objective and understanding about his father's point of view. It is surprising how effectively individuals fill the roles to which they are assigned and how realistically feelings are expressed. The leader stops the action when he or she believes the enactment has progressed far enough to provide the audience with a basis for a fruitful discussion.

Another method that has been used productively in psychodrama is for the leader to request a volunteer from the audience to come forward to set up a situation that the person wishes to portray. This person is also asked to select individuals from the audience to play the parts required and to provide the players with the necessary information about the roles they will enact. This technique focuses specifically on some personal concern of the individual who volunteered to develop the psychodramatic situation. With either of these methods, individuals from the audience may be asked to come forward to play the role of alter ego for the major characters in the psychodrama.

After the role playing is completed, the people in the audience are given an opportunity to discuss the situation they have witnessed and experienced vicariously. The participants from the audience may focus attention on various aspects of the situation and frequently present similar life experiences.

Psychodrama provides individuals with an opportunity to express feelings and concerns that relate to a personal human relations situation that is similar to, but not identical to, a personal problem of their own. Thus, psychodrama has somewhat the same therapeutic effect as **abreaction,** the lessening of emotional trauma by reenacting the situation. It also furnishes individuals with an opportunity for **catharsis,** an opportunity to express feelings freely. As in other group therapy situations, the individual is helped by the group to express feelings and consider them objectively.

The nurse is frequently involved in psychodrama as a role player or as a discussant. Skill and understanding of psychodrama are developed through continued participation in this treatment modality. Eventually the nurse may accept the role of the leader of the psychodrama sessions.

TRANSACTIONAL ANALYSIS

Transactional analysis is both a theoretical framework and a treatment method developed by Eric Berne. Its popularity and usefulness are attested to by the amount of literature available to lay persons on the subject. As a theory, transactional analysis postulates that each person has three elements of personality in greater or lesser operation at any given point in time: (1) the immature, need-gratifying aspect, referred to as the Child; (2) the moralistic, rigid, standard-setting aspect, referred to as the Parent; (3) and the mature, reality-based aspect, referred to as the Adult. The student will notice the similarity between this theoretical formulation and Freud's conception of the id, superego, and ego, respectively. Unlike Freudian theory, however, Berne's construct does not imply a judgment about the existence of these personality elements. Rather, he states that problems arise only when an incongruency exists among the elements operating when people relate with each other. This belief is the foundation for his use of the term *transactional*. The emphasis on dysfunctional interpersonal relationships as the crux of emotional problems is reminiscent of Sullivan's theories. Consequently, Berne's theory of transactional analysis is seen by many as effectively combining the salient intrapsychic features of Freudian theory and the aspects of Sullivanian theory that provide direction for therapeutic intervention.

When persons communicate and the adult elements of their personalities are operative, they probably will be effective in hearing and responding to each other. In addition, the nonverbal aspects of the process will be congruent with the verbal content, and no hidden messages will be perceived by either person. Each will reality test on the basis of feedback received, and each is likely to think that the interaction has been satisfying. This is not to imply that no differences of opinion will arise during such an interaction, but the individuals will probably believe that any differences are based on content issues rather than on covert attempts to dominate, control, or otherwise minimize the value of the other person. Adult-Adult interactions are effective and therefore desired interactional processes when the participants are engaged in problem-solving or task-oriented activities.

Another effective, desired interactional process occurs when two or more chronological adults simultaneously have the Child element of their personalities in preeminence. At these times they have fun "playing." Many adults have had the experience of spontaneously engaging in what appear to be foolish or childlike activities with another adult, such as frolicking through a park on a beautiful autumn day instead of attending a scheduled meeting. As long as this behavior does not have major irreversible consequences and does not become a persistent pattern, it can enhance the individuals' feelings of well-being and strengthen the relationship.

Problems arise when two persons characteristically relate to each other through divergent elements of their personalities. For example, a husband who relates to his wife through the Parent element of his personality will feel continuously dissatisfied with their interactions unless she responds with the Child element of her personality. If she does respond in this way, there may be little initial conflict because both their needs are superficially being met. However, neither is engaged in reality-testing behaviors, and neither can change interactional elements without open conflict emerging. Therefore, this pattern is growth stifling for both partners.

The previous situation is merely one example of a common interactional problem. The student can speculate as to the variety of interactional problems that can occur when two or more people interact from the basis of incongruent personality elements. For more detailed explanations of transactional analysis, the student is referred to the many excellent books on the subject.

Transactional analysis as a method of treatment is most effective as a form of family therapy. When this is not possible, it can be effectively implemented as a method of group therapy, in which the group members consciously and unconsciously assume characteristic familial roles.

In either the family or group setting, the participants can analyze their reactions and subsequent behavior in light of the Child-Parent-Adult framework and experience how they affect others and are affected by them. They also can experiment with using other elements of their personality and can receive immediate feedback.

Transactional analysis is also used for individual treatment. The effectiveness of this treatment modality is limited, however, since the client has only one other person with whom to interact, and feedback about behavioral changes in life situations is delayed. Nevertheless, many therapists successfully adopt some of the concepts of transactional analysis in their treatment of individuals because these concepts are seen by many clients as easy to understand and relevant to their life situations.

Regardless of setting, the primary role of the transactional therapist is to observe and comment tactfully on the discrepancies between the personality elements of those engaged in the interactional process. The therapist often suggests and supports role playing with another personality element so that the person can experience its effects. The dynamics that underlie the person's use of one personality element as opposed to the other two are not always explored. If they are discussed, it is usually done in the context of the present rather than in terms of childhood experiences.

GESTALT THERAPY

Gestalt therapy is as much a philosophy as it is an intervention technique. Its developer is Frederic S. Perls, who has trained many others in its use. The emphasis in gestalt therapy is on treatment of the person as a holistic being, placing as much importance on somatic responses as on emotional responses. Proponents of gestalt therapy believe that many persons' problems emanate from individuals having lost touch with their feelings, both physical and emotional. If one is unaware of what one is feeling, the likelihood of being able express these feelings is greatly diminished, and therefore one is unlikely to have one's needs met. Therefore, treatment consists primarily of helping individuals increase sensory awareness of their present state. Once individuals begin the process of "getting in touch" with themselves, their current relationships with others and with the environment are explored. The configuration of the holistic being in interaction with others and with the environment is referred to as the *gestalt* and is heavily based on systems theory. Although it is acknowledged that multiple factors produced the individual's current responses, the understanding of these factors is not believed to alleviate the present problems, and they are therefore not explored.

As with transactional analysis, the principles of gestalt therapy can be used in a one-to-one psychotherapeutic relationship but are most often practiced as a form of group therapy. Eight to 10 participants are seen as an ideal number for a gestalt group. The environment in which the group meets is viewed as instrumental in facilitating self-awareness. Therefore, factors such as comfortable chairs, a pleasing decor, and adequate space are seen as essential. Techniques such as role playing and ventilation are used frequently. The ultimate goal of gestalt therapy is to assist clients to fulfill their potential, and therefore it is appropriately used with individuals interested in self-growth and with persons who are emotionally disturbed.

SELECTION OF A THERAPEUTIC GROUP

The type of group activity most appropriate for persons depends on several variables, including their degree of ego strength and current insight into their problems. A person whose contact with reality is tenuous probably would benefit most from a socialization group rather than from a more formal group psychotherapy session. As clients gain more ego strength, they may be introduced into a group whose primary goal

is supportive therapy. As members progress in this type of group, the focus of the group may change to insight therapy. This is not to say that socialization groups do not have therapeutic effects, but rather that the degree of stress persons are able to tolerate should be a major determining factor in the decision as to the type of group in which they will participate. Furthermore, this determination should be made jointly by the multidisciplinary health care team, which is able to view the client from a variety of perspectives.

GROWTH AND SELF-ACTUALIZATION GROUPS

Other types of groups, such as sensitivity, encounter, and self-help groups, are well known in our society. The nature of these groups is not discussed here because expert leaders, or **facilitators,** of these groups believe that their primary goal is not and should not be therapeutic but rather educative, in the sense of self-growth, self-actualization, and increased self-awareness. Therefore, these types of groups are rarely, if ever, used with persons who have a mental illness, and the nurse is not likely to be involved with them in a professional capacity. Nevertheless, much literature is available about these groups, which the student may be interested in exploring.

KEY POINTS

1. A group is an identifiable system composed of three or more individuals who engage in certain tasks to achieve a common goal.
2. To be a group, members must relate to one another, usually around the tasks and goals of the group.
3. An effective group is large enough to fulfill all the roles necessary to achieve the group's goals and small enough so that its members can comfortably relate to one another at the same time.
4. All groups have goals; in effective groups the members are aware of and support the group's goals.

5. Individuals have great value in a group, but the result of their interactions is best appreciated when viewed from a group perspective.

6. The group needs to address the tasks necessary to achieve its goal while also maintaining its life.

7. An individual may assume different roles in different groups and different roles at different times in the same group.

8. To function effectively, groups develop norms that govern their operation. Norms with the most meaning are those that have emerged from within the group.

9. Each group has a unique identity while also sharing much with all other groups. Members modify their behavior to adapt to the group's uniqueness.

10. Before group meetings are initiated, decisions are made about the size of membership, frequency of meetings, time and place of meetings, and characteristics of members.

11. The goal of the therapeutic group is the alteration of the behavioral patterns of group members through the development of new and more effective ways of coping with stress.

12. Each group progresses through several developmental phases, including preaffiliation, power and control, working, and termination.

13. An effective group leader is essential to successful group therapy.

14. Group interaction is one of the most successful ways of stimulating persons who have lost interest in their surroundings.

15. Psychodrama is a form of group therapy that allows individuals to role-play problem situations by alternating various roles and to receive feedback from observers in the audience.

16. Transactional analysis uses the Child-Parent-Adult framework to analyze and improve interactional patterns.

17. Gestalt therapy focuses on helping persons fulfill their potential through increased sensory awareness of themselves and their relationships with others and with the environment within the context of the present.

18. The type of group activity most appropriate for persons who have a mental illness should be determined after consideration of several variables.

As each individual progresses in treatment, the type of group activity appropriate to meet his or her needs will change.

SUGGESTED SOURCES OF ADDITIONAL INFORMATION

Adrian S: A systematic approach to selecting group participants, *J Psychosoc Nurs Ment Health Serv* 18:37, February 1980.

Alley NM, Foster MC: Using self-help support groups: a framework for nursing practice and research, *J Adv Nurs* 15:1383, 1990.

Appelbaum PS, Greer A: Confidentiality in group therapy, *Hosp Community Psychiatry* 44:311, April 1993.

Bales R: *Interaction process analysis: a method for the study of small groups,* Reading, Mass, 1950, Addison-Wesley.

Beeber LS, Schmitt MH: Cohesiveness in groups: a concept in search of a definition, *Adv Nurs Sci* 9:1, 1986.

Brickhead L: The nurse as leader: group psychotherapy with psychiatric patients, *J Psychosoc Nurs Ment Health Serv* 22:24, June 1984.

Collison C: Grappling with group resistance, *J Psychosoc Nurs Ment Health Serv* 22:6, August 1984.

Ernst C, Vanderzyl S, Salinger R: Preparation of psychiatric inpatients for group therapy, *J Psychosoc Nurs Ment Health Serv* 19:28, July 1981.

Goble J: Didactic psychodrama and sociodrama, *Nurse Educ Today* 10:457, 1990.

Heiney SP, Wells LM: Strategies for organizing and maintaining successful support groups, *Oncol Nurs Forum* 16(6):803, 1989.

Hochberger JM, Fisher-James L: A discharge group for chronically mentally ill: easing the way, *J Psychosoc Nurs Ment Health Serv* 30(4):25, 1992.

Hoover R, Parnell P: An inpatient educational group on stress and coping, *J Psychosoc Nurs Ment Health Serv* 22:16, June 1984.

Klose P, Tinius T: Confidence builders: a self-esteem group at an inpatient psychiatric hospital, *J Psychosoc Nurs Ment Health Serv* 30(7):5, 1992.

Miller D: Group dynamics: handling subgroups, *Nurs Management* 22:33, December 1991.

Moreno JL: *Psychodrama,* 1946, Beacon.

Neizo B, Murphy M: Medication groups on an acute psychiatric unit, *Perspect Psychiatr Care* 21:70, April-June 1983.

Pelletier L: Interpersonal communications task group, *J Psychosoc Nurs Ment Health Serv* 21:32, September 1983.

Ribble D: Psychosocial support groups for people with HIV infection and AIDS, *Holistic Nurs Pract* 3(4):52, 1989.

Rogers C: *On encounter groups,* New York, 1970, Harper & Row.

Small LL: Finding your leadership style in groups, *Am J Nurs* 80:1301, 1980.

Von Mering O, King SH: *Remotivating the mental patient,* New York, 1957, Russell Sage Foundation.

White E, Kahn EM: Use and modifications in group psycho-

therapy with chronic schizophrenic outpatients, *J Psychosoc Nurs Ment Health Serv* 20:14, February 1982.

Yalom ID: *Inpatient group psychotherapy,* New York, 1983, Basic Books.

Yalom ID: *The theory and practice of group psychotherapy,* ed 3, New York, 1985, Basic Books.

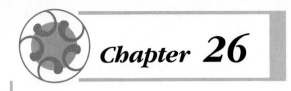

Chapter 26

Family Theory and Intervention

Christine S. Fawcett

LEARNING OBJECTIVES
After studying this chapter, the student will be able to:
* Define the term *family*.
* Discuss the functions of the family.
* Discuss the developmental stages of the family.
* Discuss the patterns of behavior characteristic of the effective family.
* Describe the characteristics of the child-abusing family as an example of the ineffective family.
* Explain the rationale underlying the use of family therapy as a treatment modality.

It has been declared that the **family** is the most prevalent of all societal institutions. This assertion stems from two factors: (1) the universal tendency of human beings to organize themselves around the family structure from which they are born and (2) the belief that the child's experiences as a family member have the most powerful influence on the type of adult he or she will become. Society as a whole is greatly affected by the family, both directly and indirectly, in both the present and the future. Other societal institutions, such as the school and the church, are fundamental to the society but are believed to be organizational structures that fulfill functions that historically have been delegated by the family. These societal institutions have developed in the belief that the collective society can fulfill certain functions more efficiently than the singular family. However, the question of whether the society can fulfill these functions more effectively than the family is the subject of continuous debate, and dynamic fluctuations of functions between the family and other societal institutions can be observed over the course of generations.

The nurse often deals not just with an individual but also with a family. This contact may be direct and formalized, as when engaging in communication with the family, or direct but informal, as when seeking information from or supplying information to family members. Some family theorists believe that even when the nurse is dealing only with an individual, it is impossible for the interaction not to affect and be affected by that individual's family. Therefore, interactions with an individual are seen as indirect interactions with that individual's family.

This view stems from the belief that the family is a system. An individual's behavior is greatly influenced by the family, and in turn, any alterations in the person's behavior will invariably affect the family. Whether one agrees with this view or not, it is difficult to deny that to be effective, the nurse needs to understand the family.

HISTORICAL PERSPECTIVE

Awareness of the family as a significant social institution has been present throughout history. However, not until the twentieth century was the family recognized as a system and studied as such. Before that time the family unit was understood to be a summation of the characteristics of its members. This view resulted in ascribing praise or blame to one or more family members for the effectiveness of the family's functioning. When a member was diagnosed as having a mental illness, it was often thought to be the parents' fault, particularly the mother's.

The family unit was not studied as a system until the escalating divorce rate after World War II created concern about the future of the family in the United States. In retrospect, it seems clear that the many divorces that occurred after World War II resulted because while husbands were serving in the Armed Forces, wives were working in factories; both evolved adaptations in the former stereotypical roles they played. When the husband returned, the lifestyles that each had evolved were not necessarily compatible, and no help was available to assist the marriage partners to regain system stability. In addition, increasing stress and economic demands impacted on the extended family system design, demanding change.

In **nonindustrial societies** the family pattern most often observed is the **extended family,** in which several generations live together and leave only for the purpose of joining another extended family through marriage. Before the Industrial Revolution, families in the United States often consisted of children, parents, and grandparents and perhaps one or more unmarried aunts or uncles. This pattern of family life provided the work force necessary for the productive management of the family business, usually the farm. When daughters married, they often left their family to join their husband's family, whereas the sons' wives were incorporated into the sons' family. This traditional family structure was also the mechanism whereby family resources, primarily land, were passed from generation to generation. Many advantages were associated with the extended family structure; physical and emotional resources were shared among a large group, and a broad division of labor was possible.

However, many disadvantages also existed. Families whose offspring were all female had to face the possibility of all the children leaving, thereby placing the elderly parents in a very vulnerable economic and social position. Furthermore, although the prescribed roles of each family member provided stability and continuity, this prescription also thwarted individuality. The eldest boy was expected to continue the family business, leaving the younger brother, who might have been more interested and capable of so doing, the choice of either striking out on his own or working at the behest of his older sibling. The image now present of the "good old days," characterized by close-knit, warm, loving families, is believed by most authorities to be a distortion of the reality of intense sibling rivalry and parental frustration.

The settlement of the western U.S. frontier, which placed great value on rugged individualism, and the Industrial Revolution both contributed greatly to a dramatic change in the typical family structure. Individuals moved from settled rural areas to the unsettled West or to industrialized urban areas with the goal of making their own fortune. A pervasive belief in both instances was that more money could be earned with less labor. Initially, that belief proved to be false, as evidenced by the hardships of western settlement and the horrors of the urban sweatshop. The mobility of American citizens, along with waves of European immigrants, combined to create cities where people lived in dense concentration. Population density and mobility militated against the perpetuation of the extended family, and the nuclear family structure became the norm.

FAMILY STRUCTURE

The **nuclear family** is defined as a two-generational family in which it is understood that the children will leave once they have achieved maturity. Therefore the nuclear family, as a family, is only a temporary arrangement. The nuclear family has the disadvantages of potential alienation from the family of origin and fewer emotional supports from within the family. However, it has the major advantage of facilitating upward social mobility because it tends not to predetermine the children's roles as inheritors of the family business.

DEFINITION OF FAMILY

A family is traditionally defined as two or more people who are related by blood or by legal ties such as marriage or adoption. However, a family also has the characteristic of identifying itself and being identified by others as such. Sharing a common surname is a manifestation of this characteristic, although it is not requisite to being a family. A family may be made up of those who share a household, hold similar values, and participate in shared goals. Another characteristic of a family is that it is a relatively permanent human affiliation. A family, therefore, has a past, present, and future.

In the complex, highly mobile, technological society in which we live, an increasing number of human groups identify themselves as a family and exist over time, but their members do not meet the traditional criteria of being related by blood or by legal ties. Therefore a more accurate, relevant definition of family may be one that reflects the functions of a family.

FUNCTIONS OF THE FAMILY

A family is a specialized group that bands together in pursuit of the common goal of growth and development of its members. This goal is achieved through certain functions. Although none of these functions is unique to the family, the combination of them is unique to this institution. The following functions are considered by most authorities to belong to the family.

Regulation of sexual activity and reproduction. The family structure provides for socially sanctioned sexual activity between spouses, while at the same time enforcing the societal taboo against incest by defining parental and sibling relationships. Survival of the culture is ensured by systematizing reproduction within a context that is capable of providing for children, who in turn become the vehicle for the transmission of **cultural values** and practices. Therefore a family conveys to its children its cultural heritage to ensure the culture's future.

Physical maintenance. The family structure provides a vehicle through which the physical needs of its members can be met. It provides an efficient means of organizing responsibility for meeting the needs of individuals for food, clothing, shelter, and health care. In this regard, the family can be seen as an economic unit.

Protection. The family structure is designed to provide both literal and figurative protection of its members by providing a model for interacting with the society in a way that protects the family members from undesirable outside influences.

Education and socialization. Some authorities believe that the family's function of providing education and socialization is the most fundamental one, since through the family, children learn how to function in and relate to the world in which they live.

Recreation. Traditionally the family has been the structure in which the individual has engaged in leisure activities that are a source of personal and group refreshment and stress management, leading to increased family cohesion. The function of recreation is feared to be rapidly waning since the advent of television and other passive or nonparticipant forms of entertainment.

Status conferring. Another traditional function of the family that seems to be undergoing fundamental alteration is status conferring. Before the advent of industrialization in a democratic society, which places emphasis on individualism, the individual was conferred social status by virtue of the family into which he or she was born. Although this is no longer strictly the case today, social status is still somewhat determined by the race and socioeconomic level of one's family of origin.

Affection giving. Only within the family can an individual be guaranteed unconditional acceptance by the mere fact of his or her relationship to that family. In all other societal interactions, acceptance of an individual is determined by such factors as the quality or speed of his or her performance, appearance, social class, or occupation. In functional families, acceptance is conveyed by a deep, enduring affection among the members.

A perusal of these family functions reveals that the family unit provides services that are essential to the survival and stability of the society.

FAMILY STAGES

Not all functions of a family are equally prominent at any given time. Each function is more specific to certain stages of family development than others and as such becomes a developmental task of the family.

Every family progresses through stages or cycles of life. These stages are predictable, orderly, and normative (Carter and McGoldrick, 1988). Each stage offers challenges and rewards and is marked by particular events, such as change in membership (e.g., birth, marriage) or change in activity (e.g., retirement).

Sociologist Evelyn Duvall (1977) outlined a series of **developmental stages** for the family. Her work was the first to define the family stages and was based on the traditional two-parent family (see the box at left below).

Carter and McGoldrick (1988) separated family development into two types of changes, normative (similar to Duvall) and paranormative (see the box at right below).

Each stage of the **normative cycle** notes a change in the structure (membership) or focus of the family system.

The **paranormative cycle** consists of stages or events that change the family's normal functioning. Although they occur frequently, they do not occur in every family.

THE CHANGING FAMILY

The structure, size, functions, and developmental stages of the family are undergoing many changes in today's society. For example, a family may consist of only one parent who is raising one or more children and fulfilling both mother and father roles. Blended, or reconstituted, families are increasing and consist of a parent who had been previously married and has children. This parent may marry another parent who also has children from a previous marriage. Such a couple may also have children of their own, so this family's task is to "blend" together three different sets of children into a functional family structure.

The number of people who are joining together to form a family group based on mutual respect and common interests rather than for the purpose of procreation also is increasing. These persons may or may not be related by blood or by law but tend to reside in the same household. The household concept, or living under the same roof, has been the criterion used by the U.S. Census Bureau to define a family. With the many family structures apparent in society, this criterion may prove to be the most applicable.

In any event, the nurst must extend the definition of family beyond the traditional nuclear or extended family structure when dealing with individuals who do not live in these structures in order to assess accurately the individual's familial associations and dynamics.

THE EFFECTIVE FAMILY

The effective family is able to facilitate the growth and development of its members while still maintaining cohesion and identity as a unit. This definition implies that these patterns of be-

---

STAGES IN DUVALL'S MODEL

Marriage of the couple. Two individuals learn to live together as husband and wife.
Childbearing. Stage begins with wife's pregnancy and changes family focus from couple to children.
Preschool-aged family. Roles expand to mother and father; priorities and activities shift.
School-aged family. Children are confronted with societal values.
Teenage years. Child confronts adolescence; family controls shift.
Launching center. Children prepare to leave home; family allows shift in control.
Middle-aged parents. Parental roles shift back to those of a couple; "empty nest syndrome" occurs.
Aging family members. Family prepares for death of one of its members.

NORMATIVE AND PARANORMATIVE STAGES AND EVENTS IN FAMILY DEVELOPMENT

Normative stages	Paranormative stages/ events
Marriage	Miscarriage
Birth of a child	Marital separation and divorce
Child enters school	Illness, disability, and death
Child enters adolescence	Relocations of household
	Changes in economic status
Birth of grandchild	Extrinsic catastrophe with
Retirement	massive dislocation of the
Senescence	family unit

havior are characteristic of an effective family:

1. The family places the emotional, physical, and social needs of its members over other concerns, such as acquisition of possessions or status.
2. The family recognizes, values, and accommodates to differences among its members.
3. The family is sufficiently flexible so that changes stemming from within and outside the system can be accommodated without loss of family stability.
4. The family seeks and uses information from relevant outside sources, simultaneously maintaining its autonomy.
5. The family makes and carries out decisions, taking into account its goals and the age and experience of its members.

An effective family is not necessarily a family without problems, conflicts, or stress. Rather, an effective family has developed a structure and pattern of functioning that enables it to deal with its problems as they arise and to learn and grow together from the problem-solving process. As with individuals, families must learn these procedures, and many authorities believe that helping young families to develop effective patterns of functioning is the crux of promoting mental health.

Most young people receive no preparation for establishing an effective family. Therefore, they unconsciously perpetuate the only patterns of familial functioning they know—the patterns they experienced in their families of origin. If such learned patterns of behavior are conducive to effective family functioning, effective families will perpetuate. If ineffective patterns are learned, the probability of perpetuating ineffective family patterns is greatly enhanced.

THE INEFFECTIVE FAMILY

Families that are unable to establish and maintain a structure and patterns of behavior conducive to effective functioning often show signs of continuous, irresolvable stress. Such stress may be manifested by the entire system, as when overt tension and hostility occur among members, or the stress may be focused on only one member who is covertly designated to assume and act out the family problems. This family member may often, although not always, be a child. This phenomenon occurs because children are likely to be more vulnerable and less powerful, since they are so highly dependent on the family and their behavioral patterns are less firmly entrenched. Bed-wetting, learning difficulties, antisocial behaviors, and chronic depression in a child may all be symptoms of an ineffective family.

It is beyond the scope of this text to discuss the many types of family dysfunction. The following discussion of abuse and violence is presented as an example of one increasingly common and very serious form of ineffective family functioning.

THE ABUSING FAMILY

The incidence of reported family violence in the form of child abuse, spouse abuse, and elder abuse has dramatically increased. However, accurate statistics are difficult to obtain because the phenomenon of **abuse** is poorly defined.

Child abusers often go to extraordinary lengths to conceal their actions, and friends, relatives, and health care providers may be hesitant to become involved. Nevertheless, it is known that the neglect or abuse of children occurs often enough to be of major concern to the legal and health care professions.

Child abuse can range from violent, physical attacks that result in severe injury to passive neglect that results in insidious malnutrition. Child abuse is not limited to physical maltreatment; it also includes emotional maltreatment such as continual yelling at and berating of the child.

Children may be the targets of family violence because they are relatively powerless and, until they reach adolescence, are certainly physically weaker than adults. The pattern of the powerless becoming victims of violence is seen not only in child abuse but also in wife battering and the tyrannization of elderly persons in their homes.

The concept of powerlessness includes social subordination as well as physical weakness. Children, women, and the elderly are all persons who traditionally have had less power in society than adult males. This situation is gradually changing. The values, needs, and rights of children, women, and elderly persons are being recognized and becoming protected by law. Therefore these persons are achieving an allotment of social power. Ironically, some authorities believe that the identification of this problem is contributing to its intensification. In other words, individuals who have no power and do not assert themselves are often not overtly abused. As children, women, and elderly persons achieve more power, they are more likely to constitute a threat and therefore be abused more often.

Table 26-1 lists physical and behavioral indicators of child abuse and neglect. The laws of most states require that health care personnel report to legal authorities situations in which child abuse or maltreatment is suspected; most state laws do not require proof before reporting child abuse or maltreatment. After a report is made, the child protective agency is responsible for the actual determination of the situation.

Many health care professionals, including nurses, are hesitant to report incidents of suspected child abuse. Frequently expressed reservations include a fear of becoming involved in legal processes and a desire to protect the familial integrity. By not reporting suspected instances of child abuse, however, the health care worker is *not* protecting the family and is also indirectly contributing to the perpetuation of physical and emotionally harmful family patterns.

Dynamics underlying abusing families

An understanding of the dynamics underlying family abuse includes societal, familial, and individual factors.

Societal factors

Sociologists believe that family violence reflects a society that endorses violence as a means of dealing with frustration and achieving goals. Much publicity has surrounded the amount of violence on television and in the movies. Some social learning theorists believe that by the time children reach age 16, they may have witnessed more than 16,000 episodes of violence either on television or in movies.

More subtle forms of violence are socially sanctioned by the national preoccupation with such sports as football and boxing. In this way, children learn that violent acts are socially acceptable outlets for anger and frustration.

Familial factors

It is a well-known fact that patterns of violence and abuse occur with generational repetition. That is, people who have themselves been abused as children may become child abusers. Therefore a multigenerational pattern of violence occurs.

In addition, many authorities believe that the nuclear family structure contributes to the incidence of domestic abuse. In this family structure, a small group of persons, the nuclear family, is often isolated from other sources of concerned support. Therefore an intensity of demands develops, and few outlets are available to meet these needs. This leads to increased tension, which may explode in the form of violence or neglect directed at a member with lesser power—the wife, the child, or the frail elder.

Individual factors

Whether or not ineffective family functioning will manifest itself by child abuse is largely determined by the dynamics of the family members and how these interact with each other. The box on p. 491 lists behavioral indicators of abusive parents. These indicators, however, fail to reflect the human pain that many child-abusing parents experience. As previously stated, these individuals are most likely to have been abused children

Table 26-1. Physical and behavioral indicators of child abuse and neglect

TYPE OF ABUSE/NEGLECT	PHYSICAL INDICATORS	BEHAVIORAL INDICATORS

Physical abuse	Unexplained bruises and welts:
	  On face, lips, mouth
	  On torso, back, buttocks, thighs
	  In various stages of healing
	  Clustered, forming regular patterns
	  Reflecting shape of article used to inflict (e.g., electric cord, belt buckle)
	  On several different surface areas
	  Regularly appear after absence, weekend, vacation
	Unexplained burns:
	  Cigar, cigarette burns, especially on soles, palms, back, buttocks
	  Immersion burns (socklike, glovelike, doughnut shaped on buttocks or genitalia)
	  Patterned resembling electric burner, iron, etc.
	  Rope burns on arms, legs, neck, torso
	  Infected burns, indicating delay in seeking treatment
	Unexplained fractures/dislocations
	  To skull, nose, facial structure
	  In various stages of healing
	  Multiple or spiral fractures
	Unexplained lacerations or abrasions:
	  To mouth, lips, gums, eyes
	  To external genitalia
	  In various stages of healing
	Bald patches on the scalp
		Feels deserving of punishment
		Wary of adult contacts
		Apprehensive when other children cry
		Behavioral extremes:
		  Aggressiveness
		  Withdrawal
		Frightened of parents
		Afraid to go home
		Reports injury by parents
		Vacant or frozen stare
		Lies very still while surveying surroundings
		Will not cry when approached by examiner
		Responds to questions in monosyllables
		Inappropriate or precocious maturity
		Manipulative behavior to get attention
		Capable of only superficial relationships
		Indiscriminately seeks affection
		Poor self-concept

Physical neglect	Underweight, poor growth pattern, failure to thrive Consistent hunger, poor hygiene, inappropriate dress Consistent lack of supervision, especially in dangerous activities or for long periods Wasting of subcutaneous tissue Unattended physical problems or medical needs	Begging, stealing food Extended stays at school (early arrival, late departure) Rare attendance at school Constant fatigue, listlessness, falling asleep in class Inappropriate seeking of affection Assuming adult responsibilities and concerns Alcohol or drug abuse

From Heindl C and others: *The nurse's role in the prevention and treatment of child abuse and neglect,* DHEW Pub No (OHDS) 79-30202, Washington, DC, 1979, US Government Printing Office.

Continued.

Table 26-1. Physical and behavioral indicators of child abuse and neglect—cont'd

TYPE OF ABUSE/NEGLECT	PHYSICAL INDICATORS	BEHAVIORAL INDICATORS
Physical neglect—cont'd	Abandonment	Delinquency (e.g., thefts)
	Abdominal distention	States there is no caretaker
	Bald patches on scalp	
Sexual abuse	Difficulty in walking or sitting	Unwilling to change for gym or partici-
	Torn, stained, or bloody underclothing	pate in physical education class
	Pain, swelling, or itching in genital area	Withdrawal, fantasy, or infantile behav-
	Pain on urination	ior
	Bruises, bleeding, or lacerations in ex-	Bizarre, sophisticated, or unusual sex-
	ternal genitalia, vaginal, or anal areas	ual behavior or knowledge
	Vaginal/penile discharge	Poor peer relationships
	Venereal disease, especially in preteens	Delinquent or runaway
	Poor sphincter tone	Reports sexual assault by caretaker
	Pregnancy	Change in school performance
Emotional maltreatment	Speech disorders	Habit disorders (sucking, biting, rock-
	Lags in physical development	ing, etc.)
	Failure to thrive	Conduct/learning disorders (antisocial,
	Hyperactive/disruptive behavior	destructive, etc.)
		Anxiety disorders (hysteria, obsession,
		compulsion, phobias, hypochon-
		driasis, sleep disturbances, inhibition
		of play, unusual fearfulness)
		Behavior extremes:
		Compliant, passive
		Aggressive, demanding
		Overly adaptive behavior:
		Inappropriately adult
		Inappropriately infantile
		Developmental lags (mental, emo-
		tional)
		Attempted suicide

themselves. Therefore, they have many unmet needs, are emotionally immature, and have limited control of their impulses. Many abusing parents, especially mothers, unconsciously look to their children as a vehicle through which their own needs can be met. When it becomes obvious that an infant or young child is very dependent or takes more than he or she can give, these parents may react with almost uncontrollable rage at once again being disappointed and deprived of their own needs. In other words, these parents have many fundamental, unmet needs themselves that they look to their children to meet. When this need fulfillment is not forthcoming, they tend to react with violence, reflecting a primitive expression of frustration.

Why is one child in a family consistently abused while others develop unscathed? This question has no definitive answer, but some hypotheses can be stated. The abused child often has characteristics that set him or her apart from others in the family. These include placement in

BEHAVIORAL INDICATORS OF ABUSIVE PARENTS

Parents of abused children may:

Lack family supports such as friends, relatives, neighbors, and community groups; consistently fail to keep appointments, discourage social contact, and never participate in school activities or events

Seem to trust no one

Have a childhood history of abuse or neglect

Be reluctant to give information about the child's injuries or condition; when questioned, are unable to explain or offer farfetched or contradictory explanations

Respond inappropriately to the seriousness of the child's condition either by overreacting, seeming hostile or antagonistic when questioned even casually, or by underreacting, showing little concern or awareness and seeming more preoccupied with their own problems than those of the child

Refuse to consent to diagnostic studies

Fail or delay to take the child for medical care, for routine checkups, for optometric or dental care, or for treatment of injury or illness; in taking an injured child for medical care, may choose a different hospital or physician each time

Be overcritical of the child; seldom if ever discuss the child in positive terms

Have unrealistic expectations of the child, expecting or demanding behavior that is beyond the child's years or ability

Believe in the necessity of harsh punishment for children

Seldom touch or look at the child; ignore the child's crying or react with impatience

Keep the child confined, perhaps in a crib or playpen, for overlong periods

Seem to lack understanding of children's physical, emotional, and psychological needs

Appear to be abusing alcohol or drugs

Be difficult or impossible to locate

Appear to lack control or fear losing control

Be of borderline intelligence, psychotic, or antisocial. Although such diagnoses are the responsibility of mental health professionals, even the lay observer can note whether the parent seems intellectually capable of childrearing, exhibits generally irrational behavior, or seems excessively cruel and sadistic.

From *Child abuse and neglect.* Vol 1, An overview of the problem; vol 2, The problem and its management, Department of Health, Education and Welfare, Washington, DC, 1975, US Government Printing Office.

birth order (youngest or oldest), physical characteristics (resembles paternal or maternal side of the family), particular skills or deficits and identifiable personality characteristics (greater or lesser intelligence), more or less assertiveness, and enjoyment of solitary activities or activities involving others.

In any event, the abused child seems to have particular significance not only to the parents but also to the siblings. The question arises as to why the abused child characteristically colludes with the family in concealing the events surrounding his or her injuries. Many social scientists believe the answer to this question is that children so desperately need attention from significant adults that they are willing to submit to abuse if this appears to be the only way they can gain this attention.

Family therapists postulate that the child knowingly assumes a role that is necessary for the family system's survival. Regardless of why it occurs, it is well known that abused children block attempts to divulge the reality of the situation.

Many women who are abused are also shameful and express the feeling of being economically trapped. The woman states she still loves her spouse and "knows" he really loves her as well. Many women are rightfully fearful of permanent injury or death should they decide to leave an abusing spouse.

The nurse's role

Because of the multifaceted dynamics operating in the ineffective family that abuses its members, treatment is very complex. The physical needs of the injured or neglected victim must be met before attempts are made to alter the family's pattern of functioning. During the time the child or adult is receiving treatment, the other family members need much support and understanding. Health care personnel, including nurses, often have great difficulty avoiding the tendency to blame one or both parents. This attitude, which may be conveyed overtly or covertly, is counterproductive, since it reinforces the guilt, shame, and sense of worthlessness the parents already feel. Such an attitude also reflects a lack of understanding that family units function as a system in which each member contributes to the unit's function or dysfunction.

The treatment of choice for the abusive family, as for all ineffective families, is family therapy. As nurses become more educationally prepared, they increasingly become responsible for using this treatment modality.

FAMILY THERAPY

The concept of **family therapy** is based on the belief that the family is a social system with its own characteristic structure and pattern of communication. Although this structure and communication pattern are certainly related to the personalities of the family members, they cannot be explained by a mere summation of the traits of the individuals who make up the family. In other words, the family as a unit is seen as a *system* and the family members as subsystems that influence the system and are in turn influenced by it.

If one accepts this concept, it becomes inappropriate to refer to one member as having a mental illness without looking at the family constellation, which, it is believed, has sanctioned the deviant behavior of one member and in turn is affected by it. In other words, the behavior of the "sick" member serves a function within the family. This belief is supported by two observations. First, it is not unusual for a person to be successfully treated for mental illness on an individual basis and for another family member to become ill, sometimes with very similar symptoms. This phenomenon suggests that the family structure and communication pattern, if they are to be maintained, require one member to be deviant, weaker, or labeled.

A second observation that supports the systems approach is the frequency with which the family members bring one member for treatment with the statement that all is well within the family except for the one member's stress-producing behavior. When that member is removed from the family, either through prolonged hospitalization or by geographical relocation, the family may enter into a state of acute disequilibrium that may manifest itself by a new type of dysfunctional behavior. This phenomenon is equally well documented in families in which a person with a chronic physical illness has died.

Recently, a growing number of mental health professionals believes that any attempt to treat individuals in isolation from their families is futile, or if helpful to the individual, is at the expense of the family system's equilibrium. Proponents of family therapy maintain that major strides in the promotion of mental illness will occur only when the individual's needs are considered within the context of the family system, which still remains as the fundamental social unit of our society. Although this may seem an extreme view, family therapy undoubtedly is the treatment of choice when the identified client is a child or adolescent, and this treatment modality should be used in other situations when possible.

The goals of family therapy are (1) to assist in resolving pathological conflicts and anxiety, (2) to strengthen the individual member against destructive forces both within the self and within the family environment, (3) to strengthen the family against critical upsets, and (4) to influence the orientation of the family identity and values toward health. When therapy commences, the therapist assembles all family members, regardless of age, and pays as much attention to their behavior toward each other as to the content of what they say. For example, the husband and wife may vehemently state how emotionally close they are while sitting as far as possible from each other. It is important for the therapist not to blame one or the other member. This pitfall can be avoided if the role of each member is seen in relation to total family functioning.

In one family therapy situation, the identified client was a 20-year-old daughter who had made numerous suicidal attempts. This girl was hospitalized, and the entire family came to the hospital once a week for family therapy. The parents maintained that they had an unusually good relationship and could not understand why their daughter tormented them with her life-threatening gestures. Several times during the course of therapy, their adolescent son took the risk of contradicting his parents by observing that the parents' relationship was highly tension laden, at which point the daughter would begin crying. Her behavior diverted the participants' attention to her and successfully prevented the parents from having to face, much less talk about, their differences. The therapist interpreted the daughter's role in the maintenance of the family's equilibrium.

It is the family's prerogative to determine its own destiny, and often the therapist's major role is to comment on the interactional process as it is observed. Bringing this process to a level of consciousness allows the family to evaluate its purpose and outcome. If the family desires a change, the therapist can be instrumental in modeling behaviors that can initiate such change.

Some family therapy sessions have been held in the home. As this trend develops, it appears likely that the role of the family therapist will become increasingly identified with the advanced practice psychiatric nurse, since she or he is comfortable in the role of family visitor, is knowledgeable about family dynamics, and is skillful in family therapy.

KEY POINTS

1. The child's experiences as a family member have the most influence on the type of adult he or she will become.

2. A nurse's interactions with an individual are indirect interactions with that individual's family because the family is a system.

3. The extended family is a type of family structure seen in nonindustrial societies and consists of several generations living together.

4. The nuclear family is a type of family structure seen in industrialized societies and consists of two generations.

5. A family is traditionally defined as two or more people who are related by blood or legal ties, although nonrelated groups are increasingly identifying themselves as families.

6. Traditional families progress through a series of developmental stages that are primarily related to role changes of their members.

7. A common change in family structure is the blended, or reconstituted, family. Nurses must expand their view of family when dealing with individuals who live in "nontraditional" structures.

8. An effective family is able to deal with problems productively when they arise.

9. Ineffective families show signs of continuous, irresolvable stress manifested either by the entire system or by one of its members.

10. Child abuse ranges from violent, physical attacks to passive neglect. Maltreatment may be physical or emotional.

11. Children are the usual victims of family violence because they are relatively powerless, being both physically weaker and socially subordinate.

12. Social, family, and individual factors must be considered to understand the dynamics of child abuse.

13. Family treatment is the treatment of choice for child-abusing families and all other ineffective families.

14. Family therapy is based on the belief that the behavior of any one family member affects and is affected by the entire family system.

15. Family therapy also is based on the belief that the treatment and prevention of mental illness will occur only when the individual's needs are considered within the context of the family system.

16. The advanced practice psychiatric nurse seems ideally suited to the role of therapist as the trend toward family therapy in the home increases.

SUGGESTED SOURCES OF ADDITIONAL INFORMATION

Battered women: issues of public policy, Washington, DC, 1978, US Commission on Civil Rights.

Berkey KM, Hanson S: *Pocket guide to family assessment and intervention,* St Louis, 1991, Mosby–Year Book.

Bowen M: *Family therapy in clinical practice,* New York, 1986, Aronson.

Cain AO: Family therapy: one role of the clinical specialist in psychiatric nursing, *Nurs Clin North Am* 21(3):483, 1986.

Campbell J, Humphreys J: *Nursing care of victims of family violence,* Reston, Va, 1984, Reston.

Carter E, McGoldrick M: *The changing family life cycle: a framework for family therapists,* ed 2, New York, 1988, Gardner.

Child abuse and neglect. Vol 1, An overview of the problem, Department of Health, Education and Welfare, Washington, DC, 1975, US Government Printing Office.

Child abuse and neglect. Vol 2, The problem and its management, Department of Health, Education and Welfare, Washington, DC, 1975, US Government Printing Office.

Coker LS: A therapeutic recovery model for the female adult incest survivor, *Issues Ment Health Nurs* 11:109, 1990.

Collison C, Futrell JA: Family therapy for the single-parent family system, *J Psychosoc Nurs Ment Health Serv* 20:16, July 1982.

deChesnay M: Father-daughter incest, *J Psychosoc Nurs Ment Health Serv* 22:24, September 1984.

Duvall EM: *Marriage and family development,* ed 5, Philadelphia, 1977, Lippincott.

Gemmill F: A family approach to the battered woman, *J Psychosoc Nurs Ment Health Serv* 20:22, September 1982.

Grossman J, Pozanski E, Bonegas M: Lunch: time to study family interactions, *J Psychosoc Nurs Ment Health Serv* 21:19, July 1983.

Hall JE, Weaver BR, editors: *Nursing of families in crisis,* Philadelphia, 1974, Lippincott.

Harter L: Multi-family meetings on the psychiatric unit, *J Psychosoc Nurs Ment Health Serv* 26(8):19, 1988.

Heindl C and others: *The nurse's role in the prevention and treatment of child abuse and neglect,* DHEW Pub No (OHDS) 79-30202, Washington, DC, 1979, US Government Printing Office.

Herrick CA, Goodykoontz L: Neuman's systems model for nursing practice as a conceptual framework for a family assessment, *J Child Parent Nurs* 2(2):61, 1989.

Johnston M: *The health of families in a culture of crisis,* Kansas City, Mo, 1981, American Nurses' Foundation.

Jones S, Dimond M: Family theory and family therapy models: comparative review with implications for nursing practice, *J Psychosoc Nurs Ment Health Serv* 20:12, October 1982.

Lantz J, Treece N: Identity operations and family treatment, *J Psychosoc Nurs Ment Health Serv* 20:20, October 1982.

Lapp CA, Diemert CA: Family-based practice: discussion of a tool merging assessment with intervention, *Fam Community Health* 12(4):21, 1990.

Martin AC, Starling BP: Managing common marital stresses, *Nurse Pract* 14:11, October 1989.

Miller SR, Winstead-Fry P: *Family systems theory in nursing practice,* Reston, Va, 1982, Reston.

Miller V, Mansfield E: Family therapy for the multiple incest family, *J Psychosoc Nurs Ment Health Serv* 19:29, April 1984.

Minuchin S: *Families and family therapy,* Cambridge, Mass, 1974, Harvard University.

Palermo E: Remarriage: parental perceptions of step-relations with children and adolescents, *J Psychosoc Nurs Ment Health Serv* 18:9, April 1980.

Richards E: Self-reports of differentiation of self and marital compatibility as related to family functioning in the third and fourth stages of the family life cycle, *Schol Inq Nurs Pract* 3(3):163, 1989.

Rose L, Finestone, K, Bass J: Group support for the families of psychiatric patients, *J Psychosoc Nurs Ment Health Serv* 23:24, December 1985.

Sedgwick R: *Family mental health: theory and practice,* St Louis, 1981, Mosby–Year Book.

So you use a systems approach in therapy: what does that mean? *Arch Psychiatr Nurs* 2:55, April 1988 (editorial).

Starkey P: Genograms: a guide to understanding one's own family system, *Perspect Psychiatr Care* 19:164, September-December 1982.

Stern PN: Conflicting family culture: an impediment to integration in stepfather families, *J Psychosoc Nurs Ment Health Serv* 20:27, October 1982.

Swanson A, Hurley P: Family systems: values and value conflicts, *J Psychosoc Nurs Ment Health Serv* 21:24, July 1983.

Tamex E: Familism, machismo and child rearing practices among Mexican Americans, *J Psychosoc Nurs Ment Health Serv* 19:21, September 1981.

Toman W: *Family therapy & sibling position,* Northvale, NJ, 1988, Aronson.

Tousley M: The use of family therapy in terminal illness and death, *J Psychosoc Nurs Ment Health Serv* 20:17, January 1982.

White J: Bulimia: utilizing individual and family therapy, *J Psychosoc Nurs Ment Health Serv* 22:22, April 1984.

Wilk J: Family environments and the young chronically mentally ill, *J Psychosoc Nurs Ment Health Serv* 26:15, October 1988.

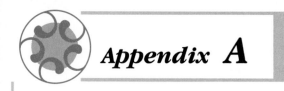

Appendix A

DSM-III-R Classification

axes I and II
categories and codes

All official DSM-III-R codes are included in ICD-9-CM. Codes followed by a * are used for more than one DSM-III-R diagnosis or subtype in order to maintain compatibility with ICD-9-CM.

A long dash following a diagnostic term indicates the need for a fifth digit subtype or other qualifying term.

The term *specify* following the name of some diagnostic categories indicates qualifying terms that clinicians may wish to add in parentheses after the name of the disorder.

NOS = Not Otherwise Specified

The current severity of a disorder may be specified after the diagnosis as:

mild
moderate
severe
} currently
meets
diagnostic
criteria

in partial remission
(or residual state)
in complete remission

DISORDERS USUALLY FIRST EVIDENT IN INFANCY, CHILDHOOD, OR ADOLESCENCE

DEVELOPMENTAL DISORDERS

Note: These are coded on Axis II.

Mental retardation

317.00	Mild mental retardation
318.00	Moderate mental retardation
318.10	Severe mental retardation
318.20	Profound mental retardation
319.00	Unspecified mental retardation

Pervasive developmental disorders

299.00	Autistic disorder
	Specify if childhood onset
299.80	Pervasive developmental disorder NOS

Specific developmental disorders
Academic Skills Disorders

315.10	Developmental arithmetic disorder
315.80	Developmental expressive writing disorder
315.00	Developmental reading disorder

Language and Speech Disorders

315.39	Developmental articulation disorder
315.31*	Developmental expressive language disorder
315.31*	Developmental receptive language disorder

Motor Skills Disorder

315.40	Developmental coordination disorder
315.90*	Specific developmental disorder NOS

Other developmental disorders

315.90*	Developmental disorder NOS

Disruptive behavior disorders

314.01	Attention-deficit hyperactivity disorder
	Conduct disorder,
312.20	group type
312.00	solitary aggressive type
312.90	undifferentiated type
313.81	Opposition defiant disorder

Anxiety disorders of childhood or adolescence

309.21   Separation anxiety disorder
313.21   Avoidant disorder of childhood or adolescence
313.00   Overanxious disorder

Eating disorders

307.10   Anorexia nervosa
307.51   Bulimia nervosa
307.52   Pica
307.53   Rumination disorder of infancy
307.50   Eating disorder NOS

Gender identity disorders

302.60   Gender identity disorder of childhood
302.50   Transsexualism
           Specify sexual history: asexual, homosexual, heterosexual, unspecified
302.85*   Gender identity disorder of adolescence or adulthood, nontranssexual type
           Specify sexual history: asexual, homosexual, heterosexual, unspecified
302.85*   Gender identity disorder NOS

Tic disorders

307.23   Tourette's disorder
307.22   Chronic motor or vocal tic disorder
307.21   Transient tic disorder
           Specify: single episode or recurrent
307.20   Tic disorder NOS

Elimination disorders

307.70   Functional encopresis
           Specify: primary or secondary type
307.60   Functional enuresis
           Specify: primary or secondary types
           Specify: nocturnal only, diurnal only, nocturnal and diurnal

Speech disorders not elsewhere classified

307.00*   Cluttering
307.00*   Stuttering

Other disorders of infancy, childhood, or adolescence

313.23   Elective mutism
313.82   Identity disorder
313.89   Reactive attachment disorder of infancy or early childhood
307.30   Stereotypy/habit disorder
314.00   Undifferentiated attention-deficit disorder

ORGANIC MENTAL DISORDERS
Dementias arising in the senium and presenium

           Primary degenerative dementia of the Alzheimer type, senile onset,
290.30   with delirium
290.20   with delusions
290.21   with depression
290.00*   uncomplicated
           (Note: code 331.00 Alzheimer's disease on Axis III)
Code in fifth digit:
1 = with delirium, 2 = with delusions, 3 = with depression, 0* = uncomplicated
290.1x   Primary degenerative dementia of the Alzheimer type presenile onset, _____
           (Note: code 331.00 Alzheimer's disease on Axis III)
290.4x   Multi-infarct dementia, _____
290.00*   Senile dementia NOS
           Specify etiology on Axis III if known
290.10*   Presenile dementia NOS
           Specify etiology on Axis III if known (e.g., Pick's disease, Jakob-Creutzfeldt disease)

Psychoactive substance-induced organic mental disorders

           Alcohol
303.00   intoxication
291.40   idiosyncratic intoxication
291.80   Uncomplicated alcohol withdrawal
291.00   withdrawal delirium

291.30	hallucinosis
291.10	amnestic disorder
291.20	Dementia associated with alcoholism

Amphetamine or similarly acting sympathomimetic

305.70*	intoxication
292.00*	withdrawal
292.81*	delirium
292.11*	delusional disorder

Caffeine

305.90*	intoxication

Cannabis

305.20*	intoxication
292.11*	delusional disorder

Cocaine

305.60*	intoxication
292.00*	withdrawal
292.81*	delirium
292.11*	delusional disorder

Hallucinogen

305.30*	hallucinosis
292.11*	delusional disorder
292.84*	mood disorder
292.89*	Posthallucinogen perception disorder

Inhalant

305.90*	intoxication

Nicotine

292.00*	withdrawal

Opioid

305.50*	intoxication
292.00*	withdrawal

Phencyclidine (PCP) or similarly acting arylcyclohexylamine

305.90*	intoxication
292.81*	delirium
292.11*	delusional disorder
292.84*	mood disorder
292.90*	organic mental disorder NOS

Sedative, hypnotic, or anxiolytic

305.40*	intoxication
292.00*	Uncomplicated sedative, hypnotic, or anxiolytic withdrawal

292.00*	withdrawal delirium
292.83*	amnestic disorder

Other or unspecified psychoactive substance

305.90*	intoxication
292.00*	withdrawal
292.81*	delirium
292.82*	dementia
292.83*	amnestic disorder
292.11*	delusional disorder
292.12	hallucinosis
292.84*	mood disorder
292.89*	anxiety disorder
292.89*	personality disorder
292.90*	organic mental disorder NOS

Organic mental disorders associated with Axis III physical disorders or conditions, or whose etiology is unknown

293.00	Delirium
294.10	Dementia
294.00	Amnestic disorder
293.81	Organic delusional disorder
293.82	Organic hallucinosis
293.83	Organic mood disorder
	Specify: manic, depressed, mixed
294.80*	Organic anxiety disorder
310.10	Organic personality disorder
	Specify if explosive type
294.80*	Organic mental disorder NOS

PSYCHOACTIVE SUBSTANCE USE DISORDERS

Alcohol

303.90	dependence
305.00	abuse

Amphetamine or similarly acting sympathomimetic

304.40	dependence
305.70*	abuse

Cannabis

304.30	dependence
305.20*	abuse

	Cocaine
304.20	dependence
305.60*	abuse
	Hallucinogen
304.50*	dependence
305.30*	abuse
	Inhalant
304.60	dependence
305.90*	abuse
	Nicotine
305.10	dependence
	Opioid
304.00	dependence
305.50*	abuse

Phencyclidine (PCP) or similarly acting arylcyclohexylamine

| 304.50* | dependence |
| 305.90* | abuse |

Sedative, hypnotic, or anxiolytic

304.10	dependence
305.40*	abuse
304.90*	Polysubstance dependence
304.90*	Psychoactive substance dependence NOS
305.90*	Psychoactive substance abuse NOS

SCHIZOPHRENIA

Code in fifth digit: 1 = subchronic, 2 = chronic, 3 = subchronic with acute exacerbation, 4 = chronic with acute exacerbation, 5 = in remission, 0 = unspecified.

Schizophrenia,

295.2x	catatonic, _____
295.1x	disorganized, _____
295.3x	paranoid, _____
	Specify if stable type _____
295.9x	undifferentiated, _____
295.6x	residual, _____
	Specify if late onset

DELUSIONAL (PARANOID) DISORDER

| 297.10 | Delusional (Paranoid) disorder |
| | *Specify* type: erotomanic |

grandiose
jealous
persecutory
somatic
unspecified

PSYCHOTIC DISORDERS NOT ELSEWHERE CLASSIFIED

298.80	Brief reactive psychosis
295.40	Schizophreniform disorder
	Specify: without good prognostic features or with good prognostic features
295.70	Schizoaffective disorder
	Specify: bipolar type or depressive type
297.30	Induced psychotic disorder
298.90	Psychotic disorder NOS (Atypical psychosis)

MOOD DISORDERS

Code current state of Major Depression and Bipolar Disorder in Fifth digit:

1 = mild
2 = moderate
3 = severe, without psychotic features
4 = with psychotic features (*specify* mood-congruent or mood-incongruent)
5 = in partial remission
6 = in full remission
0 = unspecified

For major depressive episodes, *specify* if chronic and *specify* if melancholic type.

For Bipolar Disorder, Bipolar Disorder NOS, Recurrent Major Depression, and Depressive Disorder NOS, *specify* if seasonal pattern.

Bipolar disorders

Bipolar disorder,

296.6x	mixed, _____
296.4x	manic, _____
296.5x	depressed, _____

301.13   Cyclothymia
296.70   Bipolar disorder NOS

Depressive disorders

    Major Depression,
296.2x   single episode, _____
296.3x   recurrent, _____
300.40   Dysthymia (or Depressive neurosis)
    Specify: primary or secondary type
    Specify: early or late onset
311.00   Depressive disorder NOS

ANXIETY DISORDERS (OR ANXIETY AND PHOBIC NEUROSES)

    Panic disorder
300.21   with agoraphobia
    Specify current severity of agoraphobic avoidance
    Specify current severity of panic attacks
300.01   without agoraphobia
    Specify current severity of panic attacks
300.22   Agoraphobia without history of panic disorder
    Specify with or without limited symptom attacks
300.23   Social phobia
    Specify if generalized type
300.29   Simple phobia
300.30   Obsessive compulsive disorder (or Obsessive compulsive neurosis)
309.89   Post-traumatic stress disorder
    Specify if delayed onset
300.02   Generalized anxiety disorder
300.00   Anxiety disorder NOS

SOMATOFORM DISORDERS

300.70*   Body dysmorphic disorder
300.11   Conversion disorder (or Hysterical neurosis, conversion type)
    Specify: single episode or recurrent
300.70*   Hypochondriasis (or Hypochondriacal neurosis)

300.81   Somatization disorder
307.80   Somatoform pain disorder
300.70*   Undifferentiated somatoform disorder
300.70*   Somatoform disorder NOS

DISSOCIATIVE DISORDERS (OR HYSTERICAL NEUROSES, DISSOCIATIVE TYPE)

300.14   Multiple personality disorder
300.13   Psychogenic fugue
300.12   Psychogenic amnesia
300.60   Depersonalization disorder (or Depersonalization neurosis)
300.15   Dissociative disorder NOS

SEXUAL DISORDERS
Paraphilias

302.40   Exhibitionism
302.81   Fetishism
302.89   Frotteurism
302.20   Pedophilia
    Specify: same sex, opposite sex, same and opposite sex
    Specify if limited to incest
    Specify: exclusive type or nonexclusive type
302.83   Sexual masochism
302.84   Sexual sadism
302.30   Transvestic fetishism
302.82   Voyeurism
302.90*   Paraphilia NOS

Sexual dysfunctions

    Specify: psychogenic only, or psychogenic and biogenic (Note: If biogenic only, code on Axis III)
Specify: lifelong or acquired
Specify: generalized or situational
    Sexual desire disorders
302.71   Hypoactive sexual desire disorder
302.79   Sexual aversion disorder
    Sexual arousal disorder
302.72*   Female sexual arousal disorder

302.72*	Male erectile disorder
	Orgasm disorders
302.73	Inhibited female orgasm
302.74	Inhibited male orgasm
302.75	Premature ejaculation
	Sexual pain disorders
302.76	Dyspareunia
306.51	Vaginismus
302.70	Sexual dysfunction NOS

Other sexual disorders

302.90*	Sexual disorder NOS

SLEEP DISORDERS

Dyssomnias

	Insomnia disorder
307.42*	related to another mental disorder (nonorganic)
780.50*	related to known organic factor
307.42*	Primary insomnia
	Hypersomnia disorder
307.44	related to another mental disorder (nonorganic)
780.50*	related to a known organic factor
780.54	Primary hypersomnia
307.45	Sleep-wake schedule disorder
	Specify: advanced or delayed phase type, disorganized type, frequently changing type
	Other dyssomnias
307.40*	Dyssomnia NOS

Parasomnias

307.47	Dream anxiety disorder (Nightmare disorder)
307.46*	Sleep terror disorder
307.46*	Sleepwalking disorder
307.40*	Parasomnia NOS

FACTITIOUS DISORDERS

	Factitious disorder
301.51	with physical symptoms
300.16	with psychological symptoms
300.19	Factitious disorder NOS

IMPULSE CONTROL DISORDERS NOT ELSEWHERE CLASSIFIED

312.34	Intermittent explosive disorder
312.32	Kleptomania
312.31	Pathological gambling
312.33	Pyromania
312.39*	Trichotillomania
312.39*	Impulse control disorder NOS

ADJUSTMENT DISORDER

	Adjustment disorder
309.24	with anxious mood
309.00	with depressed mood
309.30	with disturbance of conduct
309.40	with mixed disturbance of motions and conduct
309.28	with mixed emotional features
309.82	with physical complaints
309.83	with withdrawal
309.23	with work (or academic) inhibition
309.90	Adjustment disorder NOS

PSYCHOLOGICAL FACTORS AFFECTING PHYSICAL CONDITION

316.00	Psychological factors affecting physical condition
	Specify physical condition on Axis III

PERSONALITY DISORDERS

Note: These are coded on Axis II.

Cluster A

301.00	Paranoid
301.20	Schizoid
301.22	Schizotypal

Cluster B

301.70	Antisocial
301.83	Borderline
301.50	Histrionic
301.81	Narcissistic

PERSONALITY DISORDERS—cont'd

Cluster C

301.82	Avoidant
301.60	Dependent
301.40	Obsessive compulsive
301.84	Passive aggressive
301.90	Personality disorder NOS

V CODES FOR CONDITIONS NOT ATTRIBUTABLE TO A MENTAL DISORDER THAT ARE A FOCUS OF ATTENTION OR TREATMENT

V62.30	Academic problem
V71.01	Adult antisocial behavior

V40.00	Borderline intellectual functioning (Note: This is coded on Axis II.)

V71.02	Childhood or adolescent antisocial behavior
V65.20	Malingering
V61.10	Marital problem
V15.81	Noncompliance with medical treatment

V62.20	Occupational problem
V61.20	Parent-child problem
V62.81	Other interpersonal problem
V61.80	Other specific family circumstances
V62.89	Phase of life problem or other life circumstance problem
V62.82	Uncomplicated bereavement

ADDITIONAL CODES

300.90	Unspecified mental disorder (nonpsychotic)
V71.09*	No diagnosis or condition on Axis I
799.90*	Diagnosis or condition deferred on Axis I

V71.09*	No diagnosis or condition on Axis II
799.90*	Diagnosis or condition deferred on Axis II

MULTIAXIAL SYSTEM

Axis I	Clinical Syndromes V Codes
Axis II	Developmental Disorders Personality Disorders
Axis III	Physical Disorders and Conditions
Axis IV	Severity of Psychosocial Stressors
Axis V	Global Assessment of Functioning

Severity of psychosocial stressors scale: adults

CODE	TERM	EXAMPLES OF STRESSORS	
		ACUTE EVENTS	ENDURING CIRCUMSTANCES
1	None	No acute events that may be relevant to the disorder	No enduring circumstances that may be relevant to the disorder
2	Mild	Broke up with boyfriend or girlfriend; started or graduated from school; child left home	Family arguments; job dissatisfaction; residence in high-crime neighborhood
3	Moderate	Marriage; marital separation; loss of job; retirement; miscarriage	Marital discord; serious financial problems; trouble with boss; being a single parent
4	Severe	Divorce; birth of first child	Unemployment; poverty
5	Extreme	Death of a spouse; serious physical illness diagnosed; victim of rape	Serious chronic illness in self or child; ongoing physical or sexual abuse
6	Catastrophic	Death of a child; suicide of spouse; devastating natural disaster	Captivity as hostage; concentration camp experience
0	Inadequate information, or no change in condition		

Severity of psychosocial stressors scale: children and adolescents

CODE	TERM	EXAMPLES OF STRESSORS	
		ACUTE EVENTS	ENDURING CIRCUMSTANCES
1	None	No acute events that may be relevant to the disorder	No enduring circumstances that may be relevant to the disorder
2	Mild	Broke up with boyfriend or girlfriend; change of school	Overcrowded living quarters; family arguments
3	Moderate	Expelled from school; birth of sibling	Chronic disabling illness in parent, chronic parental discord
4	Severe	Divorce of parents; unwanted pregnancy; arrest	Harsh or rejecting parents; chronic life-threatening illness in parent; multiple foster home placements
5	Extreme	Sexual or physical abuse; death of a parent	Recurrent sexual or physical abuse
6	Catastrophic	Death of both parents	Chronic life-threatening illness
0	Inadequate information, or no change in condition		

Global assessment of functioning scale (GAF scale)

Consider psychological, social, and occupational functioning on a hypothetical continuum of mental health-illness. Do not include impairment in functioning due to physical (or environmental) limitations.

Note: Use intermediate codes when appropriate, e.g., 45, 68, 72.

CODE

90 | **Absent or minimal symptoms** (e.g., mild anxiety before an exam), **good functioning in all areas, interested and involved in a wide range of activities, socially effective, generally satisfied with life, no more than everyday problems or concerns** (e.g., an occasional
81 | argument with family members).

80 | **If symptoms are present, they are transient and expectable reactions to psychosocial stressors** (e.g., difficulty concentrating after family argument); **no more than slight impairment in social, occupational, or school functioning** (e.g., temporarily falling behind in
71 | school work).

70 | **Some mild symptoms** (e.g., depressed mood and mild insomnia) **OR some difficulty in social, occupational, or school functioning** (e.g., occasional truancy, or theft within the household), **but generally functioning pretty well, has some meaningful interpersonal
61 | relationships.**

60 | **Moderate symptoms** (e.g., flat affect and circumstantial speech, occasional panic attacks) **OR moderate difficulty in social, occupational, or school functioning** (e.g., few friends, con-
51 | flicts with co-workers).

50 | **Serious symptoms** (e.g., suicidal ideation, severe obsessional rituals, frequent shoplifting) **OR any serious impairment in social, occupational, or school functioning** (e.g., few friends,
41 | unable to keep a job).

40 | **Some impairment in reality testing or communication** (e.g., speech is at times illogical, obscure, or irrelevant) **OR major impairment in several areas, such as work or school, family relations, judgment, thinking, or mood** (e.g., depressed man avoids friends, neglects family, and is unable to work; child frequently beats up younger children, is defiant at
31 | home, and is failing at school).

30 | **Behavior is considerably influenced by delusions or hallucinations OR serious impairment in communication or judgment** (e.g., sometimes incoherent, acts grossly inappropriately, suicidal preoccupation) **OR inability to function in almost all areas** (e.g., stays in
21 | bed all day; no job, home, or friends).

20 | **Some danger of hurting self or others** (e.g., suicide attempts without clear expectation of death, frequent violent, manic excitement) **OR occasionally fails to maintain minimal personal hygiene** (e.g., smears feces) **OR gross impairment in communication** (e.g., largely
11 | incoherent or mute).

10 | **Persistent danger of severely hurting self or others** (e.g., recurrent violence) **OR persistent inability to maintain minimal personal hygiene OR serious suicidal act with clear ex-
1 | pectation of death.**

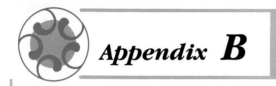

Appendix *B*

Preliminary DSM-IV Classification

Note: These codes are preliminary and are subject to further updates and modifications after additional consultations.

DISORDERS USUALLY FIRST DIAGNOSED IN INFANCY, CHILDHOOD, OR ADOLESCENCE

Mental retardation

317	Mild Mental Retardation
318.0	Moderate Retardation
318.1	Severe Mental Retardation
318.2	Profound Mental Retardation
319	Mental Retardation, Severity Unspecified

Learning disorders (academic skills disorder)

315.00	Reading Disorder (Developmental Reading Disorder)
315.1	Mathematics Disorder (Developmental Arithmetic Disorder)
315.2	Disorder of Written Expression (Developmental Expressive Writing Disorder)
315.9	Learning Disorder NOS

Reprinted with permission from the *DSM-IV Draft Criteria,* Task Force on DSM-IV, American Psychiatric Association, Copyright 1993, American Psychiatric Association.

Motor skills disorder

315.4	Developmental Coordination Disorder

Pervasive developmental disorders

299.00	Autistic Disorder
299.80	Rett's Disorder
299.10	Childhood Disintegrative Disorder
	Asperger's Disorder (? placement)
299.80	Pervasive Developmental Disorder NOS (Including Atypical Autism)

Disruptive behavior and attention-deficit disorders

	Attention-deficit/Hyperactivity Disorder
314.00	predominantly inattentive type
314.01	predominantly hyperactive-impulsive type
314.01	combined type
314.9	Attention-deficit/Hyperactivity Disorder NOS
313.81	Oppositional Defiant Disorder
312.8	Conduct Disorder
312.9	Disruptive Behavior Disorder NOS

Feeding and eating disorders of infancy or early childhood

307.52	Pica
307.53	Rumination Disorder
307.59	Feeding Disorder of Infancy or Early Childhood

Tic disorders

307.23	Tourette's Disorder
307.22	Chronic Motor or Vocal Tic Disorder
307.21	Transient Tic Disorder
307.20	Tic Disorder NOS

Communication disorders

315.31	Expressive Language Disorder (Developmental Expressive Language Disorder)
315.31	Mixed Receptive/Expressive Language Disorder (Developmental Receptive Language Disorder)

315.39	Phonological Disorder (Developmental Articulation Disorder)
307.0	Stuttering
315.39	Communication Disorder NOS

Elimination disorders

| 307.7 | Encopresis |
| 307.6 | Enuresis |

Other disorders of infancy, childhood, or adolescence

309.21	Separation Anxiety Disorder
313.23	Selective Mutism (Elective Mutism)
313.89	Reactive Attachment Disorder of Infancy or Early Childhood
307.3	Stereotypic Movement Disorder (Stereotypy/Habit Disorder)
313.9	Disorder of Infancy, Childhood, or Adolescence NOS

DELIRIUM, DEMENTIA, AMNESTIC AND OTHER COGNITIVE DISORDERS

Deliria

293.0	Delirium Due to a General Medical Condition
---.-	Substance-Induced Delirium (refer to specific substance for code)
---.-	Delirium Due to Multiple Etiologies (use multiple codes based on specific etiologies)
293.89	Delirium NOS

Dementias

---.-	Dementia of the Alzheimer's Type With Early Onset: if onset at age 65 or below.
290.10	uncomplicated
290.11	with delirium
290.12	with delusions
290.13	with depressed mood
290.14	with hallucinations
290.15	with perceptual disturbance
290.16	with behavioral disturbance

290.17	with communication disturbance With Late Onset: if onset after age 65.
290.00	uncomplicated
290.30	with delirium
290.20	with delusions
290.21	with depressed mood
290.22	with hallucinations
290.23	with perceptual disturbance
290.24	with behavioral disturbance
290.25	with communication disturbance
---.-	Vascular Dementia (D:9)
290.40	uncomplicated
290.41	with delirium
290.42	with delusions
290.43	with depressed mood
290.44	with hallucinations
290.45	with perceptual disturbance
290.46	with behavioral disturbance
290.47	with communication disturbance

Dementias due to other general medical conditions

294.9	Dementia Due to HIV Disease (Code 043.1 on Axis III)
294.1	Dementia Due to Head Trauma (Code 905.0 on Axis III)
294.1	Dementia Due to Parkinson's Disease (Code 332.0 on Axis III)
294.1	Dementia Due to Huntington's Disease (Code 333.4 on Axis III)
290.10	Dementia Due to Pick's Disease (Code 331.1 on Axis III)
290.10	Dementia Due to Creutzfeldt-Jakob Disease (Code 046.1 on Axis III)
294.1	Dementia Due to Other General Medical Condition
---.-	Substance-Induced Persisting Dementia (refer to specific substance for code)
---.-	Dementia Due to Multiple Etiologies (use multiple codes based on specific etiologies)
294.8	Dementia NOS

Amnestic disorders

294.0 Amnestic Disorder Due to a General Medical Condition

---.- Substance-induced Persisting Amnestic Disorder
(refer to specific substance for code)

294.8 Amnestic Disorder NOS

294.9 Cognitive Disorder NOS

MENTAL DISORDERS DUE TO A GENERAL MEDICAL CONDITION NOT ELSEWHERE CLASSIFIED

293.89 Catatonic Disorder Due to a General Medical Condition

310.1 Personality Change Due to a General Medical Condition

293.9 Mental Disorder NOS Due to a General Medical Condition

SUBSTANCE RELATED DISORDERS

Alcohol use disorders

303.90 Alcohol Dependence
305.00 Alcohol Abuse
303.00 Alcohol Intoxication
291.8 Alcohol Withdrawal
291.0 Alcohol Delirium
291.2 Alcohol Persisting Dementia
291.1 Alcohol Persisting Amnestic Disorder
Alcohol Psychotic Disorder
291.5 with delusions
291.3 with hallucinations
291.8 Alcohol Mood Disorder
291.8 Alcohol Anxiety Disorder
292.8 Alcohol Sexual Dysfunction
292.89 Alcohol Sleep Disorder
291.9 Alcohol Use Disorder NOS

Amphetamine (or related substance) use disorders

304.40 Amphetamine (or Related Substance) Dependence
305.70 Amphetamine (or Related Substance) Abuse

305.70 Amphetamine (or Related Substance) Intoxication
292.0 Amphetamine (or Related Substance) Withdrawal
292.81 Amphetamine (or Related Substance) Delirium
Amphetamine (or Related Substance) Psychotic Disorder
291.11 with delusions
291.12 with hallucinations
292.84 Amphetamine (or Related Substance) Mood Disorder
292.89 Amphetamine (or Related Substance) Anxiety Disorder
292.89 Amphetamine (or Related Substance) Sexual Dysfunction
292.89 Amphetamine (or Related Substance) Sleep Disorder
292.9 Amphetamine (or Related Substance) Use Disorder NOS

Caffeine use disorders

305.90 Caffeine Intoxication
292.84 Caffeine Anxiety Disorder
292.89 Caffeine Sleep Disorder
292.9 Caffeine Use Disorder NOS

Cannabis use disorders

304.30 Cannabis Dependence
305.20 Cannabis Abuse
305.20 Cannabis Intoxication
292.81 Cannabis Delirium
Cannabis Psychotic Disorder
291.11 with delusions
291.12 with hallucinations
292.89 Cannabis Anxiety Disorder
292.9 Cannabis Use Disorder NOS

Cocaine use disorders

304.20 Cocaine Dependence
305.60 Cocaine Abuse
305.60 Cocaine Intoxication
292.0 Cocaine Withdrawal
292.81 Cocaine Delirium
Cocaine Psychotic Disorder

291.11	with delusions
291.12	with hallucinations
292.84	Cocaine Mood Disorder
292.89	Cocaine Anxiety Disorder
292.89	Cocaine Sexual Dysfunction
292.89	Cocaine Sleep Disorder
292.9	Cocaine Use Disorder NOS

Hallucinogen use disorders

304.50	Hallucinogen Dependence
305.30	Hallucinogen Abuse
305.30	Hallucinogen Intoxication
292.89	Hallucinogen Persisting Perception Disorder
292.81	Hallucinogen Delirium
	Hallucinogen Psychotic Disorder
291.11	with delusions
291.12	with hallucinations
292.84	Hallucinogen Mood Disorder
292.89	Hallucinogen Anxiety Disorder
292.9	Hallucinogen Use Disorder NOS

Inhalant use disorders

304.60	Inhalant Dependence
305.90	Inhalant Abuse
305.90	Inhalant Intoxication
292.81	Inhalant Delirium
292.82	Inhalant Persisting Dementia
	Inhalant Psychotic Disorder
291.11	with delusions
291.12	with hallucinations
292.84	Inhalant Mood Disorder
292.89	Inhalant Anxiety Disorder
292.9	Inhalant Use Disorder NOS

Nicotine use disorders

305.10	Nicotine Dependence
292.0	Nicotine Withdrawal
292.9	Nicotine Use Disorder NOS

Opioid use disorders

304.00	Opioid Dependence
305.50	Opioid Abuse
305.50	Opioid Intoxication
292.0	Opioid Withdrawal

292.81	Opioid Delirium
	Opioid Psychotic Disorder
291.11	with delusions
291.12	with hallucinations
292.84	Opioid Mood Disorder
292.89	Opioid Sleep Disorder
292.89	Opioid Sexual Dysfunction
292.9	Opioid Use Disorder NOS

Phencyclidine (or related substance) use disorders

304.90	Phencyclidine (or Related Substance) Dependence
305.90	Phencyclidine (or Related Substance) Abuse
305.90	Phencyclidine (or Related Substance) Intoxication
292.81	Phencyclidine (or Related Substance) Delirium
	Phencyclidine (or Related Substance) Psychotic Disorder
291.11	with delusions
291.12	with hallucinations
292.84	Phencyclidine (or Related Substance) Mood Disorder
292.89	Phencyclidine (or Related Substance) Anxiety Disorder
292.9	Phencyclidine (or Related Substance) Use Disorder NOS

Sedative, hypnotic, or anxiolytic substance use disorders

304.10	Sedative, Hypnotic, or Anxiolytic Dependence
305.40	Sedative, Hypnotic, or Anxiolytic Abuse
305.40	Sedative, Hypnotic, or Anxiolytic Intoxication
292.0	Sedative, Hypnotic, or Anxiolytic Withdrawal
292.81	Sedative, Hypnotic, or Anxiolytic Delirium
292.82	Sedative, Hypnotic, or Anxiolytic Persisting Dementia
292.83	Sedative, Hypnotic, or Anxiolytic Persisting Amnestic Disorder

Sedative, Hypnotic, or Anxiolytic Psychotic Disorder
291.11   with delusions
291.12   with hallucinations
292.84 Sedative, Hypnotic, or Anxiolytic Mood Disorder
292.89 Sedative, Hypnotic, or Anxiolytic Anxiety Disorder
292.89 Sedative, Hypnotic, or Anxiolytic Sleep Disorder
292.89 Sedative, Hypnotic, or Anxiolytic Sexual Dysfunction
292.9 Sedative, Hypnotic, or Anxiolytic Use Disorder NOS

Polysubstance use disorder

304.80 Polysubstance Dependence (E:27)

Other (or unknown) substance use disorders

304.90 Other (or Unknown) Substance Dependence
305.90 Other (or Unknown) Substance Abuse
305.90 Other (or Unknown) Substance Intoxication
292.0 Other (or Unknown) Substance Withdrawal
292.81 Other (or Unknown) Substance Delirium
292.82 Other (or Unknown) Substance Persisting Dementia
292.83 Other (or Unknown) Substance Persisting Amnestic Disorder
Other (or Unknown) Substance Psychotic Disorder
291.11   with delusions
291.12   with hallucinations
292.84 Other (or Unknown) Substance Mood Disorder
292.89 Other (or Unknown) Substance Anxiety Disorder
292.89 Other (or Unknown) Substance Sexual Dysfunction
292.89 Other (or Unknown) Substance Sleep Disorder

292.9 Other (or Unknown) Substance Use Disorder NOS

SCHIZOPHRENIA AND OTHER PSYCHOTIC DISORDERS

Schizophrenia
295.30 paranoid type
295.10 disorganized type
295.20 catatonic type
295.90 undifferentiated type
295.60 residual type
295.40 Schizophreniform Disorder
295.70 Schizoaffective Disorder
297.1 Delusional Disorder
298.8 Brief Psychotic Disorder
297.3 Shared Psychotic Disorder (Folie a Deux)

Psychotic Disorder Due to a General Medical Condition
293.81 with delusions
293.82 with hallucinations
---.- Substance-Induced Psychotic Disorder (refer to specific substances for codes)
298.9 Psychotic Disorder NOS

MOOD DISORDERS

Code current state of Major Depressive Disorder or Bipolar Disorder in fifth digit:

0 unspecified
1 mild
2 moderate
3 severe, without psychotic features
4 severe, with psychotic features
5 in partial remission
6 in full remission

Depressive disorders

Major Depressive Disorder
296.2x single episode
296.3x recurrent
300.4 Dysthymic Disorder
311 Depressive Disorder NOS

Bipolar disorders

Bipolar I Disorder
296.0x	single manic episode
296.4	most recent episode hypomanic
296.4x	most recent episode manic
296.6x	most recent episode mixed
296.5x	most recent episode depressed
296.7	most recent episode unspecified
296.89	Bipolar II Disorder (Recurrent major depressive episodes with hypomania)
301.13	Cyclothymic Disorder
296.80	Bipolar Disorder NOS
293.83	Mood Disorder Due to a General Medical Condition
---.-	Substance-Induced Mood Disorder (refer to specific substances for codes)
296.90	Mood Disorder NOS

ANXIETY DISORDERS

Panic Disorder
300.01	Without Agoraphobia
300.21	With Agoraphobia
300.22	Agoraphobia Without History of Panic Disorder
300.29	Specific Phobia (Simple Phobia)
300.23	Social Phobia (Social Anxiety Disorder)
300.3	Obsessive-Compulsive Disorder
309.81	Posttraumatic Stress Disorder
300.3	Acute Stress Disorder
300.02	Generalized Anxiety Disorder (includes Overanxious Disorder of Childhood)
293.89	Anxiety Disorder Due to a General Medical Condition
---.-	Substance-Induced Anxiety Disorder (refer to specific substances for codes)
300.00	Anxiety Disorder NOS

SOMATOFORM DISORDERS

300.81	Somatization Disorder
300.11	Conversion Disorder
300.7	Hypochondriasis
300.71	Body Dysmorphic Disorder
	Pain Disorder
307.80	Associated with Psychological Factors
307.89	Associated with Both Psychological Factors and a General Medical Condition
300.82	Undifferentiated Somatoform Disorder
300.89	Somatoform Disorder NOS

FACTITIOUS DISORDERS

Factitious Disorder
300.16	with predominantly psychological signs and symptoms
300.17	with predominantly physical signs and symptoms
300.18	with combined psychological and physical signs and symptoms
300.19	Factitious Disorder NOS

DISSOCIATIVE DISORDERS

300.12	Dissociative Amnesia
300.13	Dissociative Fugue
300.14	Dissociative Identity Disorder (Multiple Personality Disorder)
300.6	Depersonalization Disorder
300.15	Dissociative Disorder NOS

SEXUAL AND GENDER IDENTITY DISORDERS

Sexual dysfunctions

Sexual Desire Disorders
302.71	Hypoactive Sexual Desire Disorder
?302.79	Sexual Aversion Disorder

Sexual Arousal Disorders
302.72	Female Sexual Arousal Disorder
302.72	Male Erectile Disorder

Orgasm Disorders
302.73	Female Orgasmic Disorder (Inhibited Female Orgasm)
302.74	Male Orgasmic Disorder (Inhibited Male Orgasm)

302.75 Premature Ejaculation
Sexual Pain Disorders
302.76 Dyspareunia
306.51 Vaginismus
Sexual Dysfunctions Due to a General Medical Condition
607.84 Male Erectile Disorder Due to a General Medical Condition
606.89 Male Dyspareunia Due to a General Medical Condition
625.0   Female Dyspareunia Due to a General Medical Condition
608.89 Male Hypoactive Sexual Desire Disorder Due to a General Medical Condition
625.8   Female Hypoactive Sexual Desire Disorder Due to a General Medical Condition
608.89 Other Male Sexual Dysfunction Due to a General Medical Condition
625.8   Other Female Sexual Dysfunction Due to a General Medical Condition
---.-   Substance-Induced Sexual Dysfunction (refer to specific substances for codes)
302.70 Sexual Dysfunction NOS

Paraphilias

302.4   Exhibitionism
302.81 Fetishism
?302.85 Frotteurism
302.2   Pedophilia
302.83 Sexual Masochism
302.84 Sexual Sadism
302.82 Voyeurism
302.3   Transvestic Fetishism
302.9   Paraphilia NOS

302.9   Sexual Disorder NOS

Gender identity disorders

        Gender Identity Disorder
302.6   in Children
302.85   in Adolescents and Adults
302.6   Gender Identity Disorder NOS

EATING DISORDERS

307.1   Anorexia Nervosa
307.51 Bulimia Nervosa
307.50 Eating Disorder NOS

SLEEP DISORDERS
Primary sleep disorders
Dyssomnias
307.42 Primary Insomnia
307.44 Primary Hypersomnia
347   Narcolepsy
780.59 Breathing-Related Sleep Disorder
307.45 Circadian Rhythm Sleep Disorder (Sleep-Wake Schedule Disorder)
307.47 Dyssomnia NOS
Parasomnias
307.47 Nightmare Disorder (Dream Anxiety Disorder)
307.46 Sleep Terror Disorder
307.46 Sleepwalking Disorder
?307.47 Parasomnia NOS

Sleep disorders related to another mental disorder

307.42 Insomnia related to [Axis I or Axis II Disorder]
307.44 Hypersomnia related to [Axis I or Axis II Disorder]

Other sleep disorders

        Sleep Disorder Due to a General Medical Condition
780.52   insomnia type
780.54   hypersomnia type
780.59   parasomnia type
780.59   mixed type
---.-   Substance-Induced Sleep Disorder (refer to specific substances for codes)

IMPULSE CONTROL DISORDERS NOT ELSEWHERE CLASSIFIED

312.34 Intermittent Explosive Disorder
312.32 Kleptomania

312.33	Pyromania
312.31	Pathological Gambling
?312.39	Trichotillomania
312.30	Impulse Control NOS

ADJUSTMENT DISORDERS

	Adjustment Disorder
309.24	With Anxiety
309.0	With Depressed Mood
309.3	With Disturbance of Conduct
309.4	With Mixed Disturbance of Emotions and Conduct
309.28	With Mixed Anxiety and Depressed Mood
309.9	Unspecified

PERSONALITY DISORDERS

301.0	Paranoid Personality Disorder
301.20	Schizoid Personality Disorder
301.22	Schizotypal Personality Disorder
301.7	Antisocial Personality Disorder
301.83	Borderline Personality Disorder
301.50	Histrionic Personality Disorder
301.81	Narcissistic Personality Disorder
301.82	Avoidant Personality Disorder
301.6	Dependent Personality Disorder
301.4	Obsessive-Compulsive Personality Disorder
301.9	Personality Disorder NOS

OTHER CONDITIONS THAT MAY BE A FOCUS OF CLINICAL ATTENTION

316 (Psychological Factors) Affecting Medical Condition
Choose name based on nature of factors:
Mental Disorder Affecting Medical Condition
Psychological Symptoms Affecting Medical Condition
Personality Traits or Coping Style Affecting Medical Condition
Maladaptive Health Behaviors Affecting Medical Condition
Unspecified Psychological Factors Affecting Medical Condition

Medication-induced movement disorders

332.1	Neuroleptic-induced Parkinsonism
333.92	Neuroleptic Malignant Syndrome
333.7	Neuroleptic-induced Acute Dystonia
333.99	Neuroleptic-induced Acute Akathisia
333.82	Neuroleptic-induced Tardive Dyskinesia
333.1	Medication-induced Postural Tremor
333.90	Medication-induced Movement Disorder NOS
995.2	Adverse Effects of Medication NOS

Relational problems

V61.9	Relational Problem Related to A Mental Disorder or General Medical Condition
V61.20	Parent-Child Relational Problem
V61.12	Partner Relational Problem
V61.8	Sibling Relational Problem
V62.81	Relational Problem NOS

Problems related to abuse or neglect

V61.21	Physical Abuse of Child
V61.22	Sexual Abuse of Child
V61.21	Neglect of Child
V61.10	Physical Abuse of Adult
V51.11	Sexual Abuse of Adult

Additional conditions that may be a focus of clinical attention

V62.82	Bereavement
V40.0	Borderline Intellectual Functioning
V62.3	Academic Problem
V62.2	Occupational Problem
V71.02	Childhood or Adolescent Antisocial Behavior
V71.01	Adult Antisocial Behavior
V65.2	Malingering
V62.89	Phase of Life Problem
V15.81	Noncompliance with treatment for a mental disorder
313.82	Identity Problem

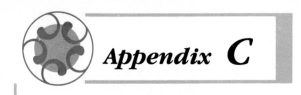

Appendix C

DEPARTMENT OF HEALTH, EDUCATION, AND WELFARE
PUBLIC HEALTH SERVICE
ALCOHOL, DRUG ABUSE,
AND MENTAL HEALTH ADMINISTRATION
NATIONAL INSTITUTE OF MENTAL HEALTH

STUDY	PATIENT	FORM	PERIOD	RATER	HOSPITAL
		117			
(1-6)	(7-9)	(10-12)	(13-15)	(16-17)	(79-80)

PATIENT'S NAME

RATER

DATE

ABNORMAL INVOLUNTARY MOVEMENT SCALE (AIMS)

INSTRUCTIONS: Complete Examination Procedure (reverse side) before making ratings.
MOVEMENT RATINGS: Rate highest severity observed.
Rate movements that occur upon activation one *less* than those observed spontaneously.

Code:
0 = None
1 = Minimal, may be extreme normal
2 = Mild
3 = Moderate
4 = Severe

CARD 01 (18-19)

		(Circle One)	
FACIAL OR ORAL MOVEMENTS:	1. Muscles of Facial Expression e.g., movements of forehead, eyebrows, periorbital area, cheeks; include frowning, blinking, smiling, grimacing	0 1 2 3 4	(20)
	2. Lips and Perioral Area e.g., puckering, pouting, smacking	0 1 2 3 4	(21)
	3. Jaw e.g., biting, clenching, chewing, mouth opening, lateral movement	0 1 2 3 4	(22)
	4. Tongue Rate only increase in movement both in and out of mouth, NOT inability to sustain movement	0 1 2 3 4	(23)
EXTREMITY MOVEMENTS:	5. Upper (*arms, wrists, hands, fingers*) Include choreic movements (i.e., rapid, objectively purposeless, irregular, spontaneous), athetoid movements (i.e., slow, irregular, complex, serpentine). Do NOT include tremor (i.e., repetitive, regular, rhythmic)	0 1 2 3 4	(24)
	6. Lower (*legs, knees, ankles, toes*) e.g., lateral knee movement, foot tapping, heel dropping, foot squirming, inversion and eversion of foot	0 1 2 3 4	(25)
TRUNK MOVEMENTS:	7. Neck, shoulders, hips e.g., rocking, twisting, squirming, pelvic gyrations	0 1 2 3 4	(26)
GLOBAL JUDGMENTS:	8. Severity of abnormal movements	None, normal 0 Minimal 1 Mild 2 Moderate 3 Severe 4	(27)
	9. Incapacitation due to abnormal movements	None, normal 0 Minimal 1 Mild 2 Moderate 3 Severe 4	(28)
	10. Patient's awareness of abnormal movements Rate only patient's report	No awareness 0 Aware, no distress 1 Aware, mild distress 2 Aware, moderate distress 3 Aware, severe distress 4	(29)
DENTAL STATUS:	11. Current problems with teeth and/or dentures	No 0 Yes 1	(30)
	12. Does patient usually wear dentures?	No 0 Yes 1	(31)

EXAMINATION PROCEDURE

Either before or after completing the Examination Procedure observe the patient unobtrusively, at rest (e.g., in waiting room).

The chair to be used in this examination should be a hard, firm one without arms.

1. Ask patient whether there is anything in his/her mouth (i.e., gum, candy, etc.) and if there is, to remove it.
2. Ask patient about the *current* condition of his/her teeth. Ask patient if he/she wears dentures. Do teeth or dentures bother patient *now*?
3. Ask patient whether he/she notices any movements in mouth, face, hands, or feet. If yes, ask to describe and to what extent they *currently* bother patient or interfere with his/her activities.
4. Have patient sit in chair with hands on knees, legs slightly apart, and feet flat on floor. (Look at entire body for movements while in this position).
5. Ask patient to sit with hands hanging unsupported. If male, between legs, if female and wearing a dress, hanging over knees. (Observe hands and other body areas.)

6. Ask patient to open mouth. (Observe tongue at rest within mouth.) Do this twice.
7. Ask patient to protrude tongue. (Observe abnormalities of tongue movement.) Do this twice.
■ 8. Ask patient to tap thumb, with each finger, as rapidly as possible for 10-15 seconds; separately with right hand, then with left hand. (Observe facial and leg movements.)
9. Flex and extend patient's left and right arms (one at a time). (Note any rigidity and rate on DOTES.)
10. Ask patient to stand up. (Observe in profile. Observe all body areas again, hips included.)
■11. Ask patient to extend both arms outstretched in front with palms down. (Observe trunk, legs, and mouth.)
■12. Have patient walk a few paces, turn, and walk back to chair. (Observe hands and gait.) Do this twice.

■Activated movements

Glossary

The following words are frequently used by the psychiatric nurse. Many of the definitions were taken from *A Psychiatric Glossary** and *Longman Dictionary of Psychology and Psychiatry*.† A larger and equally useful book is the *Psychiatric Dictionary*.‡

abreaction Lessening of emotional trauma by reenacting an emotionally painful situation.

abstinence Voluntarily denying oneself some kind of gratification; in the area of alcohol or drug dependence, being without the substance on which the subject is dependent. The abstinence syndrome is equivalent to withdrawal symptoms, and its appearance suggests the presence of physiological dependence or addiction.

abused child Child or infant who has suffered repeated injuries, which may include bone fractures, neurological and psychological damage, and sexual abuse at the hands of a parent, parents, or parent surrogates. The abuse takes place repeatedly and is often precipitated by the child's minor and normal irritating behavior.

acceptance Conveying implicit respect for and value of another by one's behavior and words.

accommodation According to Piaget, the modification of the existing body of knowledge based on newly acquired knowledge.

acrophobia Fear of heights.

acting out Expressions of unconscious emotional conflicts or feelings in actions rather than words. The person is not consciously aware of the meaning of such acts. Acting out may be harmful or, in controlled situations, therapeutic (e.g., children's play therapy).

Action for Mental Health The 1960 report of the Joint Commission on Mental Health and Mental Illness, which recommended community-based care for those with a mental illness.

adaptation In systems theory the response of a system to a stressor.

addiction Strong emotional and physiologic dependence on a chemical substance that has progressed beyond voluntary control.

addictions nursing Nursing specialty that focuses on the care of persons who are dependent upon mind-altering substances.

affect Emotional feeling tone; affect and emotional response are commonly used interchangeably.

ageism Systematic stereotyping of and discrimination against elderly people to create distance from the social plight of older people and to avoid primitive fears of aging and death. It is distinguished from gerontophobia, a specific pathological fear of old people and aging.

aggression Forceful physical, verbal, or symbolic action.

agitation Excessive motor activity, usually nonpurposeful and associated with internal tension, for example, inability to sit still, fidgeting, pacing, wringing of hands, or pulling of clothes.

agoraphobia Fear of open spaces.

akathisia Extrapyramidal side effect to antipsychotic medications, manifested by motor restlessness, inability to sit still, and pacing.

Al-Anon Organization of relatives of alcoholics operating in many communities under the philosophical and organizational structure of Alcoholics Anonymous to facilitate discussion and resolution of common problems.

---

*American Psychiatric Association: *A psychiatric glossary,* ed 5, Washington DC, 1980, The Association.
†Goldenson RM: *Longman Dictionary of Psychology and Psychiatry,* New York, 1984, Longman.
‡Campbell RJ: *Psychiatric dictionary,* ed 5, New York, 1981, Oxford University Press.

514

Alateen Organization of teenaged children of alcoholic parents operating in some communities under the philosophical and organizational structure of Alcoholics Anonymous. It provides a setting in which the children may receive group support in achieving a better understanding of their parents' problems and better methods for coping with them.

alcohol dependence (alcoholism) Physical dependence on alcohol characterized by either tolerance to the agent or development of withdrawal phenomena on cessation of, or reduction in, intake. Other aspects of the syndrome are psychological dependence and impairment in social or vocational functioning.

Alcoholics Anonymous (AA) Group of abstinent alcoholics who collectively assist other alcoholics through personal and group support.

Alzheimer's disease Degenerative brain disease of unknown cause marked by insidious onset and uniformly progressive deterioration. The disorder occurs most commonly in those over 65 but may occur as early as age 40.

ambivalence Coexistence of two opposing drives, desires, feelings, or emotions toward the same person, object, or goal; may be conscious or partially conscious.

amphetamines Central nervous system stimulants.

anal stage Second stage of psychosexual development, immediately following the oral stage, marked by a shift of libidinal energy to the anus and urethra; includes both anal-expulsive and anal-retentive phases. Many adult traits, such as stinginess, hoarding, and collecting, find their prototypes here.

anorexia nervosa Psychiatric disorder marked by severe and prolonged refusal to eat with severe weight loss, amenorrhea or impotence, disturbance of body image, an intense fear of becoming obese, and peculiar patterns of eating and handling food. Most frequently encountered in girls and young women.

anticipatory guidance Educative process to prepare the individual and family for changes likely to occur in the near future as a result of developmental changes.

antipsychotic medication Group of prescription drugs that are particularly effective in minimizing the positive symptoms of schizophrenia. This group includes the phenothiazines, thioxanthenes, butyrophenones, dihydroindolones, and dibenzoxaze-

pines. They act primarily by blocking dopamine receptors in brain tissue. Also called neuroleptic agents or major tranquilizers.

antisocial personality Personality disorder marked by a history of chronic antisocial behavior in which the rights of others are violated, with persistence into adult life of a pattern of antisocial behavior that began in adolescence, and a failure to sustain good job performance over several years. Lying, stealing, fighting, and truancy are typical early signs.

anxiety Apprehension, tension, or uneasiness that stems from the anticipation of danger, the source of which is largely unknown or unrecognized; primarily of intrapsychic origin, in distinction to fear, which is the emotional response to a consciously recognized and usually external threat or danger.

anxiolytic Ability to relieve anxiety or simple emotional tension. Medications used to treat anxiety are called anxiolytic agents.

apathy Used by Sullivan to describe the security operation whereby the individual defends against anxiety by not experiencing the emotion associated with an anxiety-producing event; there is a manifestation of extreme indifference.

assimilation According to Piaget, the adjustment of new experiences by the child so that knowledge of them can be incorporated into the child's existing body of knowledge.

assisted suicide Controversial practice of aiding an individual, usually one who is terminally ill, to kill himself or herself by providing the means or opportunity to do so.

attractiveness Value placed on a group by both members and nonmembers.

autism Developmental disability caused by a physical disorder of the brain appearing during the first 3 years of life. Symptoms include disturbances in physical, social, and language skills; abnormal responses to sensations; and abnormal ways of relating to people, objects, and events.

autistic thinking Form of thinking that attempts to gratify unfulfilled desires without due regard for reality; objective facts are distorted, obscured, or excluded in varying degrees.

autonomy Quality or state of being self-governing. The living organism does not represent merely an inactive element but is to a large extent a self-governing entity.

barbiturates Central nervous system depressants.

bargaining Third stage of the dying process, characterized by the individual's attempt to gain more time by trading off "good" behavior. This stage temporarily eases anxiety and enables the person to cope.

beliefs Thoughts held to be true but not proved to be so.

biochemistry Study of the chemical elements and their interactions within the body.

biological variations Cultural phenomenon that reflects biological differences among individuals in different cultural groups.

bipolar disorder Major affective disorder in which there are episodes of both mania and depression; formerly called manic depressive psychosis, circular or mixed type.

blocking Difficulty in recollection or the sudden interruption of a train of thought or speech resulting from emotional factors that are usually unconscious.

body image One's sense of self as presented to others.

body language Message(s) transmitted by one's body motion and facial expressions that are learned forms of communication and that have meaning within the context in which they appear.

bonding Attachment and unity of two people whose identities are significantly affected by their mutual interactions. Bonding often refers to the result of the process of attachment between the mother and her child.

bulimia nervosa Psychiatric disorder, occurring primarily in females, marked by episodic uncontrolled and rapid consumption of food over a short period of time (binges), inconspicuous eating during a binge, and termination of the binge by abdominal pain, social interruption, sleep, or self-induced vomiting.

butyrophenones Group of antipsychotic agents.

catchment area Geographical area for which a mental health program or facility has responsibility.

catecholamine hypothesis Theory that some forms of depression are associated with catecholamine deficiency, particularly norepinephrine, in the brain.

catharsis Healthful (therapeutic) release of ideas through a "talking out" of conscious material accompanied by an appropriate emotional reaction. Also, the release into awareness of repressed material from the unconscious.

cathexis Attachment, conscious or unconscious, of emotional feeling and significance to an idea, an object, or most commonly, a person.

cerea flexibilitas "Waxy flexibility" often present in catatonic schizophrenia in which the individual's arm or leg remains in the position in which it is placed.

chronic alcoholic Alcohol-dependent individual who drinks excessively and may be incapacitated most of the time.

clanging Type of thinking in which the sound of a word, rather than its meaning, gives the direction to subsequent associations; punning and rhyming may substitute for logic, and language may become increasingly a senseless compulsion to associate and decreasingly a vehicle for communication.

claustrophobia Fear of closed spaces.

cocaine Central nervous system stimulant that acts directly on the cerebral cortex and initially increases the sensation of mental and physical well-being.

cognitive Refers to the mental process of comprehension, judgment, memory, and reasoning, as contrasted with emotional and volitional processes.

cognitive development Beginning in infancy, the acquisition of intelligence, conscious thought, and problem-solving abilities. An orderly sequence in the increase in knowledge derived from sensorimotor activity has been empirically demonstrated by Piaget.

commitment Legal process for admitting a person who has a mental illness to a psychiatric treatment program. The legal definition and procedure vary from state to state, although commitment usually requires a court or judicial procedure.

communication Reciprocal exchange of information, ideas, beliefs, feelings, and attitudes between two persons or among a group of persons.

Community Mental Health Centers Act Enacted in 1963 by the U.S. Congress; sought to revolutionize the provision of mental health care by emphasizing prevention and decentralized, local community treatment for all persons with a mental illness.

Community Support Program Program mounted by the National Institute of Mental Health in 1977 to award federal money to the states for the purpose of coordinating the services offered by the variety of agencies attempting to serve individuals with a long-term mental illness.

community support system Wide range of coordinated basic community services and supports designed to enable persons with a long-term mental illness to live and function in the community.

compensation Mental mechanism, operating unconsciously, by which the individual attempts to make up for real or fancied deficiencies; conscious process by which the individual strives to make up for real or imagined defects in such areas as physique, performance, skills, or psychological attributes—the two types frequently merge.

complex Group of associated ideas that have a common strong emotional tone; these may be in part unconscious and may significantly influence attitudes and associations.

compulsion Insistent, repetitive, intrusive, and unwanted urge to perform an act that is contrary to the person's ordinary conscious wishes or standards; a defensive substitute for hidden and still more unacceptable ideas and wishes. Anxiety results from failure to perform the compulsive act.

computerized axial tomography (CAT scan) Technique for noninvasive radiologic examination of soft tissues. Scan of the intracranial contents allows visualization of the structure of the brain, including cerebrospinal fluid–filled spaces.

concept Mental image.

conceptual framework Theoretical model that attempts to logically explain and relate a discipline's phenomena of concern. The appropriateness of a conceptual framework is determined by its applicability and usefulness.

concluding phase (termination) Final stage of the nurse-client relationship. This stage is characterized by mutual feelings of loss. Its goal is to assist the client to review what was learned from the relationship and to transfer this learning to interactions with others.

condensation Psychological process often present in dreams in which two or more concepts are fused so that a single symbol represents the multiple components.

confabulation Unconscious, defensive "filling in" of actual memory gaps by imaginary or fantastic experiences, often complex, that are recounted in a detailed and plausible way as though they were factual.

confidentiality Right of clients to have their medical records held secret unless they consent to disclosure; also applies to information verbally communicated by the client to health professionals in the belief that this information will not be told to anyone else. Laws that pertain to the confidentiality of psychiatric records vary greatly among the states.

conflict Mental struggle that arises from the simultaneous operation of opposing impulses, drives, and external (environmental) or internal demands; termed intrapsychic when the conflict is between forces within the personality; extrapsychic, when it is between the self and the environment.

confusion Disturbed orientation in respect to time, place, or person; sometimes accompanied by disturbances of consciousness.

conscience Morally self-critical part of one's standards of behavior, performance, and value judgments. Commonly equated with the superego.

conscious Content of mind or mental functioning of which one is aware.

consistent Behaving in the same predictable manner in the same or similar situations.

conversion Defense mechanism, operating unconsciously, by which intrapsychic conflicts that would otherwise give rise to anxiety are instead given symbolic external expression. The repressed ideas or impulses and the psychological defenses against them are converted into a variety of somatic symptoms involving the nervous system. These may include such symptoms as paralysis, pain, or loss of sensory function.

coping mechanism Adaptation to anxiety based on conscious acknowledgment of a problem; the individual engages in reality-oriented problem-solving activities designed to reduce tension.

countertransference Therapist's conscious or unconscious emotional reaction to the client.

crack Central nervous system stimulant, derived from cocaine. Crack is generally smoked and has an immediate but short-lived, intense euphoric effect. It is highly addictive.

crisis State of disequilibrium resulting from the interaction of an event with the individual's or family's coping mechanisms, which are inadequate to meet the demands of the situation, combined with the individual's or family's perception of the meaning of the event.

cultural values Unique, individual expressions of a particular culture that have been accepted as appropriate. They guide actions and decision making that facilitate self-worth and self-esteem.

culturally diverse nursing care Nursing care that is culturally appropriate.

culture Patterned behavioral response that develops over time as a result of imprinting the mind through social and religious structure and intellectual and artistic manifestations. Culture is shaped by values, beliefs, norms, and practices that are shared by members of the same cultural group.

decompensation Deterioration of existing defenses, leading to an exacerbation of pathological behavior.

defense mechanism Unconscious intrapsychic processes serving to provide relief from emotional conflict and anxiety.

deinstitutionalization Change in locus of mental health care from traditional, institutional settings to community-based services.

delirium Acute organic mental disorder characterized by confusion and altered, possibly fluctuating, consciousness resulting from an alteration of cerebral metabolism; illusions, delusions, or hallucinations may be present. Often emotional lability, typically appearing as anxiety and agitation, is present.

delirium tremens Acute and sometimes fatal brain disorder caused by total or partial withdrawal from excessive alcohol intake. Usually develops in 24 to 96 hours after cessation of drinking.

delusion False belief out of keeping with the individual's level of knowledge and cultural group; the belief is maintained against logical argument and despite objective contradictory evidence.

delusions of grandeur Exaggerated, unrealistic ideas of one's importance or identity.

delusions of persecution Unrealistic ideas that one has been singled out for persecution.

delusions of reference Incorrect assumption that certain or unrelated remarks or the behavior of others applies to oneself.

dementia Organic mental disorder in which there is a deterioration of previously acquired intellectual abilities of sufficient severity to interfere with social or occupational functioning. Memory disturbance is the most prominent symptom.

dementia praecox Obsolete descriptive term for schizophrenia.

denial Defense mechanism, operating unconsciously, used to resolve emotional conflict and allay anxiety by disavowing thoughts, feelings, wishes, needs, or external reality factors that are consciously intolerable.

dependency needs Vital needs for mothering, love, affection, shelter, protection, security, food, and warmth. May be a manifestation of regression when they reappear openly in adults.

depersonalization Feelings of unreality or strangeness concerning the environment, the self, or both.

depression In the psychiatric sense, a morbid sadness, dejection, or melancholy; may vary in depth; to be differentiated from grief, which is realistic and proportionate to what has been lost.

derailment Pattern of speech seen most commonly in schizophrenic disorders, in which incomprehensible, disconnected, and unrelated ideas replace logical and orderly thought.

desensitization Talking about anxiety-producing subjects until they no longer cause excess emotion.

detoxification Treatment by the use of medication, diet, rest, fluids, and nursing care to restore physiological functioning after it has been seriously disturbed by the overuse of alcohol, barbiturates, or other addictive drugs.

developmental disability Handicap or impairment originating before the age of 18 that may be expected to continue indefinitely and that constitutes a substantial impairment.

developmental events Situations that occur naturally during the lifetime of an individual and the family.

developmental tasks Age-specific achievements identified by Erikson, success with which allows the individual to progress satisfactorily to the next phase of development. Largely culturally determined.

deviant Any person differing markedly from what is accepted as the norm, the average, or the usual.

dibenzoxazepines Group of antipsychotic agents.

dihydroindolones Group of antipsychotic agents.

discussion When related to the development of self-awareness, a process of having a focused conversation about one's behavior with a group or one other person.

disorientation Loss of awareness of the position of self in relation to space, time, or persons.

displacement Mental mechanism, operating unconsciously, by which an emotion is transferred or "displaced" from its original object to a more acceptable substitute object.

dissociation Psychological separation or splitting off; an intrapsychic defensive process, which operates automatically and unconsciously, through which emotional significance and affect are separated and detached from an idea, situation, or object.

dissociative disorder   Category of psychiatric disorder in which there is a sudden, temporary alteration in normally integrated functions of consciousness, identity, or motor behavior so that some part of one or more of these functions is lost.

distractibility   Inability to maintain attention; shifting from one area or topic to another with minimal provocation.

Dix, Dorothea Lynde   American educator, 1802-1887. Based on her investigations of the inhumane care of those with a mental illness, she crusaded in the press and before state legislatures for the establishment of suitable hospitals. She was successful in reforming mental health care not only in the United States but also in several other countries. She also organized the nursing forces of the Northern army during the Civil War. In 1901 the U.S. Congress cited her as "among the noblest examples of humanity in all history."

dopamine hypothesis   Theory that attempts to explain the pathogenesis of schizophrenia and other psychotic states as due to excesses in dopamine activity in various areas of the brain.

double-bind communication   Interaction in which one person demands a response to a message containing mutually contradictory signals while the other person is unable either to comment on the incongruity or to escape from the situation.

Down syndrome   Common form of mental retardation caused by a chromosomal abnormality; formerly called mongolism.

drive   Basic urge, instinct, motivation.

drug dependence   Habituation to, abuse of, and/or addiction to a chemical substance.

DSM   *Diagnostic and Statistical Manual of Mental Disorders.* A taxonomy of mental disorders developed and published by the American Psychiatric Association.

dyad   Two-person relationship, such as the therapeutic relationship between nurse and client in the nurse-client relationship.

dynamism   Methods, identified by Harry Stack Sullivan, that individuals use to meet their needs and thereby reduce tension. Certain dynamisms are characteristic of each age group, e.g., oral dynamism in infancy.

dyskinesias   Extrapyramidal side effect of antipsychotic medications manifested by involuntary rhythmic body movements.

dyslexia   Inability or difficulty in reading, including word-blindness and a tendency to reverse letters and words in reading and writing.

dysphagia   Difficult or painful swallowing.

dysphoria   Unpleasant mood.

dystonia   Acute tonic muscular spasms, often of the tongue, jaw, eyes, and neck, but sometimes of the whole body. Sometimes occurs during the first few days of antipsychotic drug administration.

Eastern Psychiatric Hospital   Built in 1773 in Williamsburg, Virginia, and believed to be the first public psychiatric hospital in America.

ego   In psychoanalytic theory, one of the three major divisions in the model of the psychic apparatus. The ego represents the sum of certain mental mechanisms, such as perception and memory, and specific defense mechanisms. It serves to mediate between the demands of primitive instinctual drives (the id), of internalized parental and social prohibitions (the superego), and of reality. The compromises between these forces achieved by the ego tend to resolve intrapsychic conflict and serve an adaptive and executive function. Psychiatric usage of the term should not be confused with common usage, which connotes self-love or selfishness.

ego defense mechanisms   Mental mechanisms to prevent awareness of anxiety. According to Freud, they emanate from the unconscious and use psychic energy derived from the ego.

ego ideal   That part of the personality comprising the aims and goals of the self; usually refers to the conscious or unconscious emulation of significant persons with whom one has identified.

elation   Affect consisting of feelings of euphoria, triumph, intense self-satisfaction, optimism; an elated although unstable mood is characteristic of mania.

electroconvulsive treatment (ECT)   Use of electric current to induce convulsive seizures. Most effective in the treatment of depression. Used with anesthetics and muscle relaxants.

emotion   State of arousal determined by a set of subjective feelings (e.g.., fear, anger, grief, joy, love), often accompanied by physiological changes, that impels one toward action.

empathic linkage   Sullivan's term for the relationship unique to infant and mothering one, whereby each is highly sensitive to the other's feeling states.

empathy Objective and insightful awareness of the feelings, emotions, and behavior of another person and their meaning and significance; to be distinguished from sympathy, which is nonobjective and usually noncritical.

energy In systems theory, the ability of the system to do work.

enlarging experience When related to developing self-awareness, the act of purposefully choosing to engage in unfamiliar activities and carefully noting one's reactions to them.

entropy In systems theory, a relatively closed system characterized by increased system disorganization leading to death of the system.

enuresis Incontinence of urine.

environment In systems theory, those elements that lie outside the boundary of the system.

environmental control Cultural phenomenon reflecting the ability of an individual or group representing a particular culture to plan activities that control nature. Also refers to the individual's perception of the ability to direct factors in the environment.

erogenous zone Area of the body particularly susceptible to erotic arousal when stimulated, especially the oral, anal, and genital areas.

ethnicity Groups whose members share a common social and cultural heritage passed on to each successive generation. Members of an ethnic group share a sense of identity with one another.

etiology Causation, particularly with reference to disease.

euphoria Exaggerated feeling of physical and emotional well-being, usually of psychological origin.

extended family Household structure in which several generations live under the same roof. Commonly seen in nonindustrial societies.

extrapyramidal side effects (EPS) Variety of signs and symptoms, including muscular rigidity, tremors, drooling, shuffling gait (parkinsonism); restlessness (akathisia); peculiar involuntary postures (dystonia); motor inertia (akinesia); and many other neurological disturbances. Results from dysfunction of the extrapyramidal system. May occur as a side effect of certain psychotropic drugs, particularly phenothiazines.

facilitated communication Technique in which autistic children use a computerized letterboard to spell words.

family System traditionally defined as individuals who have blood or legal ties. Now considered to be those persons who choose to live in the same household.

family therapy Treatment of more than one member of a family simultaneously in the same session.

fantasy Imagined sequence of events or mental images that serves to express unconscious conflicts, to gratify unconscious wishes, or to prepare for anticipated future events.

fear Emotional and physiological response to recognized sources of anger, to be distinguished from anxiety.

feedback In systems theory, a unique form of input derived from the system's output. Feedback is the message that the system receives about the degree to which it is successful in attaining a steady state and is therefore essential if the system is to adjust or regulate itself. A time lag always exists between the system's perception of the feedback and its ability to use the information in the service of self-regulation.

feelings Affective states or emotions.

fixation Arrest of psychosexual maturation at an immature level; depending on degree, may be either normal or pathological.

flight of ideas Verbal skipping from one idea to another before the preceding one has been concluded; the ideas appear to be continuous but are fragmentary and determined by chance associations.

forensic psychiatry Branch of psychiatry dealing with legal issues related to mental disorders.

free association In psychoanalytical therapy, spontaneous, uncensored verbalization by the client of whatever comes to mind.

free-floating anxiety Severe, generalized, persistent anxiety not specifically ascribed to a particular object or event and often a precursor of panic.

Freud, Sigmund Austrian neurologist and psychiatrist, 1856-1939. Demonstrated the existence of the unconscious mind and developed the discipline of psychoanalysis, considered highly controversial at the time.

gender identity Inner sense of maleness or femaleness that identifies the person as being male, female, or ambivalent. To be distinguished from sexual identity, which is biologically determined.

gender role Image a person presents to others and

to the self that declares him or her to be boy or girl, man or woman. Gender role is the public declaration of gender identity, but the two do not necessarily coincide.

general adaptation syndrome   Total, nonspecific mobilization of the organism's resources to meet situations of severe stress.

genetic(s)   In biology, pertaining to genes or to inherited characteristics. Also, in psychiatry, pertaining to the historical development of one's psychological attributes or disorders.

genital stage   Period of psychosexual development from the age of about 12 to 18 years, marked by a reactivation of libidinal energy and the focusing of this energy on the genital area.

geriatrics   Branch of medicine dealing with the aging process and diseases of the aging human being.

gerontology   Study of aging.

gestalt therapy   A philosophy and an intervention technique developed by Fritz S. Perls. Its emphasis is on treatment of the person as a holistic being.

grandiose   Exaggerated belief or claims of one's importance or identity, often manifested by delusions of great wealth, power, or fame.

grief   Normal, appropriate emotional response to an external and consciously recognized loss; usually time-limited and gradually subsides.

group cohesiveness   Heightened sense of belonging experienced by members during the third stage of group development, the working phase.

guardian   Person appointed by the court or state authorities to protect the rights and property of an individual who is deemed incapable of doing so.

halfway house   Specialized residence for individuals who do not require full hospitalization but who need an intermediate degree of care before returning to independent community living.

hallucination   False sensory perception in the absence of an actual external stimulus; may be of emotional or chemical (drugs, alcohol, etc.) origin and may occur in any of the five senses.

hallucinogen   Chemical agent that produces hallucinations.

holistic   Approach to the study of the individual in totality, rather than as an aggregate of separate physiological, psychological, and social characteristics.

homosexual panic   Acute and severe attack of anxiety based on unconscious conflicts involving homosexuality.

homosexuality   Sexual attraction or relationship between members of the same sex; active homosexuality is marked by overt activity, whereas latent homosexuality is marked by unconscious homosexual desires or conscious desires consistently denied expression.

hyperactivity   Excessive motor activity, generally purposeful. It is frequently, but not necessarily, associated with internal tension or a neurological disorder. Usually the movements are more rapid than is customary for the person.

hypertensive crisis   Sudden extreme rise in blood pressure that may result in intracranial hemorrhage.

hypomania   Psychopathological state and abnormality of mood falling somewhere between normal euphoria and mania.

id   In Freudian theory, that part of the personality structure that harbors the unconscious instinctive desires and strivings of the individual.

ideas of reference   Incorrect interpretation of casual incidents and external events as having direct reference to oneself; may reach sufficient intensity to constitute delusions.

identification   Mental mechanism, operating unconsciously, by which an individual endeavors to pattern himself or herself after another; plays a major role in the development of one's personality and specifically of one's superego (conscience).

identity crisis   Loss of the sense of the sameness and historical continuity of one's self and inability to accept or adopt the role one perceives as being expected by society.

idiopathic   Term applied to diseases of unknown cause, for example, idiopathic epilepsy.

illusion   Misinterpretation of a real external sensory experience.

impulse   Psychic striving; usually refers to an instinctual urge.

impulse control   Ability to resist an impulse, desire, or temptation.

incorporation   Primitive mental mechanism, operating unconsciously, by which another person or parts of another person are symbolically ingested and assimilated; for example, infantile fantasy that the mother's breast has been ingested and is a part of oneself.

informed consent   Right of all clients to decide whether to accept or reject treatment based on an explanation, in language they can understand, of the treatment, its intended effects, its risks, and other alternatives.

inhibition   Unconscious interference with or restriction of instinctual drives.

input   In systems theory, matter and energy that move from the environment into the system through the system's boundary.

insight   Self-understanding; a major goal of psychotherapy; the extent of the individual's understanding of the origin, nature, and mechanisms of his or her attitudes and behavior.

insomnia   Inability to fall asleep, difficulty staying asleep, or early morning awakening.

instinct   Inborn drive. The primary human instincts include self-preservation, sexuality, and—according to some authorities—aggression, the ego instincts, and herd or social instincts.

institutionalization   Syndrome in which persons become so adapted to and reliant on the hospital that they resist efforts to be discharged or cannot function outside its structured environment.

integration   Useful organization of both new and old data, experience, and emotional capacities incorporated into the personality; also refers to the organization and amalgamation of functions at various levels of psychosexual development.

intelligence   Capacity to learn and to use appropriately what one has learned. May be affected by emotions.

intelligence quotient (IQ)   Numerical rating determined through psychological testing that indicates the approximate relationship of a person's mental age (MA) to chronological age (CA). Expressed mathematically as $IQ = MA/CA \times 100$.

interdisciplinary mental health care team   Approach to treatment and rehabilitation in which professionals from all appropriate disciplines and the client and family work together to address the client's needs.

interpersonal theory   Theory of personality development developed by Sullivan, stressing the nature and quality of relationships with significant others as the most critical factor in personality development.

intrapsychic   Situated, originating, or taking place in the psyche.

introjection   Mental mechanism, operating unconsciously, whereby loved or hated external objects are taken within oneself symbolically; the converse of projection; may serve as a defense against conscious recognition of intolerable hostile impulses; for example, in severe depression the individual may unconsciously direct unacceptable hatred or aggression toward himself or herself, that is, toward the introjected object within himself or herself; related to the more primitive mechanisms of incorporation.

introspection   Process of observing one's own behavior in various situations and identifying its themes and patterns. Useful in developing self-awareness.

involuntary admission   Type of admission to a psychiatric treatment program undertaken by someone other than the client. Involuntary admission is governed by state laws that differ among the 50 states. Suicidal, violent, acute psychotic, and antisocial behaviors in persons unwilling to be treated are the usual reasons for a person to be involuntarily admitted to a psychiatric treatment program.

isolation   Mental mechanism whereby the feeling is detached from the event in an individual's memory, enabling the event to be recalled without its attendant anxiety.

Johari window   Designed by Joseph Luft and Harry Lipton, a four-quadrant model helpful in understanding the nature of self-awareness.

kinetic energy   In systems theory, energy currently being used and therefore unavailable for additional work.

kleptomania   Compulsive stealing, largely without any apparent material need for the stolen objects.

la belle indifference   Literally, "beautiful indifference." Seen in certain persons with conversion disorders who show an inappropriate lack of concern about their disabilities.

labile   Rapidly shifting emotions.

latency period   In psychoanalysis, a phase between the phallic (or oedipal) and adolescent periods of psychosexual development; characterized by a marked decrease of sexual behavior and interest in sex.

learning disability   Syndrome affecting school-age children of normal or above-normal intelligence and characterized by specific difficulties in learning to read (dyslexia), write (dysgraphia), and calculate (dyscalculia). The disorder is believed to be related to slow developmental progression of perceptual motor skills.

libido Psychic drive or energy usually associated with the sexual instinct (sexual is used here in the broad sense to include pleasure and love-object seeking); also used broadly to connote the psychic energy associated with instincts in general.

life review Process of thinking about the meaning of one's life, believed to be a universal occurrence in older persons as they face the prospect of impending death.

limit setting Nonpunitively preventing clients from physically harming themselves or others, destroying property, or causing other clients or personnel to become tense and upset by their verbalizations.

lithium carbonate Alkali metal, the salt of which is used in the treatment of acute mania and as a maintenance medication to help reduce the duration, intensity, and frequency of recurrent affective episodes, especially in bipolar disorders.

logorrhea Uncontrollable, excessive talking.

loosening of associations Disturbance of thinking in which ideas shift from one subject to another in an oblique or unrelated manner. The speaker is unaware of the disturbance. When loosening of associations is severe, speech may be incoherent.

LSD (lysergic acid diethylamide) Potent hallucinogen that produces psychotic symptoms and behavior.

lust Sullivan's term for the sexual urges first erupting in early adolescence.

magical thinking Conviction that thinking equates with doing. Occurs in dreams, in children, in primitive peoples, and in persons with some forms of mental illness. Characterized by lack of realistic relationship between cause and effect.

mainstreaming Education of physically disabled, retarded, and learning-disabled children within regular schools, but with special assistance where needed. Also, the return of persons recovered from a mental illness or deinstitutionalized individuals with a chronic mental illness to the community, where they receive rehabilitative assistance directed toward helping them achieve as full and normal a life as possible.

malnutrition State of health characterized by an improper balance of carbohydrates, fats, proteins, vitamins, and minerals in the diet with respect to energy needs as reflected in physical activity.

mania Mood disorder characterized by excessive elation, hyperactivity, agitation, and accelerated thinking and speaking.

marijuana Mind-altering substance made from the *Cannabis sativa* plant. The active ingredient is tetrahydrocannabinol. Marijuana is smoked and causes a state of exhilaration or euphoria.

Maslow's hierarchy of needs Framework developed by Abraham Maslow (1908-1970) to help understand mental health. Based on the beliefs that all humans strive to develop but all have inherent basic needs that are ordered hierarchically and that emerge only when lower-level needs have been satisfied. Also referred to as the theory of self-actualization.

matter In systems theory, anything that has mass and occupies space.

megalomania Syndrome marked by delusions of great self-importance, wealth, or power.

melancholia Pathological dejection, usually of psychotic depth.

mental disorder Illness with psychological or behavioral manifestations or impairment in functioning resulting from a social, psychological, genetic, physical/chemical, or biological disturbance. The disorder is not limited to relations between the person and society. The illness is characterized by symptoms or impairment in functioning.

mental health State of being, relative rather than absolute. The best indices of mental health are simultaneous success at working, loving, and creating with the capacity for mature and flexible resolution of conflicts between instincts, conscience, important other people, and reality.

Mental Health Study Act Enacted by Congress in 1955 to provide funds for a 5-year study of mental illness in the United States. As a result, the Joint Commission on Mental Illness was established. This commission published its report *Action for Mental Health,* a landmark document that was the basis for additional legislation leading to deinstitutionalization of those with a mental illness.

mental mechanisms Also called defense mechanisms and mental dynamisms; specific intrapsychic defensive processes, operating unconsciously, that are employed to seek resolution of emotional conflict and freedom from anxiety; conscious efforts are frequently made for the same reasons, but true mental mechanisms are out of awareness (unconscious).

mental retardation Significantly subaverage general intellectual functioning existing concurrently with deficits in adaptive behavior. Must be present before age 18.

mental status Level and style of functioning of the psyche, including a person's intellectual functioning and emotional, attitudinal, psychological, and personality aspects. The term is commonly used to refer to the results of the examination of an individual's mental status.

mental ventilation Seemingly random talk in which the client freely follows the associations that come to mind.

methadone Synthetic narcotic often used as a substitute for heroin producing a less socially disabling addiction and aiding in heroin withdrawal.

middle age Conventionally considered to occur between 40 and 60 years of age and primarily defined by psychosocial rather than by physiological events.

milieu therapy Socioenvironmental therapy in which the attitudes and behavior of the staff of a treatment service and the activities prescribed for the client are determined by the client's emotional and interpersonal needs. This therapy is an essential part of all inpatient treatment.

minority Any racial, religious, or occupational group that constitutes less than a numerical majority of the population. Also used to refer to groups that may not constitute less than a numerical majority but that are relatively socially powerless.

mood Pervasive and sustained emotion that in the extreme markedly colors the person's perception of the world. Mood is to affect as climate is to weather. Common examples of mood include depression, elation, anger, and anxiety.

moral treatment Philosophy and technique of treating persons with a mental illness that prevailed in the first half of the nineteenth century and emphasized removal of restraints, humane and kindly care, attention to religion, and performance of useful tasks in the hospital.

multiple personality Term used by Morton Prince for a type of dissociative reaction in which the person adopts two or more personalities.

mysophobia Morbid fear of dirt, germs, or contamination.

NANDA North American Nursing Diagnosis Association. The classification system of nursing diagnoses approved by NANDA, although not complete, is the most widely used.

narcissism Self-love as opposed to object-love (love of another person). In psychoanalytical theory, cathexis of the psychic representation of the self with libido. An excess interferes with relations with others. To be distinguished from egotism, which carries the connotation of self-centeredness, selfishness, and conceit. Egotism is but one expression of narcissism.

narcotic Any opiate derivative drug, natural or synthetic, that relieves pain or alters mood.

National Alliance for the Mentally Ill A national lay organization of families of persons with a mental illness. One of its major functions is the promotion of research into the causes of mental illness and improved treatment of those with a mental illness.

National Mental Health Act Federal legislation enacted in 1946 that provided for the establishment of the National Institute of Mental Health and charged this agency with promoting and financing research and training programs to prevent and treat mental illness. This act grew out of experiences during World War II, when more men in the U.S. Armed Forces were disabled by mental illness than by all the other problems related to military action.

negative symptoms When referring to schizophrenia, the absence of behavior normally expected, specifically in the dimensions of affect, definition of self, volition, interpersonal relations, and psychomotor behavior.

negentropy In systems theory, a relatively open system characterized by movement toward integration and growth.

neologism In psychiatry, a new word or condensed combination of several words coined by a client to express a highly complex meaning related to his or her conflicts; not readily understood by others; common in schizophrenia.

neuroendocrinology Study of the relationships between the nervous and endocrine systems.

neuroleptic malignant syndrome Serious, potentially fatal side effect of any medication that alters dopamine mechanisms in the central nervous system, particularly antipsychotic drugs. Risk for this syndrome is increased by the use of two or more neuroleptic agents concurrently and by depot injections of antipsychotic agents. It may be manifested by sudden onset of muscular rigidity, akinesia, and hyperthermia or gradual onset with symptoms of tachycardia, diaphoresis, and severely altered consciousness or delirium. Medications should be withheld and the physician notified as soon as the syndrome is suspected.

neurophysiology Branch of biology and medicine that is concerned with the normal and abnormal activity of nervous system functions, including the chemical activity of individual nerve cells.

NIMBY phenomenon "Not in My Back Yard." The belief of some persons that community-based group homes for persons with a mental illness are more desirable than long-term hospitalization but that such homes should not be located in their neighborhoods.

nonjudgmental Withholding of value-laden opinions, both positive and negative.

nonsummativity In systems theory, the system characteristic of the whole being greater than the sum of its parts.

nonverbal communication Messages sent and received through such means as facial expression, voice quality, physical posture, and gestures. Sometimes referred to as body language. An integral part of verbal communication, but is always present when people interact even when no words are spoken.

normative family stages Usual events in the life of a family that change its structure and focus.

norms Rules that govern the operation of a group. Norms are usually implicit.

nuclear family Two-generational family.

nurse-client relationship Specific type of nurse-client interaction over time in which the nurse becomes a significant other to the client. As a treatment intervention the nurse-client relationship has the goal of providing corrective emotional experiences for the client.

object That through which an instinct can achieve its aim; object relations theory is the psychoanalytical description of the internalization of interpersonal relations and the organizing effects of internalized human object relationships on the structure of the psyche.

observation Active goal-directed process in which the person uses all appropriate senses to become aware of the environment and the people in it.

obsession Persistent, unwanted idea or impulse that cannot be eliminated by usual logic or reasoning.

obsessive-compulsive disorder Psychiatric disorder characterized by disturbing, unwanted, intruding thoughts and ideas and repetitive impulses

to perform acts that the person may consider abnormal, undesirable, or distasteful.

Oedipus complex Situation occurring during the phallic stage of psychosexual development (approximate ages 3 to 6) in which the child shifts energies into sexual interest in parents. The child normally becomes attached to the parent of the opposite sex and develops competitive feelings toward the same-sex parent. Eventually, through identification with the same-sex parent, the child relinquishes oedipal strivings.

omnipotence Infantile perception that the outside world is part of the organism and within it, which leads to a primitive feeling of all-powerfulness. This feeling gradually becomes limited as the ego and a sense of reality develop. Similar phenomena are found in disturbed individuals who lose contact with reality.

opiate Any chemical derived from opium; relieves pain and produces a sense of well-being.

oral stage Includes both the oral-erotic and oral-sadistic phases of infantile psychosexual development, lasting from birth to 12 months or longer; oral-erotic phase is the initial pleasurable experience of nursing; oral-sadistic phase is the subsequent aggressive (biting) phase; both eroticism and sadism normally continue to later life in disguised or sublimated forms.

organic mental disorder Transient or permanent dysfunction of the brain, caused by a disturbance of physiologic functioning of brain tissue at any level of organization—structural, hormonal, biochemical, electrical, etc.

orientation Awareness of oneself in relation to time, place, and person.

orientation phase First stage in the development of the nurse-client relationship or a group. The participants initially are essentially strangers, and the goal of this stage is the development of trust. The conclusion of this stage is often characterized by testing behaviors on the part of the client or group.

output In systems theory, matter and energy that move from the system through its boundary into the environment.

panic In psychiatry, refers to an attack of acute, intense, and overwhelming anxiety, accompanied by a considerable degree of personality disorganization.

paranoia Psychotic disorder that develops slowly and becomes chronic; characterized by an intricate and internally logical system of persecutory or grandiose delusions, or both; stands by itself and does not interfere with the remainder of the personality, which continues essentially normal and apparently intact; to be distinguished from paranoid schizophrenic reactions and paranoid states.

paranoid Lay term commonly used to describe an overly suspicious person. The technical use of the term refers to people with paranoid ideation or to a type of schizophrenia or a class of disorders.

paranoid ideation Suspiciousness or nondelusional belief that one is being harassed, persecuted, or unfairly treated.

paranormative family stages or events Unanticipated events in the life of the family that change its normal functioning.

parkinsonism Extrapyramidal side effects of antipsychotic medications, manifested by muscle rigidity and tremors, a shuffling gait, excessive salivation and drooling, a masklike facial expression, and loss of muscle movement.

Parnate-cheese reaction Syndrome resulting from taking an monoamine oxidase inhibitor, particularly tranylcypromine (Parnate), and also eating a food containing tyramine. The tyramine cannot be metabolized and can cause a hypertensive crisis.

pedophilia Term used to describe adults who demonstrate a pathological sexual interest in children.

penis envy Literally, envy by the female of the penis of the male; more generally, the female's wish for male attributes, position, or advantages; believed by many to be a significant factor in female character development.

periodic alcoholic Alcohol-dependent individual who drinks excessively during certain periods but may not drink at all during other times. Also known as a cyclical alcoholic.

personality Aggregate of the physical and mental qualities of the individual as these interact in characteristic fashion with the environment.

personality disorders Deeply ingrained, inflexible, dysfunctional patterns of relating, perceiving, and thinking of sufficient severity to cause either impairment in functioning or distress. Personality disorders are generally recognizable by adolescence or earlier, continue throughout adulthood, and become less obvious in middle or old age.

personality traits Characteristics of individuals that make them unique and form the basis for the way they perceive the world and how they relate to others.

phallic stage Period of psychosexual development from the age of about 3 to 6 years during which sexual interest, curiosity, and pleasurable experience center about the penis and, in girls, to a lesser extent, the clitoris.

phencyclidine (PCP) A hallucinogen of the piperidine family. Street names are, among others, PCP, crystal, angel dust, or the peace pill. PCP is smoked, sniffed, swallowed, or injected.

phenothiazines Group of antipsychotic agents developed in the 1950s. They account for about two thirds of all antipsychotic medications and act primarily to block dopamine receptors in brain tissue.

philosophy Statement of beliefs, not facts, about the phenomena of concern.

phobia Obsessive, persistent, unrealistic fear of an external object or situation such as heights, open spaces, dirt, and animals; fear believed to arise through a process of displacing an internal (unconscious) conflict to an external object symbolically related to the conflict.

Pinel, Philippe French physician, 1745-1826. At great professional risk he removed the chains of inmates of two large asylums in Paris in 1792, demonstrating the fallacy of inhumane treatment of persons with a mental illness.

play therapy Treatment technique using the child's play as a medium for expression and communication between the child and therapist.

pleasure principle Basic psychoanalytical concept that humans instinctually seek to avoid pain and discomfort and strive for gratification and pleasure; in personality development theories, the pleasure principle antedates and subsequently comes into conflict with the reality principle.

positive symptoms When referring to schizophrenia, the presence of unusual behavior, specifically distortions in both the content and the form of thought and in perception.

posttraumatic stress disorder Develops after experiencing a psychologically distressing event. It is characterized by reexperiencing the event and by overresponsiveness to, or involvement with, stimuli that recall the event.

potential energy In systems theory, energy not currently engaged in work but available for use; stored energy.

preconscious   Thoughts that are not in immediate awareness but that can be recalled by conscious effort.

preoccupation   State of being self-absorbed or engrossed in one's own thoughts, typically to a degree that hinders effective contact with or relationship to external reality.

President's Commission on Mental Health   Established in 1977 by President Jimmy Carter for the purpose of identifying the mental health needs of the nation. Nursing was represented for the first time on such a commission by Martha Mitchell, a nurse educator and clinical specialist in psychiatric–mental health nursing. The commission's report recommended strengthening community efforts to address mental health needs, emphasized meeting the needs of undeserved and high-risk populations and areas, and recommended that coverage for mental health treatment be included in all health insurance.

pressured speech   Rapid, accelerated, frenzied speech. Sometimes it exceeds the ability of the vocal musculature to articulate, leading to jumbled and cluttered speech; at other times it exceeds the ability of the listener to comprehend as the speech expresses a flight of ideas or an unintelligible jargon.

primary gain   Relief from emotional conflict and the freedom from anxiety achieved by a defense mechanism.

primary narcissism   In Freudian terms, the exclusive focus on the self; characteristic of the stage of infancy. Self-love.

principles   Rules.

projection   Mental mechanism whereby that which is emotionally unacceptable in the self is unconsciously rejected and attributed (projected) to others.

projective tests   Psychological diagnostic tests in which the test material is unstructured so that any response will reflect a projection of some aspect of the subject's underlying personality and psychopathology.

psyche   Mind, in distinction to the soma, or body.

psychodrama   Technique of group psychotherapy in which individuals express their own or assigned emotional problems in dramatization.

psychodynamics   Systematized knowledge and theory of human behavior and its motivation, the study of which depends largely on the functional significance of emotion; psychodynamics recognizes the role of unconscious motivation in human behavior; a predictive science, based on the assumption that a person's total makeup and probable reactions at any given moment are the product of past interactions between the person's specific genetic endowment and the environment in which he or she has lived from conception onward.

psychometric tests   Psychological instruments administered to determine intelligence, manual skills, personality characteristics, interests, or other mental factors.

psychomotor overactivity   Generalized physical and emotional overactivity in response to internal or external stimuli, as in hypomania.

psychomotor retardation   Generalized slowing of physical and emotional reactions. Specifically, the slowing of movements such as eye-blinking; frequently seen in depression.

psychopathology   Study of the significant causes and processes in the development of mental disorders. Also the manifestations of mental disorders.

psychosexual development   Series of stages from infancy to adulthood, relatively fixed in time, determined by the interaction between a person's biological drives and the environment. With resolution of this interaction, a balanced, reality-oriented development takes place; with disturbance, fixation and conflict ensue. This disturbance may remain latent or give rise to characterologic or behavioral disorders.

psychosexual theory   Theory of personality development formulated by Sigmund Freud.

psychosis   Major mental disorder of organic or emotional origin in which a person's ability to think, respond emotionally, remember, communicate, interpret reality, and behave appropriately is sufficiently impaired to interfere grossly with the capacity to meet the ordinary demands of life.

psychosocial development   Progressive interaction between a person and the environment through stages beginning in infancy, as primarily described by Erikson. Specific developmental tasks involving social relations and the role of social reality are faced by a person at phase-specific developmental points. The early tasks parallel stages of psychosexual development; the later tasks extend through adulthood.

psychotherapy   Any form of treatment for mental

illness, behavioral dysfunctions, and other problems that are assumed to be of an emotional nature, in which a trained person deliberately establishes a professional relationship with a client for the purpose of removing, modifying, or retarding existing symptoms, of attenuating or reversing disturbed patterns of behavior, and of promoting positive personality development and growth.

race   Distinguishing physical features such as color, bone structure, or blood group that identify a group of people.

rapport   Confidential relationships between the client and the professional person who is in a helping relationship with the client.

rationalization   Mental mechanism, operating unconsciously, by which the individual attempts to justify or make consciously tolerable by plausible means those feelings, behaviors, and motives that would otherwise be intolerable (not to be confused with conscious evasion or dissimulation).

reaction formation   Mental mechanism, operating unconsciously, wherein attitudes and behavior are adopted that are the opposite of impulses the individual disowns either consciously or unconsciously—for example, excessive moral zeal may be the product of strong but repressed antisocial impulses.

reality orientation   Form of remotivation that aims to reduce the confusion of a person who lacks full orientation to time, place, or person. The technique consists of continual reminders to the person of who he or she is, what day it is, where he or she is, and what is happening or is about to take place.

reality principle   In Freudian theory, the concept that the pleasure principle in personality development in infancy is normally modified by the inescapable demands and requirements of external reality; the process by which this compromise is effected is technically known as reality testing, both in normal development and in psychiatric treatment.

reality testing   Ability to evaluate the external world objectively and to differentiate adequately between it and the internal world.

reassurance   Supportive approach to clients that encourages them to believe that they have value and worth as human beings and that they will be able to cope with stressful events.

regression   Partial or symbolic return to more infantile ways of gratification; most clearly seen in severe psychoses.

relatively closed system   In systems theory, a system whose boundaries have little permeability, allowing for relatively little exchange of matter or energy with the environment. Boundaries cannot be totally closed in a living system, since some exchange of matter and energy is necessary for life. The bulk of energy in a relatively closed system is in use, leaving little potential energy available to respond to input.

relatively open system   In systems theory, a system whose boundaries are semipermeable, allowing exchange of matter and energy with the system's environment. A sufficient amount of potential energy is available to use input in the service of system growth.

repression   Mental mechanism, operating unconsciously; the common denominator and unconscious precursor of all mental mechanisms in which there is involuntary relegation of unbearable ideas and impulses into the unconscious whence they are not ordinarily subject to voluntary recall but may emerge in disguised form through use of the various mental mechanisms; particularly operative in early years.

rescue fantasy   Incorrect belief, particularly common among health care professionals, that only oneself is able to be of significant help to the client.

resistance   In psychiatry, an individual's massive psychological defense against bringing repressed (unconscious) thoughts or impulses into awareness, thus avoiding anxiety.

revolving door syndrome   Phenomenon in which persons with a mental illness receive intensive care through hospitalization, are discharged to the community where adequate and appropriate care is often not available, and shortly require hospitalization again, repeating the cycle.

ritual   Repetitive activity, usually a distorted or stereotyped elaboration of some routine of daily life, employed to relieve anxiety.

role playing   Exercise in which participants enact the parts of the person involved in a real or anticipated interaction. Role playing is often useful in developing self-awareness, practicing interpersonal skills, and developing empathy for the positions of others.

Rorschach test   Psychological test, developed by the Swiss psychiatrist Hermann Rorschach (1884-1922), that seeks to disclose conscious and unconscious personality traits and emotional conflicts through eliciting the person's associations to a standard set of inkblots.

Rush, Benjamin American physician, 1745-1813. The "father" of American psychiatry, Rush practiced at the Pennsylvania Hospital beginning in 1783.

schema According to Piaget, the individual's innate knowledge structure that allows that person to organize mentally ways to behave in the environment.

schizophrenia, catatonic Type of schizophrenia characterized by immobility with muscular rigidity or inflexibility; alternating periods of physical hyperactivity and excitability may occur; generally there is marked inaccessibility to ordinary methods of communication.

schizophrenia, disorganized Type of schizophrenia characterized by incoherence and flat, incongruous, or silly affect, with no systematized delusions.

schizophrenia, paranoid Type of schizophrenia marked by a feeling that external reality has altered; suspiciousness; ideas of reference; hallucinations; delusions of persecution or grandiosity.

schizophrenia, residual Condition of being without gross psychotic symptoms following a psychotic schizophrenic episode.

schizophrenia, undifferentiated Type of schizophrenia characterized by prominent delusions, hallucinations, incoherence, or grossly disorganized behavior that cannot be classified in one of the other categories.

secondary gain External gain derived from any illness, such as personal attention and service, monetary gains, disability benefits, and release from unpleasant responsibility.

security operations Sullivan's term for mechanisms such as apathy and selective inattention that, no matter how rational at first glance, are defenses against recognizing or experiencing anxiety.

selective inattention Term for a security operation identified by Sullivan, whereby anxiety-producing aspects of a situation are not allowed into awareness.

self-care Ability of a person to engage in the usual activities of daily living, especially those related to personal hygiene, grooming, nutrition, and elimination.

self-concept According to Sullivan, the view of self that develops from the reflected appraisals of significant others during infancy.

self-help programs Banding together of individuals with a particular disorder for purposes of emotional support, morale-boosting, and practical assistance. Some programs are for families only, and some have the additional purpose of influencing public policy about the disorder.

self-help trend Current tendency of people to believe that professionals do not necessarily have all the answers. Reflected in the numerous newspaper and magazine articles and books on health. Has resulted in a population that is increasingly well educated about health matters and therefore demands accountability from health professionals.

self-perception Awareness of the various components that constitute the self, that is, one's unique feelings, impulses, aspirations, and personality characteristics.

sensorium Synonymous with consciousness. Includes the special sensory perceptive powers and their central correlation and integration in the brain. A clear sensorium conveys the presence of a reasonably accurate memory together with orientation for time, place, and person.

separation-individuation Psychological awareness of one's separateness, described by Margaret Mahler as a phase in the mother-child relationship that follows the symbiotic stage. In the separation-individuation stage, the child begins to perceive himself or herself as distinct from the mother and develops a sense of individual identity and an image of the self as object.

shame Emotion resulting from the failure to live up to self-expectations.

sibling rivalry Competition between siblings for the love of a parent or for other recognition or gain.

simple phobia Persistent fear of a specific object or situation. Also known as specific phobia.

situational events Situations that do not inevitably occur to all individuals or families and therefore are unexpected.

social ineptitude Inability of an adult to relate comfortably to others in a culturally appropriate manner.

social organization Cultural phenomenon referring to the manner in which a cultural group organizes itself around the family unit.

social phobia Persistent fear of any group situation in which persons believe they are the focus of attention and in which they fear they will act in a way that will be humiliating or embarrassing. The most common social phobia is the fear of public speaking.

social support   Assistance provided by others, usually not in the immediate family.

socializing agent   One function of the psychiatric nurse in which the nurse helps clients to participate with others in informal group activities such as discussions and group games.

soma   Body; the physical aspect of a human as distinguished from the psyche.

somatic therapy   In psychiatry, the biological treatment of mental disorders (e.g., electroconvulsive therapy, psychopharmacological treatment).

somatization   Automatic physiological reaction to emotional conflicts or stress.

somnolent detachment   Sullivan's term for the security operation with its origin in infancy, whereby the individual falls asleep when confronted by a highly-threatening, anxiety-producing experience.

space   Cultural phenomenon referring to the area that surround the person's body.

speech disturbance   Any disorder of verbal communication that is not due to faulty innervation of speech muscles or organs of articulation.

stereotypy   Persistent, mechanical repetition of an activity; common in schizophrenia.

stress   Condition in which the human system responds to input that has disturbed its steady state. It is neither positive or negative but may have positive or negative effects. It is a subjective phenomenon that must be inferred from the person's response.

stressor   In terms of stress and adaptation theory, the stressor is any system input, which may have either positive or negative effects, depending on the way it is processed; may be classified as situational (untoward events) or developmental (anticipated events related to growth and maturation).

stupor   State in which a person does not react to or is unaware of the surroundings. Caused by neurological as well as psychiatric disorders. In catatonic stupor, the unawareness is more apparent than real.

subconscious   Freudian term referring to that part of the mind in which partially forgotten ideas and reactions are stored. Material stored in the subconscious can usually be brought into conscious awareness if the individual concentrates on recall. Also known as the preconscious.

subgroups   Small offshoots of larger groups; usually form because the original group is too large to fulfill its functions. Sometimes referred to as cliques.

sublimation   Mental mechanism, operating unconsciously, through which consciously unacceptable instinctual drives are diverted into personally and socially acceptable channels.

substance abuse   Pathological use of agents modifying mood, behavior, and cognition, creating an impairment in social or occupational functioning.

substance dependence   Increased tolerance to a mind-altering substance along with behaviors, thought processes, and other symptoms that indicate a lack of control of substance use despite its negative consequences.

substitution   Mental mechanism, operating unconsciously, by which an unattainable or unacceptable goal, emotion, or object is replaced by one that is more attainable or acceptable.

subsystem   In systems theory, one element of a system.

suggestion   Process of influencing a client to accept an idea, belief, or attitude suggested by the therapist.

superego   In Freudian theory, that part of the mind that unconsciously identifies itself with important and esteemed persons from early life, particularly parents; the supposed or actual wishes of these significant persons are taken over as part of one's own personal standards to help form the "conscience."

supportive psychotherapy   Type of psychotherapy that aims to reinforce a client's defenses and help suppress disturbing psychological material. Supportive psychotherapy uses such measures as inspiration, reassurance, suggestion, persuasion, counseling, and reeducation. It avoids probing the client's emotional conflicts in depth.

suppression   Conscious effort to overcome unacceptable thoughts or desires by forcing them out of the conscious mind.

symbiosis   Mutually reinforcing relationship between two persons who are dependent on each other. A normal characteristic of the relationship between the mothering one and infant child.

symbolization   Mental mechanism, operating unconsciously, in which a person forms an abstract representation of a particular object, idea, or constellation. The symbol carries, in more or less disguised form, the emotional feelings vested in the initial object or ideas.

system   In systems theory, a complex of elements in interaction wherein a relationship between these elements and their properties can be theoretically demonstrated. Delineated by an artificially established boundary that is conceptualized as semipermeable, allowing matter and energy to pass to and from the system's environment.

tangentiality Replying to a question in an oblique or irrelevant way.

tardive dyskinesia Serious side effect of antipsychotic medication characterized by grimacing, choreiform, or athetoid movements of the arms, fingers, ankles, and toes, and tonic contractions of the neck and back muscles. At present it is irreversible.

target symptom Specific problem on which treatment is focused. It is most desirable for the problem to be one identified by the client as distressing to him or her.

thanatology Study of death and dying.

therapeutic community Term of British origin, now widely used, for a specially structured environment that encourages clients to function within the range of social norms.

therapeutic foster care Living arrangements for a child within a foster family chosen for its potential to have a positive influence on the child.

therapeutic window Range of blood levels associated with clinical response to certain drugs.

thioxanthenes Group of antipsychotic agents.

thought disorder Disturbance of speech, communication, or content of thought, such as delusions, ideas of reference, poverty of thought, flight of ideas, perseveration, loosening of association, etc.

thought processes Thinking or symbolic process involved in such activities as judgments, imagination, problem solving, and drawing inferences.

throughput In systems theory, the transformation of matter and energy that takes place as these are processed by the system.

time Cultural phenomenon referring to the perspective held by a cultural group regarding time. Most cultures are past, present, or future oriented in regard to time.

toxic psychosis Psychosis resulting from the toxic effect of chemicals and drugs, including those produced in the body.

tranquilizer Medication that decreases anxiety and agitation. Preferred terms are antianxiety or anxiolytic and antipsychotic medications.

transactional analysis Theoretical framework and treatment method developed by Eric Berne. Postulates that each person has three elements of personality: the Child, the Parent, and the Adult. Problems arise when an incongruency exists among the elements operating when people relate with each other.

transference Unconscious attachment to others of feelings and attitudes that were originally associated with important figures (parents, siblings, etc.) in one's early life. The transference relationship follows roughly the pattern of its prototype; the therapist uses the phenomenon as a therapeutic tool to help the client understand his or her emotional problems and their origin; in the client-therapist relationship the transference may be negative (hostile) or positive (affectionate).

tyramine Precursor to norepinephrine naturally found in a number of foods and beverages such as aged cheese, meat and fish that has been aged without refrigeration, beef and chicken livers, certain fruits and vegetables, and alcoholic beverages. Causes increase in blood pressure and, when combined with monoamine oxidase inhibitors, can result in a hypertensive crisis (severe headache, severe chest pain, nausea and vomiting, diarrhea, changes in pulse rate, and diaphoresis).

unconscious In Freudian theory, that part of the mind or mental functioning the content of which is only rarely subject to awareness; a repository for data that have never been conscious (primary repression) or that may have become conscious briefly and were then repressed (secondary repression).

uncovering or insight psychotherapy Exploration and bringing to consciousness the source of repressed and suppressed conflicts and experiences that operate at unconscious levels to cause anxiety. Uncovering psychotherapy gives meaning to abnormal or irrational feelings and dysfunctional behaviors. Clients with available ego strength, a viable support system, and at least average intelligence often can benefit from this form of therapy.

undoing Primitive defense mechanism, operating unconsciously, by which something unacceptable and already done is symbolically acted out in reverse, usually repetitiously, in the hope of "undoing" it and thus relieving anxiety.

verbal communication Words exchanged by two or more people.

vocational therapy Process of developing or restoring the productivity of persons with a mental or physical disability through vocational guidance, testing, training, and adjustment to the work situation.

volition Will.

voluntary admission Type of admission to a psychiatric treatment program in which the individual is willing to be hospitalized and treated and indicates this by signing appropriate documents.

Ward Atmosphere Scale (WAS) Tool to measure the ward atmosphere. Consists of 10 subscales that both staff and clients complete in terms of their perception of ward atmosphere as it actually exists and what they believe should exist.

wholeness In systems theory, the concept that each subsystem interacts directly or indirectly with all other subsystems by exchanging matter and energy.

withdrawal Pathological retreat from people or the world of reality, often seen in schizophrenia.

withdrawal symptoms Physical and mental effects of withdrawing addictive substances from clients who have become habituated or addicted to them.

word salad Mixture of words and phrases that lacks comprehensive meaning or logical coherence, commonly seen in schizophrenic states.

working phase (maintenance) Second stage in the development of a nurse-client relationship. The goal of this stage is to address the problems and issues that are unique to the client.

working through Exploration of a problem by client and therapist until a satisfactory solution has been found or until a symptom has been traced to its unconscious sources.

York Retreat Asylum in England, established by the Quakers in the eighteenth century, that implemented humane care of persons with a mental illness.

Index

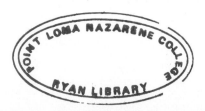

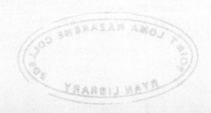